Handbook of Neuroimaging Data Analysis

Handbook of Neuroimaging Data Analysis

Editor: Emery Peterson

AMERICAN
MEDICAL PUBLISHERS
www.americanmedicalpublishers.com

AMERICAN
MEDICAL PUBLISHERS
www.americanmedicalpublishers.com

Cataloging-in-Publication Data

Handbook of neuroimaging data analysis / edited by Emery Peterson.
p. cm.
Includes bibliographical references and index.
ISBN 979-8-88740-152-2
1. Brain--Imaging. 2. Brain--Imaging--Statistical methods. 3. Nervous system--Imaging.
4. Diagnostic imaging. 5. Nervous system--Radiography. I. Peterson, Emery.
RC386.6.D52 H36 2023
616.804 754--dc23

American Medical Publishers,
41 Flatbush Avenue,
1st Floor, New York,
NY 11217, USA

ISBN 979-8-88740-152-2 (Hardback)

Contents

Preface

This book has been an outcome of determined endeavour from a group of educationists in the field. The primary objective was to involve a broad spectrum of professionals from diverse cultural background involved in the field for developing new researches. The book not only targets students but also scholars pursuing higher research for further enhancement of the theoretical and practical applications of the subject.

Neuroimaging is the use of quantitative methods to study the structure and function of the central nervous system. It is basically developed for scientifically studying the healthy human brain in a non-invasive manner. It is utilized for quantitative studies of psychiatric illness and brain diseases. It can be categorized into structural imaging and functional imaging. Structural imaging is used for quantifying the structure of the brain utilizing voxel based morphometry, whereas in functional imaging, brain function is studied by utilizing techniques such as MEG and PET. Techniques of functional brain imaging such as functional magnetic resonance imaging are commonly utilized techniques in neuroimaging. Medical imaging of the brain has various distinguishing features, which increases the difficulty in the assessment. Various artificial intelligence techniques like expert systems, machine learning, knowledge representation, robotics and perception, deep neural networks, reinforcement learning, and evolutionary computation can be used for better interpretation of the brain images. This book unravels the recent studies on neuroimaging data analysis. It is a resource guide for experts as well as students.

It was an honour to edit such a profound book and also a challenging task to compile and examine all the relevant data for accuracy and originality. I wish to acknowledge the efforts of the contributors for submitting such brilliant and diverse chapters in the field and for endlessly working for the completion of the book. Last, but not the least; I thank my family for being a constant source of support in all my research endeavours.

Editor

1

Multiple Sclerosis Identification by 14-Layer Convolutional Neural Network With Batch Normalization, Dropout, and Stochastic Pooling

Shui-Hua Wang [1,2†], *Chaosheng Tang* [1†], *Junding Sun* [1†], *Jingyuan Yang* [3†], *Chenxi Huang* [4*], *Preetha Phillips* [5*] and *Yu-Dong Zhang* [1,6*†]

[1] *School of Computer Science and Technology, Henan Polytechnic University, Jiaozuo, China,* [2] *School of Architecture Building and Civil Engineering, Loughborough University, Loughborough, United Kingdom,* [3] *The Faculty of Computer Science and Engineering, Xi'an University of Technology, Xi'an, China,* [4] *Department of Computer Science and Technology, Tongji University, Shanghai, China,* [5] *West Virginia School of Osteopathic Medicine, Lewisburg, WV, United States,* [6] *Department of Informatics, University of Leicester, Leicester, United Kingdom*

***Correspondence:**
Chenxi Huang
1710051@tongji.edu.cn
Preetha Phillips
pphillips@osteo.wvsom.edu
Yu-Dong Zhang
yudongzhang@ieee.org

† *These authors have contributed equally to this work*

Aim: Multiple sclerosis is a severe brain and/or spinal cord disease. It may lead to a wide range of symptoms. Hence, the early diagnosis and treatment is quite important.

Method: This study proposed a 14-layer convolutional neural network, combined with three advanced techniques: batch normalization, dropout, and stochastic pooling. The output of the stochastic pooling was obtained via sampling from a multinomial distribution formed from the activations of each pooling region. In addition, we used data augmentation method to enhance the training set. In total 10 runs were implemented with the hold-out randomly set for each run.

Results: The results showed that our 14-layer CNN secured a sensitivity of 98.77 ± 0.35%, a specificity of 98.76 ± 0.58%, and an accuracy of 98.77 ± 0.39%.

Conclusion: Our results were compared with CNN using maximum pooling and average pooling. The comparison shows stochastic pooling gives better performance than other two pooling methods. Furthermore, we compared our proposed method with six state-of-the-art approaches, including five traditional artificial intelligence methods and one deep learning method. The comparison shows our method is superior to all other six state-of-the-art approaches.

Keywords: multiple sclerosis, deep learning, convolutional neural network, batch normalization, dropout, stochastic pooling

INTRODUCTION

Multiple sclerosis (abbreviated as MS) is a condition that affects the brain and/or spinal cord (Chavoshi Tarzjani et al., 2018). It will lead to a wide range of probable symptoms, likely with balance (Shiri et al., 2018), vision, movement, sensation (Demura et al., 2016), etc. It has two main types: (i) relapsing remitting MS and (ii) primary progressive MS. More than eight out of every ten diagnosed MS patients are of the "relapsing remitting" type (Guillamó et al., 2018).

MS diagnosis may be confused with other white matter diseases, such as neuromyelitis optica (NMO) (Lana-Peixoto et al., 2018), acute cerebral infarction (ACI) (Deguchi et al., 2018), acute disseminated encephalomyelitis (ADEM) (Desse et al., 2018), etc. Hence, accurate diagnosis of MS is important for patients and following treatments. In this study, a preliminary study that identifies MS from healthy controls with the help of magnetic resonance imaging (MRI) was investigated and implemented.

Recently, researchers tend to use computer vision and image processing (Zhang and Wu, 2008, 2009; Zhang et al., 2009a,b, 2010a,b) techniques to accomplish MS automatic-identification tasks. For instances, Murray et al. (2010) proposed to use multiscale amplitude modulation and frequency modulation (AM-FM) to identify MS. Nayak et al. (2016) presented a novel method, combining AdaBoost with random forest (ARF). Wang et al. (2016) combined biorthogonal wavelet transform (BWT) and logistic regression (LR). Wu and Lopez (2017) used four-level Haar wavelet transform (HWT). Zhang et al. (2017) proposed a novel MS identification system based on Minkowski-Bouligand Dimension (MBD).

Above methods secured promising results. Nevertheless, their methods need to extract features beforehand, and they need to validate their hand-extracted features effective (Chang, 2018a,b,c; Lee et al., 2018). Recently, convolutional neural network (CNN) attracts the research interest of scholars, since it can mechanically develop the features by its early layers. CNN has already been applied to many fields, such as biometric identification (Das et al., 2019), manipulation detection (Bayar and Stamm, 2018), etc. Zhang et al. (2018) is the first to apply CNN to identify MS, and their method achieved an overall accuracy of 98.23%.

This study is based on the CNN structure of Zhang et al. (2018). We proposed two other improvements: batch normalization and stochastic pooling. In addition, we used dynamic learning rate to accelerate the convergence. Learning rate is a parameter to control how quickly the proposed model converge to a local minimal. Low learning rate means a slow speed toward the downward slope. However, it can certain that we won't miss the local minimum but a long time to converge. Therefore, in our research, we set the learning rate a large value and reduce it by every given number of epochs instead of the fixed small learning rate until achieve convergence.

The rest of this paper is organized as follows: section Data Preprocessing described the data processing including data sources and data preprocessing. Section Methodology illustrates the method used in our research. Section Experiments, Results, and Discussions provided the experiment result and discussion.

DATA PREPROCESSING

Two Sources

The dataset in this study were obtained from Zhang et al. (2018). First, MS images were obtained from the eHealth laboratory (2018). All brain lesions were identified and delineated by experienced MS neurologists, and were confirmed by radiologists. Second, the healthy controls were used from 681 slices of 26 healthy controls provided in Zhang et al. (2018). **Table 1** shows the demographic characteristics of two datasets.

Figure 1A shows the original slice, and **Figure 1B** shows the delineated results with four plaques, Areas surrounded by red line denotes the plaque. **Figures 1C,D** presents two slices from healthy controls.

Contrast Normalization

The brain slices are from two different sources; hence, the scanner machines may have different hardware setting (scanning sequence) and software settings (reconstruction from k-space, the store format, etc.). It is necessary to match the two sources of images in terms of gray-level intensities. This is also called contrast normalization, with aim of achieving consistency in dynamic range of various sources of data.

Histogram stretching (HS) method (Li et al., 2018) was chosen due to ease of implementation. HS aims to enhance the contrast by stretching the range of intensity values of two sources of

TABLE 1 | Demographic characteristics of two datasets.

Dataset	Source	# Subjects	Number of Slice	Age	Gender (m/f)
Multiple sclerosis (2018)	eHealth	38	676	34.1 ± 10.5	17/21
Healthy control (Zhang et al., 2018)	private	26	681	33.5 ± 8.3	12/14

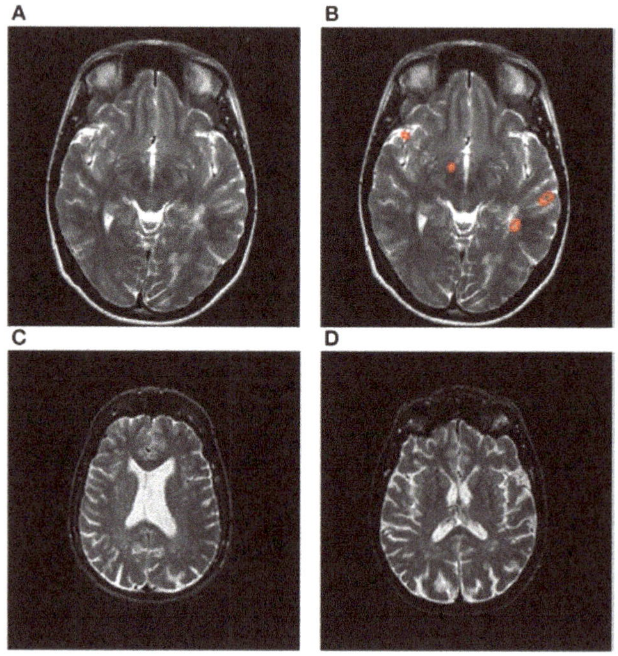

FIGURE 1 | Samples of our dataset. **(A)** Original MS image. **(B)** MS image with plaque delineated. **(C)** Healthy control image I. **(D)** Healthy control image II.

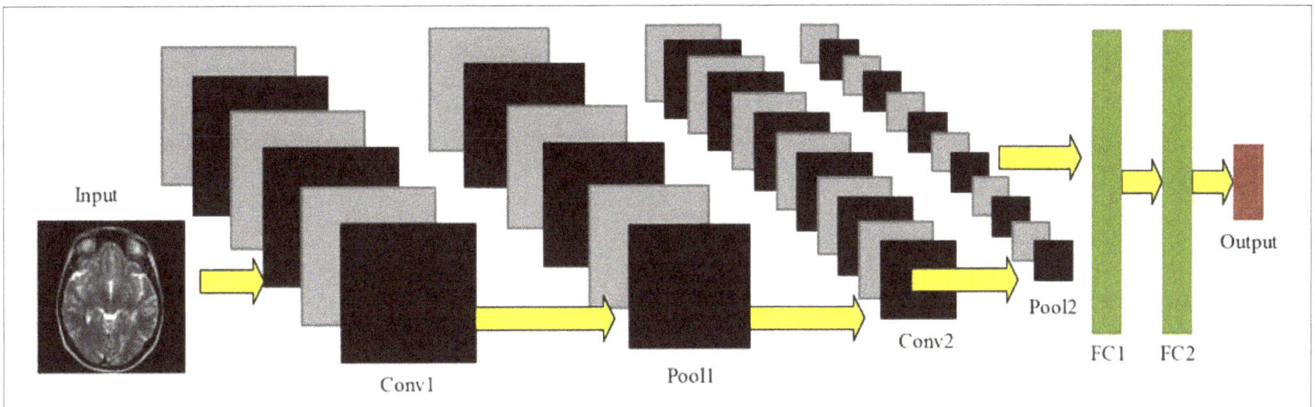

FIGURE 2 | Pipeline of convolutional neural network.

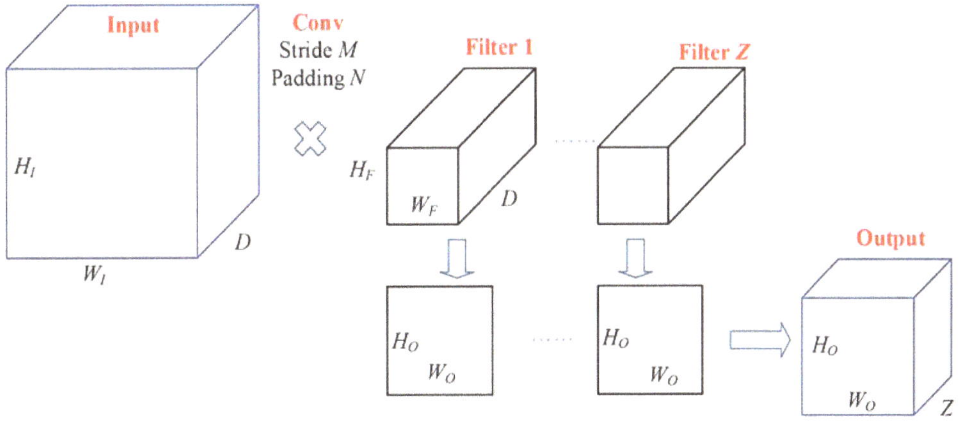

FIGURE 3 | Pipeline of conv layer.

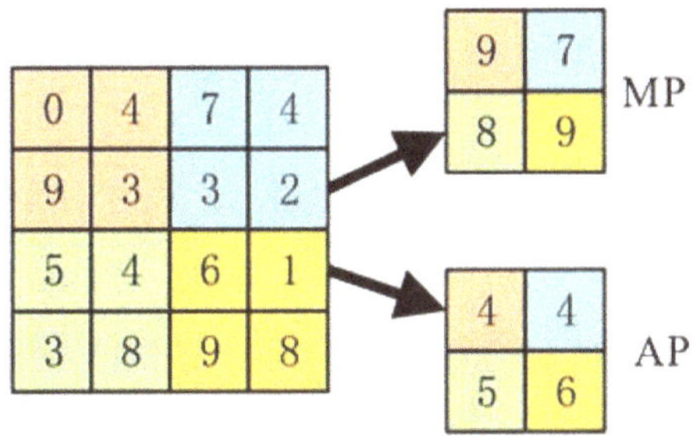

FIGURE 4 | A toy example of max pooling and average pooling.

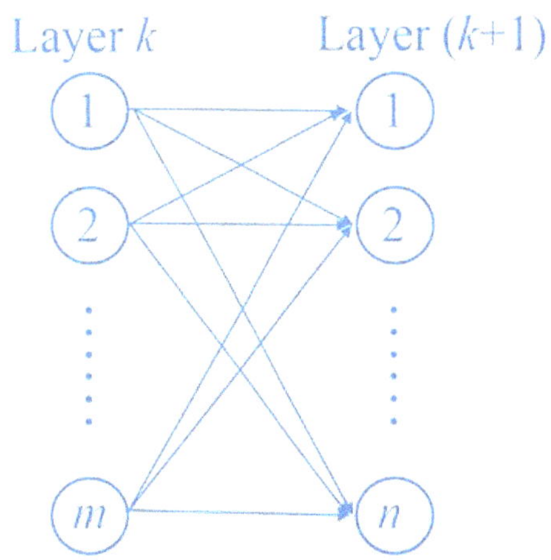

FIGURE 5 | Structure of FC layer.

images to the same range, providing the effect of inter-scan normalization.

The contrast normalization is implemented in following way. Let us assume μ is the original brain image, and φ is the contrast-normalized image, the process of HS can be described as

$$\varphi(x, y) = \frac{\mu(x, y) - \mu_{\min}}{\mu_{\max} - \mu_{\min}} \tag{1}$$

where (x, y) represents the coordinate of pixel, $\mu_{\min}$ and $\mu_{\max}$ represents the minimum and maximum intensity values of original brain image μ.

$$\mu_{\min} = \min_x \min_y \left(\mu(x, y)\right) \tag{2}$$

$$\mu_{\max} = \max_x \max_y \left(\mu(x, y)\right) \tag{3}$$

We do contrast normalization for both two data of different sources, and finally combine them together, forming a 676+681 = 1,357-image dataset.

METHODOLOGY

Convolutional neural network is usually composed of conv layers, pooling layer, and fully connected layers. **Figure 2** gives a toy example that consists of two conv layers, two pooling layers, and two fully connected layers. CNN can achieve comparable or even better performance than traditional AI approaches, while it does not need to manual design the features (Zeng et al., 2014, 2016a,b, 2017a,b).

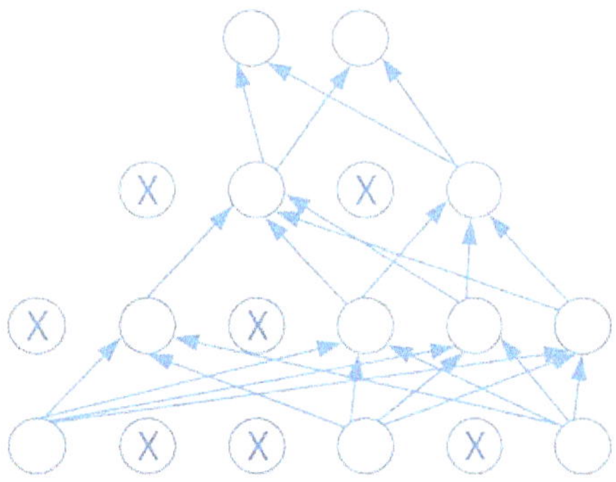

FIGURE 6 | An example of dropout neural network.

TABLE 2 | Variables used in batch normalization.

Parameter	Meaning
z	The output of a layer
z_{norm}	The normalization of z
~li	Input of the non-linearity layer
α	Mean value of the minibatch
δ^2	Variance of the minibatch
l	Layer index
i	i^{th} data in the mini batch
ε	A small constant
m	The number of samples of the minibatch

Conv Layer

The conv layers performed Two-dimensional convolution along the width and height directions (Yu et al., 2018). It is worth noting that the weights in CNN are learned from backpropagation, except for initialization that weights are given randomly. **Figure 3** shows the pipeline of data passing through a conv layer. Suppose there is an input with size of

$$\text{Input}: H_I \times W_I \times D \tag{4}$$

where H_I, W_I, and C represent the height, width, and channels of the input, respectively.

Suppose the size of filter is

$$\begin{aligned}&\text{Filter } 1: H_F \times W_F \times D\\&\ldots\\&\text{Filter } Z: H_F \times W_F \times D\end{aligned} \tag{5}$$

where H_F and W_F are height and width of each filter, and the channels of filter should be the same as that of the input. Z denotes the number of filters. Those filters move with stride of M and padding of N, then the channels of output activation map should be Z. The output size is:

$$\text{Output}: H_O \times W_O \times Z \tag{6}$$

where H_O and W_O are the height and width of the output. Their values are:

$$H_O = 1 + \left\lfloor \frac{2N + H_I - H_F}{M} \right\rfloor \tag{7}$$

$$W_O = 1 + \left\lfloor \frac{2N + W_I - W_F}{M} \right\rfloor \tag{8}$$

where $\lfloor\rfloor$ denotes the floor function. The outputs of conv layer are usually passed through a non-linear activation function, which normally chooses as rectified linear unit (ReLU) function.

TABLE 3 | Hold-out validation setting.

	Training	Test
MS	350	326
HC	350	331
Total	700	657

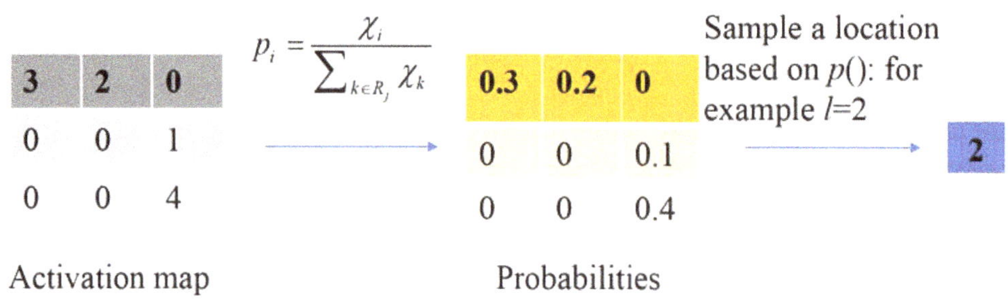

FIGURE 7 | A toy example of stochastic pooling.

Pooling Layer

The activation map contains too much features which can lead to overfitting and computational burden. Pooling layer is often used to implement dimension reduction. Furthermore, pooling can help to obtain invariance to translation. There are two commonly-used pooling methods: average pooling (AP), max pooling (MP).

The average pooling (Ibrahim et al., 2018) is to calculate the average value of the elements in each pooling region, while the max pooling is to select the max value of the pooling region. Suppose the region R contains pixelsχ , the average pooling and max pooling are defined as:

$$AP:\{y_j = \chi_i / \sum_{i \in R_j} \chi_i \} \tag{9}$$

$$MP:\{y_j = \max_{i \in R_j} \chi_i\} \tag{10}$$

Figure 4 shows the difference, where the kernel size equals 2 and stride equals 2. The max pooling finally outputs the maximum values of all four quadrants, while the average pooling outputs the average values.

Softmax and Fully-Connected Layer

In fully connected (FC) layer, each neuron connects to all neurons of the previous layer, which makes this layer produce many parameters in this layer. The fully connected layer multiplied the input by a weight matrix and added to a bias vector. Suppose layer k contains m neurons, layer $(k+1)$ contains n neurons. The weight matrix will be of size of $m \times n$, and the bias vector will be size of $1 \times n$. **Figure 5** shows the structure of FC layer.

Meanwhile, fully connected layer is often followed by a softmax function used to convert the input to a probability distribution. Here the "softmax" in this study only denotes the softmax function. While some literature will add a fully-connected layer before the softmax function and call the both layers as "softmax function."

Dropout

Deep neural network provides strong learning ability even for very complex function which is hard to understand by human. However, one problem often happened during the training of the deep neural network is overfitting, which means the error based on the training set is very small, but the error is large when the test data is provided to the neural network. We name it as bad generation to new dataset.

Dropout was proposed to overcome the problem of overfitting. Dropout works as randomly set some neurons to zero in each forward pass. Each unit has a fixed probability p independent of the other units to be dropped out. The probability p is commonly set as 0.5. **Figure 6** shows an example of dropout neural network, where the empty circle denotes a normal neuron, and a circle with X inside denotes a dropout neuron. It is obvious using dropout can reduce the links and make the neural network easy to train.

Batch Normalization

As the change of each layer's input distribution caused by the updating of the parameter in the previous layer, which is called as internal covariate shift, can result the slow training. Thus, to solve this problem, we employ the batch normalization to normalizes the layer's inputs over a mini batch to make the input layer have a uniform distribution. All the variables are listed in **Table 2**, then the batch normalization can be implemented as follows:

$$\alpha^l = \frac{1}{m} \sum_i z^{li} \tag{11}$$

$$\sigma^{l2} = \frac{1}{m} \sum_i (z^{li} - \alpha^l)^2 \tag{12}$$

$$z^{li}_{norm} = \frac{z^{li} - \alpha^l}{\sqrt{\delta^{l2} + \varepsilon}} \tag{13}$$

$$\tilde{z}^{li} = \lambda^l z^{li}_{norm} + \beta^l \tag{14}$$

Here, ε is employed to improve numerical stability while the mini-batch variance is very small. Usually is set as default value e^{-5}. However, the offset β and scale factor γ are updated during training as learnable parameters.

Stochastic Pooling

The stochastic pooling is proposed to overcome the problems caused by the max pooling and average pooling. The average pooling has a drawback, that all elements in the pooling region are considered, thus it may down-weight strong activation due to many near-zero elements. The max pooling solves this problem,

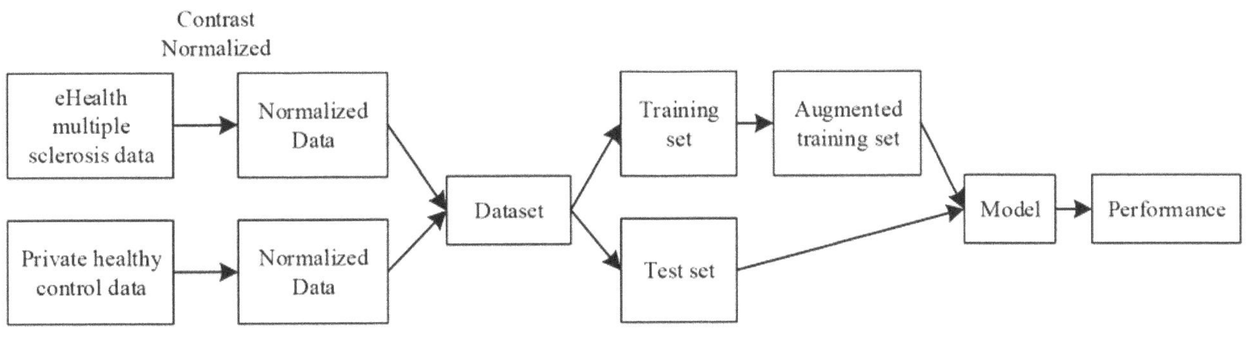

FIGURE 8 | Pipeline of data preprocessing.

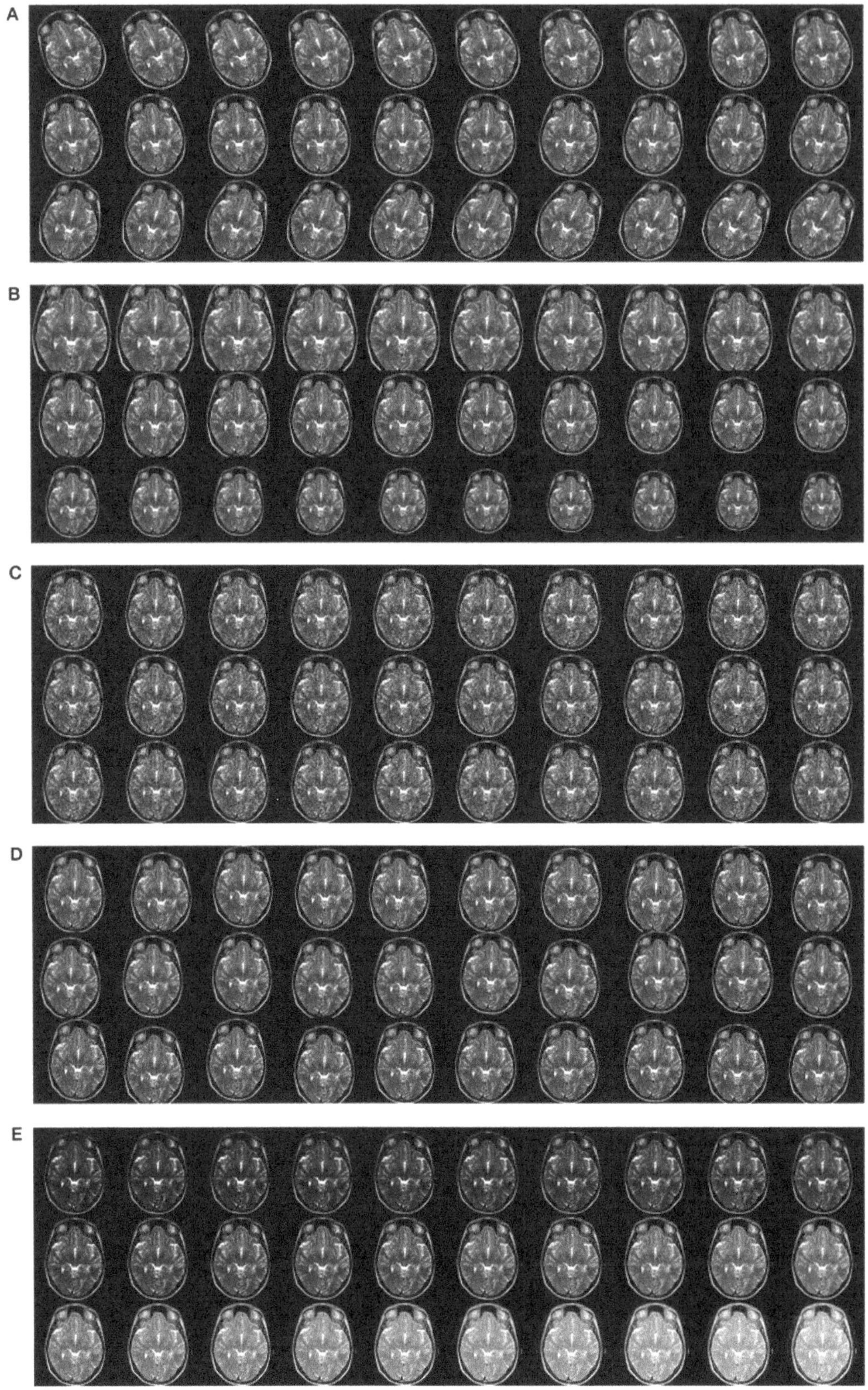

FIGURE 9 | Results of data augmentation. **(A)** Rotation. **(B)** Scaling. **(C)** Noise injection. **(D)** Random translation. **(E)** Gamma correction.

but it easily overfits the training set. Hence, max pooling does not generalize well to test set.

Instead of calculating the mean value or the max value of each pooling region, the output of the stochastic pooling is obtained via sampling from a multinomial distribution formed from the activations of each pooling region R_j. The procedure can be expressed as follows:

(1) Calculate the probability p of each element χ within the pooling region.

$$p_i = \frac{\chi_i}{\sum_{k \in R_j} \chi_k} \tag{15}$$

in which, k is the index of the elements within the pooling region.

TABLE 4 | Hyperparameters of Conv layers.

Layer	Filter size	# Channel	# Filters	Stride
Conv_1	3 × 3	1	8	2
Pool_1	3 × 3			2
Conv_2	3 × 3	8	8	2
Pool_2	3 × 3			2
Conv_3	3 × 3	8	16	1
Conv_4	3 × 3	16	16	1
Conv_5	3 × 3	16	16	1
Pool_3	3 × 3			2
Conv_6	3 × 3	16	32	1
Conv_7	3 × 3	32	32	1
Conv_8	3 × 3	32	32	1
Conv_9	3 × 3	32	64	1
Conv_10	3 × 3	64	64	1
Conv_11	3 × 3	64	64	1
Pool_4	3 × 3			2

TABLE 5 | Hyperparameters of Fully-connected layers.

Layer	Weights	Bias	Probability
FCL_1	20 × 1024	20 × 1	
DO_1			0.5
FCL_2	10 × 20	10 × 1	
DO_2			0.5
FCL_3	2 × 10	2 × 1	

(2) Pick a location l within the pooling region according to the probability p. It is calculated by scanning the pooling region from left to right and up to bottom.

$$A_j = \chi_l, l \sim P(p_1, \ldots, p_{|R_j|}) \tag{16}$$

Instead of considering the max values only, stochastic pooling may use non-maximal activations within the pooling region. **Figure 7** shows a toy example of using stochastic pooling. We first output the probabilities of the input matrix, then the roulette wheel falls within the pie of 0.2. Hence the location l is finally chosen as 2, and the output is the value at second position.

EXPERIMENTS, RESULTS, AND DISCUSSIONS

Division of the Dataset

Hold-out validation method (Monteiro et al., 2016) was used to divide the dataset. In the training set, there are 350 MS images and 350 HC images. In the test set, we have 326 MS images and 331 HC images. **Table 3** presents the setting hold-out validation method.

The dataset is divided into two parts without validation dataset for our research: training dataset and test dataset as shown in **Table 3**. The missing of validation set is mainly because of following reasons: First, according to the past research, validation

TABLE 6 | Statistical analysis of 10 runs.

Run	Sensitivity	Specificity	Precision	Accuracy
1	98.77	98.19	98.17	98.48
2	98.47	97.58	97.57	98.02
3	98.47	98.79	98.77	98.63
4	98.16	98.79	98.77	98.48
5	99.08	98.79	98.78	98.93
6	98.77	98.79	98.77	98.78
7	99.39	99.40	99.39	99.39
8	99.08	98.49	98.48	98.78
9	98.77	99.40	99.38	99.09
10	98.77	99.40	99.38	99.09
Average	98.77 ± 0.35	98.76 ± 0.58	98.75 ± 0.58	98.77 ± 0.39

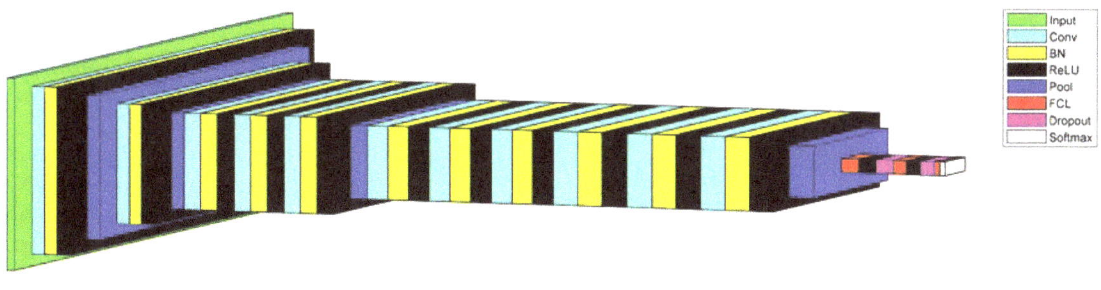

FIGURE 10 | Activation map of proposed CNN model.

$$\begin{bmatrix} 322 & 4 \\ 6 & 325 \end{bmatrix} \quad \begin{bmatrix} 321 & 5 \\ 8 & 323 \end{bmatrix} \quad \begin{bmatrix} 321 & 5 \\ 4 & 327 \end{bmatrix} \quad \begin{bmatrix} 320 & 6 \\ 4 & 327 \end{bmatrix} \quad \begin{bmatrix} 323 & 3 \\ 4 & 327 \end{bmatrix}$$

(a) run 1 (b) run 2 (c) run 3 (d) run 4 (e) run 5

$$\begin{bmatrix} 322 & 4 \\ 4 & 327 \end{bmatrix} \quad \begin{bmatrix} 324 & 2 \\ 2 & 329 \end{bmatrix} \quad \begin{bmatrix} 323 & 3 \\ 5 & 326 \end{bmatrix} \quad \begin{bmatrix} 322 & 4 \\ 2 & 329 \end{bmatrix} \quad \begin{bmatrix} 322 & 4 \\ 2 & 329 \end{bmatrix}$$

(f) run 6 (g) run 7 (h) run 8 (i) run 9 (j) run 10

FIGURE 11 | Confusion matrixes of each run.

TABLE 7 | Ten random runs of MP and AP methods.

	Sensitivity (%)	Specificity (%)	Precision (%)	Accuracy (%)
MP				
R1	97.87	97.87	97.89	97.87
R2	98.63	98.63	98.66	98.63
R3	98.18	98.18	98.20	98.17
R4	96.04	96.04	96.11	96.04
R5	96.80	96.80	96.86	96.80
R6	98.78	98.78	98.81	98.78
R7	98.63	98.63	98.65	98.63
R8	97.86	97.86	97.88	97.87
R9	99.24	99.24	99.25	99.24
R10	98.63	98.63	98.64	98.63
Average	98.07 ± 0.93	98.07 ± 0.98	98.10 ± 0.96	98.07 ± 0.98
AP				
1	97.41	97.41	97.55	97.41
2	96.65	96.66	96.67	96.65
3	98.33	98.32	98.37	98.33
4	97.41	97.41	97.42	97.41
5	96.65	96.65	96.65	96.65
6	97.87	97.87	97.88	97.87
7	97.56	97.57	97.58	97.56
8	97.87	97.87	97.92	97.87
9	98.48	98.48	98.52	98.48
10	98.48	98.47	98.51	98.48
Average	97.67 ± 0.64	97.67 ± 0.67	97.71 ± 0.68	97.67 ± 0.67

TABLE 8 | Pooling method comparison and *p*-values of singed-rank test.

Pooling	Sensitivity (%)	Specificity (%)	Precision (%)	Accuracy (%)
MP	98.33 ± 0.75	98.33 ± 0.79	98.34 ± 0.79	98.33 ± 0.80
p-value (SP-MP)	0.0645	**0.0469**	0.0605	**0.0430**
AP	97.67 ± 0.64	97.67 ± 0.67	97.71 ± 0.68	97.67 ± 0.67
p-value (SP-AP)	**0.0020**	**0.0020**	**0.0020**	**0.0020**
SP (Ours)	98.77 ± 0.35	98.76 ± 0.58	98.75 ± 0.58	98.77 ± 0.39

Bold means the p-values are less than 0.05.

TABLE 9 | Comparison of the approach with and without data augmentation.

Approach	Sensitivity (%)	Specificity (%)	Precision (%)	Accuracy (%)
No augmentation	98.22 ± 0.71	98.19 ± 1.03	98.18 ± 1.01	98.20 ± 0.77
Data augmentation	98.77 ± 0.35	98.76 ± 0.58	98.75 ± 0.58	98.77 ± 0.39

set error rate may tend to overestimate the test error rate for the model fit on the entire data set (Bylander, 2002; Whiting et al., 2004). Second, as in order to avoid the overfitting, in addition of the training and test datasets, the validation dataset is necessary to tune the classification parameters. However, in this paper, we employed the drop out to overcome the problem of overfitting. The experiment result showed that there is no overfitting existing. Therefore, validation dataset is not used in our research.

Data Augmentation Results

The deep learning usually needs a large amount of samples. However, ass it is a well-known challenge to collect biomedical data so as to generate more data from the limited data. Meanwhile, data augmentation has been shown to overcome the overfitting and increase the accuracy of classification tasks (Wong et al., 2016; Velasco et al., 2018). Therefore, in this study, we employed five different data augmentation (DA) methods to enlarge the training set (Velasco et al., 2018). First, we used image rotation. The rotation angle θ was set from -30 to 30° in step of 2°. The second DA method was scaling. The scaling factors varied from 0.7 to 1.3 with step of 0.02. The third DA method was noise injection. The zero-mean Gaussian noise with variance of 0.01 was added to the original image to generate 30 new noise-contaminated images due to the random seed. The fourth DA method used was random translation by 30 times for each original image. The value of random translation t falls within the range of [0, 15] pixels, and obeys uniform distribution. The fifth DA method was gamma correction. The gamma-value r varied from 0.4 to 1.6 with step of 0.04.

The original training is presented in **Figures 1A**, **8** shows the pipeline of the data preprocessing, where the augmented training set is used to create a deep convolutional neural network model, and this trained model was tested over the test set, with final performance reported in **Table 6**. **Figure 9A** shows the results of image rotation. **Figure 9B** shows the image scaling results. **Figures 9C–E** shows the results of noise injection, random

TABLE 10 | Comparison to traditional AI approaches.

Approach	Sensitivity (%)	Specificity (%)	Precision(%)	Accuracy (%)
Multiscale AM-FM (Murray et al., 2010)	94.08	93.64	91.91	93.83
ARF (Nayak et al., 2016)	96.23 ± 1.18	96.32 ± 1.48	N/A	96.28 ± 1.25
BWT-LR (Wang et al., 2016)	97.12 ± 0.14	98.25 ± 0.16	N/A	97.76 ± 0.10
4-level HWT (Wu and Lopez, 2017)	N/A	N/A	N/A	87.65 ± 1.79
MBD (Zhang et al., 2017)	97.78 ± 1.29	97.82 ± 1.60	N/A	97.80 ± 1.40
CNN-DO-BN-SP (Ours)	98.77 ± 0.35	98.76 ± 0.58	98.75 ± 0.58	98.77 ± 0.39

TABLE 11 | Comparison to deep learning approaches.

Approach	Sensitivity (%)	Specificity (%)	Precision (%)	Accuracy (%)
CNN-PReLU-DO (Zhang et al., 2018)	98.22	98.24	N/A	98.23
CNN-DO-BN-SP (Ours)	98.77 ± 0.35	98.76 ± 0.58	98.75 ± 0.58	98.77 ± 0.39

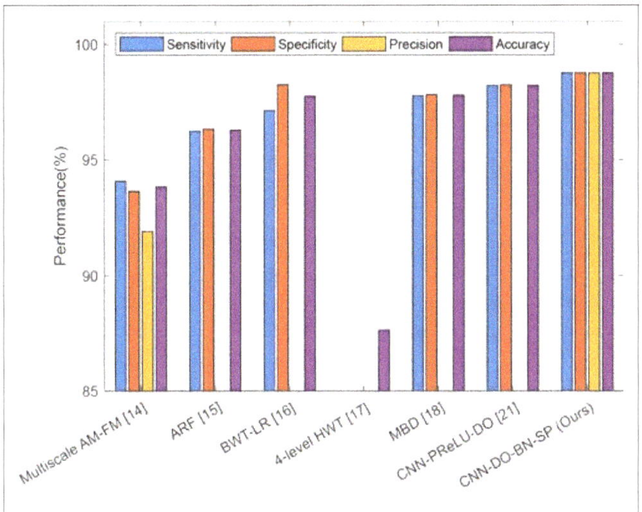

FIGURE 12 | Comparison plot.

translation, and Gamma correction, respectively. As is shown, one training image can generate 150 new images, and thus, the data-augmented training image set is now 151x size of original training set.

Structure of Proposed CNN

We built a 14-layer CNN model, with 11 conv layers and 3 fully-connected layers. Here we did not the number of other layers as convention. The hyperparameters were fine-tuned and their values were listed in **Tables 4**, **5**. The padding values of all layers are set as "same." **Figure 10** shows the activation map of each layer. It is obvious that the height of width of output of each layer shrinks as going to the late layers.

Statistical Results

We used our 14-layer CNN with "DO-BN-SP." We ran the test 10 times, each time the hold-out division was updated randomly. The results over 10 runs are shown in **Table 6**. The average of sensitivity, specificity, and accuracy are 98.77 ± 0.35, 98.76 ± 0.58, and 98.77 ± 0.39, respectively. The confusion matrix of all runs are listed in **Figure 11**.

Pooling Method Comparison

In this experiment, we compared the stochastic pooling (SP) with max pooling (MP) and average pooling (AP). All the other settings are fixed and unchanged. The results of 10 runs of MP and AP are shown in **Table 7**.

We performed Wilcoxon signed rank test (Keyhanmehr et al., 2018) between the results of SP and those of MP, and between the results of SP and those of AP. The results are listed in **Table 8**. It shows SP are significantly better than MP in terms of specificity and accuracy. Meanwhile, SP are significantly better than AP in all four measures.

In this section, Wilcoxon signed rank test was utilized instead of two-sample *t*-test (Jafari and Ansari-Pour, 2018) and chi-square test (Kurt et al., 2019) based on following reasons: two-sample *t*-test supposes the data comes from independent random samples of normal distributions, the same for chi-square goodness-of-fit test. However, our sensitivity/specificity/precision/accuracy data do not meet the condition of gaussian distribution.

Validation of the Data Augmentation

We compared the training process with and without data augmentation to explore the augmentation strategies. The data augmentation methods including: image rotation, scaling, noise injection, random translation and gamma correction as stated in section Data Augmentation Results. The respective performance is shown in **Table 9**. Training with data augmentation could provide better performance, particularly reducing the range of standard deviation.

Comparison to State-Of-The-Art Approaches

In this experiment, we compared our CNN-DO-BN-SP method with traditional AI methods: Multiscale AM-FM (Murray et al., 2010), ARF (Nayak et al., 2016), BWT-LR (Wang et al., 2016), 4-level HWT (Wu and Lopez, 2017), and MBD (Zhang et al., 2017). The results were presented in **Table 10**. Besides, we compared our method with a modern CNN method, viz., CNN-PReLU-DO (Zhang et al., 2018). The results were listed in **Table 11**. We can observe that our method achieved superior performance than all six state-of-the-art approaches, as shown in **Figure 12**.

The reason why our method is the best among all seven algorithms lies in four points. (i) We used data augmentation, to enhance the generality of our deep neural network. (ii) The batch normalization technique was used to resolve the internal covariate shift problem. (iii) Dropout technique was used to avoid overfitting in the fully connected layers. (iv) Stochastic pooling was employed to resolve the down-weight issue caused by average pooling and overfitting problem caused by max pooling.

The bioinspired-algorithm may help the design or initialization of our model. In the future, we shall try particle swarm optimization (PSO) (Zeng et al., 2016c,d) and other methods. The hardware of our model can be optimized using specific optimization method (Zeng et al., 2018).

In this paper, we employed data augmentation, the main benefits mainly as follows: As it is a well-know challenge to collect biomedical data so as to generate more data from the limited data. Second, data augmentation has been shown to overcome the overfitting and increase the accuracy of classification tasks (Wong et al., 2016; Velasco et al., 2018).

CONCLUSION

In this study, we proposed a novel fourteen-layer convolutional neural network with three advanced techniques: dropout, batch normalization, and stochastic pooling. The main contributes are list as follows:

(1) In this paper, we first applied CNN with stochastic pooling for the Multiple sclerosis detection whose early diagnosis is important for patients' following treatment.
(2) In order to overcome the problems happened in the traditional CNN, such as the internal co shift invariant and overfitting, we utilized batch normalization and dropout.
(3) Considering the size of the dataset, data augmentation was employed in our research for the train set.
(4) The proposed method has the best performance compared to the other state of art methods in terms of sensitivity, specificity, precision and accuracy.

The results showed our method is superior to six state-of-the-art approaches: five traditional artificial intelligence methods and one deep learning method. The detail explanation is provided in section Comparison to State-of-the-art approaches. In the future, we shall try to test other pooling variants, such as pyramid pooling. The dense-connected convolutional networks will also be tested for our task. Meanwhile, we will also work on finding more ways to accelerate convergence (Liao et al., 2018).

AUTHOR CONTRIBUTIONS

S-HW conceived the study. CT and JS designed the model. CT and Y-DZ analyzed the data. S-HW, PP, and Y-DZ acquired the preprocessed the data. JY and JS wrote the draft. CH, PP, and Y-DZ interpreted the results. All authors gave critical revision and consent for this submission.

ACKNOWLEDGMENTS

This paper is supported by Natural Science Foundation of China (61602250), National key research and development plan (2017YFB1103202), Henan Key Research and Development Project (182102310629), Open Fund of Guangxi Key Laboratory of Manufacturing System & Advanced Manufacturing Technology (17-259-05-011K).

REFERENCES

(2018). *MRI Lesion Segmentation in Multiple Sclerosis Database, in eHealth laboratory*. University of Cyprus. Available online at: http://www.medinfo.cs.ucy.ac.cy/index.php/facilities/32-software/218-datasets

Bayar, B., and Stamm, M. C. (2018). Constrained convolutional neural networks: a new approach towards general purpose image manipulation detection. *IEEE Trans. Inform. Forensics Security* 13, 2691–2706. doi: 10.1109/TIFS.2018.2825953

Bylander, T. (2002). Estimating generalization error on two-class datasets using out-of-bag estimates. *Mach. Learn.* 48, 287–297. doi: 10.1023/A:1013964023376

Chang, V. (2018a). An overview, examples, and impacts offered by emerging services and analytics in cloud computing virtual reality. *Neural Comput. Appli.* 29, 1243–1256. doi: 10.1007/s00521-017-3000-1

Chang, V. (2018b). A proposed social network analysis platform for big data analytics. *Technol. Forecast. Soc. Change* 130, 57–68. doi: 10.1016/j.techfore.2017.11.002

Chang, V. (2018c). Data analytics and visualization for inspecting cancers and genes. *Multimed. Tools Appl.* 77, 17693–17707. doi: 10.1007/s11042-017-5186-8

Chavoshi Tarzjani, S. P., Shahzadeh Fazeli, S. A. H., Sanati, M. H., and Nabavi, S. M. (2018). Heat shock protein 70 and the risk of multiple sclerosis in the iranian population. *Cell J.* 20, 599–603. doi: 10.22074/cellj.2019.5620

Das, R., Piciucco, E., Maiorana, E., and Campisi, P. (2019). Convolutional neural network for finger-vein-based biometric identification. *IEEE Trans. Inform. Forensics Security* 14, 360–373. doi: 10.1109/TIFS.2018.2850320

Deguchi, I., Tanahashi, N., and Takao, M. (2018). Clinical Study of Intravenous, low-dose recombinant tissue plasminogen activator for acute cerebral infarction: comparison of treatment within 3 hours versus 3-4.5 hours. *J. Stroke Cerebrovasc. Dis.* 27, 1033–1040. doi: 10.1016/j.jstrokecerebrovasdis.2017.11.009

Demura, Y., Kinoshita, M., Fukuda, O., Nose, S., Nakano, H., Juzu, A., et al. (2016). Imbalance in multiple sclerosis and neuromyelitis optica: association with deep sensation disturbance. *Neurol. Sci.* 37, 1961–1968. doi: 10.1007/s10072-016-2697-4

Desse, N., Sellier, A., Bernard, C., and Dagain, A. (2018). Fatal acute disseminated encephalomyelitis (ADEM) after third ventricle colloid cyst resection with ultrasonic aspirator during neuroendoscopic procedure. *Acta Neurochir.* 160, 1789–1792. doi: 10.1007/s00701-018-3631-8

Guillamó, E., Cobo-Calvo, Á., Oviedo, G. R., Travier, N., Álamo, J., Niño-Mendez, O. A., et al. (2018). Feasibility and effects of structured physical exercise interventions in adults with relapsing-remitting multiple sclerosis: a pilot study. *J. Sports Sci. Med.* 17, 426–436.

Ibrahim, A., Peter, S., and Yuntong, S. (2018). Comparison of a vertically-averaged and a vertically-resolved model for hyporheic flow beneath a pool-riffle bedform. *J. Hydrol.* 557, 688–698. doi: 10.1016/j.jhydrol.2017.12.063

Jafari, M., and Ansari-Pour, N. (2018). Why, When and How to adjust your p values? *Cell J.* 20, 604–607. doi: 10.22074/cellj.2019.5992

Keyhanmehr, A. S., Movahhed, M., Sahranavard, S., Gachkar, L., Hamdieh, M., Afsharpaiman, S., et al. (2018). The effect of aromatherapy with rosa damascena essential oil on sleep quality in children. *Res. J. Pharmacognosy* 5, 41–46.

Kurt, M. N., Yilmaz, Y., and Wang, X. (2019). Real-time detection of hybrid and stealthy cyber-attacks in smart grid. *IEEE Trans. Inform. Forensics Security* 14, 498–513. doi: 10.1109/TIFS.2018.2854745

Lana-Peixoto, M. A., Pedrosa, D., Talim, N., Amaral, J. M., Horta, A., and Kleinpaul, R. (2018). Neuromyelitis optica spectrum disorder associated with dengue virus infection. *J. Neuroimmunol.* 318, 53–55. doi: 10.1016/j.jneuroim.2018.02.003

Lee, J., Hong, B., Jung, S., and Chang, V. (2018). Clustering learning model of CCTV image pattern for producing road hazard meteorological information. *Fut. Generat. Comp. Syst.* 86, 1338–1350. doi: 10.1016/j.future.2018.03.022

Li, X., Hu, H., Zhao, L., Wang, H., Yu, Y., Wu, L., et al. (2018). Polarimetric image recovery method combining histogram stretching for underwater imaging. *Sci. Rep.* 8:12430. doi: 10.1038/s41598-018-30566-8

Liao, D., Sun, G., Yang, G., and Chang, V. (2018). Energy-efficient virtual content distribution network provisioning in cloud-based data centers. *Fut. Gener. Comp. Syst.* 83, 347–357. doi: 10.1016/j.future.2018.01.057

Monteiro, J. M., Rao, A., Shawe-Taylor, J., and Mourão-Miranda, J. (2016). A multiple hold-out framework for sparse partial least squares. *J. Neurosci. Methods* 271, 182–194. doi: 10.1016/j.jneumeth.2016.06.011

Murray, V., Rodriguez, P., and Pattichis, M. S. (2010). Multiscale AM-FM demodulation and image reconstruction methods with improved accuracy. *IEEE Trans. Image Process.* 19, 1138–1152. doi: 10.1109/TIP.2010.2040446

Nayak, D. R., Dash, R., and Majhi, B. (2016). Brain MR image classification using two-dimensional discrete wavelet transform and AdaBoost with random forests. *Neurocomputing* 177, 188–197. doi: 10.1016/j.neucom.2015.11.034

Shiri, V., Emami, and, M., and Shiri, E. (2018). Investigating the relationship between selective attention and cognitive flexibility with balance in patients with relapsing-remitting multiple sclerosis. *Arch. Rehabil.* 18, 296–305. doi: 10.21859/jrehab.18.4.4

Velasco, J. M., Garnica, O., Lanchares, J., and Botella, M. (2018). Combining data augmentation, EDAs and grammatical evolution for blood glucose forecasting. *Memetic Comp.* 10, 267–277. doi: 10.1007/s12293-018-0265-6

Wang, S., Zhan, T. M., Chen, Y., Zhang, Y., Yang, M., Lu, H. M., et al. (2016). Multiple sclerosis detection based on biorthogonal wavelet transform, RBF kernel principal component analysis, and logistic regression. *IEEE Access* 4, 7567–7576. doi: 10.1109/ACCESS.2016.2620996

Whiting, P., Rutjes, A. W., Reitsma, J. B., Glas, A. S., Bossuyt, P. M., and Kleijnen, J. (2004). Sources of variation and bias in studies of diagnostic accuracy: a systematic review. *Ann. Intern. Med.* 140, 189–202. doi: 10.7326/0003-4819-140-3-200402030-00010

Wong, S. C., Gatt, A., Stamatescu, V., and McDonnell, M. D. (2016). "Understanding data augmentation for classification: when to warp?" in *International Conference on Digital Image Computing: Techniques and Applications (DICTA)* (Gold Coast, QLD), 1–6.

Wu, X., Lopez, M. (2017). Multiple sclerosis slice identification by haar wavelet transform and logistic regression. *Adv. Eng. Res.* 114, 50–55. doi: 10.2991/ammee-17.2017.10

Yu, B., Yang, L., and Chen, F. (2018). Semantic segmentation for high spatial resolution remote sensing images based on convolution neural network and pyramid pooling module. *IEEE J. Selected Topics in Appl. Earth Observ. Remote Sens.* 11, 3252–3261. doi: 10.1109/JSTARS.2018.2860989

Zeng, N., Wang, Z., Zineddin, B., Li, Y., Du, M., Xiao, L., et al. (2014). Image-based quantitative analysis of gold immunochromatographic strip via cellular neural network approach. *IEEE Trans. Med. Imag.* 33, 1129–1136. doi: 10.1109/TMI.2014.2305394

Zeng, N. Y., Wang, Z., and Zhang, H. (2016b). Inferring nonlinear lateral flow immunoassay state-space models via an unscented Kalman filter. *Sci. China-Inform. Sci.* 59:112204. doi: 10.1007/s11432-016-0280-9

Zeng, N. Y., Wang, Z., Zhang, H., and Alsaadi, F. E. (2016c). A novel switching delayed PSO algorithm for estimating unknown parameters of lateral flow immunoassay. *Cognit. Comput.* 8, 143–152. doi: 10.1007/s12559-016-9396-6

Zeng, N. Y., Wang, Z., Zhang, H., Liu, W., and Alsaadi, F. E. (2016a). Deep belief networks for quantitative analysis of a gold immunochromatographic Strip. *Cognit. Comput.* 8, 684–692. doi: 10.1007/s12559-016-9404-x

Zeng, N. Y., Yi, Y., Lusheng, X., Hong, Z., Lishan, Y., Wenxing, H., et al. (2018). A new imaged-based quantitative reader for the gold immunochromatographic assay. *Optik* 152, 92–99. doi: 10.1016/j.ijleo.2017.09.109

Zeng, N. Y., Zhang, H., and Chen, Y. (2016d). Path planning for intelligent robot based on switching local evolutionary PSO algorithm. *Assem. Automat.* 36, 120–126. doi: 10.1108/AA-10-2015-079

Zeng, N. Y., Zhang, H., Li,., Y., and Liang, J., Dobaie, A. M. (2017a). Denoising and deblurring gold immunochromatographic strip images via gradient projection algorithms. *Neurocomputing* 247, 165–172. doi: 10.1016/j.neucom.2017.0 3.056

Zeng, N. Y., Zhang, H., Liu, W., Liang, J., and Alsaadi, F. E. (2017b). A switching delayed PSO optimized extreme learning machine for short-term load forecasting. *Neurocomputing* 240, 175–182. doi: 10.1016/j.neucom.2017.01.090

Zhang, Y., Jun, Y., Wei, G., and Wu, L. (2010a). Find multi-objective paths in stochastic networks via chaotic immune PSO. *Expert Syst. Appl.* 37, 1911–1919. doi: 10.1016/j.eswa.2009.07.025

Zhang, Y., and Wu, L. (2008). Pattern recognition via PCNN and tsallis entropy. *Sensors* 8, 7518–7529. doi: 10.3390/s8117518

Zhang, Y., and Wu, L. (2009). Segment-based coding of color images. *Sci. China Series F-Inform. Sci.* 52, 914–925. doi: 10.1007/s11432-009-0019-7

Zhang, Y., Wu, L., Neggaz, N., Wang, S., and Wei, G. (2009a). Remote-sensing image classification based on an improved probabilistic neural network. *Sensors* 9, 7516–7539. doi: 10.3390/s90907516

Zhang, Y., Wu, L., Wang, S., and Wei, G. (2010b). Color image enhancement based on HVS and PCNN. *Sci. China Informat. Sci.* 53, 1963–1976. doi: 10.1007/s11432-010-4075-9

Zhang, Y., Wu, L., and Wei, G. (2009b). A new classifier for polarimetric SAR images. *Prog. Electromag. Res.* 94, 83–104. doi: 10.2528/PIER09041905

Zhang, Y-D., Pan, C., Sun, J., and Tang, C. (2018). Multiple sclerosis identification by convolutional neural network with dropout and parametric ReLU. *J. Comput. Sci.* 28, 1–10. doi: 10.1016/j.jocs.2018.07.003

Zhang, Y. D., Zhang, Y., Phillips, P., Dong, Z., and Wang, S. (2017). Synthetic minority oversampling technique and fractal dimension for identifying multiple sclerosis. *Fractals* 25:1740010. doi: 10.1142/S0218348X174 00102

2

Supervised Brain Tumor Segmentation Based on Gradient and Context-Sensitive Features

Junting Zhao [1], Zhaopeng Meng [1,2], Leyi Wei [3], Changming Sun [4], Quan Zou [5] and Ran Su [1*]*

[1] School of Computer Software, College of Intelligence and Computing, Tianjin University, Tianjin, China, [2] Tianjin University of Traditional Chinese Medicine, Tianjin, China, [3] School of Computer Science and Technology, College of Intelligence and Computing, Tianjin University, Tianjin, China, [4] CSIRO Data61, Sydney, NSW, Australia, [5] Institute of Fundamental and Frontier Sciences, University of Electronic Science and Technology of China, Chengdu, China

***Correspondence:**
Quan Zou
zouquan@nclab.net
Ran Su
ran.su@tju.edu.cn

Gliomas have the highest mortality rate and prevalence among the primary brain tumors. In this study, we proposed a supervised brain tumor segmentation method which detects diverse tumoral structures of both high grade gliomas and low grade gliomas in magnetic resonance imaging (MRI) images based on two types of features, the gradient features and the context-sensitive features. Two-dimensional gradient and three-dimensional gradient information was fully utilized to capture the gradient change. Furthermore, we proposed a circular context-sensitive feature which captures context information effectively. These features, totally 62, were compressed and optimized based on an mRMR algorithm, and random forest was used to classify voxels based on the compact feature set. To overcome the class-imbalanced problem of MRI data, our model was trained on a class-balanced region of interest dataset. We evaluated the proposed method based on the 2015 Brain Tumor Segmentation Challenge database, and the experimental results show a competitive performance.

Keywords: brain tumor segmentation, gradient, context-sensitive, random forest, mRMR, class-imbalanced

1. INTRODUCTION

Gliomas, the most common brain tumors in adults, have the highest mortality rate and prevalence among the primary brain tumors (DeAngelis, 2001). They can be classified into high grade gliomas (HGG) and low grade gliomas (LGG). HGG is more aggressive and infiltrative than LGG, thus patients with HGG have a shorter life expectancy (Louis et al., 2007). Magnetic resonance imaging (MRI) with multiple sequences, such as T_2-weighted fluid attenuated inversion recovery (Flair), T_1-weighted (T_1), T_1-weighted contrast-enhanced (T_1c), and T_2-weighted (T_2) provides detailed and valuable information of the brain, and thus is commonly used to diagnose brain diseases, plan the medical treatment strategies, and monitor tumor progression (Bauer et al., 2013; Zeng et al., 2018a). However, gliomas from MRI are difficult to localize as they invade into almost everywhere in the brain with various shapes and sizes and heterogeneous growth patterns (Zhao et al., 2018); they have similar appearances with other diseases such as stroke or inflammation observed in the images; and they are also tangled with surrounding tissues, causing the boundaries diffusive and blurry (Goetz et al., 2016). Furthermore, the scale of MRI voxels is not uniform as the X-ray computed tomography (CT) scans, causing the same tumors to have different gray values, especially when the scans are obtained at different institutions (Sapra et al., 2013). Manual segmentation requires expertise and manually labeling each voxel is laborious and time-consuming (Gordillo et al., 2013). Meanwhile, a variability of 20% and 28% for intra- and inter-rater respectively has been reported for manually segmentation of brain tumors (Mazzara et al., 2004; Goetz et al., 2016). For these reasons, automatic methods instead of manual segmentation with high accuracy and less time-consumption is in high demand.

In this paper, our goal is to propose an automatic method to detect the three different regions of interest (ROI): complete tumor, tumor core, and enhancing tumor from the brain MRI. Our main contributions can be summarized as following:

1. A group of features named circular context-sensitive (CCS) features were proposed. The CCS features fully utilize the histogram information of rays along various orientations and with various lengths.
2. Gradient information was fully utilized by extracting two-dimensional and three-dimensional features. A total of 62 features were extracted to detect and classify the brain tumors.
3. We used an mRMR feature selection algorithm, which could select features that have minimum redundancy and maximum relevance with each others. This is used to significantly reduce the computational cost and increase the efficiency.

The paper is organized as follows: we give a brief literature review of related work in section 2. Then the methods are described in details in section 3. We give the experimental results in section 4, followed by the conclusions in section 5.

2. RELATED WORK

Numerous methods of brain tumor detection and segmentation including semi-automatic methods and full-automatic techniques have been proposed (Tang et al., 2017). These segmentation techniques can be roughly divided into 4 categories: threshold-based techniques, region-based techniques, model-based techniques, and pixel/voxel classification techniques.

The threshold-based techniques, region-based techniques, and pixel classification techniques are commonly used for two-dimensional image segmentation (Vijayakumar and Gharpure, 2011). Model-based techniques and voxel classification methods are usually used for three-dimensional image segmentation. We will review the four types of methods in the following subsections.

2.1. Threshold-Based Techniques

Threshold-based method is a simple and computationally efficient approach to segment brain tumors because only intensity values need to be considered. The objects in the image are classified by comparing their intensities with one or more intensity threshold values (Gordillo et al., 2013). The Otsu algorithm (Otsu, 1979), Bernsen algorithm (Bernsen, 1986), and Niblack algorithm (Niblack, 1986) are simple and commonly used algorithms.

Gibbs et al. proposed an unsupervised approach using a global threshold to segment. The ROI for the tumor extraction task from the MRI images (Gibbs et al., 1996). Stadlbauer et al. used the Gaussian distribution of intensity values as the threshold to segment tumors in brain T_2-weighted MRI (Stadlbauer et al., 2004). However, if the information in the image is too complex, the threshold-based algorithm is not suitable. It is also limited to extract enhanced tumor areas.

2.2. Region-Based Techniques

Region-based methods divide an image into several regions that have homogeneity properties according to a predefined criterion (Adams and Bischof, 1994). Region growing and watershed methods are the most commonly used region-based methods for brain tumor segmentation.

Ho et al. proposed a region competition method which modulates the propagation term with a signed local statistical force to reach a stable state (Ho et al., 2002). Salman et al. examined the seeded region growing and active contour to be compared against experts' manual segmentations (Salman et al., 2005). Sato et al. proposed a Sobel gradient magnitude-based region growing algorithm which solves the partial volume effect problem (Sato et al., 2000). Deng proposed a region growing method which was based on the gradients and variances along and inside of the boundary curve (Deng et al., 2010).

Letteboer et al. and Dam et al. described multi-scale watershed segmentation (Letteboer et al., 2001; Dam et al., 2004). Letteboer et al. proposed a semi-automatic multi-scale watershed algorithm for brain tumor segmentation in MR images (Letteboer et al., 2001). Region-based techniques are used commonly in brain tumor segmentation. However, region-based segmentation has the over-segmentation problem and there is considerable difficulty in marker extraction when using marker-based watershed segmentation. Li and Wan solved these problems by proposing an improved watershed segmentation method with an optimal scale based on ordered dither halftone and mutual information (Li and Wan, 2010).

2.3. Model-Based Techniques

Model-based segmentation techniques could be divided into parametric deformable and geometric deformable approaches. There are a number of studies on image segmentation based on active contours, which is a popular parametric deformable method (Boscolo et al., 2002; Amini et al., 2004). Snake is one of the most commonly used geometric deformable algorithm for brain tumor segmentation. Luo et al. proposed a deformable model to segment brain tumors (Luo et al., 2003). This method combined the adaptive balloon force and the gradient vector flow (GVF) force to increase the GVF snake's capture range and convergence speed. Ho et al. proposed a new region competition method for automatic 3D brain tumor segmentation based on level-set snakes which overcome the difficulty in initialization and the missing boundary problems by modulating the propagation term with a signed local statistical force (Ho et al., 2002).

2.4. Pixel/Voxel Classification Techniques

Voxel-based classification usually uses voxel attributes for each voxel in the image such as gray level and color information. In brain tumor segmentation, voxel-based techniques are classified as unsupervised classifiers and supervised classifiers to cluster each voxel in the feature space (Gordillo et al., 2013).

Juang and Wu proposed a color-converted segmentation approach with the K-means clustering technique for MRI which converts the input gray-level MRI image into a color space image and the image is labeled by cluster indices (Juang and Wu, 2010). Selvakumar et al. implemented a voxel classification method which combined K-means clustering and fuzzy C-means (FCM) segmentation (Selvakumar et al., 2012). Vasuda and Satheesh improved the conventional FCM by implementing data compression including quantization and aggregation to significantly reduce the dimensionality of the input (Vasuda and Satheesh, 2010). Comparing to the conventional FCM, the modified FCM has a higher convergence rate. Ji et al. proposed a modified possibilistic FCM clustering of MRI utilizing local contextual information to impose local spatial continuity to reduce noise and resolve classification ambiguity (Ji et al., 2011). Autoencoders were used in Vaidhya et al. and Zeng et al. work for brain tumor segmentation and other imaging tasks (Vaidhya et al., 2015; Zeng et al., 2018b). Zhang et al. proposed a hidden Markov random field model and the expectation-maximization algorithm for brain segmentation on MRI (Zhang et al., 2001).

For the voxel-classification MRI processing techniques, proper depiction of voxels is required as a criteria to accurately classify each voxel. In the previous studies, Zulpe et al. used gray-level co-occurrence matrix (GLCM) textural features to detect the brain tumors (Zulpe and Pawar, 2012); Context-sensitive features were used in Meier et al.'s study to classify tumors and non-tumors (Meier et al., 2014). Meanwhile, a feature selection algorithm also requires good designs to select a compact set of features in order to reduce the computation cost (Zou et al., 2016a,b; Su et al., 2018), considering the huge data size of the MRI. In our study, one set of informative features and efficient feature selection algorithm were proposed. The experimental results have demonstrated that promising brain tumor segmentation performance can be achieved using the proposed method.

3. METHODOLOGY

In this paper, we extracted various types of features from the brain MRI and used for classification. And an mRMR feature selection method was used to reduce the feature dimension and select the best feature set. The whole pipeline was depicted in **Figure 1**. Firstly, the MRI sequences were pre-processed with smoothing and normalization operations. Secondly, we extracted two types of features, gradient-based features and context-sensitive features. Thirdly, we used an mRMR feature selection method to select the optimal feature set with minimal redundancy and maximal relevance. We will explain the whole process in detail later.

3.1. Data

We used the training data of BraTS 2015 as our training and test data (Menze et al., 2015). It provides 4 sequences T_1, T_1c, T_2, and Flair. The image data contains 220 HGG (anaplastic astrocytomas and glioblastoma multiforme tumors) MR scans and 54 LGG (histological diagnosis: astrocytomas or oligoastrocytomas) cases. The "ground truth" are labeled by manual annotations with 0-5 with four types of tumoral structures labeled as the following: "necrotic (or fluid-filled) core" is labeled 1, "edema" is labeled 2 , "non-enhancing(solid) core" is labeled 3, and "enhancing core" is labeled 4. The normal tissue is labeled 0. We evaluated our work within three regions: complete tumor (which contains necrotic core, edema, non-enhancing core and enhancing core), tumor core (which contains necrotic core, non-enhancing, and enhancing core) and enhancing tumor.

3.2. Pre-processing

We carried out smoothing and normalization on the MRI sequences to reduce the impact of image noise and to enhance image quality for further processing. As for smoothing, we chose the Gaussian filter which has been widely used in image processing and computer vision for noise suppression (Bergholm, 1987; Deng and Cahill, 1993; Kharrat et al., 2009; Zeng et al., 2017).

For further processing, MRI sequences are sensitive to all the acquisition conditions such as MR protocols, MR scanners, and MR adjustments (Sled et al., 1998). Even for the same tissue information acquired with the same conditions, there will be a variation because MRI intensities do not have a tissue specific value. In order to eliminate the impact of the variation for further image processing which is based on image intensity, we normalized the smoothed value to the range from 0 to 1. The normalization was calculated as in Equation (1)

$$X^* = \frac{X - X_{\min}}{X_{\max} - X_{\min}} \tag{1}$$

where X^* and X are the normalized and raw gray value respectively; $X_{\max}$ is the maximal gray value, and $X_{\min}$ is the minimal gray values.

3.3. Gradient Based Features

The gradient value represents the rate of change in the direction of the largest possible intensity change. In our study, we used the central difference gradient as the gradient operator. For each voxel p, the derivative at one direction is the mean of the two voxels adjacent to p in that particular direction. Here we calculated two sets of gradient-based features within the ROI. The first set calculated the gradient along each coordinate plane, which we named as Gradient2D. The Gradient2D of one image in each coordinate plane has two components: the x-derivative and the y-derivative. In Equation (2), we take the x-derivative as an example (I is the input image). The second set, the Gradient3D, is based on the three-dimensional gradient magnitude. We further divide the Gradient3D into five subsets, the GM, rMean, rVar, seqMean, and seqVar, and we show them in **Table 1**.

The GM feature consists of the three-dimensional gradient magnitude, which is calculated based on Equation (3). G_x is the directional gradient along the x-axis, G_y is the directional gradient along the y-axis and G_z is the directional gradient along the z-axis. In our study, we also used the central difference gradient as gradient operator to extract the GM feature for

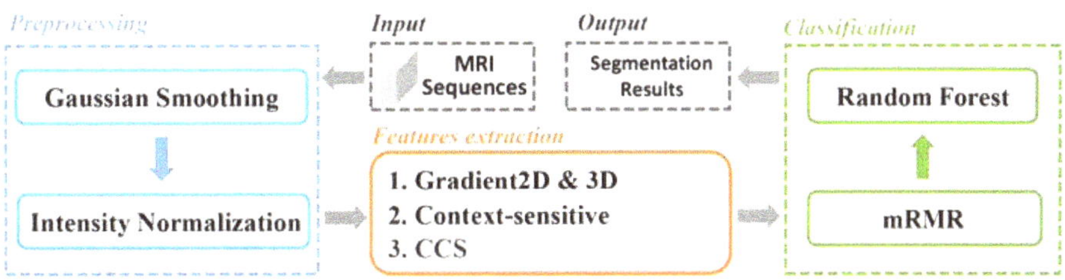

FIGURE 1 | The pipeline of our proposed method.

TABLE 1 | The five feature subsets in Gradient3D.

Feature name	Modality	Cube size
GM	Flair, T_1, T_1c, T_2	–
rMean	Flair, T_1, T_1c, T_2	3, 5, 7
rVar	Flair, T_1, T_1c, T_2	3, 5, 7
seqMean	all modalities	3, 5, 7
seqVar	all modalities	3, 5, 7

each respective MRI image sequence. The operator is given in Equation (2).

$$dI/dx = \frac{I(x+1) - I(x-1)}{2} \tag{2}$$

$$mag(G_x, G_y, G_z) = \sqrt{G_x^2 + G_y^2 + G_z^2} \tag{3}$$

We further extracted the rMean and rVar features by calculating the mean and variance of the GM feature over a cube-shaped neighborhood with sizes 3^3, 5^3, 7^3 for each GM feature of each respective sequence. Meanwhile, we extracted seqMean and seqVar by calculating the mean and variance of the GM features over the sequences in cube-shaped neighborhoods.

3.4. Circular Context-Sensitive Feature

Meier et al. proposed context-sensitive features for brain tumor segmentation which extracts ray features in plane by calculating the histogram using intensity values from T_1 and Flair-weighted images after atlas-normalization (Meier et al., 2014). The rationale of this method is that the intensity range of T_1 and Flair-weighted modalities is larger than that of the healthy tissues. Based on this method, we proposed a circular context-sensitive (CCS) feature to capture more details in various sizes.

In context-sensitive features, every voxel sends out four rays with radius $r \in \{10, 20\}$ and orienting at $ang \in \{0, \pi/2, \pi, 2\pi/3\}$. In order to obtain more information and extract features in multiple scales, we made several improvements to the original context-sensitive features. Firstly, instead of utilizing only voxel information in the horizontal or vertical directions, we used rays evenly distributed on a circle to swipe all the orientations, which are denser. The directions are calculated using the following equation:

$$\begin{aligned} ang &= \beta + n * \beta_\theta, n \in N, \\ \beta_\theta &= 2\pi / N_\beta \end{aligned} \tag{4}$$

where β is the initial angle, β_θ is the step size rotating around the center point, and N_β is the total number of directions. Secondly, in order to capture context features with all the scales, we used a continuous radius to cover the neighboring voxel information as much as possible. The radius r is defined as:

$$\begin{aligned} r &= r_0 + n * r_\theta, n \in N^*, \\ r_\theta &= (r_{\max} - r_{\min})/N_r \end{aligned} \tag{5}$$

where r_0 is the initial radius, where r_θ is the step size moving toward the outermost circle, $r_{\min}$ and $r_{\max}$ are the minimum and maximum of the radius, and N_r is the total number of rays. We show the comparison between the original context-sensitive features and the circular context-sensitive features in **Figure 2**. The original context-sensitive sends out four rays in four directions. The CCS features, however, send out rays along all the orientations and with all the radius, which is supposed to capture rich context information. In our studies, we used 8 rays evenly distributed on 45 circles ranging from 10 to 20 with even numbers to capture the context-sensitive features.

In the MRI, the slice thickness varies considerably which will affect the feature extraction results so the features are considered only for the T_1 and Flair-weighted in-plane images. In summary, our CCS feature extraction is summarized as the following:

1. For one voxel i, we calculated r and ang of all the rays, based on Equations (4, 5).
2. Using T_1 and Flair images, we computed the histograms and obtained the maximal $H_{\max}$ and minimal $H_{\min}$ histogram values.
3. The mean values of each ray was calculated using $H_{\max}$ and $H_{\min}$ as the CCS feature values.

In summary, we extracted 12 Gradient2D features, 34 Gradient3D features, 4 context-sensitive features, and 12 CCS features, as shown in **Table 2**. In the next section, we will show the voxel-based classification and feature selection to label different regions of the brain MR images.

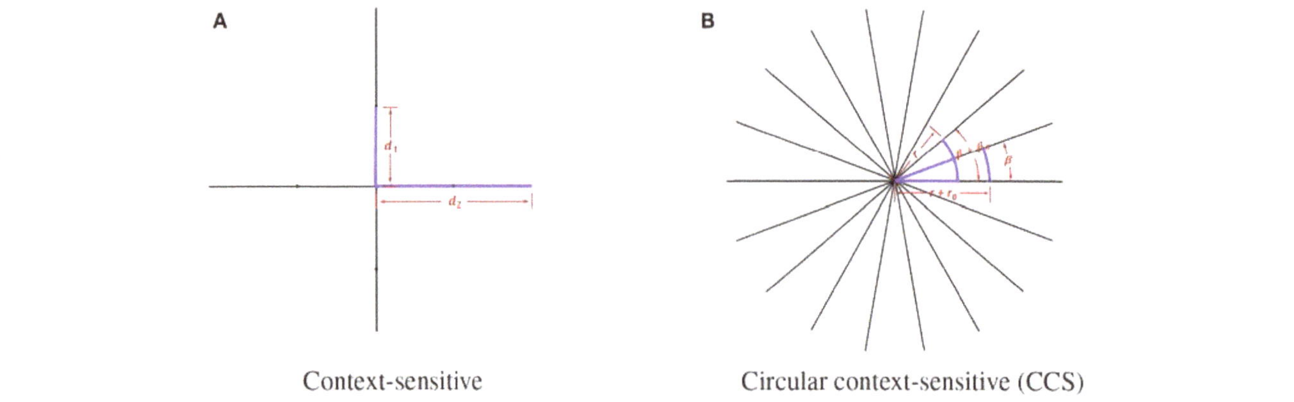

FIGURE 2 | The original context-sensitive features and the circular context-sensitive (CCS) features. **(A)** shows the original context-sensitive features. **(B)** shows the CCS features. In this example, the center voxel sends out 18 rays of length $r + n * r_\theta$ with an angle $\beta + n * \beta_\theta$. The CCS can fully extract context information instead of only voxel information in horizontal or vertical directions.

TABLE 2 | Number of features in each feature group.

Feature type	Counts
Gradient2D	12
Gradient3D	34
Context-sensitive	4
CCS	12
Total	62

3.5. Feature Selection Based on mRMR

We classified the brain MRI images into five categories: normal tissue, edema, non-enhancing core, necrotic core, and enhancing core. Random forests (RF) (Breiman, 2001) is an ensemble learning method for classification, regression, and other tasks, and has been widely used in image analysis (Jin et al., 2014; Liu et al., 2015). It consists of multitude of decision trees and outputs the votes over each tree. They are able to handle multi-class problems, and they provide a probabilistic output instead of hard label separations. However, due to the large volume of MRI images, direct classification based on the extracted features (as shown in **Table 2**) is time-consuming. A proper feature selection algorithm will greatly reduce the computational cost and increase the efficiency.

Minimal Redundancy maximal Relevance(mRMR) was proposed by Peng et al. which can select features that have minimum redundancy and maximum relevance with each other (Peng et al., 2005) . We use Equation (6) to search for features which have the maximum relevance, and use the minimal redundancy condition as the Equation (7) to select mutually exclusive features. Equation (8) gives mRMR features. x_i represents the $i-$ th feature in feature set S with target class c. Φ means the combination of D and R.

$$maxD(S,c), D = \frac{1}{|S|}\sum_{x_i \epsilon S} I(x_i; c) \tag{6}$$

$$minR(S), R = \frac{1}{|S|^2}\sum_{x_i, x_j \epsilon S} I(x_i, x_j) \tag{7}$$

$$max\Phi(D,R), \Phi = D - R \tag{8}$$

In order to avoid over-learning and under-learning, we evaluated our RF classifier by 5-fold cross validation with the measurements in section 3.7. In detail, we divided the subcases into 5 roughly equal parts. For each $k = 1, 2, ..., 5$, we fit the RF model to the other 4 parts, and predict the kth part with the fitted RF model. The final outcome equals to the mean of the results of the 5-folds. In our study, we used the mRMR feature selection method to select the minimal feature set which reduces the computational cost without performance degradation. The raw 62-dimensional feature set is shown in **Table 2**. The mRMR feature selection details are as follows:

1. Train the RF classifier with top f features which are ranked by mRMR from the raw feature set and test the model with 5-fold cross validation. Here, we set $f = 62 - 5n, n = 0, 1, 2, ..., 12$.
2. Rank the performance in step 1. Set the final feature set with f_m dimension as the features which achieve the best performance among all the f-dimensional features. Here, f_m is the dimension of the final feature set.

3.6. Solution to the Class-Imbalance Problem

The "BraTS" data is seriously unbalanced, with less than 1% of voxels being tumor voxels. Training on them would result in problems such as higher mis-classification rate for the minority class data. Thus, we carried out three steps to overcome the class-imbalance problem.

1. Detect the boundary of ROI: We used a plane to move along each axis's direction until it detected a voxel labeled with none-zero. Then the plane in the current position was used as the boundary in that direction.

TABLE 3 | Performance of feature sets with different dimension.

The nth training	Feature Dimension	Measurements	Dice			PPV			Sensitivity			Specificity		
		ROI	Complete	Core	Enhancing	Complete	Core	Enhancing	Complete	Core	Enhancing	Complete	Core	Enhancing
1	62	HGG&LGG	0.91	0.62	0.61	0.94	0.63	0.64	0.89	0.61	0.58	0.79	0.81	0.92
		HGG	0.92	0.63	0.61	0.94	0.65	0.64	0.89	0.62	0.59	0.79	0.82	0.92
		LGG	0.86	0.54	–	0.91	0.56	–	0.83	0.55	–	0.76	0.55	–
2	57	HGG&LGG	0.91	0.62	0.61	0.94	0.63	0.64	0.88	0.61	0.58	0.78	0.80	0.92
		HGG	0.92	0.63	0.61	0.94	0.64	0.64	0.89	0.61	0.58	0.79	0.82	0.92
		LGG	0.87	0.55	–	0.91	0.55	–	0.84	0.57	–	0.75	0.57	–
3	52	HGG&LGG	0.91	0.62	0.61	0.94	0.63	0.64	0.88	0.61	0.58	0.78	0.80	0.92
		HGG	0.91	0.63	0.61	0.94	0.64	0.64	0.89	0.61	0.58	0.79	0.82	0.92
		LGG	0.87	0.55	–	0.91	0.55	–	0.83	0.57	–	0.74	0.57	–
4	47	HGG&LGG	0.91	0.62	0.61	0.94	0.63	0.64	0.88	0.61	0.58	0.78	0.80	0.92
		HGG	0.91	0.63	0.61	0.94	0.64	0.64	0.89	0.61	0.58	0.79	0.81	0.92
		LGG	0.87	0.56	–	0.91	0.55	–	0.83	0.57	–	0.74	0.57	–
5	42	HGG&LGG	0.91	0.62	0.61	0.94	0.63	0.64	0.88	0.61	0.58	0.78	0.80	0.92
		HGG	0.91	0.63	0.61	0.94	0.64	0.64	0.89	0.61	0.58	0.79	0.81	0.92
		LGG	0.87	0.55	–	0.91	0.55	–	0.83	0.56	–	0.74	0.56	–
6	37	HGG&LGG	0.91	0.61	0.60	0.94	0.63	0.64	0.88	0.61	0.58	0.78	0.80	0.92
		HGG	0.91	0.63	0.60	0.94	0.64	0.64	0.89	0.61	0.58	0.79	0.82	0.92
		LGG	0.86	0.55	–	0.92	0.56	–	0.82	0.54	–	0.76	0.54	–
7	32	HGG&LGG	0.91	0.62	0.61	0.94	0.62	0.64	0.88	0.61	0.58	0.76	0.79	0.92
		HGG	0.91	0.63	0.61	0.94	0.64	0.63	0.89	0.62	0.58	0.77	0.80	0.92
		LGG	0.87	0.55	–	0.91	0.55	–	0.83	0.57	–	0.72	0.57	–
8	27	HGG&LGG	0.91	0.62	0.61	0.93	0.62	0.64	0.89	0.62	0.58	0.76	0.78	0.92
		HGG	0.91	0.63	0.61	0.94	0.64	0.63	0.89	0.62	0.58	0.77	0.80	0.92
		LGG	0.87	0.55	–	0.90	0.54	–	0.83	0.57	–	0.71	0.57	–
9	22	HGG&LGG	0.91	0.62	0.61	0.93	0.62	0.64	0.89	0.62	0.58	0.75	0.77	0.92
		HGG	0.91	0.63	0.61	0.94	0.63	0.63	0.89	0.63	0.58	0.76	0.79	0.92
		LGG	0.87	0.56	–	0.90	0.54	–	0.84	0.58	–	0.71	0.58	–
10	17	HGG&LGG	0.91	0.62	0.61	0.93	0.61	0.64	0.89	0.62	0.58	0.73	0.76	0.92
		HGG	0.91	0.63	0.61	0.93	0.62	0.64	0.89	0.63	0.58	0.74	0.78	0.92
		LGG	0.86	0.55	–	0.90	0.54	–	0.84	0.57	–	0.70	0.57	–
11	12	HGG&LGG	0.91	0.61	0.60	0.92	0.59	0.63	0.89	0.63	0.57	0.70	0.74	0.92
		HGG	0.91	0.62	0.60	0.93	0.61	0.63	0.90	0.63	0.57	0.71	0.76	0.91
		LGG	0.87	0.56	–	0.89	0.54	–	0.85	0.59	–	0.67	0.59	–
12	7	HGG&LGG	0.90	0.58	0.55	0.91	0.56	0.59	0.89	0.61	0.52	0.67	0.70	0.91
		HGG	0.90	0.59	0.55	0.92	0.57	0.59	0.89	0.62	0.52	0.68	0.72	0.91
		LGG	0.86	0.54	–	0.88	0.52	–	0.84	0.56	–	0.65	0.56	–
13	2	HGG&LGG	0.86	0.48	0.34	0.85	0.44	0.36	0.87	0.53	0.33	0.42	0.52	0.86
		HGG	0.87	0.48	0.36	0.86	0.44	0.38	0.89	0.54	0.34	0.42	0.54	0.86
		LGG	0.81	0.43	–	0.83	0.44	–	0.80	0.42	–	0.41	0.42	–

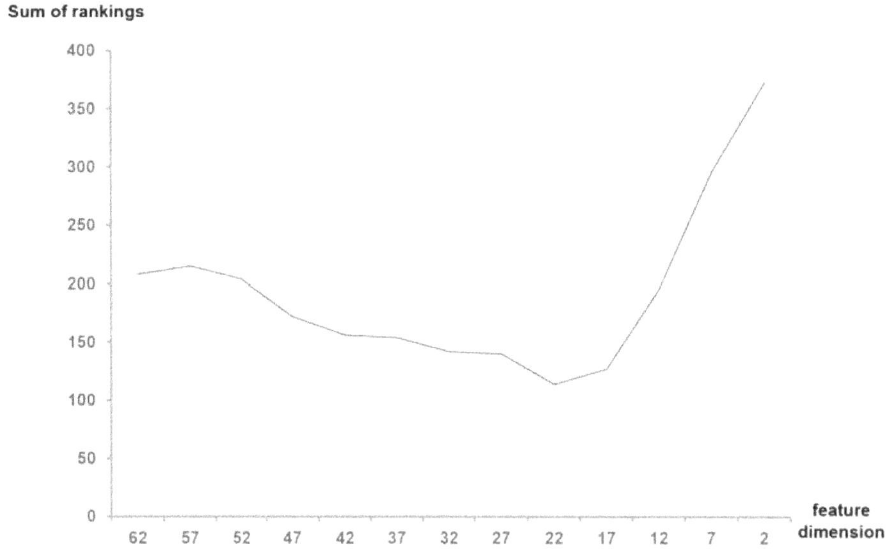

FIGURE 3 | Sum of rankings for each feature dimension *f*. The ranking rules are defined as follows: In each feature set with dimension *f*, we observed the three metrics (Dice, sensitivity and specificity) in three ROIs (Complete, enhancing and core) of HGG, LGG and both, totally 32 values in **Table 3**. We ranked the corresponding values across all the *f*. If equal values appeared, we took another metric, the size of the feature set into account. Then we summed all the rankings of each *f* and plotted the curve.

2. Split the ROI: After step 1, each raw MR image would have a total of 6 boundaries in the xyz space. We split out a cuboid as our ROI using the boundaries. This removed a large number of zero label voxels and voxels inside each ROI contained all the categories.
3. Equally select voxels for each category: Within the segmented ROI, the label with the least number of voxels was recorded. We randomly picked the equal number of voxels in the ROI to form a balanced data.

3.7. Performance Measurements

To show the performance of our segmentation approach, we use Dice, positive predictive value (PPV), Sensitivity, Specificity to evaluate HGG and LGG tumor regions segmentation. TP represents the number of "true positive," where "true positive" is the event that the test makes a positive prediction, and the subject has a positive ground truth. FP is the number of "false positive," where "false positive" is the event that the test makes a positive prediction, and the subject has a negative ground truth. FN is the number of "false negative" and TN indicateds the size of "true negative" set.

1. Dice

$$Dice = \frac{TP}{((TP + FP) + (TP + FN))/2}$$

The Dice score normalizes the number of true positives to the average size of the two segmented areas. It is identical to the F-score (the harmonic mean of the precision recall curve) and can be transformed monotonously to the Jaccard score.

2. Positive predictive value (PPV)

$$PPV = \frac{TP}{TP + FP}$$

The PPV represents the proportions of positive results in tests that are true positive results.

3. Sensitivity

$$Sensitivity = \frac{TP}{TP + FN}$$

Sensitivity measures the proportion of actual positives that are correctly identified as such.

4. Specificity

$$Specificity = \frac{TN}{FP + TN}$$

Specificity (also called the true negative rate) measures the proportion of actual negatives that are correctly identified as such.

4. EXPERIMENTAL RESULTS

In our experiments, we extracted four groups of features after pre-processing: Gradient2D features, Gradient3D features, context-sensitive features, and CCS features, including totally 62 features (as shown in **Table 2**). The Gradient3D set contains five subsets: the GM, rMean, rVar, seqMean, and seqVar. We used the mRMR feature selection method to select a compact set of features and built the random forest classifier.

TABLE 4 | Performance of different feature groups.

Feature type	Feature Dimension	Measurements	Dice			PPV			Sensitivity			Specificity		
		ROI	Complete	Core	Enhancing	Complete	Core	Enhancing	Complete	Core	Enhancing	Complete	Core	Enhancing
Gradient2D	12	HGG&LGG	0.89	0.54	0.41	0.87	0.47	0.49	0.90	0.63	0.35	0.50	0.56	0.92
		HGG	0.89	0.55	0.40	0.88	0.48	0.49	0.90	0.64	0.34	0.51	0.57	0.91
		LGG	0.85	0.54	–	0.84	0.48	–	0.87	0.62	–	0.47	0.62	–
Gradient3D	34	HGG&LGG	0.90	0.61	0.60	0.92	0.60	0.63	0.89	0.62	0.57	0.71	0.75	0.92
		HGG	0.91	0.62	0.60	0.93	0.61	0.63	0.90	0.63	0.57	0.72	0.76	0.91
		LGG	0.85	0.51	–	0.88	0.50	–	0.83	0.55	–	0.62	0.55	–
Context-sensitive	4	HGG&LGG	0.86	0.51	0.14	0.87	0.44	0.23	0.85	0.60	0.11	0.51	0.48	0.91
		HGG	0.87	0.51	0.16	0.87	0.44	0.24	0.86	0.60	0.12	0.51	0.47	0.90
		LGG	0.79	0.45	–	0.83	0.43	–	0.76	0.47	–	0.52	0.47	–
CCS	12	HGG&LGG	0.86	0.54	0.13	0.89	0.47	0.25	0.84	0.62	0.09	0.62	0.57	0.94
		HGG	0.87	0.53	0.16	0.90	0.48	0.27	0.85	0.61	0.11	0.62	0.56	0.92
		LGG	0.80	0.48	–	0.86	0.47	–	0.75	0.48	–	0.64	0.48	–

TABLE 5 | Comparison between Meier et al.'s method and the proposed method.

Method	Measurements	Dice			PPV			Sensitivity			Specificity		
	ROI	Complete	Core	Enhancing	Complete	Core	Enhancing	Complete	Core	Enhancing	Complete	Core	Enhancing
Meier et al.;s method	HGG&LGG	0.83	0.66	0.58	0.85	0.74	0.66	0.83	0.66	0.54	–	–	–
	HGG	0.84	0.73	0.68	0.80	0.80	0.72	0.89	0.70	0.70	–	–	–
The proposed method	HGG&LGG	0.91	0.62	0.61	0.93	0.62	0.64	0.89	0.62	0.58	0.75	0.77	0.92
	HGG	0.91	0.62	0.61	0.93	0.62	0.64	0.89	0.62	0.58	0.75	0.77	0.92
	LGG	0.87	0.56	–	0.90	0.54	–	0.84	0.58	–	0.71	0.58	–

Firstly, we built the random forest classifier using the top f feature set ranked by mRMR respectively. We used f to denote the dimension of the feature set, where $f = 62 - 5n, n = 0, 1, 2, ..., 12$. Secondly, we compared the performance of feature sets with diverse f. The best feature dimension f_m is the f which has the best performance. We recorded this f_m-dimensional feature set as the optimal feature set. Here we present the performance comparisons between diverse fs; Then we show the performance comparisons among different feature groups. Next, we compared our results with Meier et al.'s method (Meier et al., 2014). Lastly, we show the segmentation results marked with different colors.

4.1. Comparison Between Feature Sets With Different Dimensions

In this step, we trained our model with different numbers of features as shown in **Table 3**. For the n-th training, we selected the top f-dimensional feature set ranked by the mRMR feature selection method according to their relevance and redundancy, where $f = 62 - 5n, n = 0, 1, 2, ..., 12$. Here we used random forest as our classifier and set the number of trees in the forest to 100. For every n, we evaluated the model by the measurements in section 3.7 within three regions: complete tumor, tumor core, and enhancing tumor. The HGG&LGG, HGG, and LGG MR scans subsets were tested.

As shown in **Table 3**, the difference between the results of two adjacent experiments is very small. It is difficult to distinguish which dimension f has the best performance. In order to obtain an intuitive feature selection outcome, we provide an overall ranking of the performances for each f and show the results in **Figure 3**. It can be seen that 22-dimensional feature set achieves the best performance among all the tested feature sets.

4.2. Comparison Between Different Feature Groups

In our studies, We have tested four different types of features. In order to learn which feature group is more informative for classification, we trained the model with each feature group and compared the performances of each feature group in **Table 4**. The table shows that the Gradient3D group performed far better than the other groups. It obtained a high Dice score (0.91) for complete tumor in HGG and a high PPV (0.92) for complete tumor in HGG&LGG datasets. And the CCS features performs slightly better than the context-sensitive features. However, compared with using all the 62 features, using a single group cannot achieve a better performance, which shows that each group is useful for classification and the integration of all the four groups is more helpful for classification.

4.3. Comparison With Other Method

We compared our methods with another method which was proposed by Meier et al. (2014). They extracted appearance-sensitive and context-sensitive features and also used random forest as a classifier.

As shown in **Table 5**, Meier et al. evaluated the classifier with three ROIs: complete tumor, tumor core, and enhancing

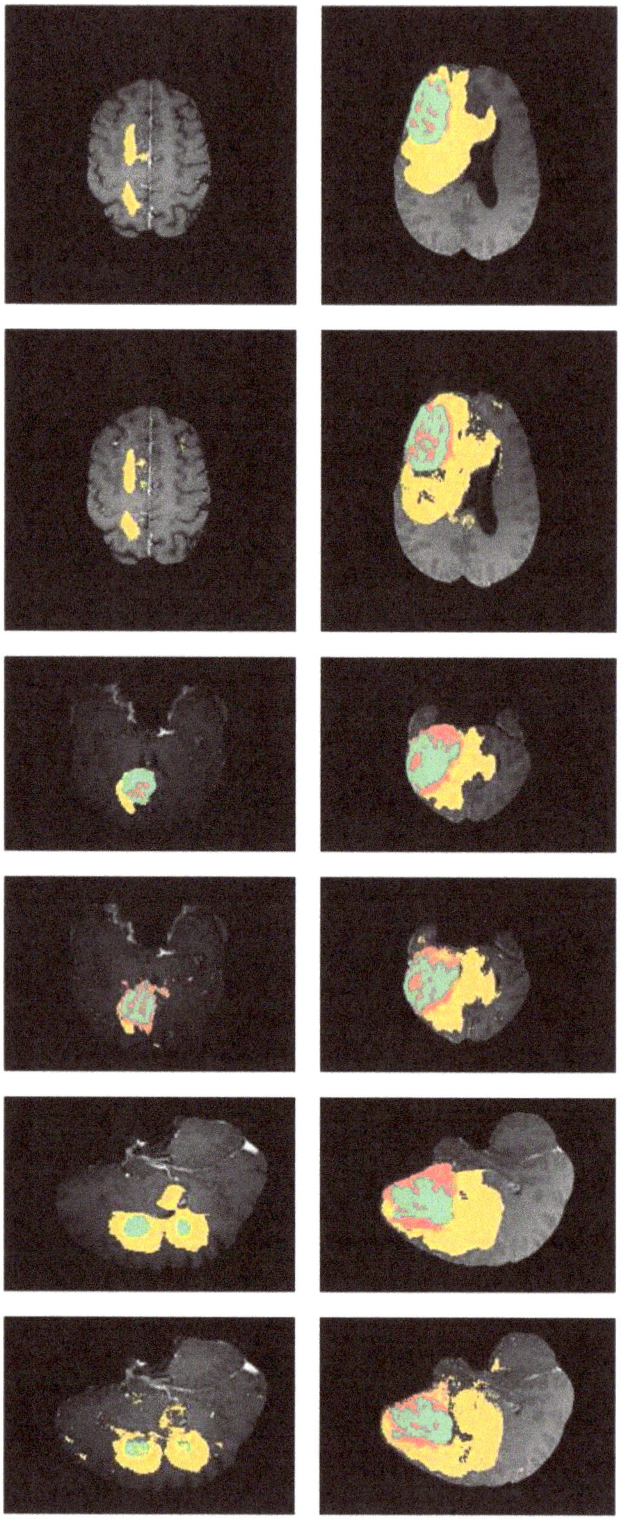

FIGURE 4 | Examples the brain tumor segmentation results using the proposed method. The rows 1,3,5 are the axial, sagittal, and coronal slices of the ground truth. Rows 2,4,6 are the axial, sagittal, and coronal slices of our results. The labels of the tumor structure: enhancing tumor (green), tumor core(green and red), complete tumor (green, red, and yellow).

tumor. However, the LGG performance was not mentioned. In our experiments, we trained the HGG&LGG, HGG, and LGG models and tested our models with three ROIs. As shown in **Table 3**, we had better performance especially for complete tumor. Compared to Meier et al.'s method, we not only extract the context-sensitive features, but we also made improvements and proposed the circular context-sensitive features, which considered multiple scales and multiple directions.

4.4. Performance of Brain Tumor Segmentation

In **Figure 4**, the axial, sagittal, and coronal slices of the ground truth are shown in rows 1, 3, and 5, respectively. The corresponding slices of the segmentation results are shown in rows 2, 4, and 6, respectively. As shown in **Figure 4**, our segmentation results are consistent with the ground truth. And we have good performance in all axial, sagittal, and coronal directions.

5. CONCLUSIONS

In our study, we proposed a supervised brain tumor segmentation method for MRI scans. We extracted four types of feature groups named Gradient2D set, Gradient3D set, context-sensitive features, and circular context-sensitive features, totally 62 features. Then we selected a set of the most informative feature set based on the mRMR algorithm and used them to build the random forest in order to distinguish different regions of brain tumors. We presented the performance comparisons among different dimensions of feature sets for feature selection, comparisons among different feature subgroups and comparisons with other tumor segmentation approaches. The results show that the proposed method is competitive in segmenting brain tumors.

AUTHOR CONTRIBUTIONS

JZ conducted the experiements. ZM, LW, and CS participated the manuscript writing. QZ and RS designed the experiments and edited the manuscript.

REFERENCES

Adams, R., and Bischof, L. (1994). Seeded region growing. *IEEE Trans. Pattern Anal. Mach. Intell.* 16, 641–647. doi: 10.1109/34.295913

Amini, L., Soltanian-Zadeh, H., Lucas, C., and Gity, M. (2004). Automatic segmentation of thalamus from brain MRI integrating fuzzy clustering and dynamic contours. *IEEE Trans. Biomed. Eng.* 51, 800–811. doi: 10.1109/TBME.2004.826654

Bauer, S., Wiest, R., Nolte, L.-P., and Reyes, M. (2013). A survey of MRI-based medical image analysis for brain tumor studies. *Phys. Med. Biol.* 58:R97. doi: 10.1088/0031-9155/58/13/R97

Bergholm, F. (1987). "Edge focusing," in *IEEE Transactions on Pattern Analysis and Machine Intelligence*, 726–741.

Bernsen, J. (1986). Dynamic thresholding of grey level images. in *Proceedings of the Eighth International Conference on Pattern Recognition* (Paris).

Boscolo, R., Brown, M. S., and McNitt-Gray, M. F. (2002). Medical image segmentation with knowledge-guided robust active contours. *Radiographics* 22, 437–448. doi: 10.1148/radiographics.22.2.g02mr26437

Breiman, L. (2001). Random forests. *Mach. Learn.* 45, 5–32. doi: 10.1023/A:1010933404324

Dam, E., Loog, M., and Letteboer, M. (2004). "Integrating automatic and interactive brain tumor segmentation," in *Proceedings of the 17th International Conference on Pattern Recognition. ICPR 2004*, Vol. 3 (Cambridge: IEEE), 790–793.

DeAngelis, L. M. (2001). Brain tumors. *N. Engl. J. Med.* 344, 114–123. doi: 10.1056/NEJM200101113440207

Deng, G., and Cahill, L. (1993). "An adaptive Gaussian filter for noise reduction and edge detection," in *Nuclear Science Symposium and Medical Imaging Conference, 1993 IEEE Conference Record* (San Francisco, CA: IEEE), 1615–1619.

Deng, W., Xiao, W., Deng, H., and Liu, J. (2010). " MRI brain tumor segmentation with region growing method based on the gradients and variances along and inside of the boundary curve," in *2010 3rd International Conference on Biomedical Engineering and Informatics*, Vol. 1 (Yantai), 393–396.

Gibbs, P., Buckley, D. L., Blackband, S. J., and Horsman, A. (1996). Tumour volume determination from MR images by morphological segmentation. *Phys. Med. Biol.* 41, 2437. doi: 10.1088/0031-9155/41/11/014

Goetz, M., Weber, C., Binczyk, F., Polanska, J., Tarnawski, R., Bobek-Billewicz, B., et al. (2016). DALSA: Domain adaptation for supervised learning from sparsely annotated MR images. *IEEE Trans. Med. Imaging* 35, 184–196. doi: 10.1109/TMI.2015.2463078

Gordillo, N., Montseny, E., and Sobrevilla, P. (2013). State of the art survey on MRI brain tumor segmentation. *Magn. Reson. Imaging* 31, 1426–1438. doi: 10.1016/j.mri.2013.05.002

Ho, S., Bullitt, E., and Gerig, G. (2002). "Level-set evolution with region competition: automatic 3-D segmentation of brain tumors," in *Proceedings of 16th International Conference on Pattern Recognition*, Vol. 1 (Quebec City, QC: IEEE), 532–535.

Ji, Z.-X., Sun, Q.-S., and Xia, D.-S. (2011). A modified possibilistic fuzzy c-means clustering algorithm for bias field estimation and segmentation of brain MR image. *Comput. Med. Imaging Graph.* 35, 383–397. doi: 10.1016/j.compmedimag.2010.12.001

Jin, M., Govindarajan, L. N., and Cheng, L. (2014). "A random-forest random field approach for cellular image segmentation," in *2014 IEEE 11th International Symposium on Biomedical Imaging (ISBI)* (Beijing: IEEE), 1251–1254.

Juang, L.-H., and Wu, M.-N. (2010). MRI brain lesion image detection based on color-converted k-means clustering segmentation. *Measurement* 43, 941–949. doi: 10.1016/j.measurement.2010.03.013

Kharrat, A., Benamrane, N., Messaoud, M. B., and Abid, M. (2009). "Detection of brain tumor in medical images," in *2009 3rd International Conference on Signals, Circuits and Systems* (Medenine: IEEE), 1–6.

Letteboer, M., Niessen, W., Willems, P., Dam, E. B., and Viergever, M. (2001). "Interactive multi-scale watershed segmentation of tumors in MR brain images," in *Proceedings of the IMIVA Workshop of MICCAI* (Berlin, Heidelberg).

Li, G., and Wan, Y. (2010). "Improved watershed segmentation with optimal scale based on ordered dither halftone and mutual information," in *IEEE International Conference on Computer Science and Information Technology*, Vol. 9 (Chengdu: IEEE), 296–300.

Liu, J., Narayanan, D., Chang, K., Kim, L., Turkbey, E., Lu, L., et al. (2015). "Automated segmentation of the thyroid gland on CT using multi-atlas label fusion and random forest," in *Biomedical Imaging (ISBI), 2015 IEEE 12th International Symposium on* (New York City, NY: IEEE), 1114–1117.

Louis, D. N., Ohgaki, H., Wiestler, O. D., Cavenee, W. K., Burger, P. C., Jouvet, A., et al. (2007). *The 2007 WHO Classification of Tumours of the Central Nervous System*. International Agency for Research on Cancer.

Luo, S., Li, R., and Ourselin, S. (2003). "A new deformable model using dynamic gradient vector flow and adaptive balloon forces," in *APRS Workshop on Digital Image Computing* (Brisbane, QLD) 9–14.

Mazzara, G. P., Velthuizen, R. P., Pearlman, J. L., Greenberg, H. M., and Wagner, H. (2004). Brain tumor target volume determination for radiation treatment planning through automated MRI segmentation. *Int. J. Radiat. Oncol. Biol. Phys.* 59, 300–312. doi: 10.1016/j.ijrobp.2004.01.026

Meier, R., Bauer, S., Slotboom, J., Wiest, R., and Reyes, M. (2014). "Appearance-and context-sensitive features for brain tumor segmentation," in *MICCAI BraTS Workshop* (Boston, MA).

Menze, B., Jakab, A., Bauer, S., Kalpathy-Cramer, J., Farahani, K., Kirby, J., et al. (2015). The multimodal brain tumor image segmentation benchmark (BRATS). *IEEE Trans. Med. Imaging* 34, 1993–2024. doi: 10.1109/TMI.2014.2377694

Niblack, W. (1986). *An Introduction to Digital Image Processing*, Vol. 34. Englewood Cliffs, NJ: Prentice-Hall.

Otsu, N. (1979). A threshold selection method from gray-level histograms. *IEEE Trans. Syst. Man Cybern.* 9, 62–66. doi: 10.1109/TSMC.1979.4310076

Peng, H., Long, F., and Ding, C. (2005). Feature selection based on mutual information criteria of max-dependency, max-relevance, and min-redundancy. *IEEE Trans. Pattern Anal. Mach. Intell.* 27, 1226–1238. doi: 10.1109/TPAMI.2005.159

Salman, Y. M., Assal, M. A., Badawi, A. M., Alian, S. M., and El-Bayome, M. El. (2005). "Validation techniques for quantitative brain tumors measurements," in *Proceedings of 2005 IEEE Engineering in Medicine and Biology 27th Annual Conference* (Shanghai), 7048–7051.

Sapra, P., Singh, R., and Khurana, S. (2013). "Brain tumor detection using neural network," in *International Journal of Science and Modern Engineering (IJISME)*, 2319–6386.

Sato, M., Lakare, S., Wan, M., Kaufman, A., and Nakajima, M. (2000). "A gradient magnitude based region growing algorithm for accurate segmentation," in *Proceedings 2000 International Conference on Image Processing (Cat. No.00CH37101)*, Vol. 3 (Vancouver, BC), 448–451.

Selvakumar, J., Lakshmi, A., and Arivoli, T. (2012). "Brain tumor segmentation and its area calculation in brain MR images using K-mean clustering and fuzzy c-mean algorithm," in *International Conference on Advances in Engineering, Science and Management* (IEEE), 186–190.

Sled, J. G., Zijdenbos, A. P., and Evans, A. C. (1998). A nonparametric method for automatic correction of intensity nonuniformity in MRI data. *IEEE Trans. Med. Imaging* 17, 87–97. doi: 10.1109/42.668698

Stadlbauer, A., Moser, E., Gruber, S., Buslei, R., Nimsky, C., Fahlbusch, R., et al. (2004). Improved delineation of brain tumors: an automated method for segmentation based on pathologic changes of 1H-MRSI metabolites in gliomas. *Neuroimage* 23, 454–461. doi: 10.1016/j.neuroimage.2004.06.022

Su, R., Wu, H., Xu, B., Liu, X., and Wei, L. (2018). "Developing a multi-dose computational model for drug-induced hepatotoxicity prediction based on toxicogenomics data," in *IEEE/ACM Transactions on Computational Biology and Bioinformatics*, doi: 10.1109/TCBB.2018.2858756.

Tang, W., Wan, S., Yang, Z., Teschendorff, A. E., and Zou, Q. (2017). Tumor origin detection with tissue-specific miRNA and DNA methylation markers. *Bioinformatics* 34, 398–406. doi: 10.1093/bioinformatics/btx622

Vaidhya, K., Thirunavukkarasu, S., Alex, V., and Krishnamurthi, G. (2015). "Multi-modal brain tumor segmentation using stacked denoising autoencoders," in *International Workshop on Brainlesion: Glioma, Multiple Sclerosis, Stroke and Traumatic Brain Injuries* (Springer), 181–194.

Vasuda, P. and Satheesh, S. (2010). Improved fuzzy C-means algorithm for MR brain image segmentation. *Int. J. Comput. Sci. Eng.* 2, 1713–1715.

Vijayakumar, C., and Gharpure, D. C. (2011). Development of image-processing software for automatic segmentation of brain tumors in MR images. *J. Med. Phys. Assoc. Med. Phys. India* 36, 147–158. doi: 10.4103/0971-6203.83481

Zeng, N., Qiu, H., Wang, Z., Liu, W., Zhang, H., and Li, Y. (2018a). A new switching-delayed-PSO-based optimized SVM algorithm for diagnosis of Alzheimer's disease. *Neurocomputing* 320, 195–202. doi: 10.1016/j.neucom.2018.09.001

Zeng, N., Zhang, H., Li, Y., Liang, J., and Dobaie, A. M. (2017). Denoising and deblurring gold immunochromatographic strip images via gradient projection algorithms. *Neurocomputing* 247, 165–172. doi: 10.1016/j.neucom.2017.03.056

Zeng, N., Zhang, H., Song, B., Liu, W., Li, Y., and Dobaie, A. M. (2018b). Facial expression recognition via learning deep sparse autoencoders. *Neurocomputing* 273, 643–649. doi: 10.1016/j.neucom.2017.08.043

Zhang, Y., Brady, M., and Smith, S. (2001). Segmentation of brain MR images through a hidden Markov random field model and the expectation-maximization algorithm. *IEEE Trans. Med. Imaging* 20, 45–57. doi: 10.1109/42.906424

Zhao, X., Wu, Y., Song, G., Li, Z., Zhang, Y., and Fan, Y. (2018). A deep learning model integrating FCNNs and CRFs for brain tumor segmentation. *Med. Image Anal.* 43, 98–111. doi: 10.1016/j.media.2017.10.002

Zou, Q., Wan, S., Ju, Y., Tang, J., and Zeng, X. (2016a). Pretata: predicting TATA binding proteins with novel features and dimensionality reduction strategy. *Bmc Syst. Biol.* 10(Suppl. 4):114. doi: 10.1186/s12918-016-0353-5

Zou, Q., Zeng, J., Cao, L., and Ji, R. (2016b). A novel features ranking metric with application to scalable visual and bioinformatics data classification. *Neurocomputing* 173, 346–354. doi: 10.1016/j.neucom.2014.12.123

Zulpe, N., and Pawar, V. (2012). GLCM textural features for brain tumor classification. *Int. J. Comput. Sci. Issues* 9:354.

3

Cerebral Micro-Bleeding Detection Based on Densely Connected Neural Network

Shuihua Wang[1†], Chaosheng Tang[1†], Junding Sun[1*] and Yudong Zhang[1,2*†]*

[1] School of Computer Science and Technology, Henan Polytechnic University, Jiaozuo, China, [2] Department of Informatics, University of Leicester, Leicester, United Kingdom

***Correspondence:**
Shuihua Wang
shuihuawang@ieee.org
Junding Sun
sunjd@hpu.edu.cn
Yudong Zhang
yudongzhang@ieee.org*

† These authors have contributed equally to this work

Cerebral micro-bleedings (CMBs) are small chronic brain hemorrhages that have many side effects. For example, CMBs can result in long-term disability, neurologic dysfunction, cognitive impairment and side effects from other medications and treatment. Therefore, it is important and essential to detect CMBs timely and in an early stage for prompt treatment. In this research, because of the limited labeled samples, it is hard to train a classifier to achieve high accuracy. Therefore, we proposed employing Densely connected neural network (DenseNet) as the basic algorithm for transfer learning to detect CMBs. To generate the subsamples for training and test, we used a sliding window to cover the whole original images from left to right and from top to bottom. Based on the central pixel of the subsamples, we could decide the target value. Considering the data imbalance, the cost matrix was also employed. Then, based on the new model, we tested the classification accuracy, and it achieved 97.71%, which provided better performance than the state of art methods.

Keywords: DenseNet, CMB detection, transfer learning, cost matrix, deep learning

INTRODUCTION

Cerebral micro-bleeding (CMB) are small chronic brain hemorrhages that can be caused by structural abnormalities of the small vessels of the brain. According to the recent research reports, the causes of CMBs also can be some other common reasons, including high blood pressure, head trauma, aneurysm, blood vessel abnormalities, liver disease, blood or bleeding disorders and brain tumors (Martinez-Ramirez et al., 2014). It also can be caused by some unusual etiologies, such as cocaine abuse, posterior reversible encephalopathy, brain radiation therapy, intravascular lymphomatosis, thrombotic thrombocytopenic purpura, moyamoya disease, infective endocarditis, sickle cell anemia/β-thalassemia, proliferating angio-endotheliomatosis, cerebral autosomal dominant arteriopathy subcortical infarcts, leukoencephalopathy (CADASIL), genetic syndromes, or obstructive sleep apnea (Noorbakhsh-Sabet et al., 2017). The patients suffering from CMBs can have symptoms where the corresponding area that is controlled by the bleeding area malfunctions, resulting in a rise in intracranial pressure due to the large mass putting pressure on the brain and so on. CMBs could be easily ignored as the similar symptoms and signs of the subarachnoid hemorrhages, unless the patients have more obvious symptoms, such as a headache followed by vomiting. Those symptoms can eventually become worse or occur suddenly, based on the distribution and intensity of the CMBs. Patients suffering from CMBs can result in cognitive impairment, neurologic dysfunction and long-term disability. CMBs could also induce side effects from medication or treatments. The worse thing is that the death is possible and can happen quickly. Therefore, the early and prompt diagnosis of CMBs is essential and helpful in timely medical treatment.

Due to the paramagnetic susceptibility of the hemosiderin (Allen et al., 2000), CMBs can be visualized by T2*-gradient recalled echo (GRE) imaging or susceptibility weighted imaging (SWI). Traditionally, CMBs are manually interpreted based on criteria including shapes, diameters and signal characteristics after imaging. However, the criteria were varied as reported in different studies (Cordonnier et al., 2007), until 2009 when Greenberg et al. (2009) published the consensus on standard criteria for CMB identification. However, manual detection methods involve the human interventions, which can bring biases. Meanwhile, the manual detection is labor intensive, hard to reproduce and difficult to exclude the mimics, which can lead to misdiagnosis.

Therefore, the development of automatic CMB detection is important and essential for the accurate detection and early diagnosis of CMBs. Due to the benefits of advanced imaging technologies, massive computer vision aided systems have been developed for automatic CMB detection. For example, Ateeq et al. (2018) proposed a system based on an ensemble classifier. Their system consisted of three steps: first the brain was extracted, then the initial candidates were detected based on the filter and threshold, and finally, feature extraction and classification model were built to remove the false alarms. Fazlollahi et al. (2015) proposed using a multi-scale Laplacian of Gaussian (msLoG) technique to detect the potential CMB candidates, followed by extracting a set of 3-dimensional Radon and Hessian based shape descriptors within each bounding box to train a cascade of binary random forests. Barnes et al. (2011) proposed a statistical thresholding algorithm to recognize the potential hypo-intensities. Then, a supervised classification model based on the support vector machine was employed to distinguish true CMBs from other marked hypo-intensities. van den Heuvel et al. (2016) proposed an automatic detection system for microbleeds in MRIs of patients with trauma based on twelve characteristics related with the dark and spherical characteristics of CMBs and the random forest classifier. Bian et al. (2013) proposed a 2D fast radial symmetry transform (RST) based method to roughly detect the possible CMBs. Then the 3D region growing on the possible CMBs was utilized to exclude the falsely identified CMBs. Ghafaryasl et al. (2012) proposed a computer aided system based on following three steps: skull-stripping, initial candidate selection and reduction of false-positives (FPs) by a two-layer classifier. Zhang et al. (2017) proposed voxel-vise detection based on a single hidden layer feed-forward neural network with scaled conjugate gradient. Chen (2017) proposed a seven-layer deep neural network based on the sparse autoencoder for voxel detection of CMBs. Seghier et al. (2011) proposed a system named MIDAS for automatic CMB detection.

All above methods have reached great progress in CMB detection. However, their detection accuracy and robustness are still in need of improvement.

Therefore, in this paper, we employed the SWI for CMB imaging, which was because SWI could provide high resolution as reported in Haacke et al. (2009) and work as the most sensitive techniques to visualize CMBs. Considering the limited amounts of labeled images, and knowledge to recognize representative characters about the medical images, we considered utilizing the DenseNet as the basic algorithm for transfer learning. The reason for this is because the amount of labeled CMB images is typically very limited, and it is hard to effectively train a classifier to get high detection accuracy. In summary, we proposed using transfer learning of DenseNet for CMB detection based on the collected images, which means we use the knowledges obtained from training the related tasks by DenseNet for CMB detection.

The remainder of this paper is organized in a structure as follows: "Materials and Methods" section describes the method used in this research, "Transfer Learning" section explains why we employed the transfer learning, "CMB Detection Based on the Transfer Learning and DenseNet" section describes the research materials used in this paper, including the training set and test set, and also offers the experiment results, and finally, "Discussion" section provides the conclusion and discussion.

MATERIALS AND METHODS

In recent years, Deep Learning (DL) has achieved great progress in object recognition (Tong et al., 2019; Xie et al., 2019), prediction (Yan et al., 2018; Hao et al., 2019), speech analysis (Cummins et al., 2018), noise reduction (Islam et al., 2018), monitoring (Li et al., 2018; Wang et al., 2018), medicine (Raja et al., 2015; Safdar et al., 2018), the recommendation system (Zhang and Liu, 2014), biometrics (Xing et al., 2017) and so on. Traditionally, DL consists of multiple layers of non-linear processing units to obtain the features. The cascaded layers take the output from their previous layer as input. In order to explore the potential of DL, many researchers tried to make the network deeper and wider. However, it suffers from either exploding or the vanishing gradient problem (VGP). Therefore, multiple different structures of DL were proposed. For example, AlexNet, the winner of ImageNet Large Scale Visual Recognition Competition (ILSVRC) 2012, was proposed by Krizhevsky et al. (2012) and has the same structure as LeNet but has max pooling and ReLU non-linearity. VGGNet, proposed by Karen Simonyan (2015), won the second place in ILSVRC 2014 and consisted of deeper networks (19 layers) compared to AlexNet. GoogLeNet, the winner of ILSVRC 2014, provides a deeper and wider network that incorporates 1×1 convolutions to reduce the dimensionality of the feature maps before expensive convolutions, together with parallel paths with different receptive field sizes to capture sparse patterns of correlations in the feature map stacks. ResNet, the winner of ILSVRC 2015, offers a 152-layer network that introduces a skip at least two layers or shortcut connections (He et al., 2016). Huang et al. (2017) proposed DenseNet where each layer takes the output from all previous layers in a feed-forward fashion and offers $L(L+1)/2$ connections for L layers, while traditional convolution networks with L layers provide L connections. According to the report in Huang et al. (2017), DenseNet can beat the state-of-the-art ResNet structure on ImageNet classification task.

Considering the outstanding performance of DenseNet, we proposed employing DenseNet for cerebral microbleed detection in this paper. The detail of DenseNet was introduced as follows. However, before providing the illustration of the DenseNet, we would first introduce the traditional convolution neural network (CNN) and figure out the difference between CNN and DenseNet later.

Traditional Convolution Neural Network

The traditional CNN usually includes convolution layer, ReLU Layer, pooling layer, fully connected layer and softmax layer (Zeng et al., 2014, 2016a,c, 2017a,b). The functions of different layers are introduced as follows:

> Convolution layer works as the core session of a CNN. The feature maps are generated via the convolution of the input with different kernels. Mathematically, it can be expressed as **Figure 1**, which shows a toy example of convolution operation.

Then, following the convolution layer, we have non-linear activation function, named ReLU, which works to obtain the non-linear features. The purpose of the ReLU layer is to introduce non-linearity into the network. The mathematic expression of ReLU is shown as Eq. 1:

$$f(x) = x^+ = \max(0, x) \tag{1}$$

The pooling layer works by resizing the feature maps spatially to decrease the number of parameters, memory footprint and to make the computation less intensive in the network. The pooling function works on each feature map, the main approaches used for pooling are max pooling as Eq. 2, average pooling as Eq. 3:

$$a_j = \max_{i \in R_j}(M_i) \tag{2}$$

$$a_j = \frac{1}{|R_j|} \sum_{i \in R_j} M_i \tag{3}$$

In which M stands for the pooling region and Rj represents for the number of elements within the pooling region.

Fully connected layers will calculate the confidential scores, which are stored in a volume of size $1 \times 1 \times n$. Here, n means the number of categories, and each element stands for class scores. Every neuron of the fully connected layer is connected to all the neurons in the earlier layers.

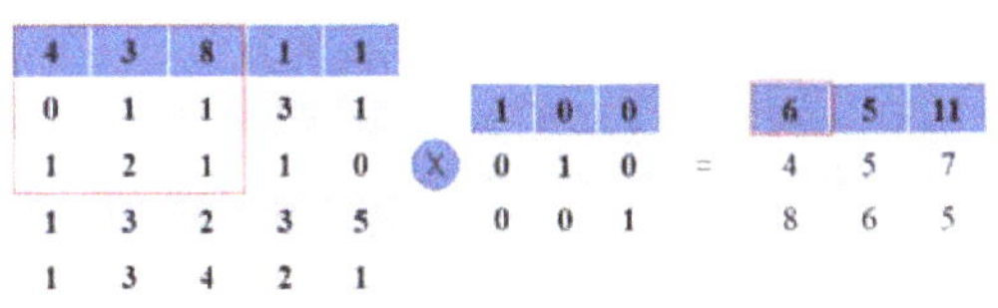

FIGURE 1 | A toy example of convolution operation in CNN with stride size as 1, in which, the left matrix means the input, the second matrix means the kernel, and the right matrix stands for the generated feature map after convolution operation. It is different from the convolution defined in purely mathematic terms.

Structure Revision of the CNN

In the traditional CNN, all layers are connected gradually as in Eq. 4:

$$x_l = H_l(x_{l-1}) \tag{4}$$

However, as the network becomes deeper and wider, the networks may suffer from either exploding or gradient vanishing. Therefore, researchers proposed different network structures to overcome this problem. For example, ResNet revised this behavior by short connection, and the equation is reformulated as (5).

$$x_l = H_l(x_{l-1}) + x_{l-1} \tag{5}$$

Instead of making the sum of the output feature maps of the layer with the incoming feature maps, DenseNet concatenates them sequentially. The expression is reformulated into Eq. 6:

$$x_l = H_l([x_0, x_1, x_2, ..., x_{l-1}]) \tag{6}$$

In which l means the index of the layer number, H stands for a non-linear operation and x_l stands for the output of the lth layer.

DenseNet

As expressed in Eq. 6, DenseNet introduces straight forward connections from any layers to all following layers. In other words, the lth layer receives feature-maps from all previous $l-1$ layers. However, if the feature maps' size changes, the concatenation operation is not feasible. Therefore, down-sampling to change the size of the feature maps are introduced. In order to make the down-sampling in the structure of DenseNet possible, multiple densely connected dense blocks are introduced to divide the network. The layers between the blocks are named as transition layers that have batch normalization, convolution and pooling operations, as shown in **Figure 2**. **Figure 2** describes a case of DenseBlock, in which the layer number is 5 and the growth rate is set as k. Each layer receives feature maps from all earlier layers.

For each operation H_l, it generates k feature maps, which is defined as growth rate. Therefore, the l_{th} layer will have $k_0 + k(l-1)$ feature maps, and k_0 is the number of channels in the

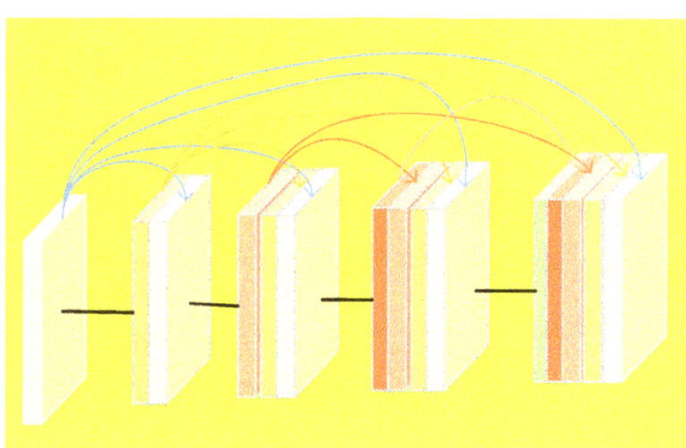

FIGURE 2 | Structure of the DenseBlock (5 layers and each layer takes feature maps from all previous layers).

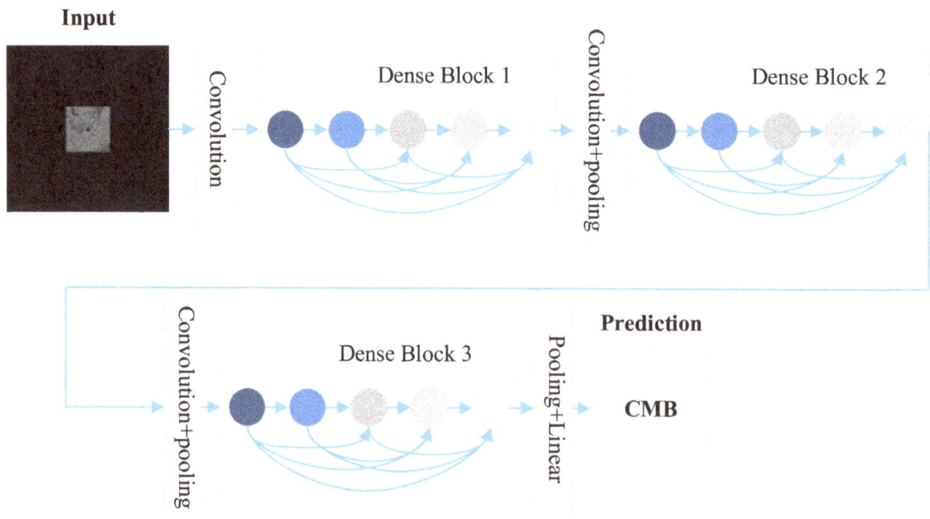

FIGURE 3 | The structure of the DenseNet.

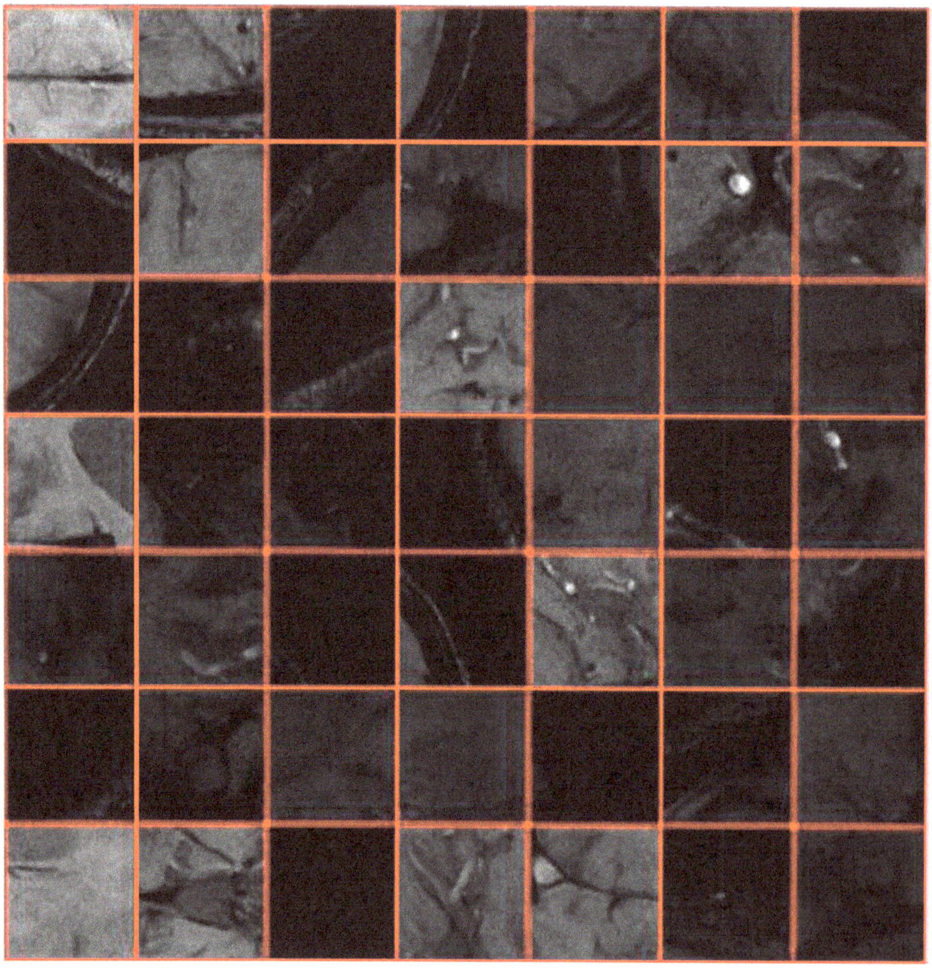

FIGURE 4 | Non-CMB samples.

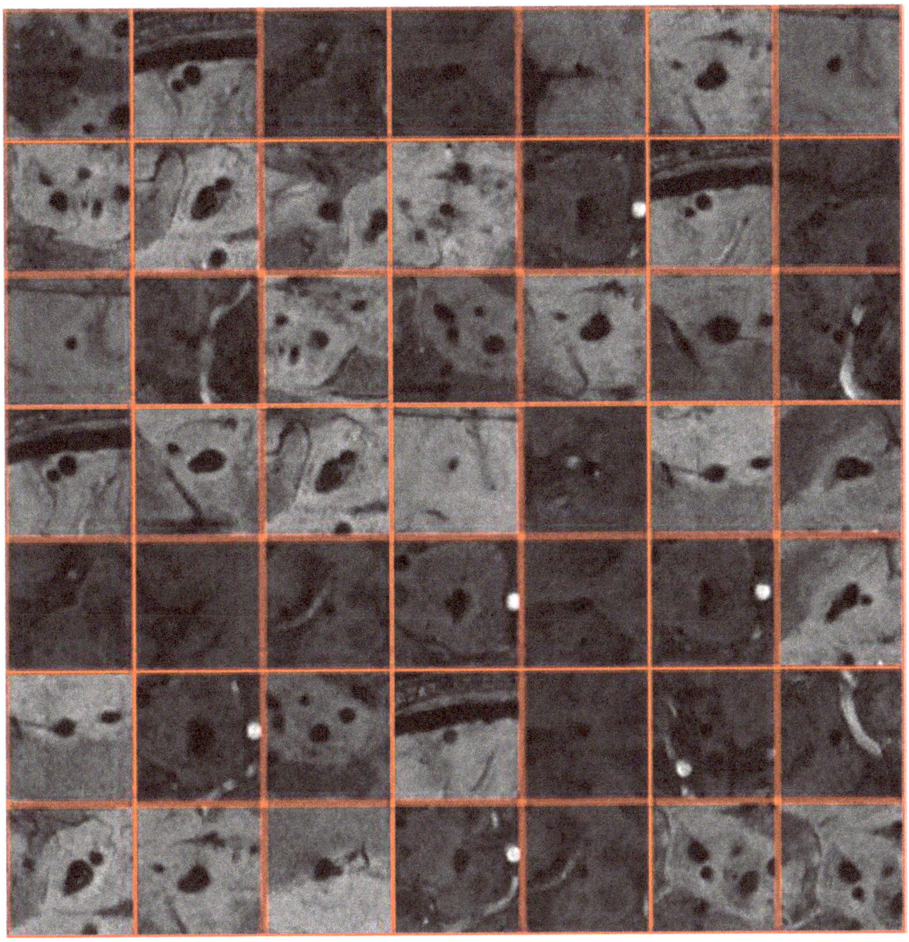

FIGURE 5 | CMB samples.

input layer. As the network typically has a large number of inputs, a 1×1 convolution is employed as the bottleneck layer before the 3×3 convolution layer to reduce the feature maps and improve the computation efficiency.

To further compress the model to improve the model compactness, the feature maps are further reduced by the transition layer. For example, if a dense block generates m feature maps and the compression factor is set as $\theta \in (0, 1]$, then the feature maps will be reduced to $\lfloor \theta m \rfloor$ via the followed transition layer. If $\theta = 1$, the number of feature maps will be the same. **Figure 3** shows the structure of DenseNet, which is composed of three DenseBlocks, an input layer and transition layers. The cropped samples are used as the input, the final layer will tell us whether it is CMB or Non-CMB in this research.

TRANSFER LEARNING

DenseNet has been widely applied in the medical research. For example, Gottapu and Dagli (2018) proposed using DenseNet for Anatomical Brain Segmentation. Khened et al. (2019) proposed cardiac segmentation based on fully convolutional multi-scale residual DenseNets. Wang H. et al. (2019) offered a system for recognition of mild cognitive impairment (MCI) and Alzheimer's disease (AD), based on the ensemble of 3D densely connected convolution network. Considering the limited amounts of labeled training samples, it is far way from enough to retrain the whole network of DenseNet from scratch to get a high classification accuracy. Therefore, in this paper, we proposed transfer learning, which means frozen the earlier layers and retrain the later layers of DenseNet for CMB detection task. The structure of DenseNet used here is DenseNet 201.

In order to make the pretrained DenseNet 201 for CMB detection feasible, which was a binary classification of CMB or non-CMB, the fully connected (FC) layer with

TABLE 1 | Dividing of the dataset for training and testing.

	Train	Test
CMB	58, 847	10000
Non-CMB	56, 572, 536	10000

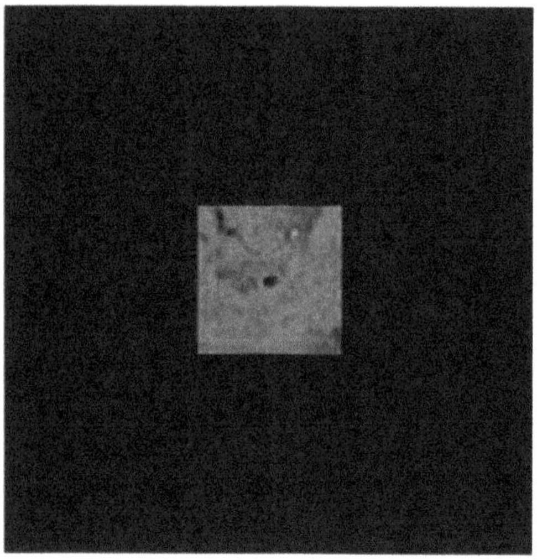

FIGURE 6 | Images padded for DenseNet.

1000 neuron was replaced by a new FC layer with 2 neurons. The structure of the remaining part of DenseNet 201 was unchanged.

CMB DETECTION BASED ON THE TRANSFER LEARNING AND DENSENET

Materials

The subjects used in this research are ten healthy controls and ten patients of CADASIL. Twenty 3D volumetric images were obtained from the 20 patients. Then, Software Sygno MR B17 was utilized to rebuild the 3D volumetric image. Each 3D volumetric image's size is uniformly set as 364*448*48.

In order to mark the CMBs from the subjects manually, we employed three neuron-radiologists with more than twenty-years' experience. The rules were set as follows: (1) via tracking the neighbor slices, blood vessels were first excluded, (2) lesions should be smaller than 10 mm in diameter. The potential CMBs were labeled as either "possible" or "Definite," Otherwise, regarded as non-CMB voxels. In case of the conflictions, we proposed to obey the rule that the minority should be subordinate to the majority.

The sample images were generated from the original image. We applied the sliding window whose size is set as 61 by 61 to the original image. The border pixels were discarded due to the fat and brain skull. All the pixels located within a sliding window were used as one input, and the point located in the center of the sliding window was used as the target value. It means that if the central pixel is true or 1, then the target value is 1, otherwise, the

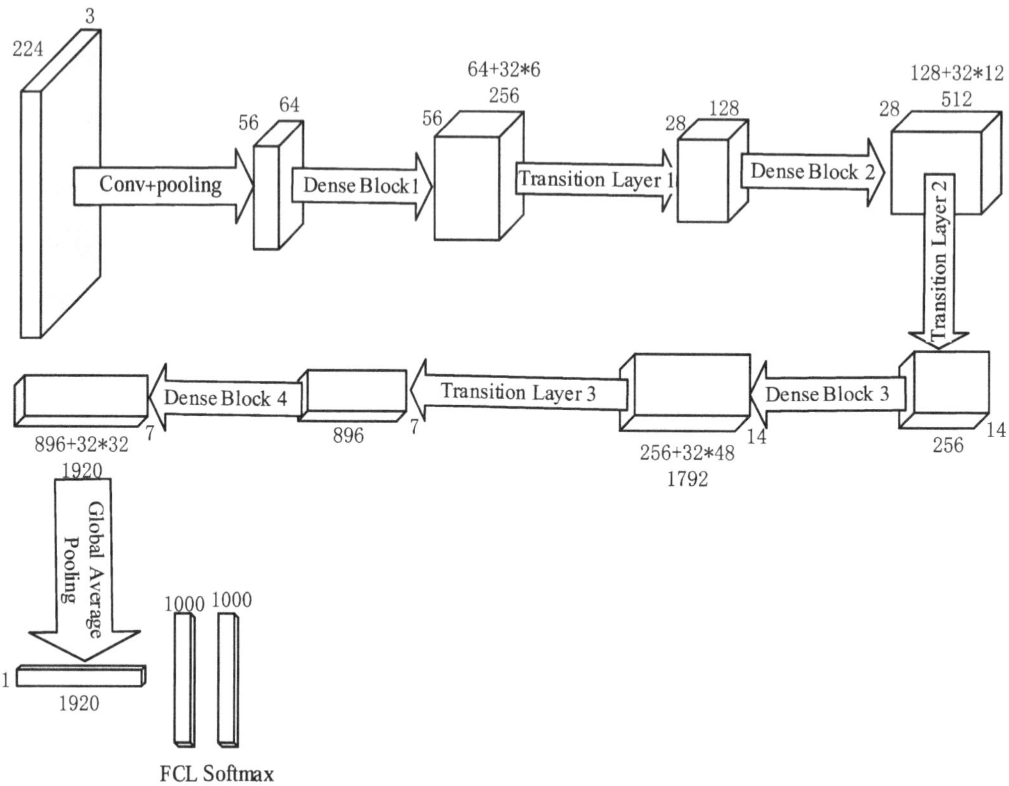

FIGURE 7 | Flowchart of DenseNet 201.

target label is set as 0. It is expressed in the Eqs 7 and 8:

$$I = W(p) \tag{7}$$

$$Ou = \begin{cases} 1, & \text{Central pixel } p \text{ is true (CMB)} \\ 0, & \text{Central pixel } p \text{ is false (non} - \text{CMB)} \end{cases} \tag{8}$$

Where I stands for the cropped sample images generated via the sliding window, p represents for the central pixel, $W(p)$ means the pixels which centered on pixel p and were located inside the sliding window, and Ou means the label value. **Figures 4, 5** show the sample of CMB and non-CMB centered images.

The sliding window was supposed to cover the image from left to right and top to bottom with the stride size as 1. Therefore, we got the total CMB voxels as 68, 847 and non-CMB voxels as 56, 582, 536. The training and test set was divided as **Table 1**. We randomly selected 10000 images for each category of the test, and the remaining images were used for training.

To make the images suitable for DenseNet, which should be resized as 224 × 224 × 3, we padded the images with zero. The preprocessed image sample is shown as **Figure 6**. Then, **Figure 7** shows the flowchart of the DenseNet, including number of feature maps generated by each layer.

From **Table 1**, we can find that the Non-CMB training data dominates the majority type CMB, which will cause the classifier more bias toward to the Non-CMB. Therefore, it may cause difficulties in controlling false positives and false negatives, which means the model is hard to find the CMB samples. Therefore, in order to overcome this challenge, we introduced cost matrix (Wu and Kim, 2010). The cost ratio ct was set as 961 via Eq. 9:

$$ct = N_{non-CMB}/N_{CMB} \tag{9}$$

In which $N_{non-CMB}$ means the number of non-CMB training samples and N_{CMB} stands for number of CMB training samples. The reason for why we employ the cost matrix instead of over sampling or down sampling is mainly because we have more concerns about the false positives and false negatives, therefore it is better to highlight the imbalanced learning problem by using cost matrices instead of creating a balanced data distribution forcefully.

Experiment Design

The goal of this research is to identify the input image as either CMB or Non-CMB. In order to achieve this goal, we proposed using DenseNet 201 as the basic algorithm for transfer learning, based on the excellent performance of DenseNet on ImageNet classification task. Section "Materials" stated the materials used in this research. Based on the original images, we created 68, 847 CMB subsamples and 56, 582, 536 Non-CMB subsamples. 10000 samples were randomly selected as test samples. The remaining sub-samples were used for training. In order to overcome the problem of data imbalance, we proposed cost matrix to show the more concerns in false positive and false negatives. The experiment is carried on by Matlab on the Windows 10 Operation System with 2.88 GHz processor and 8 GB memory. The following experiments were carried out: (1) CMB detection based on DenseNet. The measurements used here include accuracy, sensitivity and specificity. The definition of the measurements can be found in Zhang et al. (2018b). (2) Different cutting points of transfer learning. (3) In order to show the performance of proposed methods, we compared with other state of art work. Considering the measurements provided in other research, we only used sensitivity, specificity and accuracy.

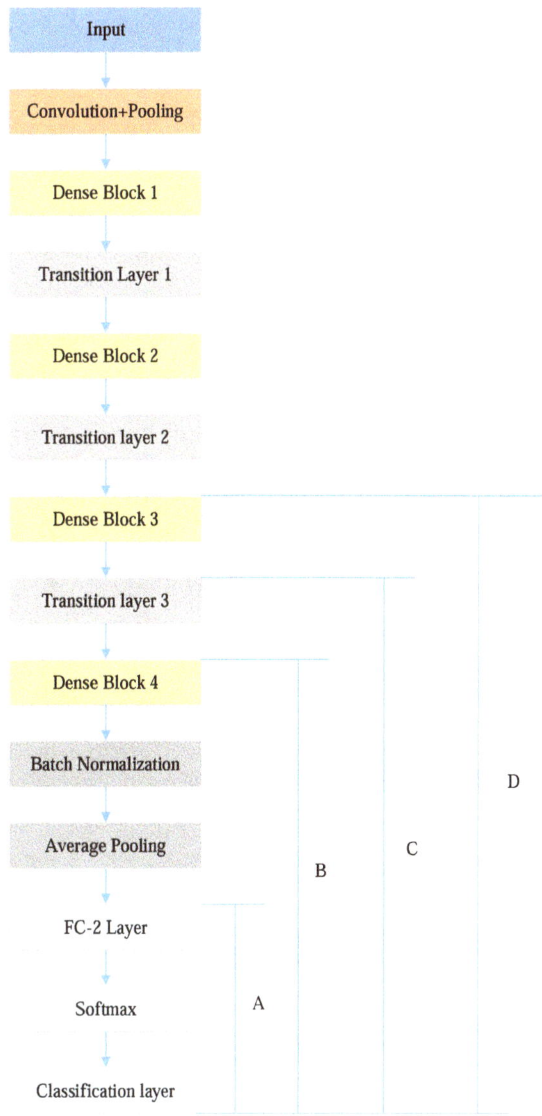

FIGURE 8 | Different cases of transfer learning (the original fully connected layer with 1000 neurons was replaced by a new fully connected layer with 2 neurons).

TABLE 2 | Confusion matrix of detected CMB and Non-CMB.

	Predicted	
Actual	**CMBs**	**Non-CMBs**
CMBs (10000)	9777	223
Non-CMBs (10000)	236	9764

In order to provide better illustration of DenseNet, we added a flowchart with feature map size, learnable weights of each layer. As we only noted the size of the width, the length should be same with the width.

CMB Detection Result Based on DenseNet

The rebuilt network was composed of four DenseBlocks, one input layer, three transition layers, one fully connected layer with two neurons, a softmax layer and a classification layer, as described in **Figure 8**.

Table 2 provides the detection result. The correctly detected CMBs were 9777, and for Non-CMB they were 9764. 236 non-CMBs were incorrectly detected as CMBs, and 223 CMBs were wrongly detected as non-CMBs. The sensitivity was achieved as 97.78%, the specificity was 97.64%, the accuracy was 97.71% and the precision was 97.65%. Above measurements were obtained based on the average of 10 runs as shown in **Table 3**.

Comparison to the Different Cases of Transfer Learning

In order to achieve the best performance of transfer learning, different cutting points for transfer learning were designed as shown in **Figure 8**. Due to the limited subjects, we mainly focused on retraining the later layers of DenseNet. Therefore, in case A, the DenseNet 201 except for the last three layers, was used as the feature extractor for this research, and we retrained the newly added three layers.

In case B, C, and D, we included extra layers for retraining. For example, case B retrained the DenseBlock 4, Batch normalization, Average pooling, Fully connected (FC) layer, softmax layer and classification layer. It was implemented via setting the learning rate to 0 for earlier layers and setting learning rate factor to 10 for layers to be retrained. **Table 4** illustrates the comparison results.

From **Table 4**, we can find that Case A performed slightly better than the other three cases in the terms of sensitivity and

TABLE 3 | Measurements value CMB detection based on transfer learning of DenseNet (Units: %).

Measurements	Sensitivity	Specificity	Accuracy	Precision
R 1	96.69	96.73	96.71	96.72
R 2	97.82	97.87	97.84	97.90
R 3	98.71	98.51	98.61	98.52
R 4	96.71	96.27	96.49	96.29
R 5	96.69	96.19	96.44	96.22
R 6	96.93	96.99	96.96	97.00
R 7	98.44	98.40	98.42	98.39
R 8	98.77	98.58	98.67	98.58
R 9	98.71	98.62	98.67	98.62
R 10	98.30	98.22	98.26	98.22
	97.78 ± 0.88	97.64 ± 0.94	97.71 ± 0.90	97.65 ± 0.93

TABLE 4 | Comparison of different cases of transfer learning (Unit: %).

	Sensitivity	Specificity	Accuracy	Precision
Case A	97.78 ± 0.88	97.64 ± 0.94	97.71 ± 0.90	97.65 ± 0.93
Case B	97.56 ± 0.83	97.65 ± 0.76	97.60 ± 0.79	97.67 ± 0.76
Case C	97.36 ± 1.05	97.66 ± 0.8	97.51 ± 0.92	97.66 ± 0.82
Case D	97.61 ± 0.63	97.54 ± 0.65	97.58 ± 0.64	97.57 ± 0.65

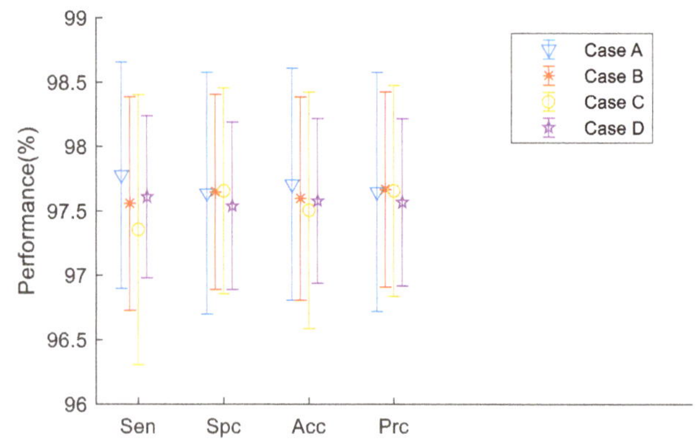

FIGURE 9 | Error bar.

TABLE 5 | Comparison to the state of art methods.

Method	Sensitivity	Specificity	Accuracy
SNP+SLFN+LReLU (Zhang et al., 2018c)	93.05	93.06	93.06
4-layer SAE (Zhang et al., 2016)	93.20 ± 1.37	93.25 ± 1.38	93.22 ± 1.37
7-layer SAE (Zhang et al., 2018d)	95.13 ± 0.84	93.33 ± 0.84	94.23 ± 0.84
CNN + RAP (Wang et al., 2017)	96.94	97.18	97.18
CNN (Lu et al., 2017)	97.29	92.23	96.05
NBC (Bao et al., 2018)	74.53 ± 0.96	74.51 ± 1.05	74.52 ± 1.00
GA-BPNN (Cloutie, 2018)	72.90 ± 1.38	72.89 ± 1.18	72.90 ± 1.28
CNN-SP (Wang S. et al., 2019)	97.22	97.35	97.28
Our method	97.78 ± 0.88	97.64 ± 0.94	97.71 ± 0.90

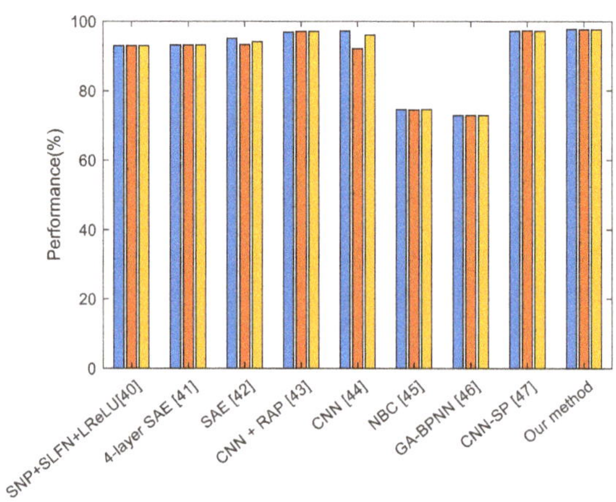

FIGURE 10 | Comparison of the state of art methods (Blue means the sensitivity, red means the specificity, and yellow means the accuracy).

accuracy. Considering that in medical research, we focus more on the sensitivity and accuracy than on the other two terms, we thought Case A provided the best performance among all the cases. **Figure 9** shows the error bar of the measurement values. From the point of storage consuming, all four cases take about the same RAM as we did when not using the precomputation method.

Comparison to the State of Art Work

In order to validate our proposed method, we compared different state of the art methods, including traditional machine learning methods and DL methods.

From **Table 5**, we compared our method with single-hidden layer feed-forward neural-network (SLFN)+ (leaky) rectified linear unit, 4-layer sparse encoder, 7-layer sparse encoder, different layers of CNN, Naive Bayesian Classifier and so on. We can find that our proposed method offers the best performance. DenseNet works as a logical extension of ResNet but provides more compact models and fully uses the features.

Figure 10 shows the bar chart of the comparison of the state of the state of art methods. It shows that our proposed method performs slightly better than the current best method, but largely improved compared to the traditional method naïve Bayes classifier (NBC).

DISCUSSION

In this paper, we proposed to employ DenseNet to detect CMBs in patients with CADASIL. DenseNet was proposed by Huang et al. (2017) and competed the other DL methods for ImageNet classification task because of its model compactness and fully used features. DenseNet are quite similar with ResNet, however, instead of the summation, DenseNet proposed the concatenation of all feature maps from previous layers, which encourages the feature reuse, the VGP alleviation, and the decreased number of parameters.

Therefore, in this paper, we proposed using DenseNet for CMB detection by supposing CMB detection has similarity with ImageNet classification. However, because of the data imbalance, we utilized cost matrix to avoid the model bias toward non-CMB, which means the model would be hard to find CMBs if trained under the imbalanced dataset. As there are some other methods for data imbalance, such as over sampling and down sampling, we have more concerns about the false negatives or false positives. Therefore, instead of enforcing the data into balanced distribution, we employed the cost matrix. In order to check the best cutting point, we test different cases of transfer learning and the results are shown in **Table 4**, however, the difference is not so obvious. On the other hand, training less layers can help us save time and decrease the computation cost if we import the strategy of precomputation.

In the future, we will try to collect more samples and test more different structures for CMB detection. Meanwhile, the training cost long term is very high (Zeng et al., 2018), therefore it is necessary to optimize the algorithm to make the training fast (Zeng et al., 2016b,d). We will consider other precomputation and some optimization methods (Zhang et al., 2018a).

ETHICS STATEMENT

This research was approved by Institutional Review Board (IRB) of the First Affiliated Hospital of Nanjing Medical University. We obtained written informed consent from the participants of this study.

AUTHOR CONTRIBUTIONS

SW proposed the study and wrote the draft. CT and JS designed the model and interpreted the results. CT and YZ analyzed the data. SW and YZ acquired the preprocessed data. All authors gave critical revision and consent for this submission.

FUNDING

This project was financially supported by Natural Science Foundation of Jiangsu Province (No. BK20180727).

REFERENCES

Allen, P. D., St Pierre, T. G., Chua-anusorn, W., Ström, V., and Rao, K. V. (2000). Low-frequency low-field magnetic susceptibility of ferritin and hemosiderin. *Biochim. Biophys. Acta* 1500, 186–196. doi: 10.1016/s0925-4439(99)00104-0

Ateeq, T., Majeed, M. N., Anwar, S. M., Maqsood, M., Rehman, Z.-U., Lee, J. W., et al. (2018). Ensemble-classifiers-assisted detection of cerebral microbleeds in brain MRI. *Comput. Electr. Eng.* 69, 768–781. doi: 10.1016/j.compeleceng.2018.02.021

Bao, F., Shen, M., and Macdonald, F. (2018). Voxelwise detection of cerebral microbleed in CADASIL patients by naïve Bayesian classifier. *Adv. Intel. Syst. Res.* 148, 176–180.

Barnes, S. R. S., Haacke, E. M., Ayaz, M., Boikov, A. S., Kirsch, W., and Kido, D. (2011). Semiautomated detection of cerebral microbleeds in magnetic resonance images. *Mag. Reson. Imag.* 29, 844–852. doi: 10.1016/j.mri.2011.02.028

Bian, W., Hess, C. P., Chang, S. M., Nelson, S. J., and Lupo, J. M. (2013). Computer-aided detection of radiation-induced cerebral microbleeds on susceptibility-weighted MR images. *NeuroImage Clin.* 2, 282–290. doi: 10.1016/j.nicl.2013.01.012

Chen, H. (2017). Seven-layer deep neural network based on sparse autoencoder for voxelwise detection of cerebral microbleed. *Multimedi. Tools Appl.* 77, 10521–10538. doi: 10.1007/s11042-017-4554-8

Cloutie, R. S. (2018). Voxelwise detection of cerebral microbleed in CADASIL patients by genetic algorithm and back propagation neural network. *Adv. Comput. Sci. Res.* 65, 101–105.

Cordonnier, C., Al-Shahi Salman, R., and Wardlaw, J. (2007). Spontaneous brain microbleeds: systematic review, subgroup analyses and standards for study design and reporting. *Brain* 130, 1988–2003. doi: 10.1093/brain/awl387

Cummins, N., Baird, A., and Schuller, B. W. (2018). Speech analysis for health: current state-of-the-art and the increasing impact of deep learning. *Methods* 151, 41–54. doi: 10.1016/j.ymeth.2018.07.007

Fazlollahi, A., Meriaudeau, F., Giancardo, L., Villemagne, V. L., Rowe, C. C., Yates, P., et al. (2015). Computer-aided detection of cerebral microbleeds in susceptibility-weighted imaging. *Comput. Med. Imag. Graph.* 46, 269–276. doi: 10.1016/j.compmedimag.2015.10.001

Ghafaryasl, B., Lijn, F. V. D., Poels, M., Vrooman, H., Ikram, M. A., Niessen, W. J., et al. (2012). "A computer aided detection system for cerebral microbleeds in brain MRI," in *Proceedings of the 2012 9th IEEE International Symposium on Biomedical Imaging (ISBI)*, Barcelona, 138–141.

Gottapu, R. D., and Dagli, C. H. (2018). DenseNet for anatomical brain segmentation. *Proc. Comput. Sci.* 140, 179–185. doi: 10.1016/j.compmedimag. 2018.09.009

Greenberg, S. M., Vernooij, M. W., Cordonnier, C., Viswanathan, A., Al-Shahi Salman, R., Warach, S., et al. (2009). Cerebral microbleeds: a guide to detection and interpretation. *Lancet Neurol.* 8, 165–174. doi: 10.1016/S1474-4422(09) 70013-4

Haacke, E. M., Mittal, S., Wu, Z., Neelavalli, J., and Cheng, Y.-C. N. (2009). Susceptibility-weighted imaging: technical aspects and clinical applications, part 1. *Am. J. Neuroradiol.* 30, 19–30. doi: 10.3174/ajnr.a1400

Hao, Y. X., Usama, M., Yang, J., Hossain, M. S., and Ghoneim, A. (2019). Recurrent convolutional neural network based multimodal disease risk prediction. *Fut. Gener. Comput. Syst.* 92, 76–83. doi: 10.1016/j.future.2018.09.031

He, K., Zhang, X., Ren, S., and Sun, J. (2016). "Deep Residual Learning for Image Recognition," in *Proceedings of the 2016 IEEE Conference on Computer Vision and Pattern Recognition (CVPR)*, (Las Vegas, NV: IEEE).

Huang, G., Liu, Z., Maaten, L. V. D., and Weinberger, K. Q. (2017). "Densely Connected Convolutional Networks," in *Proceedings of the 2017 IEEE Conference on Computer Vision and Pattern Recognition (CVPR)*, (Las Vegas, NV: IEEE), 2261–2269.

Islam, M. T., Mahbubur Rahman, S. M., Omair Ahmad, M., and Swamy, M. N. S. (2018). Mixed gaussian-impulse noise reduction from images using convolutional neural network. *Signal Process. Image Commun.* 68, 26–41. doi: 10.1016/j.image.2018.06.016

Karen Simonyan, Z. (2015). "Very Deep Convolutional Networks for Large-Scale Image Recognition," in *Proceedings of the Conference Paper at ICLR*, New Orleans.

Khened, M., Kollerathu, V. A., and Krishnamurthi, G. (2019). Fully convolutional multi-scale residual DenseNets for cardiac segmentation and automated cardiac diagnosis using ensemble of classifiers. *Med. Image Anal.* 51, 21–45. doi: 10. 1016/j.media.2018.10.004

Krizhevsky, A., Sutskever, I., and Hinton, G. E. (2012). "ImageNet classification with deep convolutional neural networks," in *Proceedings of the 25th International Conference on Neural Information Processing Systems*, Lake Tahoe.

Li, S., Sun, W., Zhang, Y., and Liu, H. (2018). Reliability analysis for multipath communications in mobile cloud computing architectures. *Wirel. Commun. Mob. Comput.* 2018:8539307.

Lu, S., Lu, Z., Hou, X., Cheng, H., and Wang, S. (2017). "Detection of cerebral microbleeding based on deep convolutional neural network," in *Proceedings of the 14th International Computer Conference on Wavelet Active Media Technology and Information Processing (ICCWAMTIP)*, Chengdu, 93–96.

Martinez-Ramirez, S., Greenberg, S. M., and Viswanathan, A. (2014). Cerebral microbleeds: overview and implications in cognitive impairment. *Alzheimer's Res. Ther.* 6:33. doi: 10.1186/alzrt263

Noorbakhsh-Sabet, N., Pulakanti, V. C., and Zand, R. (2017). Uncommon causes of cerebral microbleeds. *J. Stroke Cerebrovasc. Dis.* 26, 2043–2049. doi: 10.1016/ j.jstrokecerebrovasdis.2017.07.012

Raja, K. B., Raghavendra, R., Vemuri, V. K., and Busch, C. (2015). Smartphone based visible iris recognition using deep sparse filtering. *Patt. Recogn. Lett.* 57, 33–42. doi: 10.1016/j.patrec.2014.09.006

Safdar, S., Zafar, S., Zafar, N., and Khan, N. F. (2018). Machine learning based decision support systems (DSS) for heart disease diagnosis: a review. *Artific. Intel. Rev.* 50, 597–623. doi: 10.1007/s10462-017-9552-8

Seghier, L., Kolanko, M. A., Leff, A. P., Jäger, H. R., Gregoire, S. M., and Werring, D. J. (2011). Microbleed detection using automated segmentation (MIDAS): a new method applicable to standard clinical MR images. *PLoS One* 6:e17547. doi: 10.1371/journal.pone.0017547

Tong, S., Fu, Y., and Ling, H. (2019). Gait recognition with cross-domain transfer networks. *J. Syst. Arch.* 93, 40–47. doi: 10.1016/j.sysarc.2019.01.002

van den Heuvel, T. L., van der Eerden, A. W., Manniesing, R., Ghafoorian, M., Tan, T., Andriessen, T. M., et al. (2016). Automated detection of cerebral microbleeds in patients with traumatic brain injury. *NeuroImage Clin.* 12, 241–251. doi: 10.1016/j.nicl.2016.07.002

Wang, H., Shen, Y., Wang, S., Xiao, T., Deng, L., Wang, X., et al. (2019). Ensemble of 3D densely connected convolutional network for diagnosis of mild cognitive impairment and Alzheimer's disease. *Neurocomputing* 333, 145–156. doi: 10. 1016/j.neucom.2018.12.018

Wang, S., Jiang, Y., Hou, X., Cheng, H., and Du, S. (2017). "Cerebral Micro-Bleed Detection Based on the Convolution Neural Network With Rank Based Average Pooling," in *Proceedings of the IEEE Access*, Chengdu, 16576–16583. doi: 10.1109/access.2017.2736558

Wang, S., Liu, L., Qu, L., Yu, C., Sun, Y., Gao, F., et al. (2018). Accurate Ulva prolifera regions extraction of UAV images with superpixel and CNNs for ocean environment monitoring. *Neurocomputing* (in press).

Wang, S., Sun, J., Mehmood, I., Pan, C., Chen, Y., and Zhang, Y.-D. (2019). Cerebral micro-bleeding identification based on nine-layer convolutional neural network with stochastic pooling. *Concurr. Comput. Pract. Exp.* e5130. doi: 10.1002/cpe.5130

Wu, M., and Kim, C. (2010). A cost matrix agent for shortest path routing in ad hoc networks. *J. Netw. Comput. Appl.* 33, 646–652. doi: 10.1016/j.jnca.2010. 03.013

Xie, C., Li, C., Zhang, B., Pan, L., Ye, Q., and Chen, W. (2019). Hierarchical residual stochastic networks for time series recognition. *Inform. Sci.* 471, 52–63. doi: 10.1016/j.ins.2018.08.065

Xing, J. H., Li, K., Hu, W. M., Yuan, C. F., and Ling, H. B. (2017). Diagnosing deep learning models for high accuracy age estimation from a single image. *Patt. Recogn.* 66, 106–116. doi: 10.1016/j.patcog.2017.01.005

Yan, M., Li, M., He, H., and Peng, J. (2018). Deep learning for vehicle speed prediction. *Energy Proc.* 152, 618–623. doi: 10.1016/j.egypro.2018. 09.220

Zeng, N. Y., Wang, Z. D., and Zhang, H. (2016a). Inferring nonlinear lateral flow immunoassay state-space models via an unscented Kalman filter. *Sci. China Inform. Sci.* 59:10.

Zeng, N. Y., Wang, Z. D., Zhang, H., and Alsaadi, F. E. (2016b). A novel switching delayed PSO algorithm for estimating unknown parameters of lateral flow immunoassay. *Cogn. Comput.* 8, 143–152. doi: 10.1007/s12559-016-9396-6

Zeng, N. Y., Wang, Z. D., Zhang, H., Liu, W. B., and Alsaadi, F. E. (2016c). Deep belief networks for quantitative analysis of a gold immunochromatographic strip. *Cogn. Comput.* 8, 684–692. doi: 10.1007/s12559-016-9404-x

Zeng, N. Y., Zhang, H., Chen, Y. P., Chen, B. Q., and Liu, Y. R. (2016d). Path planning for intelligent robot based on switching local evolutionary PSO algorithm. *Assemb. Automat.* 36, 120–126. doi: 10.1108/aa-10-2015-079

Zeng, N. Y., Wang, Z. D., Zineddin, B., Li, Y. R., Du, M., Xiao, L., et al. (2014). Image-based quantitative analysis of gold immunochromatographic strip via cellular neural network approach. *IEEE Trans. Med. Imag.* 33, 1129–1136. doi: 10.1109/TMI.2014.2305394

Zeng, N. Y., You, Y., Xie, L. S., Zhang, H., Ye, L. S., Hong, W. X., et al. (2018). A new imaged-based quantitative reader for the gold immunochromatographic assay. *Optik* 152, 92–99. doi: 10.1016/j.ijleo.2017.09.109

Zeng, N. Y., Zhang, H., Li, Y. R., Liang, J. L., and Dobaie, A. M. (2017a). Denoising and deblurring gold immunochromatographic strip images via gradient projection algorithms. *Neurocomputing* 247, 165–172. doi: 10.1016/ j.neucom.2017.03.056

Zeng, N. Y., Zhang, H., Liu, W. B., Liang, J. L., and Alsaadi, F. E. (2017b). A switching delayed PSO optimized extreme learning machine for short-term load forecasting. *Neurocomputing* 240, 175–182. doi: 10.1016/j.neucom.2017. 01.090

Zhang, Y., and Liu, H. (2014). DCFRS: A cloud-based distributed collaborative filtering recommender system for mobile users. *ICIC Expr. Lett.* 8, 1889–1895.

Zhang, Y., Su, Y., Weigang, L., and Liu, H. (2018a). Rumor and authoritative information propagation model considering super spreading in complex social networks. *Phys. A Stat. Mech. Appl.* 506, 395–411. doi: 10.1016/j.physa.2018. 04.082

Zhang, Y., Wang, S., Sui, Y., Yang, M., Liu, B., Cheng, H., et al. (2018b). Multivariate approach for alzheimer's disease detection using stationary wavelet entropy and predator-prey particle swarm optimization. *J. Alzheimers Dis.* 65, 855–869. doi: 10.3233/JAD-170069

Zhang, Y. D., Hou, X. X., Chen, Y., Chen, H., Yang, M., Yang, J., et al. (2018c). Voxelwise detection of cerebral microbleed in CADASIL patients by leaky rectified linear unit and early stopping. *Multimed. Tools Appl.* 77, 21825–21845. doi: 10.1007/s11042-017-4383-9

Zhang, Y. D., Zhang, Y., Hou, X. X., and Chen, H. (2018d). Seven-layer deep neural network based on sparse autoencoder for voxelwise detection of cerebral microbleed. *Multimed. Tools Appl.* 77, 10521–10538. doi: 10.1007/s11042-017-4554-8

Zhang, Y. D., Hou, X. X., Chen, Y., Chen, H., Yang, M., Yang, J., et al. (2017). Voxelwise detection of cerebral microbleed in CADASIL patients by leaky rectified linear unit and early stopping*. *Multimed. Tools Appl.* 77, 1–21.

Zhang, Y. D., Hou, X. X., Lv, Y. D., Chen, H., Zhang, Y., and Wang, S. H. (2016). "Sparse Autoencoder based deep neural network for voxelwise detection of cerebral microbleed," in *Proceedings of the 22nd International Conference on Parallel and Distributed Systems**, Wuhan, 1229–1232.

4

A U-Net Deep Learning Framework for High Performance Vessel Segmentation in Patients With Cerebrovascular Disease

Michelle Livne[1,2*], *Jana Rieger*[1], *Orhun Utku Aydin*[1], *Abdel Aziz Taha*[3], *Ela Marie Akay*[1], *Tabea Kossen*[1,2], *Jan Sobesky*[2,4], *John D. Kelleher*[5], *Kristian Hildebrand*[6], *Dietmar Frey*[1] *and Vince I. Madai*[1,2]

[1] Predictive Modelling in Medicine Research Group, Department of Neurosurgery, Charité - Universitätsmedizin Berlin, Berlin, Germany, [2] Centre for Stroke Research Berlin, Charité - Universitätsmedizin Berlin, Berlin, Germany, [3] Research Studios Data Science, Research Studios Austria, Salzburg, Austria, [4] Department of Neurology, Johanna-Etienne Hospital Neuss, Neuss, Germany, [5] Information, Communication and Entertainment Institute (ICE), Dublin Institute of Technology, Dublin, Ireland, [6] Department VI Computer Science and Media, Beuth University of Applied Sciences, Berlin, Germany

***Correspondence:**
Michelle Livne
michelle.livne@charite.de

Brain vessel status is a promising biomarker for better prevention and treatment in cerebrovascular disease. However, classic rule-based vessel segmentation algorithms need to be hand-crafted and are insufficiently validated. A specialized deep learning method—the U-net—is a promising alternative. Using labeled data from 66 patients with cerebrovascular disease, the U-net framework was optimized and evaluated with three metrics: Dice coefficient, 95% Hausdorff distance (95HD) and average Hausdorff distance (AVD). The model performance was compared with the traditional segmentation method of graph-cuts. Training and reconstruction was performed using 2D patches. A full and a reduced architecture with less parameters were trained. We performed both quantitative and qualitative analyses. The U-net models yielded high performance for both the full and the reduced architecture: A Dice value of ~0.88, a 95HD of ~47 voxels and an AVD of ~0.4 voxels. The visual analysis revealed excellent performance in large vessels and sufficient performance in small vessels. Pathologies like cortical laminar necrosis and a rete mirabile led to limited segmentation performance in few patients. The U-net outperfomed the traditional graph-cuts method (Dice ~0.76, 95HD ~59, AVD ~1.97). Our work highly encourages the development of clinically applicable segmentation tools based on deep learning. Future works should focus on improved segmentation of small vessels and methodologies to deal with specific pathologies.

Keywords: cerebrovascular disease, deep learning, medical imaging, segmentation, U-net

INTRODUCTION

Stroke is a world disease with extreme impact on patients and healthcare systems. Approximately 15 million people suffer from an ischemic stroke each year worldwide[1]. A third of the patients die, making stroke a leading cause of death. Since stroke is a cerebrovascular disease, more detailed information about arterial vessel status may play a crucial role for both the

[1]WHO EMRO Stroke, Cerebrovascular Accident | Health Topics. Available online at: http://www.emro.who.int/health-topics/stroke-cerebrovascular-accident/index.html (Accessed July 14, 2018).

prevention of stroke and the improvement of stroke therapy. It thus has potential to become a biomarker for new personalized medicine approaches for stroke prevention and treatment (Hinman et al., 2017). Considering that vessel imaging is a routine procedure in the clinical setting, vessel information could be easily integrated in the clinical workflow, if segmentations are available and processed.

Currently, however, vessel imaging is only visually—qualitatively—assessed in the clinical routine. Technical challenges of extracting brain arteries and quantifying their parameters have prevented this information from being applied in the clinical setting. If done at all, segmentations of brain vessels are to date still done predominantly manually or semi-manually and are not quantified. Additionally, (semi-) manual vessel segmentation is very time-consuming and has proven to be fairly inaccurate owing to high interrater-variability making it unfeasible for the clinical setting (Phellan et al., 2017). Consequently, research has focused on developing faster and more accurate automatic vessel segmentation methods. Many different rule-based methods exploiting various features of vessel images, such as vessel intensity distributions, geometric models, and vessel extraction schemes have been proposed for this purpose in the previous decades (Lesage et al., 2009; Zhao et al., 2017). These methods, however, are predominantly manually engineered in nature utilizing hand-crafted features and are—additionally—insufficiently validated (Lesage et al., 2009; Phellan et al., 2017). In fact, due to lack of validation and the necessary performance none of the suggested methods has found any broad use in the clinical setting or in research so far. Thus, crucial information about arterial vessel status and subsequent personalized treatment recommendation are not available. The doctor on site lacks a tool to assess this information for the potential benefit of cerebrovascular disease patients.

Deep neural network architectures are a natural choice to overcome this technological roadblock (Zhao et al., 2017). They have shown tremendous success in the last 5 years for image classification and segmentation tasks in various fields (LeCun et al., 2015; Chen et al., 2016; Badrinarayanan et al., 2017; Krizhevsky et al., 2017), and particularly in neuroimaging (Zaharchuk et al., 2018). In the peer reviewed literature for arterial brain vessel segmentation, Phellan et al. (2017) explored a relatively shallow neural net in magnetic resonance images of 5 patients (Phellan et al., 2017). While showing promising preliminary results, the small sample size and shallow net led to limited performance. Here, one of the most promising deep learning frameworks for segmentation tasks is the U-net (Ronneberger et al., 2015). It is a specialized convolutional neural net (CNN) with an encoding down-sampling path and an up-sampling decoding path similar to an autoencoder architecture. It was specifically designed for segmentation tasks and has shown high performance for the segmentation of biomedical images (Fabijanska, 2018; Huang et al., 2018; Norman et al., 2018).

In this context our central contribution is a modified U-net architecture for fully automated arterial brain vessel segmentation evaluated on a dataset of 66 magnetic resonance (MR) images of patients with cerebrovascular disease. We performed a thorough qualitative and quantitative assessment to assess performance with a special focus on performance for pathological cases. Lastly, we compared our results to a traditional standard method of the graph cut approach (Chen and Pan, 2018).

METHODS

Patients

We retrospectively used data from patients from the PEGASUS study that enrolled patients with steno-occlusive cerebrovascular disease [at least 70% stenosis and/or occlusion of one middle cerebral artery (MCA) or internal carotid artery (ICA)]. The study details have been published previously (Mutke et al., 2014; Martin et al., 2015). As additional test-sets to assess generalization we included patients with cerebrovascular disease from the 7UP study. Both the 7UP study as well as the PEGASUS study were carried out in accordance with the recommendations of the authorized institutional ethical review board of the Charité-Universitätsmedizin Berlin with written informed consent from all subjects. All subjects gave written informed consent in accordance with the Declaration of Helsinki. The protocol was approved by the authorized institutional ethical review board of the Charité-Universitätsmedizin Berlin.

Of 82 patients in total, 4 did not have vessel imaging and 6 patients were not yet processed at the time of the study. Of the 72 patients remaining, 6 were excluded due to low quality vessel images owing to patient motion leading to 66 patient scans available for our study. The test-sets from the 7UP study comprised 10 patients each with cerebrovascular disease (stroke in the past) with Time-of-Flight (TOF)-angiography from a different scanner and different parameters, and a different angiography modality, i.e. MPRAGE-angiography (Dengler et al., 2016).

Data Accessibility

At the current time-point the imaging data cannot be made publicly accessible due to data protection, but the authors will make efforts in the future, thus this status might change. Researchers interested in the code and/or model can contact the authors and the data will be made available (either through direct communication or through reference to a public repository).

Imaging

For the PEGASUS patients, scans were performed on a clinical 3T whole-body system (Magnetom Trio, Siemens Healthcare, Erlangen, Germany; in continuation referred to as Siemens Healthcare) using a 12-channel receive radiofrequency (RF) coil (Siemens Healthcare) tailored for head imaging.

Time-of-Flight (TOF) vessel imaging was performed with the following parameters: voxel size = $(0.5 \times 0.5 \times 0.7)$ mm^3; matrix size: $312 \times 384 \times 127$; TR/TE = 22 ms/3.86 ms; time of acquisition: 3:50 min, flip angle = 18 degrees.

For the additional 7UP test-sets, scans were performed on a clinical 3T whole-body system (Magnetom Verio, Siemens Healthcare) and a 12 channel RF receive coil (Siemens Healthcare) for TOF-imaging and a 7T whole-body system (Magnetom 7.0 T, Siemens Healthcare) with a 90 cm bore magnet (Magnex Scientific, Oxfordshire, United Kingdom), an avanto gradient system (Siemens Healthcare) and a 1/24 channel transmit/receive coil (NovaMedical, Wakefield, MA) was used for MPRAGE-angiography.

The parameters were:

TOF imaging: voxel size = $(0.6 \times 0.6 \times 0.6)$ mm^3; matrix size: $384 \times 384 \times 160$; TR/TE = 24 ms/3.60 ms; time of acquisition: 5:54 min, flip angle = 18 degrees.

MPRAGE imaging: voxel size = $(0.7 \times 0.7 \times 0.7)$ mm^3; matrix size: $384 \times 384 \times 240$; TR/TE = 2,750 ms/1.81 ms; time of acquisition: 5:40 min, flip angle = 25 degrees.

Data Postprocessing

The raw PEGASUS study TOF images were denoised using the oracle-based 3D discrete cosine transform filter (ODCT3D) implemented in matlab (Manjón et al., 2012). Non-uniformity correction (NUC) was performed with the *mri_nu_correct.mni* tool integrated in freesurfer (website: Freesurfer mri_nu_correct.mni)[2]. Corresponding whole-brain masks were automatically generated using the *Brain Extraction Tool (BET)* of FSL (website: BET/UserGuide-FslWiki)[3]. Both NUC and FSL-BET post-processing were performed with the *Nipype* wrapper implemented in Python[4]. The post-processing parameters were as follows: ODCT Filter: Patch size $3 \times 3 \times 3$ voxels, Search volume size: $7 \times 7 \times 7$ voxels, Rician noise model; Freesurfer mnibias correction: iterations = 6, protocol_iterations = 1,000, distance = 50; FSL BET: frac = 0.05.

The additional 7UP TOF and MPRAGE imaging test-set image pipeline differed in these points: non-local means denoising implemented in Nipype (patch radius = 1, block radius = 5, and Rician noise model) and MPRAGE-BET parameters (frac 0.15).

Data Labeling

For PEGASUS TOF data, ground-truth labels of the brain vessels were generated semi-manually using a standardized pipeline. Pre-labeling of the vessels was performed by a thresholded region-growing algorithm using the *regiongrowingmacro* module implemented in MeVisLab (website: MeVisLab)[5]. To tackle inter-rater variability in label generation, these pre-labeled data were thoroughly manually corrected by either OUA and EA (both junior raters) and then cross-checked by the other rater. These labels were then checked subsequently both by VIM (9 years experience in stroke imaging) and DF (11 years experience in stroke imaging). Thus, each ground-truth was eventually checked by 4 independent raters, two of them senior raters. The total labeling time with this framework amounted to 60–80 min per patient.

Additional test-set label data (TOF and MPRAGE imaging) was generated using the U-net model in a first step instead of the *regiongrowingmacro* framework, followed by the above described thorough manual correction steps. Images were reviewed in the final step by VIM.

Data Splitting

For U-net training, both PEGASUS TOF images and ground-truth labels were skull-stripped using the whole-brain masks. The data was split into training, validation, and test-sets with 41, 11, and 14 patients-scans, respectively. For illustration of the extracted data see **Figure 1**.

Random Patch Extraction

In order to successfully train our deep neural network we needed to consider two challenges. First, the brain slices, with 312×384 voxels, are very large and cannot processed at once due to the limited GPU memory. Second, the distribution of vessels within a slice is largely skewed as only 0.9% of brain voxels are vessels. To solve these problems we extracted 1,000 quadratic patches per patient: 500 random patches with a vessel in the center and 500 random patches without a vessel in the center. The model was trained using 4 different patch sizes (16×16, 32×32, 64×64, 96×96 voxels) and was later tested for best results against the validation set as part of the optimization process. Due to computational limitation the maximal patch size was set to 96×96 voxels. Testing the effect of different patch sizes on the model performance would reveal important information about the relevant spatial scope for a reliable vessel detection. The data was normalized patch-wise using zero-mean and unit-variance normalization.

Network Architecture and Training

Network Architecture

The U-net CNN model architecture was adapted from the framework presented by Ronneberger et al. (2015). The U-net model architecture is shown in **Figure 2**. The network is based on a convolutional neural network (CNN) and consists of an encoding and a decoding part. The contracting path, i.e., encoding part (left side) repeatedly applies two (padded) 3×3 convolutional layers with stride 1, each followed by a rectified linear unit (ReLU) and a 2×2 max-pooling operation with stride 2 on 4 levels. A dropout layer is applied following the first convolutional layer. At each down-sampling step the dimensions of the input image is reduced by half and the number of feature channels is doubled. The bottom level includes two 3×3 convolutional layers without pooling layer. The expansive path, i.e., decoding part (right side) recovers the original dimensions of the input images by up-sampling the feature map, a concatenation with the corresponding feature channels from the contractive path and two 3×3 convolutional layers, the first followed by ReLU and a dropout-layer and the second followed by ReLU. The final layer is a 1×1 convolution for mapping the feature vector to the binary prediction (i.e., vessel vs. non-vessel).

A variation of the U-net model architecture was applied, where the number of channels in each layer was consistently reduced to half. For simplicity, the additional architecture is therefore termed throughout this work as "half U-net."

[2]https://surfer.nmr.mgh.harvard.edu/fswiki/mri_nu_correct.mni (Accessed February 7, 2019).

[3]https://fsl.fmrib.ox.ac.uk/fsl/fslwiki/BET/UserGuide (Accessed July 14, 2018).

[4]Neuroimaging in Python-Pipelines and Interfaces-Nipy Pipeline and Interfaces Package. Available online at: https://nipype.readthedocs.io/en/latest/ (Accessed July 14, 2018).

[5]https://www.mevislab.de/ (Accessed July 14, 2018).

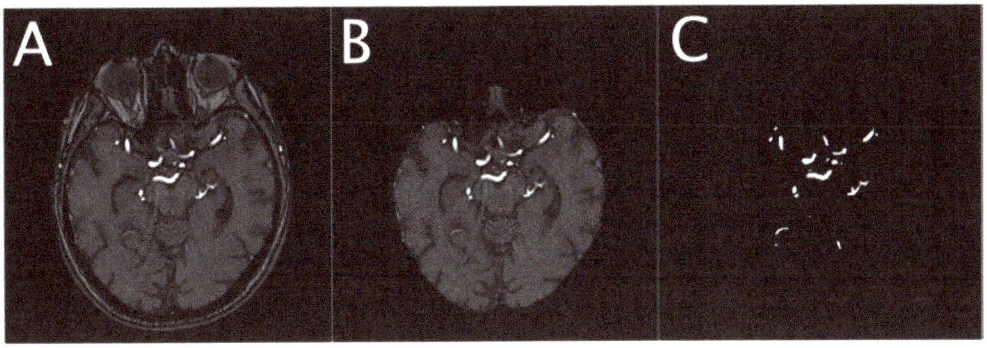

FIGURE 1 | Illustration of the dataset for a representative patient. The Figure shows an illustration of the denoised TOF image of a representative patient **(A)**, the corresponding masked brain image **(B)** and the corresponding ground-truth image of the brain vessels **(C)**.

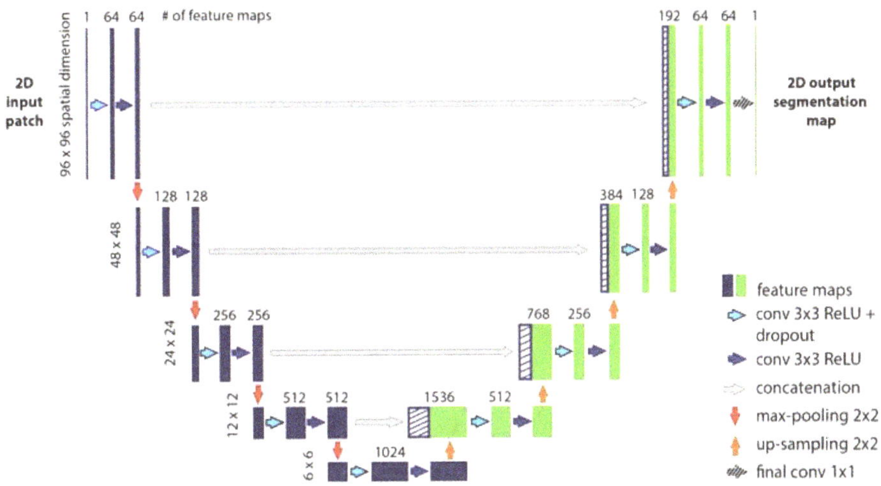

FIGURE 2 | Illustration of the U-net architecture. The figure illustrates the U-net architecture with the largest patch-size of 96 × 96 voxels. The displayed U-net is an encoder-decoder network with a contracting path (encoding part, left side) that reduces the height and width of the input images and an expansive path (decoding part, right side) that recovers the original dimensions of the input images. Each box corresponds to a multi-channel feature map. The dashed boxes stand for the concatenated copied feature maps from the contractive path. The arrows stand for the different operations as listed in the right legend. The number of channels is denoted on top of the box and the image dimensionality (x-y-size) is denoted on the left edge. The half U-net is constructed likewise, with the only difference given by the halved number of channels throughout the network.

The network is fed with 2D image patches and returns the 2D segmentation probability map for each given patch.

Model Training

The skull-stripped denoised TOF input images and the corresponding ground-truth segmentation maps were used to train the U-net using the Keras implementation of Adam optimizer (Kingma and Ba, 2014).

In the model, the energy function is computed by a pixel-wise sigmoid over the final feature map combined with the Dice coefficient loss function. The sigmoid is defined as $p(x) = 1/\left(1+\exp\left(a(x)\right)\right)$ Where $a(x)$ denotes the activation in the final feature channel at the voxel position $x \in \Omega$ with $\Omega \in Z^2$ and $p(x)$ is the approximated probability of a voxel x to be a vessel. The Dice coefficient D between two binary volumes is officially defined as $D = \frac{2TP}{2TP+FP+FN}$ Where TP is the number of true-positive voxels, FP is the number of false positive voxels and FN is the number of false negative voxels. Using the following derivation:

$$D = \frac{2TP}{2TP+FP+FN}$$
$$= \frac{2\sum_{x\in\Omega} p_x g_x}{2\sum_{x\in\Omega} p_x g_x + \sum_{x\in\Omega}\left(p_x^2 - p_x g_x\right) + \sum_{x\in\Omega}\left(g_x^2 - p_x g_x\right)}$$

The Dice coefficient can be written as:

$$D = \frac{2\sum_{x\in\Omega} p_x g_x + s}{\sum_{x\in\Omega} p_x^2 + \sum_{x\in\Omega} g_x^2 + s}$$

Where $p_x \in P : \Omega \rightarrow \{0, 1\}$ is the predicted binary segmentation volume, $g_x \in G : \Omega \rightarrow \{0, 1\}$ is the ground-truth binary volume and $s = 1$ is an additive smoothing factor (i.e., Laplace smoothing). The Dice coefficient then penalizes at each position j the deviation of p_x from the true label g_x using the differentiated gradient:

$$\frac{\partial D}{\partial p_j} = 2\left[\frac{g_j\left(\sum_{x\in\Omega} p_x^2 + \sum_{x\in\Omega} g_x^2\right) - 2p_j\left(\sum_{x\in\Omega} p_x g_x\right)}{\left(\sum_{i\in\Omega} p_x^2 + \sum_{x\in\Omega} g_x^2 + s\right)}\right]$$

(Milletari et al., 2016)

The choice of the Dice coefficient as the loss function allows to handle the skewed ground-truth labels without sample weighting.

A constructive initialization of the weights is necessary to ensure gradient convergence, while preventing the situation of "dead neurons," i.e., parts of the network that do not contribute to the model at all. This is particularly true for the case of deep neural networks with many convolutional layers and many different paths through the network. Here we applied the commonly used heuristic with ReLU activation function, the Glorot uniform initializer where the initial weights are drawn from a uniform distribution within the range $[-L, L]$ where $L = \sqrt{6/\left(f_{in} + f_{out}\right)}$, f_{in} is the number of input units in the weight tensor and f_{out} is the number of output units in the weight tensor (Glorot and Bengio, 2010).

The models were tuned in the validation process to optimize the hyperparameters learning-rate, batch-size, and dropout-rate in addition to the optimization of the patch-size as described above.

Data Augmentation

Augmentation methods introduce variance to the training data which allows the network to become invariant to certain transformations. While CNNs and U-net in specific are very good in integration of spatial information which is essential to imaging segmentation tasks, they are not equivariant to transformations such as scale and rotation (Goodfellow et al., 2016). Data augmentation methods like rotations and flips yield the desired invariance and robustness properties of the resulted network. Additionally to flips and rotations, the data augmentation included shears as a derivative of elastic deformations which are recommended as general best practice for convolutional neural networks (Ronneberger et al., 2015). The augmentation was applied on-the-fly on the patch-level using the *ImageDataGenerator* function implemented in Keras.

TABLE 1 | Model parametrization.

Optimized performance measure/ Hyperparameter	Dice coefficient	95% Hausdorff distance	Averaged Hausdorff distance
U-NET MODEL PARAMETRIZATION			
Learning rate	1e-4	1e-4	1e-5
Batch size	16	64	8
Dropout rate	0	0	0
HALF U-NET MODEL PARAMETRIZATION			
Learning rate	1e-4	1e-4	1e-4
Batch size	64	32	32
Dropout rate	0.1	0.2	0.1
GRAPH CUT PARAMETRIZATION			
Hyperparameter	**Value**		
Weights	10		

Method Comparison

For comparison we used the graph cut implementation in the PyMaxFlow Python library in Version 1.2.11 (Neila, 2018). This method is tailored for binary segmentation problems, where the combination of Markov Random Fields (MRF) with Bayesian maximum a posteriori (MAP) estimation turns the segmentation task into a graph based minimization problem. Then, the graph cut methodology provides a computationally efficient solution to the minimization problem (Chen and Pan, 2018). We tuned the *weights* hyperparameter, representing the uniform capacity of the edges, on the validation set to determine the optimal setting. With this setting the algorithm was applied on the 14 patients of the test-set to produce segmentation images. We applied both patch wise segmentation with a patch size of 96 as well as segmentation whole slice by slice.

Performance Assessment

Quantitative Assessment

The model performance was assessed based on three different measures: The Dice coefficient, 95HD and the AVD. While the Dice coefficient serves as a general common measure for segmentation tasks, the 95HD and AVD metrics allow to capture more accurate estimation of performance with relation to the boundary error of the branched and complex structure of brain vessels. In contrast to the Hausdorff distance which relates to the maximum of the distance metrics, the 95HD and AVD are calculated as the 95% percentile- and the average distance, respectively.

Therefore, 95HD and AVD are stable and not sensitive to outliers which is typically an important quality measure in medical images analysis. While the Dice coefficient ranges from [0,1] unitless values where the larger the value, the better performance it indicates, the units of 95HD and AVD represent real distances with voxels as a unit, hence the smaller the value is, the better the performance is. The measures were calculated using the EvaluateSegmentation tool provided by Taha and Hanbury (2015), Taha (2018). We identified three final models for performance comparison: Since we based our assessment on three different metrics—the Dice coefficient, the 95HD and the AVD—we chose a model that optimized each of the metrics based on the validation set. The performance was assessed as an average of the measures of all fully reconstructed vasculatures of the patients in the test-set as well as on the segmentations resulting from the graph cut approach.

Qualitative Assessment

For qualitative assessment the predicted segmentation masks as well as the graph cut results of the 14 patients in the test-set were transformed by an in-house python code where true positives (TP), false positives (FP), and false negatives (FN) were assigned different voxel values (True negatives (TN) remained labeled with 0). The images were then visualized by overlaying these new masks with the original scans using ITK-Snap (website: ITK-SNAP)[6]. By adjusting the opaqueness, it was possible to qualitatively assess which structures were correctly identified and which anatomical structures

[6]http://www.itksnap.org/pmwiki/pmwiki.php (Accessed July 14, 2018).

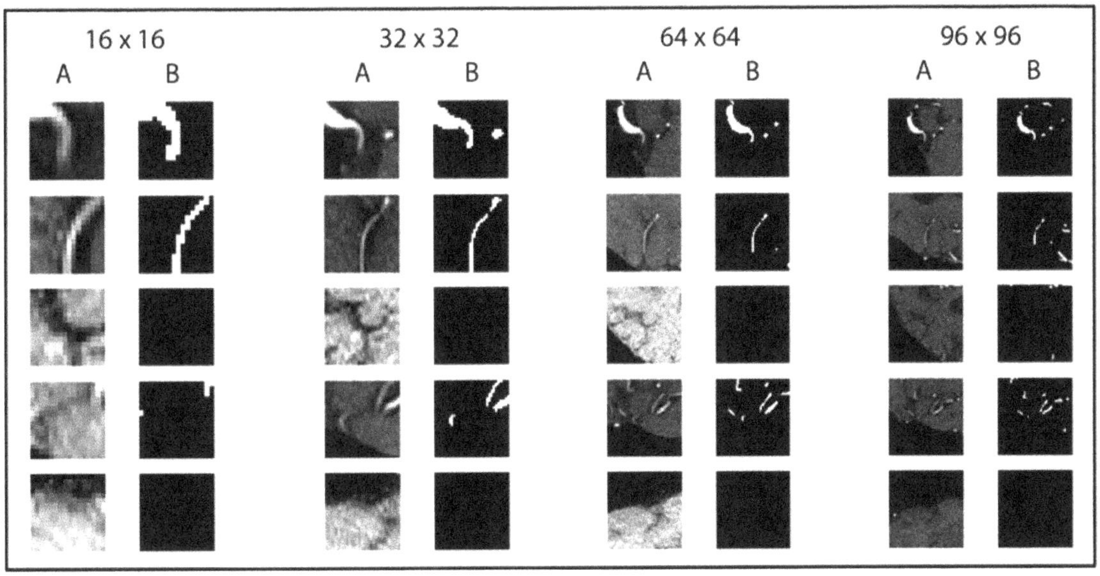

FIGURE 3 | Exemplary patches used for training. Five pairs of random patches with increasing patch size from left to right are shown. "A" columns indicate the MRA-TOF-scans, whereas "B" columns indicate the ground truth label.

dominated with errors. For each architecture and each model (2 architectures × 3 models = 6) VIM visually assessed per patient the images based on a predefined scheme. Large vessels were defined as the all parts of the ACA and the M1, A1, and P1 segments of the three large brain arteries. All other parts were considered small vessels. The results of the visual analysis are summarized qualitatively in the results section. The scheme was the following:

Large vessels, overall impression (bad, sufficient, good); Small vessels, overall impression (bad, sufficient, good); Large vessels, errors (FP or FN dominating); Small vessels, errors (FP or FN dominating); Pathology detected (yes/no); Other tissues type segmentation errors (yes/no).

TABLE 2 | Summary of test-set performance measures.

Model architecture/Performance measure	U-net	Half U-net	Graph cut (patch/whole slice)
Dice coefficient	0.891	0.892	0.758/0.758
95% Hausdorff distance (voxels)	47.277	47.099	58.79/59.24
Averaged Hausdorff distance (voxels)	0.342	0.385	1.965/1.974

*Detailed performance measures of the two Dice-optimized U-net model architectures and the baseline graph-cuts segmentation model as the averaged value over the 14 test patients. For the detailed models parametrization, see **Table 1**.*

Generalization Assessment

All 6 models were applied on the additional 10 7UP patients with different TOF parameters as well as 10 patients with a different angiography modality (7T MPRAGE angiography). Segmentation quality was compared vs. the semimanual gold-standard labels as described above quantitatively with the EvaluateSegmentation framework using as metrics Dice, 95HD and AVD.

Hardware

All trainings ran on a GPU workstation with 16 GB RAM, Intel(R) Xeon(R) CPU E3-1231 v3 @ 3.40GHz and a NVidia TITAN X (Pascal) GPU with 12 GB VRAM.

RESULTS

The U-net model was trained on 81,000 extracted and augmented patches of 41 patients, validated using 11 full patient volumes and assessed for performance using the test-set of 14 full patient volumes. The U-net architecture resulted in 31,377,793 parameters, while the half U-net resulted in 7,846,081 parameters. For the U-net and half U-net, respectively, model training ran for ∼100 and 50 min, while segmentation of a previously unseen volume took about 20 and 10 s. The optimal patch-size was identified as 96 × 96 voxels for both suggested architectures. The model parametrization can be found in **Table 1**. Exemplary patches used for training can be seen in **Figure 3**.

The U-net model yielded high performance in terms of the three measures that were comparable for both the full and the half architecture: The models optimized for the Dice coefficient had a Dice value of 0.89. The 95HD value was 47 voxels and the AVD models yielded results around 0.35 voxels. The detailed performance assessment of the finalized models is presented in **Table 2**. A representative overview of the visual analysis can be found in **Figure 4**.

The visual analysis of the three full models showed that consistently in all 14 patients the large vessels were segmented excellently. Only very few false positive voxels in the border zones of the vessels were present (see **Figure 5**). Small vessels were segmented well in half of the patients, in the other patients small vessels were segmented less well (see **Figure 6**). In 12 patients, we found false positive labeling of small parts of meningeal arteries present in the image or of venous structures (sinus and central veins) (see **Figures 4**, **6**). In one patient, tissue in an old

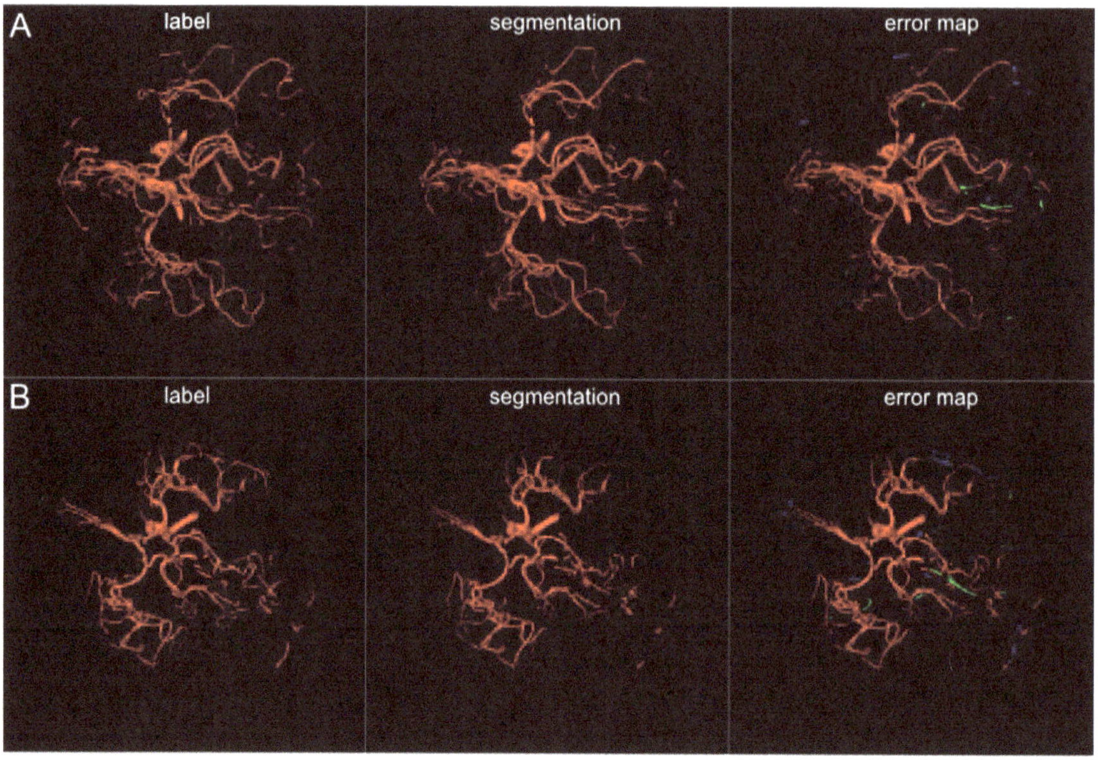

FIGURE 4 | 3D projections of segmentation results. The figure illustrates exemplary segmentation results as 3D projections for two representative patients **(A,B)**. Labels are shown in the first column and exemplary segmentation results are shown in the second column. The third column shows the error map, where red voxels indicate true positives, green voxels false positives, and blue voxels false negatives. Overall a high performance segmentation could be achieved. In the error maps it can be seen that false positives mainly presented as central venous structures and parts of meningeal arteries. (3D view is meant for an overall overview. Due to 3D interpolation, very small structures may appear differently in the images. This does not translate to real voxel-to-voxel differences. For direct voxel-wise comparison please use the 2D-images in **Figures 5–8**).

infarct presented as cortical laminar necrosis with hyperintense elongated tissue against the dark cerebrospinal fluid. These parts were partially labeled as vessels (see **Figure 7A**). In another patient, a rete mirabile, a vessel network of small arteries developing due to occlusion, was present. The rete mirabile was only partially segmented (see **Figure 7B**).

A comparison of the three models showed comparable performance and consistent artifacts as described above. There was a tendency, however, for 95HD and AVG models to have less false positively labeled meningeal and venous structures than the Dice-optimized model. The visual comparison of the full and the half architecture showed comparable performance in the large vessels. We saw a tendency for slightly worse performance in smaller vessels in the half architectures. Vessel pathologies (stenosis/occlusion) were depicted in all patients and all models.

Graph cut results showed inferior performance to the U-net models with the following results (patch/whole slice): Dice 0.76/0.76, 95 HD 58.8/59.2, and AVD 1.97/1.97 (Detailed results can be found in **Table 2** and a visual example in **Figure 8**).

Generalization assessment showed a very good performance of the Dice optimized models for the intra-modal comparison with 3T TOF images with a Dice of 0.86 / 0.92, 95 HD of 64.5 / 50.0, and AVD of 1.591 / 0.650 for the full U-net and half U-net, respectively. We found insufficient performance for inter-modal comparison with 7T MPRAGE angiography (Dice around 0.60, 95 HD around 50, and AVD around 3.5). Detailed results can be found in **Table 3**.

DISCUSSION

We present in the current work a U-net deep learning framework for fully automated brain arterial vessel segmentation from TOF-images of patients with cerebrovascular disease. Our framework demonstrated a very high quantitative performance based on three validation metrics. A lighter architecture—half U-net—achieved comparable quantitative performance. Visual inspection showed excellent performance in large vessels and sufficient to good performance in small vessels as well as comparable performance between the full architecture and the half-net. Special cerebrovascular pathologies presented challenges for the network and need to be addressed in the future.

Applying a modified U-net framework as suggested by Ronneberger et al. (2015), we achieved a very high quantitative performance for the segmentation of arterial brain vessels in patients with cerebrovascular disease. To the best of our knowledge, our work is the first study to show the value of a U-net architecture for fully automated arterial brain vessel segmentation in cerebrovascular disease. Our results are therefore highly encouraging for the

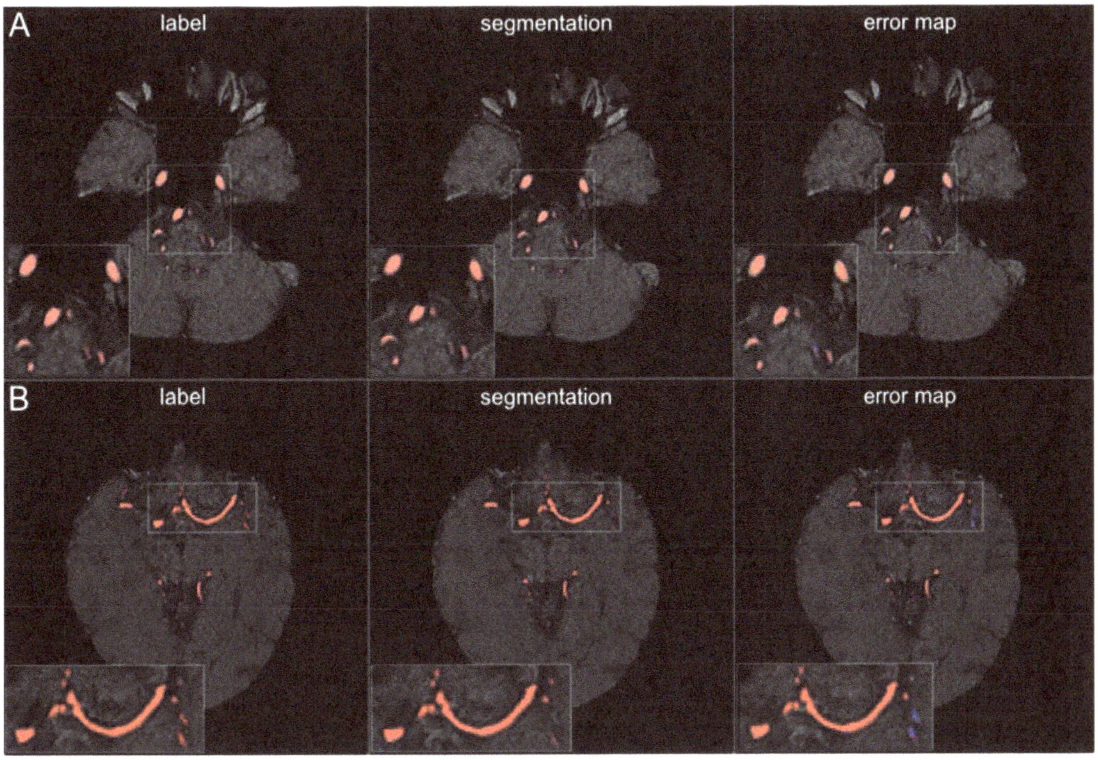

FIGURE 5 | Segmentation results for large vessels. The figure illustrates exemplary segmentation results for large vessels for two representative patients **(A,B)**. Labels are shown in the first column and exemplary segmentation results are shown in the second column. The third column shows the error map, where red voxels indicate true positives, green voxels false positives, and blue voxels false negatives. Only few false positive voxels can be seen in the border zones of the vessels.

further development of automated clinical vessel segmentation tools for cerebrovascular disease. In contrast to the so called "rule-based" non-neural-net attempts of the past, deep learning based networks do not require hand-crafted features or prior feature selection (Lesage et al., 2009; Zhao et al., 2017). The main reason for this is the inherent ability of U-nets to efficiently extract the relevant features in the training process. Confirming the broad consensus that deep learning based approaches constitute the new state-of-the-art in medical segmentation, the U-Net architecture clearly outperformed the traditional graph-cut based segmentation method.

Next to a quantitative assessment, an experienced medical professional also visually assessed the quality of the segmentations. We found that also in the visual analysis the performance of the networks was very high. However, while we saw excellent performance for large vessels, the performance in smaller vessels was less pronounced. While future networks should be improved regarding small vessel segmentation, the clinically most relevant vessels are the large vessels. Thus, we present evidence that already a relatively simple U-net architecture shows clinically highly relevant performance. Even higher performance can be expected using newer segmentation architectures, e.g., the MS-net (Shah et al., 2018). Also, when confronted with pathological cases, like cortical laminar necrosis and a rete mirabile, the performance of the network was limited. Here, there is a need for specifically tailored datasets being incorporated in the training samples. Taken together, the high quantitative and qualitative performance of the U-net are very promising for the development of new individualized precision medicine tools for stroke and cerebrovascular disease in the clinical setting. Vessel parameters could augment predictive models in cerebrovascular disease (Feng et al., 2018; Livne et al., 2018; Nielsen et al., 2018).

Our results confirm previous works in the field of vessel segmentation. Recently, pre-prints on ArXiv.org have explored deep neural nets architectures for brain vessel segmentation in healthy subjects (Chen et al., 2017; Tetteh et al., 2018). The reported performance measures were comparable to our results. This confirms the advantages of deep learning approaches for vessel segmentation tasks. A current limitation, however, is the lack of a standardized labeled vessel imaging dataset. For other segmentation tasks, labeled datasets have been published in the past, usually within public competitions (website: grand-challenges)[7]. A big advantage of such datasets and the competition framework is that it makes models comparable. If different datasets and especially different types of labeling are used, results can be roughly compared qualitatively, but a direct quantitative comparison cannot be performed. If, however, models cannot be compared, the translation of these new methodologies into clinically usable tools is strongly hampered. Thus, the medical machine learning community needs to address this issue by providing standardized datasets of vessels both with and without pathology for segmentation tasks in the established form of

[7] https://grand-challenge.org/All_Challenges/ (Accessed July 14, 2018).

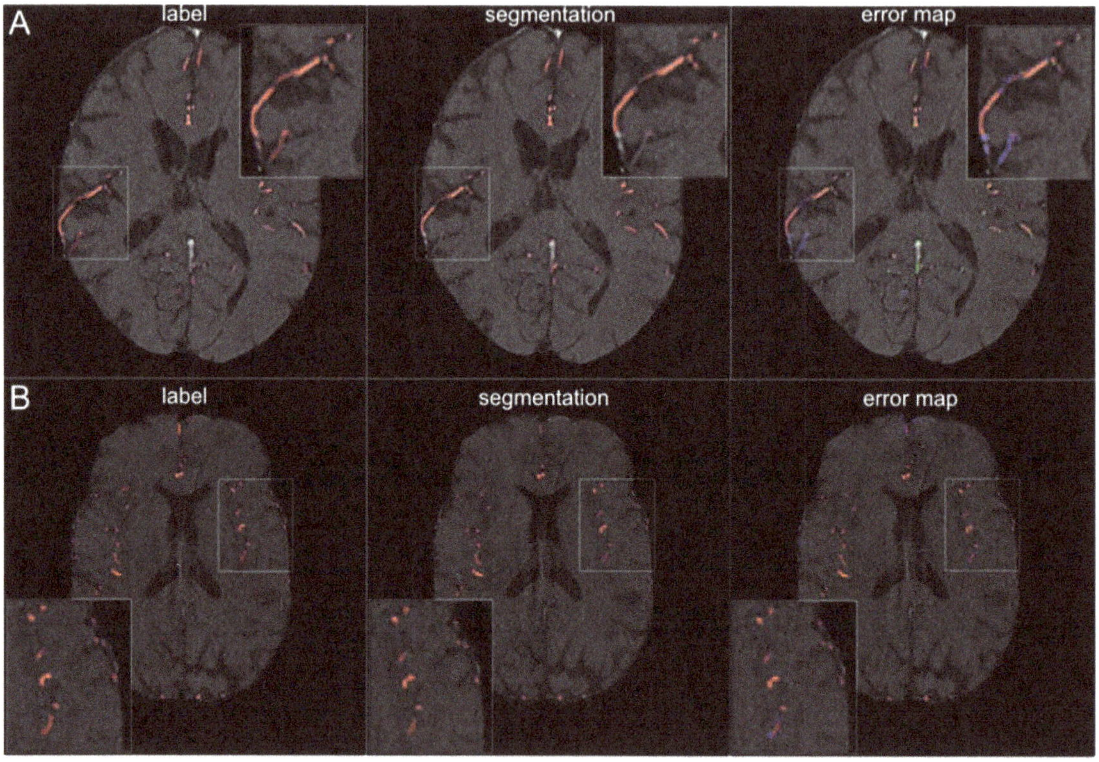

FIGURE 6 | Segmentation results for small vessels. The figure illustrates exemplary segmentation results for small vessels for two representative patients **(A,B)**. Labels are shown in the first column and exemplary segmentation results are shown in the second column. The third column shows the error map, where red voxels indicate true positives, green voxels false positives and blue voxels false negatives. In 7 patients (50%) also small vessels were segmented well, with only few false negatives **(B)**. In the other patients, the small vessels were segmented only sufficiently, with both false positives and false negatives **(A)**.

competitions to allow proper benchmarking of methods. The authors of this study would happily contribute to such an effort.

We chose a simple architecture that closely followed the suggested U-net by Ronneberger et al. This resulted in roughly 30 million parameters. Promisingly, we found that a U-net with half of the convolution channels—coined half U-net—showed comparable performance, and yet consisted of only roughly 8 million trainable parameters. Naturally, the training of the half U-net can be done much faster, in our case in 50% of the time. This might be attributable to a limited variability of brain vessels as captured by the dataset that allows less complex architectures to perform comparably. This is also shown by the fact that we used a simple 2D-patch approach with success. It seems that certain segmentation tasks do not necessarily need complex models and 3D approaches to reach sufficient performance. However, a systematic assessment of the necessary model complexity, particularly the number of feature channels, and 2.5D and 3D approaches is warranted in future studies to find the optimal approach for vessel segmentation. Especially for small vessels detection, such approaches might be promising. The optimal patch-size was identified for both architectures as the largest tested value of 96 $\times$ 96 voxels. This may imply that a larger patch-size may be more beneficial for the segmentation task. Such future optimization could be potentially done using advanced hardware or by increasing the patch-size on the expanse of the batch-size.

An important part of the model training is the augmentation of the data. CNNs—and the encoder part of the U-net utilizes convolutional layers—are not equivariant to certain transformations, especially not rotations. It is thus absolutely essential to perform augmentations, especially when (relatively) few training examples are available (Ronneberger et al., 2015). The main principle of augmentation is that the newly generated data represents new information that would occur in the same domain where the original images stem from. We chose in our work the *ImageDataGenerator* implemented in Keras. It is a multi-purpose augmentation tool, that on one hand will generate helpful new training examples with high likelihood, but on the other hand will be naturally less specific than individually tailored augmentation strategies. Here, a highly promising approach is the application of Generative Adversarial Networks (GANs) for data augmentation, e.g., by Antoniou et al. (2017). The adversarial generative and discriminative networks ensure—if mode collapse can be avoided—that a large variety of new data is generated which all lie in the same domain as the original data. Such images would allow ideal augmentation for any segmentation task.

Generalization of our findings to other vessel segmentation tasks signifies an important implication of our work. While it is possible to achieve high performance for vessel segmentation with hand-crafted features and parameters optimized for a special case, e.g., for CT-angiographies (Meijs et al., 2017), the development of such methods is time-consuming and a transfer of these results to images from other sources and other organs is hard to perform. In the case of a well-trained U-net, the convolutional layers have already learned the

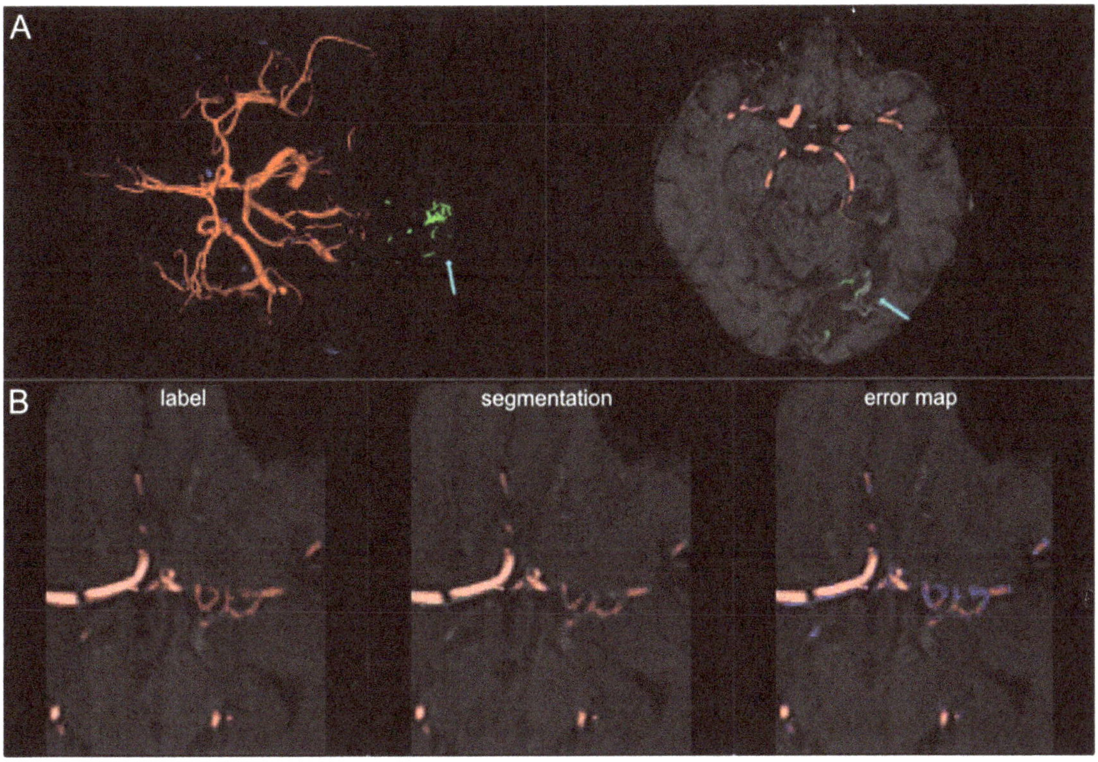

FIGURE 7 | False labeling of specific cerebrovascular pathologies. **(A)** The error map of a 3D projection on the left shows falsely labeled structures in the posterior part of the brain (arrow). On a transversal slice (on the right) false labeling of parts of cortical laminar necrosis can be identified as the cause (arrow). **(B)** The rete mirabile network of small vessels was only partially depicted (false negative labeling in blue in the error map). A rete mirabile is a relatively rare occurrence, only 3 patients of 66 in our study presented with one (2 in the training set and one in the test-set).

features necessary for the detection of vessels. Thus, it is possible to train new highly performant models for so far unseen vessel images by freezing the convolutional layers and by focusing the training on the rest of the model. This method is called "transfer learning" (Oquab et al., 2014) and requires only a few labeled datasets for each new source. Consequently, potential new tools can easily be adapted to various scanner settings, imaging modalities and even new organs, which is necessary for broad clinical adaptation and multicenter imaging studies.

We assessed model performance based on three different measures: First, the Dice coefficient. Mathematically it is equivalent to the F1 measure and thus the harmonic mean of precision and recall (Taha and Hanbury, 2015). It is a widely used measure for segmentation tasks and its popularity is explained by its insensitivity to background voxels, its easy interpretability and its customizability to improve learning in hard-to-segment regions (Shah et al., 2018). Together with patch extraction, the use of the Dice coefficient allowed us to alleviate the imbalanced sample distribution in our dataset, as only 0.9% of all voxels in the brain depict vessels. However, based on theoretical considerations, the Dice coefficient is limited when assessing the validity of vessel segmentations (Taha and Hanbury, 2015). For example, since vessels are narrow and elongated, segmentations errors can quickly lead to loss of overlap. However, once no overlap exists, the Dice coefficient cannot distinguish whether a segmented vessel is closer (better segmentation) or further away (worse segmentation) from the ground truth. Here, distance based measures are better suited (Taha and Hanbury, 2015), as they take into account the spatial position of voxels. Thus, we used two additional distance-based measures, the 95HD and the AVG. The plain Hausdorff distance was avoided due to its sensitivity to outliers. Promisingly, we saw a tendency that the models optimized by distance-based measures show improved results. It can thus be anticipated that customized loss functions incorporating distance-based measures will improve the performance of deep learning models for segmentation. Thus, future works should first systematically assess which metrics are best suited for brain vessel segmentation and then develop a customized loss function for vessel segmentation.

A special focus of our work was the selection of the dataset. First, we used patients with pathology, in our case cerebrovascular disease. The vessels of such patients are more challenging to segment owing to stenoses and occlusions, old infarcts and small vascular networks ("rete mirabile"). Thus, our results are more representative of the clinical challenges than the results of works using the data of healthy patients. And indeed, we found that special pathological cases like cortical laminar necrosis and a rete mirabile were challenging for the network and need to be focused in future works. In summary, our work serves as the starting point to develop new pathology-tailored models which are applicable in the clinical setting. In their training, random patch extraction should

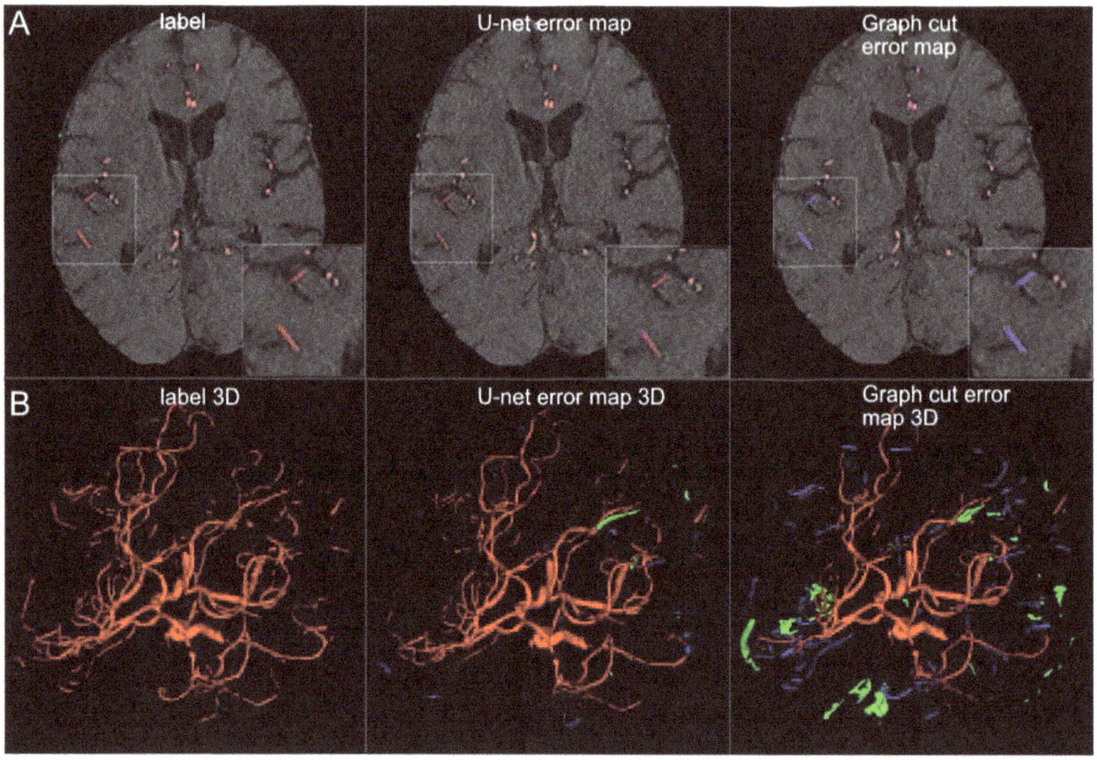

FIGURE 8 | Comparison of U-net and graph cut segmentations. **(A)** 2D comparison and **(B)** 3D comparison of labels, U-net error maps and graph cut error maps. The quantitative results are confirmed by visual inspection. The graph cut segmentation shows more false negatively (blue) and false positively (green) segmented voxels.

be avoided, and patch selection should be focused on the special cases identified in our study. Second, we labeled 66 patients, which is—in medical imaging—a large number of patients. This number is roughly double to triple of the number of the datasets used by Ronneberger et al. in their original U-net paper (Ronneberger et al., 2015). Since the U-net is tailored for use with limited data, our number of patients should allow for strong generalization and this is reflected by our high performance. Lastly, we invested a large effort into the labeling of the dataset. Every patient scan was labeled by a medical researcher and independently checked by 3 others medical researchers, 2 amongst them expert readers. It is very encouraging that two-digit numbers of high-quality labeled medical imaging data are sufficient to achieve very strong segmentation results with modern deep learning architectures. Labeling of such a number of patient scans is achievable in a justifiable time and opens the door for the development of high-performance models for the clinical setting for any medical segmentation task. It is to be expected that such models will soon be translated into applicable tools and will be available for research and the clinical setting.

Our study has several limitations. First, we used a monocentric dataset. Thus, imaging parameters and scanner parameters were fixed. In an intra-modal analysis, i.e., TOF-images from a different scanner with different parameters, the generalization performance was very good. In the inter-modal analysis, however, applying the models on MPRAGE-angiography images, the performance was considerably inferior. For the applicability in the clinical setting, two different strategies can be envisioned: (1) Since clinical on-site postprocessing is tied to the scanner-vendor and software, segmentation products tuned for vendor-specific sequences and parameter-ranges are possible and lack of generalization is unproblematic. (2) For development of a vendor-independent pipelines, clinical segmentation algorithms need to cover a much broader range of image variability. Here, a large number of varied datasets needs to be used for training of single models or model zoos in the future. Second, we reconstructed the images on the patch level and did not perform an algorithm-based optimization of the whole reconstructed vessel tree. Here, future works can explore for example recurrent neural networks,

TABLE 3 | Summary of generalization assessment results.

	U-net	Half U-net
3T TOF ANGIOGRAPHY:		
Dice coefficient	0.858	0.921
95% Hausdorff distance (voxels)	64.535	50.015
Averaged Hausdorff distance (voxels)	1.591	0.650
7T MPRAGE ANGIOGRAPHY:		
Dice coefficient	0.594	0.661
95% Hausdorff distance (voxels)	54.598	48.414
Averaged Hausdorff distance (voxels)	3.467	3.489

Detailed performance measures of the two tested model architectures as the averaged value over 10 test patients each for 3T TOF and 7T MPRAGE angiography. The results for the two Dice optimized models are shown. The half U-net architecture exhibited better generalization performance.

especially architectures with long short-term memory (LSTM) layers. Applying these techniques, an increase of small vessel segmentation performance might be possible. Third, also, the patch size was limited due to hardware constraints potentially reducing the performance of the network where more context is needed. Fourth, we performed an exploratory qualitative visual analysis by one medical expert. Future clinical assessments of different models should include a systematic quantitative rating by multiple medical expert readers, which exceeded the scope of the present work.

CONCLUSION

In conclusion, a U-net deep learning framework yielded high performance for vessel segmentation in patients with cerebrovascular disease. Future works should focus on improved segmentation of small vessels and removal of artifacts resulting from specific cerebrovascular pathologies.

AUTHOR CONTRIBUTIONS

ML, TK, JS, JDK, KH, DF, and VM: concept and design; VM and JS: acquisition of data; ML, JR, AT, JDK, KH, and VM: model design; ML, JR, OA, EA, DF, and VM: data analysis; ML, JR, AT, TK, JS, JDK, KH, DF, and VM: data interpretation; ML, JR, OA, AT, EA, TK, JS, JDK, KH, DF, and VM: manuscript drafting and approval.

FUNDING

This work has received funding by the German Federal Ministry of Education and Research through (1) the grant Centre for Stroke Research Berlin and (2) a Go-Bio grant for the research group PREDICTioN2020 (lead: DF). For open access publication, we acknowledge support from the German Research Foundation (DFG) via the Open Access Publication Fund of Charité - Universitätsmedizin Berlin.

REFERENCES

Antoniou, A., Storkey, A., and Edwards, H. (2017). *Data Augmentation Generative Adversarial Networks. ArXiv171104340 Cs Stat.* Available online at: http://arxiv.org/abs/1711.04340 (Accessed December 14, 2017).

Badrinarayanan, V., Kendall, A., and Cipolla, R. (2017). SegNet: a deep convolutional encoder-decoder architecture for image segmentation. *IEEE Trans. Pattern Anal. Mach. Intell.* 39, 2481–2495. doi: 10.1109/TPAMI.2016.2644615

Chen, L., Xie, Y., Sun, J., Balu, N., Mossa-Basha, M., Pimentel, K., et al. (2017). *Y-net: 3D Intracranial Artery Segmentation Using a Convolutional Autoencoder. ArXiv171207194 Cs Eess.* Available online at: http://arxiv.org/abs/1712.07194 (Accessed May 28, 2018).

Chen, L.-C., Papandreou, G., Kokkinos, I., Murphy, K., and Yuille, A. L. (2016). *DeepLab: Semantic Image Segmentation with Deep Convolutional Nets, Atrous Convolution, and Fully Connected CRFs. ArXiv160600915 Cs.* Available online at: http://arxiv.org/abs/1606.00915 (Accessed July 14, 2018).

Chen, X., and Pan, L. (2018). A survey of graph cuts/graph search based medical image segmentation. *IEEE Rev. Biomed. Eng.* 11, 112–124. doi: 10.1109/RBME.2018.2798701

Dengler, N. F., Madai, V. I., Wuerfel, J., von Samson-Himmelstjerna, F. C., Dusek, P., Niendorf, T., et al. (2016). Moyamoya vessel pathology imaged by ultra-high-field magnetic resonance imaging at 7.0 T. *J. Stroke Cerebrovasc. Dis.* 25, 1544–1551. doi: 10.1016/j.jstrokecerebrovasdis.2016.01.041

Fabijanska, A. (2018). Segmentation of corneal endothelium images using a U-Net-based convolutional neural network. *Artif. Intell. Med.* 88, 1–3. doi: 10.1016/j.artmed.2018.04.004

Feng, R., Badgeley, M., Mocco, J., and Oermann, E. K. (2018). Deep learning guided stroke management: a review of clinical applications. *J. NeuroInt. Surg.* 10, 358–362. doi: 10.1136/neurintsurg-2017-013355

Glorot, X., and Bengio, Y. (2010). "Understanding the difficulty of training deep feedforward neural networks," in *Proceedings of the Thirteenth International Conference on Artificial Intelligence and Statistics*, 249–256. Available online at: http://proceedings.mlr.press/v9/glorot10a.html (Accessed July 14, 2018).

Goodfellow, I., Bengio, Y., and Courville, A. (2016). *Deep Learning*, ed F. Bach (The MIT Press:Cambridge).

Hinman, J. D., Rost, N. S., Leung, T. W., Montaner, J., Muir, K. W., Brown, S., et al. (2017). Principles of precision medicine in stroke. *J. Neurol. Neurosurg. Psychiatry* 88, 54–61. doi: 10.1136/jnnp-2016-314587

Huang, Q., Sun, J., Ding, H., Wang, X., and Wang, G. (2018). Robust liver vessel extraction using 3D U-Net with variant dice loss function. *Comput. Biol. Med.* 101, 153–162. doi: 10.1016/j.compbiomed.2018.08.018

Kingma, D. P., and Ba, J. (2014). *Adam: A Method for Stochastic Optimization. ArXiv14126980 Cs.* Available online at: http://arxiv.org/abs/1412.6980 (Accessed July 14, 2018).

Krizhevsky, A., Sutskever, I., and Hinton, G. E. (2017). ImageNet classification with deep convolutional neural networks. *Commun. ACM* 60, 84–90. doi: 10.1145/3065386

LeCun, Y., Bengio, Y., and Hinton, G. (2015). Deep learning. *Nature* 521, 436–444. doi: 10.1038/nature14539

Lesage, D., Angelini, E. D., Bloch, I., and Funka-Lea, G. (2009). A review of 3D vessel lumen segmentation techniques: models, features and extraction schemes. *Med. Image Anal.* 13, 819–845. doi: 10.1016/j.media.2009.07.011

Livne, M., Boldsen, J. K., Mikkelsen, I. K., Fiebach, J. B., Sobesky, J., and Mouridsen, K. (2018). Boosted tree model reforms multimodal magnetic resonance imaging infarct prediction in acute stroke. *Stroke* 49, 912–918. doi: 10.1161/STROKEAHA.117.019440

Manjón, J., Coupé, P., Buades, A., Collins, D. L., and Robles, M. (2012). New methods for MRI denoising based on sparseness and self-similarity. *Med. Image Anal.* 16, 18–27. doi: 10.1016/j.media.2011.04.003

Martin, S. Z., Madai, V. I., Samson-Himmelstjerna, F. C., von Mutke, M. A., Bauer, M., Herzig, C. X., et al. (2015). 3D GRASE pulsed arterial spin labeling at multiple inflow times in patients with long arterial transit times: comparison with dynamic susceptibility-weighted contrast-enhanced MRI at 3 tesla. *J. Cereb. Blood Flow Metab.* 35, 392–401. doi: 10.1038/jcbfm.2014.200

Meijs, M., Patel, A., Leemput, S. C., Prokop, M., Dijk, E. J., Leeuw, F.-E., et al. (2017). Robust segmentation of the full cerebral vasculature in 4D CT of suspected stroke patients. *Sci. Rep.* 7:15622. doi: 10.1038/s41598-017-15617-w

Milletari, F., Navab, N., and Ahmadi, S.-A. (2016). *V-Net: Fully Convolutional Neural Networks for Volumetric Medical Image Segmentation. ArXiv160604797 Cs.* Available online at: http://arxiv.org/abs/1606.04797 (Accessed July 27, 2018).

Mutke, M. A., Madai, V. I., von Samson-Himmelstjerna, F. C., Zaro Weber, O., Revankar, G. S., Martin, S. Z., et al. (2014). Clinical evaluation of an arterial-spin-labeling product sequence in steno-occlusive disease of the brain. *PLoS ONE* 9:e87143. doi: 10.1371/journal.pone.0087143

Neila, P. M. (2018). *PyMaxflow: A mincut/maxflow package for Python.* Available online at: https://github.com/pmneila/PyMaxflow (Accessed January 9, 2019).

Nielsen, A., Hansen, M. B., Tietze, A., and Mouridsen, K. (2018). Prediction of tissue outcome and assessment of treatment effect in acute ischemic stroke using deep learning. *Stroke* 49, 1394–1401. doi: 10.1161/STROKEAHA.117.019740

Norman, B., Pedoia, V., and Majumdar, S. (2018). Use of 2D u-net convolutional neural networks for automated cartilage and meniscus segmentation of knee MR imaging data to determine relaxometry and morphometry. *Radiology* 288, 177–185. doi: 10.1148/radiol.2018172322

Oquab, M., Bottou, L., Laptev, I., and Sivic, J. (2014). *Learning and Transferring Mid-level Image Representations Using Convolutional Neural Networks. IEEE* 1717–1724. doi: 10.1109/CVPR.2014.222

Phellan, R., Peixinho, A., Falcão, A., and Forkert, N. D. (2017). "Vascular Segmentation in TOF MRA Images of the Brain Using a Deep Convolutional Neural Network," in *Intravascular Imaging and Computer Assisted Stenting, and Large-Scale Annotation of Biomedical Data and Expert Label Synthesis*, eds J. Cardoso, T. Arbel, S.-L. Lee, V. Cheplygina, S. Balocco, D. Mateus, G. Zahnd, L. Maier-Hein, S. Demirci, E. Granger, L. Duong, M.-A. Carbonneau, S. Albarqouni, and G. Carneiro (Cham, Lecture Notes in Computer Science), 39–46. doi: 10.1007/978-3-319-67534-3

Ronneberger, O., Fischer, P., and Brox, T. (2015). "U-Net: Convolutional Networks for Biomedical Image Segmentation," in *Medical Image Computing and Computer-Assisted Intervention – MICCAI 2015*, eds N. Navab, J. Hornegger, W. Wells, and A. Frangi (Cham, Lecture Notes in Computer Science), 234–241. doi: 10.1007/978-3-319-24574-4_28

Shah, M. P., Merchant, S. N., and Awate, S. P. (2018). "MS-Net: Mixed-Supervision Fully-Convolutional Networks for Full-Resolution Segmentation," in *Medical Image Computing and Computer Assisted Intervention - MICCAI 2018*, eds. A. F. Frangi, J. A. Schnabel, C. Davatzikos, C. Alberola-López, and G. Fichtinger (Cham: Springer International Publishing), 379–387.

Taha, A. A. (2018). *EvaluateSegmentation: A Program to Evaluate the Quality of Image Segmentations.* Visceral-Project Available online at: https://github.com/Visceral-Project/EvaluateSegmentation (Accessed July 14, 2018).

Taha, A. A., and Hanbury, A. (2015). Metrics for evaluating 3D medical image segmentation: analysis, selection, and tool. *BMC Med. Imaging* 15:29. doi: 10.1186/s12880-015-0068-x

Tetteh, G., Efremov, V., Forkert, N. D., Schneider, M., Kirschke, J., Weber, B., et al. (2018). *DeepVesselNet: Vessel Segmentation, Centerline Prediction, and Bifurcation Detection in 3-D Angiographic Volumes. ArXiv180309340 Cs.* Available online at: http://arxiv.org/abs/1803.09340 (Accessed July 14, 2018).

Zaharchuk, G., Gong, E., Wintermark, M., Rubin, D., and Langlotz, C. P. (2018). Deep Learning in Neuroradiology. *Am. J. Neuroradiol.* 39, 1776–1784. doi: 10.3174/ajnr.A5543

Zhao, F., Chen, Y., Hou, Y., and He, X. (2017). Segmentation of blood vessels using rule-based and machine-learning-based methods: a review. *Multimed. Syst.* 1–10. doi: 10.1007/s00530-017-0580-7

5

Prediction and Classification of Alzheimer's Disease Based on Combined Features From Apolipoprotein-E Genotype, Cerebrospinal Fluid, MR, and FDG-PET Imaging Biomarkers

Yubraj Gupta, Ramesh Kumar Lama, and Goo-Rak Kwon

Department of Information and Communication Engineering, Chosun University, Gwangju, South Korea

***Correspondence:**
Goo-Rak Kwon
grkwon@chosun.ac.kr

† For information on the Alzheimer's Disease Neuroimaging Initiative please see the Acknowledgments section

Alzheimer's disease (AD), including its mild cognitive impairment (MCI) phase that may or may not progress into the AD, is the most ordinary form of dementia. It is extremely important to correctly identify patients during the MCI stage because this is the phase where AD may or may not develop. Thus, it is crucial to predict outcomes during this phase. Thus far, many researchers have worked on only using a single modality of a biomarker for the diagnosis of AD or MCI. Although recent studies show that a combination of one or more different biomarkers may provide complementary information for the diagnosis, it also increases the classification accuracy distinguishing between different groups. In this paper, we propose a novel machine learning-based framework to discriminate subjects with AD or MCI utilizing a combination of four different biomarkers: fluorodeoxyglucose positron emission tomography (FDG-PET), structural magnetic resonance imaging (sMRI), cerebrospinal fluid (CSF) protein levels, and Apolipoprotein-E (APOE) genotype. The Alzheimer's Disease Neuroimaging Initiative (ADNI) baseline dataset was used in this study. In total, there were 158 subjects for whom all four modalities of biomarker were available. Of the 158 subjects, 38 subjects were in the AD group, 82 subjects were in MCI groups (including 46 in MCIc [MCI converted; conversion to AD within 24 months of time period], and 36 in MCIs [MCI stable; no conversion to AD within 24 months of time period]), and the remaining 38 subjects were in the healthy control (HC) group. For each image, we extracted 246 regions of interest (as features) using the Brainnetome template image and NiftyReg toolbox, and later we combined these features with three CSF and two APOE genotype features obtained from the ADNI website for each subject using early fusion technique. Here, a different kernel-based multiclass support vector machine (SVM) classifier with a grid-search method was applied. Before passing the obtained features to the classifier, we have used truncated singular value decomposition (Truncated SVD) dimensionality reduction technique to reduce high dimensional features into a lower-dimensional feature. As a result, our combined method achieved an area under the receiver operating characteristic (AU-ROC) curve of 98.33, 93.59, 96.83, 94.64, 96.43, and 95.24% for AD vs. HC, MCIs vs. MCIc, AD vs. MCIs, AD vs. MCIc, HC vs. MCIc, and HC vs. MCIs subjects which are high relative to single modality results and other state-of-the-art approaches. Moreover, combined multimodal methods have improved the classification performance over the unimodal classification.

Keywords: Alzheimer's disease, MCIs (MCI stable), MCIc (MCI converted), sMRI, FDG-PET, CSF, apolipoprotein-E (APOE) genotype, support vector machine

INTRODUCTION

Alzheimer's disease (AD) is an age-related neurodegenerative disorder that is commonly seen in the aging population. Its prevalence is expected to increase greatly in the coming years as it affects one out of nine people over the age of 65 years (Bain et al., 2008). AD involves progressive cognitive impairment, commonly associated with early memory loss, leading patients to require assistance for activities of self-care during its advanced stages. AD is characterized by the accumulation of amyloid-beta (Aβ) peptide in amyloid plaques in the extracellular brain parenchyma and by intra-neuronal neurofibrillary tangles caused by the abnormal phosphorylation of the tau protein (De Leon et al., 2007). Amyloid deposits and tangles are necessary for the postmortem diagnosis of AD. A prediction of an AD dementia in a predictable time-period, i.e., within 1–2 years, appears much more pertinent in a clinical outlook than a prediction of AD dementia in the faraway future, e.g., in 10–20 years. Individual classified to be at "short-term risk" can receive more active treatment and counseling. Mild cognitive impairment (MCI) is a prodromal (predementia) stage of AD, and recent studies have shown that individuals with amnestic MCI tend to progress to probable AD at a rate of ~10–15% per year (Braak and Braak, 1995; Braak et al., 1998). Thus, accurate diagnosis of AD, and especially MCI, is of great size for prompt treatment and likely delay of the progression of the disease. MCI patients who do not progress to AD either develop another form of dementia, retain a stable condition or revert to a non-demented state. Therefore, predicting which MCI patients will develop AD in the short-term and who will remain stable is extremely relevant to future treatments and is complicated by the fact that both AD and MCI affect the same structures of the brain. In subjects with MCI, the effects of cerebral amyloidosis and hippocampal atrophy on the progression to AD dementia differ, e.g., the risk profile is linear with hippocampal atrophy but reaches a ceiling with higher values for cerebral amyloidosis (Jack et al., 2010). In subsequent investigations, biomarkers of neural injury appeared to best predict AD dementia from MCI subjects at shorter time intervals (1–2 years) in particular (Dickerson, 2013). This demonstrates the great importance of developing a sensitive biomarker that can detect and monitor early changes in the brain. The ability to diagnose and classify AD or MCI at an early stage allows clinicians to make more knowledgeable decisions at a later period regarding clinical interventions or treatment planning, thus having a great impact on reducing the cost of longtime care.

Over the past several years, several classification methods have been implemented to overcome these problems using only a single modality of biomarkers. For example, many high-dimensional classification techniques use only the sMR images for classification of AD and MCI. sMRI captures the disease-related structure patterns by measuring the loss of brain volumes and decreases in cortical thickness (Davatzikos et al., 2008; Cuingnet et al., 2011; Salvatore et al., 2015; Beheshti et al., 2016, 2017; Jha et al., 2017; Lama et al., 2017; Long et al., 2017) for the early prediction of AD and MCI. A number of studies, covering volume of interest, region of interest (ROI), shape analysis and voxel-based morphometry, have reported that the amount of atrophy in several sMRI brain regions, such as the entorhinal cortex, hippocampus, parahippocampal gyrus, cingulate, and medial temporal cortex (Cuingnet et al., 2011; Moradi et al., 2015; Beheshti et al., 2016; Gupta et al., 2019), are sensitive to the disease progression and prediction of MCI conversion. In addition to the sMRI, another important modality of biomarkers thoroughly established neuroimaging tool in the diagnosis of neurodegenerative dementia (AD or MCI) is 18F-FDG-PET image, which mainly measures hypometabolism, reflecting neuronal dysfunction (Minoshima et al., 1997; Foster et al., 2007; Li et al., 2008; Förster et al., 2012; Nozadi et al., 2018; Samper-González et al., 2018). With FDG-PET image, some recent studies have reported the reduction of glucose metabolism or an alternations of hypometabolism occurs in the posterior cingulated cortex, precuneus, and posterior parietal temporal association cortex (Förster et al., 2012), and it usually precedes cortical atrophy (Minoshima et al., 1997; Li et al., 2008) and clinical cognitive symptoms in AD patients. Besides these neuroimaging biomarkers, there are also some biochemical (blood-protein level) and genetic (gene-protein level) biomarkers for the diagnosis of AD and MCI subjects. Biochemical changes in the brain are reflected in the cerebrospinal fluid (CSF) (Chiam et al., 2014; Zetterberg and Burnham, 2019), decreased CSF levels of amyloid-beta (Aβ) 1 to 42 peptide ($A\beta_{1--42}$; a marker of amyloid mis-metabolism) (Blennow, 2004; Shaw et al., 2009; Frölich et al., 2017), and elevations of total tau (t-tau) and hyperphosphorylated tau at the threonine181 (p-tau_{181p}) protein (markers of axonal damage and neurofibrillary tangles) (Andreasen et al., 1998; Anoop et al., 2010; Fjell et al., 2010), are considered to be CSF best established predictive biomarkers of AD dementia in patients with MCI. Recent studies have shown that alternation or reduction of polymorphism (genetics) also play a vital role in AD and MCI patients (Gatz et al., 2006; Spampinato et al., 2011; Dixon et al., 2014). Perhaps, the most commonly considered polymorphism in cognitive and neurodegenerative aging is apolipoprotein E (APOE; rs7412; rs429358). It involved in lipid transfer, cell metabolism, repair of neuronal injury due to oxidative stress, amyloid-beta peptide accumulation, and in elderly process. A gene on chromosome 19 in a locus synthesizes APOE with three alleles (ε2, ε3, and ε4) and it is expressed in the central nervous system in astrocytes and neurons. The APOE ε4 allele has been consistently linked to normal cognitive decline in MCI and AD dementia patients (Luciano et al., 2009; Brainerd et al., 2011; Alzheimer's Disease Neuroimaging Initiative et al., 2016; Sapkota et al., 2017). It is also said that especially APOE ε4 is the strongest genetic risk factor that increases the occurrence with a 2-to 3-fold risk for AD, and it lowers the age of onset AD. These all research focuses using only a single modality of biomarkers and their proposed algorithm performance is low compared to a recently published multimodal method (Zhang et al., 2011; Suk et al., 2014; Ritter et al., 2015; Frölich et al., 2017; Li et al., 2017; Gupta et al., 2019). These studies suggest that classification performance will improve when combining all different modalities of biomarkers into one form because different biomarkers offer a piece of different complementary information (or capture disease information from different outlooks) which are useful for the early classification of the AD and MCI patients.

Recently, Jack et al. (2016, 2018) proposed the A/T/N system, as shown in **Table 1**, in which seven major AD biomarkers are divided into three binary categories based on the nature of the pathophysiology that each subject exhibits.

Based on the above system, we propose to combine four different modalities of biomarkers, fluorodeoxyglucose positron emission tomography (FDG-PET), structural magnetic resonance imaging (sMRI), cerebrospinal fluid (CSF) protein levels, and the apolipoprotein E (APOE) genotype, of each patient. Over the past few years, several techniques have been proposed using either a combination of two or three different biomarker modalities, such as the combination of MRI and CSF biomarkers (Vemuri et al., 2009; Fjell et al., 2010; Davatzikos et al., 2011); MRI and FDG-PET biomarkers (Chetelat et al., 2007; Li et al., 2008, 2017; Shaffer et al., 2013); MRI, FDG-PET, and CSF (Walhovd et al., 2010; Zhang et al., 2011; Shaffer et al., 2013; Ahmed et al., 2014; Ritter et al., 2015); and MRI, FDG-PET, and APOE (Young et al., 2013). Although these published approaches have utilized a combination of different types of biomarkers to develop neuroimaging biomarkers for AD, the above methods may be limited. They have used brain atrophy from a few manually extracted regions as a feature for sMRI and PET images to classify different groups. However, using only a small number of brain regions as features from any imaging modality may not be able to reflect the spatiotemporal pattern of structural and physiological abnormalities in their entirety (Fan et al., 2008). Furthermore, by only increasing the number of biomarkers, their combination did not lead to an increase in predictive power. As Heister et al. (2011) explained, a combination of impaired learning ability with medial temporal atrophy was associated with the greatest risk of developing AD in a group of MCI patients.

TABLE 1 | A/T/N biomarker grouping.

A	T	N
Aggregated Aβ or associated pathological state	Aggregated tau (neurofibrillary tangles) or associated pathological state	Neurodegeneration or neural injury
CSF Aβ42, or Aβ42/Aβ40 ratio	CSF phosphorylated tau	Anatomical MRI
Amyloid PET	Tau PET	FDG-PET, CSF total tau

In this study, we propose a novel approach for the early detection of AD with other groups and to differentiate the most similar clinical entities of MCIs and MCIc by combining biomarkers from two imaging modalities (sMRI, FDG-PET) with CSF (biochemical protein level) and APOE genotype biomarkers obtained from each patient. As the A/T/N system defines that each modality of biomarkers offers a different complementary information, which is useful for the early classification of AD and MCI subjects, so in our study we have used four different modalities of biomarkers, sMRI, FDG-PET, CSF (biochemical protein level), and APOE genotype for the early prediction of AD and MCI subjects. Moreover, using early fusion method we have combined the measurement from all four (sMRI, FDG-PET, CSF, and APOE) different biomarkers to discriminate between AD and HC, MCIc and MCIs, AD and MCIs, AD and MCIc, HC and MCIs, and HC and MCIc. We compare classification performance for different groups using typical measures of gray matter atrophy (from sMR image), average intensity of each region (from FDG-PET image), t-tau, p-tau$_{181p}$, and Aβ_{42} scores (from biochemical level), and ε3/ε4, ε4/ε4 values from APOE genotype biomarker. To distinguish between these groups, we used a different kernel-based multiclass SVM classifier with a 10-fold stratified cross-validation technique that helps to find the optimal hyperparameter for this classifier. Our experiment results show that the grouping of different measurements from four different modalities of biomarkers exhibits much better performance for all classification groups than using the best individual modality of the biomarkers.

MATERIALS AND METHODS

Participants

Data used in the preparation of this article were obtained from the Alzheimer's Disease Neuroimaging Initiative (ADNI) database (http://adni.loni.usc.edu/ADNI). The ADNI was launched in 2003 as a public-private partnership led by Principal Investigator, Michael W. Weiner, MD. The primary goal of the ADNI has been to test whether serial magnetic resonance imaging (MRI), positron emission tomography (PET), other biological markers, and clinical and neuropsychological assessment can be combined to measure the progression of mild cognitive impairment (MCI) and early Alzheimer's disease (AD). For up-to-date information, see https://www.adni-info.org.

In total, we included 158 different subjects from the ADNI database. Included subjects were African-American, Asian, and white who stay in America and their age were between 50 and 89 years and spoke either Spanish or English. Patients with specific psychoactive medications have been excluded from the study while taking scans and the general inclusion/exclusion norms were as follows: for an HC subject, a Clinical Dementia Rating (CDR) (Morris, 1993) of 0, Mini-Mental State Examination (MMSE) score must be between 24 and 30 (inclusive), non-MCI, non-depressed, and non-demented. MCI subjects had a CDR level of 0.5, MMSE scores between 24 and 30 (inclusive), a slight memory complaint, having objective memory loss measured by education adjusted scores on Wechsler Memory Scale Logical Memory II (Elwood, 1991), absence of significant levels of impairment in other cognitive domains, essentially preserved activities of daily living, and an absence of dementia, and for an AD patients the MMSE scores between 20 and 26, CDR level of 0.5 or 1.0, and meets the National Institute of Neurological and Communicative Disorders and Stroke and the Alzheimer's Disease and Related Disorders Association (NINCDS/ADRDA) criteria for probable AD. We selected all subjects for whom all four modalities of biomarkers were available. The four obtained biomarkers were 1.5-T T1-weighted sMRI, FDG-PET, CSF measures of three protein levels (t-tau, p-tau$_{181p}$, and Aβ_{42}), and APOE genotype. Of the 158 subjects, 38 subjects were in the AD group (MMSE $\leq$ 24), 82 subjects in the MCI group (46 with MCIc [converted to AD within 24 months of the time-period] and 36 with MCIs [patients who did not convert to AD within 24 months of the time-period]) (MMSE $\leq$ 28). The remaining 38 subjects were healthy controls (MMSE $\leq$ 30).

Table 2 shows the neuropsychological and demographic information for the 158 subjects. To measure the statistically important difference in demographics and clinical features, Student's *t*-test was applied using age data, were the significance value was set to 0.05. No any significant differences were found for any groups. In all groups, the number of male subjects was higher than the number of female subjects. Compared to the other groups, the HC group had higher scores on the MMSE. Healthy subjects had a significantly lower Geriatric Depression Scale (GDS) scores than the other groups. The Functional Activities Questionnaire (FAQ) was higher for the AD group than the other groups.

TABLE 2 | Demographical and neuropsychological characteristics of the studied sample.

Groups	AD	MCIs	MCIc	HC
No. of Subjects	38	36	46	38
Male/female	22/16	26/10	29/17	25/13
Age	77.15* ± 6.88	74.22* ± 5.65	76.71* ± 7.71	76.68* ± 5.01
MMSE	21.21* ± 4.45	26.91* ± 2.43	26.19* ± 2.79	29.05* ± 1.23
FAQ	17.42* ± 6.92	3.80* ± 4.06	7* ± 5.90	0.315* ± 1.02
Subject weight	73.90* ± 13.18	78.44* ± 14.64	73.51* ± 13.17	74.43* ± 14.38
GDS	1.68* ± 1.52	1.58* ± 1.58	1.63* ± 1.50	0.86* ± 1.12

Values are presented as mean ± and standard deviation (SD).

MRI and FDG-PET Datasets

MRI Protocol

Structural MRI scans were acquired from all data centers using Philips, GE, and Siemens scanners. Since the acquisition protocols were different for each scanner, an image normalization step was performed by the ADNI. The imagining sequence was a 3-dimensional sagittal part magnetization prepared of rapid gradient-echo (MPRAGE). This sequence was repeated consecutively to increase the likelihood of obtaining at least one decent quality of MPRAGE image. Image corrections involved calibration, geometry distortion, and reduction of the intensity of non-uniformity applied on each image by the ADNI. More details concerning the sMRI images is available on the ADNI homepage (http://adni.loni.usc.edu/methods/mri-tool/mri-analysis/). We used 1.5-T sMRI T1-weighted images from the ADNI website. Briefly, raw (NIFTY) sMRI scans were downloaded from the ADNI website. All scans were 176 × 256 × 256 resolution with 1 mm spacing between each scan.

FDG-PET Protocol

The FDG-PET dataset was acquired from the ADNI website. A detailed explanation of the FDG-PET image acquisition is available on the ADNI homepage (http://adni.loni.usc.edu/pet-analysis-method/pet-analysis/). Briefly, FDG-PET images were acquired from 30 to 60 min post-injection. First, images were averaged and then spatially aligned. Next, these images were interpolated to a standard voxel size, and later intensity normalization was performed. Finally, images were smoothed to a common surface of 8 mm (FWHM) full width at half maximum. First, the FDG-PET images were downloaded in the Digital Imagining and Communication in Medicine (DICOM) format. In the second step, we use the dcm2nii (Li et al., 2016) converter to convert DICOM images into the Nifty format. All scans were 160 × 160 × 96 resolution with 1.5 mm spacing between each scan.

CSF and APOE Genotype

CSF

We downloaded the required CSF biomarker values for each selected MRI and FDG-PET image from the ADNI website. A brief description regarding the collection procedure is available on the ADNI website. As the manual describes, a 20-ml volume was obtained from each subject using a lumbar puncture with a 24 or 25 gauge atraumatic needle around the time of their baseline scans. Subsequently, all samples were stored on dry ice on the same day and later they were sent to the University of Pennsylvania AD Biomarker Fluid Bank Laboratory where the levels of proteins (Aβ_{42}, total tau, and phosphorylated tau) were measured and recorded. In this study, the three protein levels, Aβ_{42}, t-tau, and p-tau$_{181p}$, were used as features.

APOE Genotype

APOE genotype is known to affect the risk of developing sporadic AD in carriers. Basically, there are three types of the APOE gene, called alleles: APOE$_2$, APOE$_3$, and APOE$_4$. Everyone has two copies of gene and their combination (ε2/ε2, ε2/ε3, ε2/ε4, ε3/ε3, ε3/ε4, and ε4/ε4) determines our APOE genotype score. The APOE (ε2) allele is the rarest form of APOE and carrying even one copy appears to reduce the risk of developing AD by up to 40%. APOE (ε3) is the most common allele and doesn't seem to influence risk whereas APOE (ε4) allele which present in ~10–15% of people, and having one copy of ε4 (ε3/ε4) can increase the risk of having AD by 2–3 times while having the two copies (ε4/ε4) of APOE ε4 can increase the risk by 12 times. The APOE genotype of each subject was recorded as a pair of numbers representing which two alleles were present in the blood. The APOE genotype was obtained from 10 ml of a blood sample taken at the time of the scan and sent immediately to the University of Pennsylvania AD Biomarker Fluid Bank Laboratory for analysis. The APOE genotype value was available for all subjects for whom we had imagining data.

Overview of Proposed Framework

The proposed framework consists of three processing stages: feature extraction and fusion of multiple features into the single form using early fusion technique, optimal feature subset selection using truncate SVD dimensionality reduction method, and classification. **Figure 1** illustrates the block diagram of the proposed framework. The set of participants were randomly split into two groups in a 75:25 ratios as a training and testing sets, respectively, before passing them to the kernel-based multiclass SVM classifier. Moreover, during the training stage, a gray matter atrophy (from sMR image) and average intensity of each region (from FDG-PET image) which had automatically extracted using NiftyReg toolbox, as well as a set of t-tau, p-tau$_{181p}$, and Aβ_{42} (from biochemical level) CSF scores, and (ε3/ε4, ε4/ε4) values from APOE genotype biomarker, were downloaded from the ADNI website. Here, we have used random tree embedding (Geurts et al., 2006; Moosmann et al., 2008) method to transform low dimensional data into a higher dimensional state, to make sure that the complementary information found across all modalities is still used while classifying AD subjects. In addition, we have used an early fusion technique for the combination of different features into one form before passing them to the feature selection process. Moreover, a feature selection technique using truncate SVD was employed to select the optimal subsets of features from the bunch of features, including the sMRI, FDG-PET, CSF, and APOE extracted features to train the classifiers to distinguish between AD and HC, MCIc and MCIs, AD and MCIs, AD and MCIc, HC and MCIs, and HC and MCIc groups. In the testing stage, a remaining 25% of the dataset is then passed to the kernel-based multiclass SVM classifier to measure the performance of our proposed method.

Image Analysis and Feature Extraction

Image preprocessing was performed for all sMR and FDG-PET images. First, we performed anterior commissure (AC)–posterior commissure (PC) correction for all subjects. Afterward, we used N4 bias field correction using ANTs toolbox (Tustison et al., 2010) to correct the intensity of inhomogeneity for each image. In our pipeline, skull striping was not necessary as images were already preprocessed. Therefore, we reduced the total number of required pre-processing steps for the original images. Later high-dimensional data from the images were preserved for the feature extraction step. For sMR images, we first aligned them to the MNI152 T1-weighted standard image using SPM12 (Ashburner and Friston, 2000) toolbox in Matlab 2018b. For the purpose of anatomical segmentation or parcellation of whole-brain into anatomic regions and to quantify the features of each specific regions of interest (ROI) from each sMR image, we have used NiftyReg toolbox (Modat et al., 2010) with 2-mm Brainnetome atlas template (Fan et al., 2016) image, which is already segmented into 246 regions, 210 cortical and 36 subcortical regions. Moreover, we processed the sMRI image using open source software, NiftyReg (Modat et al., 2010), which is an automated registration toolkit that performs fast diffeomorphic non-rigid registration. After the registration process, we gained the subject-labeled image based on a 2-mm Brainnetome atlas template with 246 segmented regions. For the 246 ROI in the labeled sMR images, we computed the volume of gray matter tissues in that ROI and used it as a feature. For the FDG-PET images, the first step was to register the FDG-PET image to its corresponding sMRI T1-weighted image, using the reg_aladin command from the NiftyReg software. Once the FDG-PET images were registered with their respective MR images, we again used NiftyReg toolbox for non-rigid registration between processed FDG-PET image and the 2-mm Brainnetome atlas template image. After registration, we obtained 246 segmented regions for each FDG-PET image. Again, we computed the average intensity of each region for the ROI and used it as a feature for classification. **Figure 2** shows the pipeline for extraction of 246 regions from sMRI and FDG-PET image.

Therefore, for each subject, we obtained 246 ROI's features for each sMRI image, another 246 features for each FDG-PET image. Three features from CSF biomarkers for each subject, and two feature values from APOE genotype for all selected images.

Combining Multimodality of Biomarkers

After assessing the performance for each individual modality, we combined different modalities in order to study possible improvements in classification performance. Here, a general framework based on an early fusion (or straightforward feature concatenation) method which use special combination rules to combine (or to concatenate) complementary information from different modalities of biomarker into single feature vector is used, and later we have used kernel-based multiclass SVM classifier to train that single feature vector. In this context, various authors have combined sMRI-based features with the features calculated from FDG-PET, DTI, and fMRI (Zhang et al., 2011, 2012; Young et al., 2013; Schouten et al., 2016; Bron et al., 2017; Bouts et al., 2018) for early classification of AD subjects. Moreover, in our case, we have combined four (sMRI, FDG-PET, CSF, and APOE) modality of biomarkers into one form using early fusion technique for the early classification of AD and MCI subjects. Here, the value of the features for the APOE and CSF are of small dimensional compared to the sMRI and FDG-PET extracted features values. Therefore, if classification algorithms trained on (high + low) dimensional combined features then it may produce prediction models that effectively ignore the low dimensional features. Moreover, to overcome this problem, we have transformed low dimensional extracted features into a high dimensional state using random tree embedding method, which ensures that the complementary information found across all modalities is still used while classifying several groups. This step

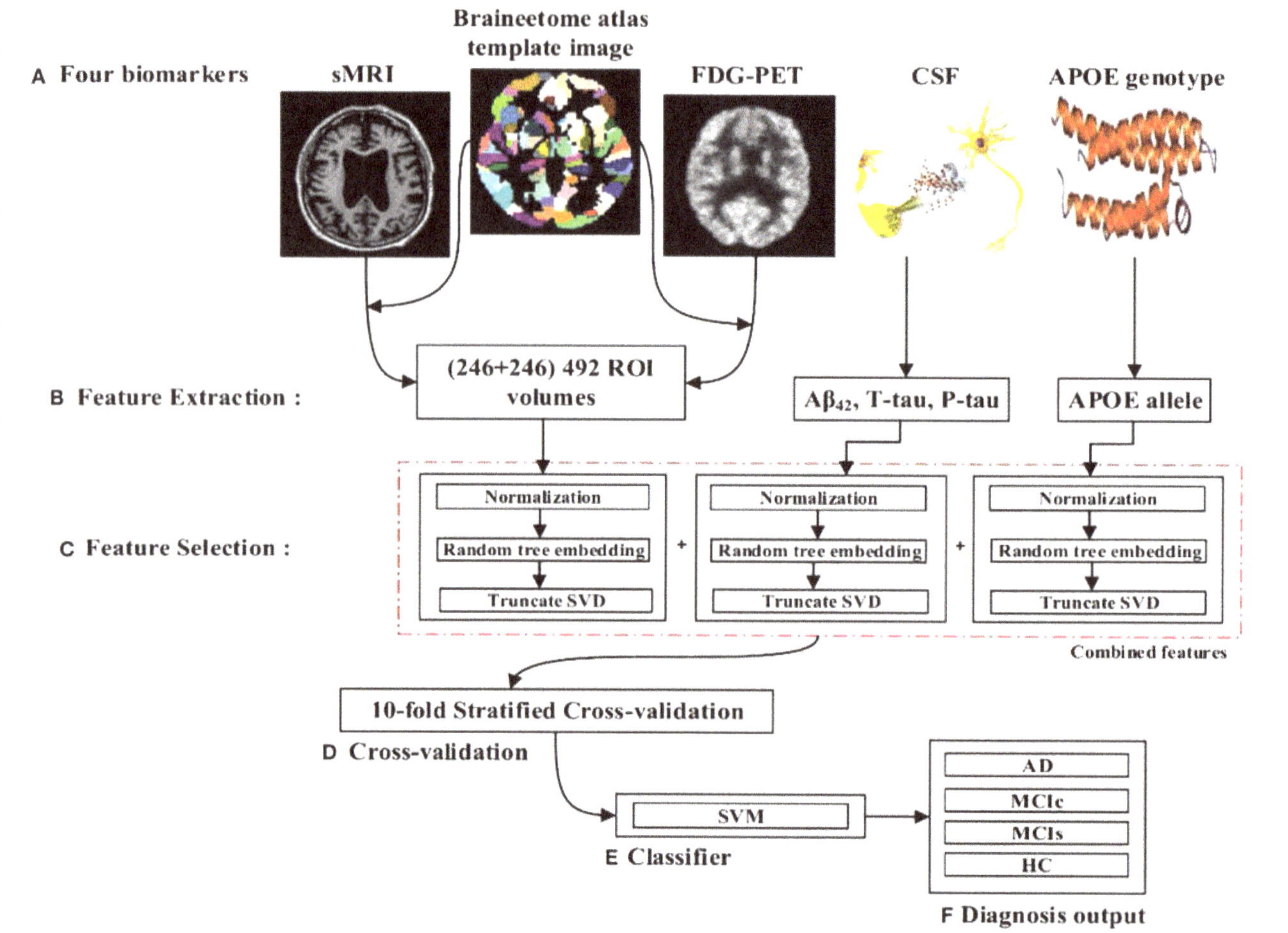

FIGURE 1 | Overview of the proposed framework. **(A)** Selection of four (sMRI, FDG-PET, CSF, and APOE) important biomarkers. **(B)** Feature extraction using NiftyReg toolbox for sMRI and FDG-PET image. **(C)** Feature selection using truncate SVD method. **(D)** Ten-fold stratified cross-validation method. **(E)** Kernel-based multiclass SVM classifier. **(F)** Diagnosis output.

is followed for every classification problem. **Figure 3** shows the early fusion pipeline. Moreover, here 1st (APOE), 2nd (CSF), 3rd (sMRI), and 4th (FDG-PET) features are concatenated with each other using early fusion technique before passing them further. We assessed the classification performance for individual and combined modalities by calculating the AUC for each group.

Feature Selection

With the help of automated feature extraction methods, we extracted 246 ROIs from each sMRI and FDG-PET image. As in the neuroimaging analysis, the number of features per subjects is very high relative to the number of patients, a phenomenon normally referred to as the curse of dimensionality. Furthermore, because of the computational difficulties of dealing with high dimensional data, dealing with many features can be a challenging task, which may result in overfitting. Feature selection is an additional helpful stage prior to the classification problem, which helps to reduce the dimensionality of a feature by selecting proper features and omitting improper features. This step helps to speed up the classification process by decreasing computational time for the training and testing datasets and increases the performance of classification accuracy. At first, we normalized the extracted features using the standard scalar function from Scikit-learn library (0.19.2) (Pedregosa et al., 2011), which transforms the dataset in such way that its distribution will have a mean of 0 and unit variance of 1 to reduce the redundancy and dependency of the data. After that, we performed high dimensional transformation of the data using random tree embedding (Geurts et al., 2006; Moosmann et al., 2008) from Scikit-learn library (0.19.2) (Pedregosa et al., 2011) and a dimensionality reduction process using truncated singular value decomposition (SVD) method. Random tree embedding system works based on the decision tree ensemble learning (Brown, 2016) system that execute an unsupervised data transformation algorithm to solve a random tree embedding task. It uses a forest of complete random trees, that encodes the data by the indices of the leaves where a data sample point

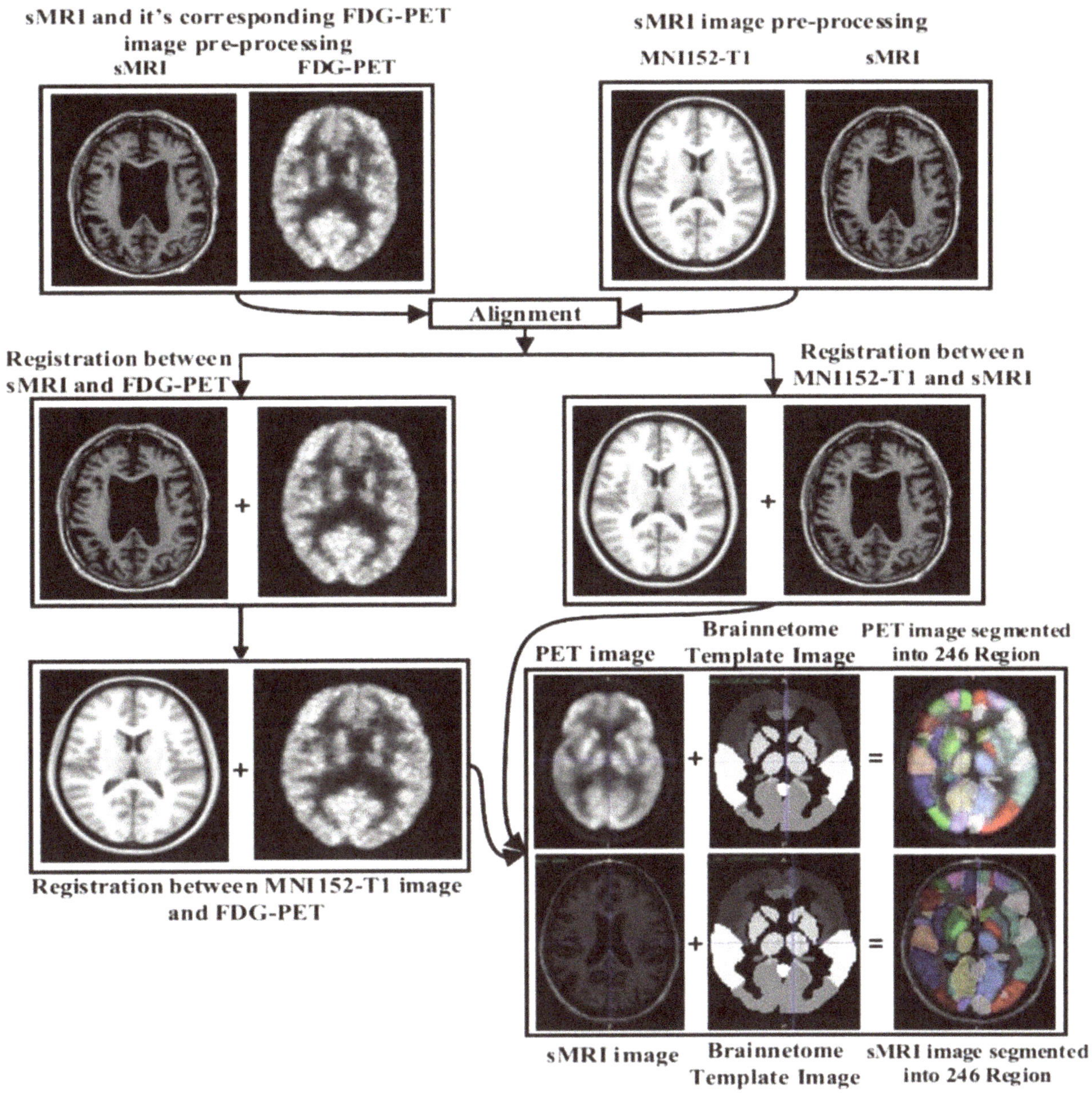

FIGURE 2 | Overview of the feature extraction pipeline for sMRI and FDG-PET image. Here, NiftyReg toolbox is used for the image registration and as well as for the non-linear registration between the (sMRI and FDG-PET) image with 2 mm Brainnetome template image. Above pipeline shows that, we have successfully extracted 246 ROI's from each (sMRI and FDG-PET) images.

ends up. This index is then encoded in a one-of-k encoder, which maps the data into a very high-dimensional state which might be beneficial for the classification process. The mapping process is completely unsupervised and very efficient for any dataset. After mapping the dataset into the very high dimensional state, we applied the truncated SVD function for dimensionality reduction purposes, which only selects the important features from the complete set of features. The truncated SVD is similar to principal component analysis (PCA) but differs in that it works on the sample matrices X directly instead of working on their covariance matrices. When performed column-wise (per-feature), i.e., means of X are deducted from the value of the feature, the truncated SVD of the resulting matrix corresponds to PCA. Truncated SVD implements an irregular SVD that only calculates the k largest singular values, where k is a user-specified parameter. Mathematically, the truncated SVD can be applied to train data X, which produces a low-rank approximation of X:

$$X = X_k = U_k \Sigma_k V_k^T \tag{1}$$

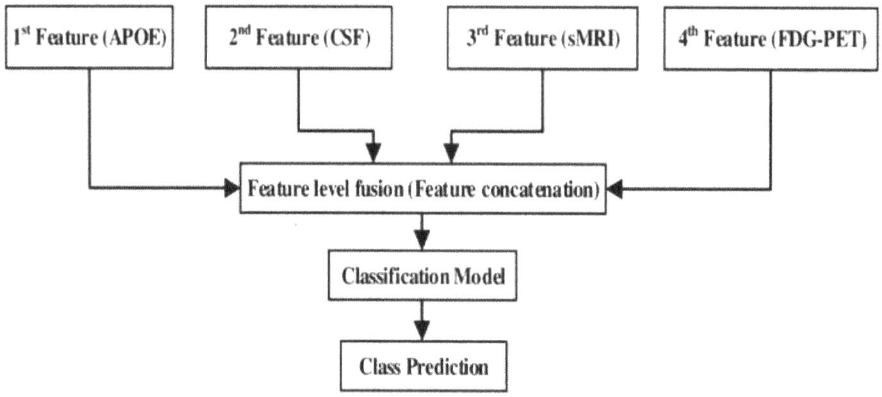

FIGURE 3 | Multimodal fusion pipeline shows the fusion of four modality of biomarkers, from which two biomarkers sMRI and FDG-PET belongs to imaging modality, CSF biomarker from biochemical, and APOE biomarker from genetics.

After this process, $U_k\Sigma_k^T$ is transformed into the training set with k features. To transform a test set X, we can multiply it by V_k:

$$X' = XV_k \tag{2}$$

In this way, we can perform the truncated SVD method on the training and testing dataset.

Classification

Support Vector Machine

SVM is a supervised learning method. SVM (Cortes and Vapnik, 1995) works by finding a hyperplane that best separates two data groups. It is trained by training data in n-dimensional training space after which test subjects are classified according to their position in n-dimensional feature space. It has been used in several neuroimaging areas (Cui et al., 2011; Zhang et al., 2011; Young et al., 2013; Collij et al., 2016) and is known to be one of the most powerful machine learning tools in the neuroscience field in recent research. In mathematical representation, for a 2D space, a line can discriminate the linearly separable data. The equation of a line is $y = ax + b$. By renaming x with x_1 and y with x_2, the equation will change to $a(x_1 - x_2) + b = 0$. If we stipulate $X = (x_1, x_2)$ and $w = (a, -1)$, we get $w.x + b = 0$, which is an equation of hyperplane. The linearly separable output with the hyperplane equation has the following form:

$$f(y) = z^T\varnothing.(y) + b \tag{3}$$

Where y is an input vector, $z^T$is a hyperplane parameter, and $\varnothing(y)$ is a function used to map feature vector y into a higher-dimensional space. The parameters z and b are scaled suitably by the same quantity, the decision hyperplane given by the Equation (2) remains unchanged. Moreover, in order to make any decision boundary surface (hyperplane) correspond to the exclusive pair of (z, b), the following constraints are familiarized:

$$min\left|z^T\varnothing.(y_i) + b\right| = 1, \qquad i = 1, \ldots, N, \tag{4}$$

Where $y_1, y_2, y_3, \ldots, y_N$ are the given training points. Equation (4) hyperplanes are known as the canonical hyperplanes. For a given hyperplane (or decision surface) which is described with the equation;

$$z^T\varnothing.(y) + b = 0, \text{which is same as } z^T\varnothing.\left(y\right) = 0 \text{ (which has more dimensions)} \tag{5}$$

And, for a vector x that does not belong to the hyperplane, the following equation is satisfied (Cortes and Vapnik, 1995, Madevska-Bogdanova et al., 2004, Cui et al., 2011):

$$z^T\varnothing.(x) + b = \pm s\,\|z\| \tag{6}$$

Where s is the distance of a point x to the given hyperplane. The different signs determine the vector's x side of the hyperplane. Therefore, the output $f\left(y\right)$ (or predictive value) of the SVM is truly proportional to the norm of vector z and the distance $s(x)$ from the chosen hyperplane. Moreover, in our study, we have used kernel-support vector machine, which is used to solve the non-linear problem with the use of linear classifier and involved in exchanging linearly non-separable data into linearly separable data. The idea behind this concept is linearly non-separated data in n-dimensional space might be linearly separated in higher m-dimensional space. Mathematically, the kernel is indicated as,

$$K\left(a, b\right) = < F\left(a\right), F\left(b\right) > \tag{7}$$

Where, K is a kernel function and a, b are inputs in n-dimensional space. F is a mapping function which maps from n-dimensional to m-dimensional space (i.e., m > n). Moreover, in our case, we have used three different kinds of kernel function which is defined as follow:

- Polynomial type: It represents the resemblance of vectors (training samples) in a feature space over the polynomials of the original variables, allowing the learning of non-linear models. A Polynomial kernel is defined as;

$$K\left(x, y\right) = (x,\ y)^d \tag{8}$$

Where x and y are vectors in the input space. d is the kernel parameter.

- Gaussian radial basis type: Radial basis functions mostly with Gaussian form and it is represented by;

$$K(x,y) = \exp(-\frac{\|x-y\|^2}{2\sigma^2}) \quad (9)$$

Where, x and y are the two input samples, which represented as a feature vector in input space. $\|x-y\|^2$ may be seen as a squared Euclidean distance between two feature vectors. σ is a kernel parameter.

- Sigmoid type: It comes from the neural networks field, where the bipolar sigmoid function is often used as an activation function for an artificial neuron. And, it is represented by;

$$K(x,y) = \tanh(\propto x^T y + c) \quad (10)$$

Where, x and y are vectors in the input space and $\propto$, c are the kernel parameters.

For our study, we used a different kernel-based multiclass SVM from Scikit-learn 0.19.2 library (Pedregosa et al., 2011). Scikit-learn library internally use LIBSVM (Chang and Lin, 2011) to handle all computations. The hyperparameter of the kernel-based SVM must be tuned to measure how much maximum performance can be augmented by tuning it. It is important because they directly control the behavior of the training algorithm and have a significant impact on the performance of the model is being trained. Moreover, a good choice of hyperparameter can really make an algorithm smooth. Therefore, to find an optimal hyperparameter for the kernel-based multiclass SVM, C (explains the SVM optimization and percentage of absconding the misclassified trained data. For high C values, training data will classify accurately by a hyperplane; similarly, for low C values, optimizer looks for a higher margin separating hyperplane while it will misclassify the more data points) and γ (Gaussian kernel width describes the impact of specific training data. The high gamma values result in consideration of datasets that are near to separation line. Likewise, for low gamma values, datasets that are away from the separation line, will also be taken into consideration while in the calculation line) parameters are optimized using a grid search and a ten-fold stratified cross-validation (CV) method on the training dataset. This validation technique gives an assurance that our trained model got most of the patterns from the training dataset. Moreover, CV works by randomly dividing training dataset into 10 parts, one of which was left as a validation set, while the remaining nine were used by a training set. In this study, ten-fold stratified cross-validation was performed 100 times to obtain more accurate results. Finally, we computed the arithmetic mean of the 100 repetitions as the final result. Note that, as a different feature had different scales, so in our case, we linearly ascend each training feature to imitate to a range between 0 and 1; the same scaling technique was then applied to the test dataset. As the number of selected features is small, in our case the RBF kernel performs better than other kernels.

Measuring the Classification Performance

To assess the classification performance of each group we have applied two method: (i) ROC-AUC curve analysis and (ii) Statistical analysis using Cohen's kappa method.

ROC-AUC Analysis

The ROC-AUC is a fundamental graph in the evaluation of diagnostic tests and is also often used in biomedical research to test classification problem performance and prediction models for decision support, prognosis, and diagnosis. ROC analysis examines the accuracy of a proposed model to separate positive and negative cases or distinguish AD patients from different groups. It is particularly useful in assessing predictive models since it records the trade-off between specificity and sensitivity over that range. In a ROC curve, the true positive rate (known as the sensitivity) is arranged as a function of a false positive rate (known as the 1-specificity) for different cut-off values of parameters. Each point's level of the ROC curve characterizes a sensitivity/specificity pair, which corresponds to a specific decision threshold. This is generally depicted in a square box for convenience and it's both axes are from 0 to 1. The area under curve (AUC) is an effective and joint measure of sensitivity and specificity for assessing inherent validity of a diagnostic test. AUC curve shows us how well a factor can differentiate between two binary diagnostic groups (diseased/normal). A result with perfect discrimination has a 100% sensitivity, 100% specificity ROC curve. Therefore the closer the ROC curve to the upper left corner, the higher the overall accuracy of the test as suggested by Greiner et al. (2000). The AUC is commonly used to visualize the performance of binary classes, producing a classifier with two possible output classes. Accuracy is measured using the AUC. Here, an AUC of one signifies a perfect score, and an area of 0.5 represents a meaningless test.

The AUC plot provides two parameters:

1. True positive rate (TPR): the TPR is a performance measure of the whole positive part of a dataset.
2. False positive rate (FPR): the FPR is a performance measure of the whole negative part of a dataset.

Moreover, classification accuracy measures the effectiveness of predicting the true class label, but in our case, it should be noted that the number of subjects was not the same in each group, so only calculating accuracy may result in a misleading estimation of the performance. Therefore, four more performance metrics have been calculated, namely specificity, sensitivity, precision, and F1-score. We have reported the accuracy, specificity, sensitivity, precision, and F1-score values corresponding to the ideal point of the ROC curve.

$$Accuracy = \frac{TP + TN}{TP + FP + FN + TN} \quad (11)$$

$$F1 - score = 2* \left[\frac{precision*recall}{precision + recall} \right] \quad (12)$$

where,

$$Precision = \frac{TP}{TP + FP}; \; Recall = Specificity = \frac{TP}{TP + FN} \quad (13)$$

TABLE 3 | Obtained best CV score for six classification groups.

Group	Regularization constant (c)	Gamma (g or γ)	Best CV score
AD vs. HC	7	0.00316227766017	0.98742
AD vs. MCIs	5	0.01	0.96207
AD vs. MCIc	6	0.004	0.92201
MCIs vs. MCIc	9	0.001	0.94782
HC vs. MCIc	4	0.001	0.94036
HC vs. MCIs	9	0.001	0.93103

With TP, FP, TN, and FN denoting true positive, false positive, true negative, and false negative, respectively. Specificity (true negative rate) provides a amount for those not in the class, i.e., it is the percentage of those not in the class that were found not to be in the class. Precision [which is also termed as positive predictive value (PPV)] is the fraction of relevant incidences among the retrieved incidences, and F1-score (which is also called F-score or F-measure) is a amount related to a test's accuracy. Moreover, in our case, we have repeated the procedure 100 times, the reported AUC-ROC, accuracy, sensitivity, specificity, precision, and F1-score are the average over the 10 repetitions of the 10-fold stratified cross-validation procedure. We have followed this method for every classification groups.

Statistical Analysis Using Cohen's Kappa Method

Cohen's kappa statistic value for each classification problem was computed. This function calculates Cohen's kappa score, which demonstrate the level of agreement between two annotators or the level of agreement between two dissimilar groups in a binary classification problem defined as,

$$k = (p_o - p_e)/(1 - p_e) \tag{14}$$

where, p_o is the empirical probability of an agreement on the label assigned to any example (the observed agreement ratio), and, p_e is the predictable agreement when both annotators assign labels randomly. Here, p_e was assessed using a per-annotator empirical prior over the class labels. The kappa statistic value is always between −1 and 1. The maximum value means complete agreement between two groups, zero or lower value means a low probability of agreement.

RESULTS

Here, all classification problems were performed using Ubuntu 16.04 LTS, running python 3.6, and using Scikit-learn library version 0.19.2. In this study, there were four classes of data, AD, MCIc, MCIs, and HC, separated using four different types of biomarker, sMRI and FDG-PET for imaging modalities, and CSF as a biochemical (or fluid vessel) that show results reflecting the formation of amyloid plaques inside the brain, and APOE genotypes as genetic features. Thus, we validated our proposed method on six different types of classification problem, i.e., six binary class problem (AD vs. HC, MCIc vs. MCIs, AD vs. MCIc, HC vs. MCIs, HC vs. MCIc, and AD vs. MCIs). At first, we extracted the featured from each sMRI and FDG-PET images by using the NiftyReg registration process with 2-mm Brainnetome atlas template image. In total, we obtained 497 features for a single image, 246 ROI-based features from the sMRI and FDG-PET images, three feature values from the CSF data, and two features from the APOE genotype data. Moreover, we have applied a random tree embedding method which transformed obtained low dimension features into a higher dimensional state, after that an early fusion technique is processed to combine the multiple features into single form before passing them for further process. Additionally, we have also applied a feature selection technique using a truncated SVD dimensionality reduction method, which will select the effective features from all 497 high dimensional features and send these selected features to the classifier, to measure the performance of identifying each group. In our case, we used a kernel-based multiclass SVM as a classifier from a Scikit-learn library (0.19.2).

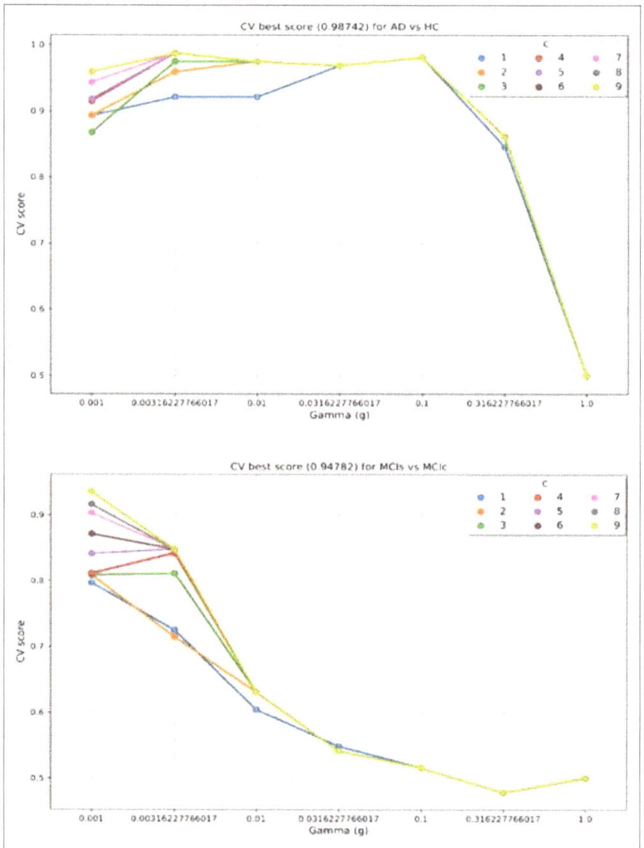

FIGURE 4 | CV best score obtained for AD vs. HC and MCIs vs. MCIc groups. Best CV score is computed by taking the average of 10 folds CV values. CV score, Cross-validation score; C, regularization constant; and *g or* γ, gamma, C and γ are the hyperparameter value for the kernel-based multiclass SVM.

In order to attain unbiased estimates of performance, the set of participants were randomly split into two groups in a 75:25 ratios as training and testing sets, respectively.

In the training set, to find the right values for the hyperparameter (C and γ) is very difficult, and their values influence the classification result. Moreover, we know that the parameter *C*, trades off the misclassification of training samples against the simplicity of a decision surface, a small *C* value makes the decision surface flat, while a high *C* value aims to classify all training samples correctly. Moreover, a γ value shows how much influence a single training sample has. The larger γ is, the closer other samples must be to be affected. Therefore, we have used cross-validation technique to get good optimal hyperparameter values for the regularization constant (*C*) and gamma (γ). We can't know the best value for a model hyperparameter on a given problem. With the right values of hyperparameters will eliminate the chances of overfitting and underfitting. Therefore, to find the optimal hyperparameter values for a kernel-based SVM, have used a grid-search (which perform a comprehensive search over the specified parameter values for an estimator) and ten-fold stratified cross-validation technique on the training set. The grid search was performed over the ranges of $C = 1$ to 9 and $\gamma = $ 1e-4 to 1. For each method, the gained optimized value of the hyperparameter was then used to train the classifier using the training set, and later the performance of the resulting classifier was then evaluated on the remaining 25% of data in the testing dataset, which was not used during the training step. The obtained optimized hyperparameter (*C* and γ) value and their best CV accuracy are shown in **Table 3**. **Figure 4** is a plot of the classifier's CV accuracy with respect to (*C* and γ) for AD vs. HC and MCIc vs. MCIs groups. In **Figure 4**, we can see the impact of having different *C* and γ values on the model. Moreover, the best found optimal hyperparameter combination for an AD vs. HC are $C = 7$, $\gamma = 0.00316227766017$ and for MCIs vs. MCIc are $C = 9$, $\gamma = 0.001$, these tuned optimal hypermeter values are automatically chosen from the given range of $C = 1$ to 9 and $\gamma = $ 1e-4 to 1 with the help of grid search and ten-fold CV. In this way, we achieved unbiased estimates of the performance for each classification problem. In our experiment, the number of subjects was not the same in each group. Therefore, only calculating accuracy does not enable a comparison of the performances of the different classification experiments. Thus, we have considered five measures. For each group, we have calculated the accuracy, sensitivity, specificity, precision, and F1-score performance measure values. **Table 4** show the classification results for AD vs. HC, MCIc vs. MCIs, AD vs. MCIs, AD vs. MCIc, HC vs. MCIc, and HC vs. MCIs.

We conduct the AD vs. HC experiment using extracted APOE, CSF, FDG-PET, and sMRI features, and the classification outcome is shown in **Table 4**. For AD vs. HC classification, we had 38 AD and 38 HC subjects and only sMRI individual biomarker performed well while compared to other individual modalities of biomarkers. Moreover, the early fusion technique that we used to combine features from different modalities resulted in an AUC of 98.33, 98.42% of accuracy, 100% of sensitivity, 96.47% of specificity, 97.89% of precision, and 98.42% of F1-score. Furthermore, Cohen's kappa value is 0.93 for the combined method, which is very close to 1. Likewise, for the MCIs vs. MCIc classification problem, 82 subjects were included. Forty-six were in the MCIc group and the remaining 36 patients were in the MCIs group. **Table 4** shows the computed performance measure for this classification problem. Compared to other classification group problem this classification group (MCIs vs. MCIc) is difficult to classify because both groups show similar brain structure; however, there are slight differences in structure. For this group, APOE genotype individual biomarker performed well while compared to other individual modalities of biomarkers. Moreover, our proposed method has performed even better than the best output obtained by individual biomarkers for this group and the achieved measures are AUC of 93.59%, with 94.86% accuracy, 100% sensitivity, 88.71% specificity, 89.62% precision, and an F1-score of 91.67% compared to those of the single modalities. For MCIs vs. MCIc, Cohen's kappa value was 0.86, which is better than those of the single modalities. Our proposed method has performed very well when classifying this group. For AD vs. MCIs group, there were 38 AD and 36 MCIs subjects. First, we extracted the features from each subject and then we combined both imaging (PET and MRI) feature values with the other two (CSF and APOE genotype) feature values to measure the performance of AD vs. MCIs classification. **Table 4** shows the results from passing obtained features to the kernel-based multiclass SVM classifier. As can be seen from **Table 4**, our proposed method to combine all four modalities of a biomarker for distinguishing between AD and MCIs achieved good results compared to single modality biomarkers. For this classification problem, our proposed method achieved 96.65% of accuracy with a Cohen's kappa of 0.91. For AD vs. MCIc group, there were 38 AD and 46 MCIc. We trained kernel-based multiclass SVM classifiers using dimensionality-reduced features from truncated SVD to measures the performance of AD vs. MCIc group. The best performance was attained using a combination of four modalities of features, i.e., sMRI, FDG-PET, APOE and CSF, which had an accuracy of 92.26%, a sensitivity of 91.67%, a specificity of 92.86%, and an AUC of 94.64% with Cohen's kappa of 0.84. For the HC vs. MCIc distinction, our proposed method achieved 96.43% AUC, 94.13% accuracy, 94.75% sensitivity, 100% of specificity and precision, and 96.72% of F1-score. **Table 4** shows the classification performance result for HC vs. MCIc classification. In this case, the obtained Cohen's kappa index value is 0.88, which is near to the maximum level agreement value of 1. For the HC vs. MCIs classification problem, 74 subjects were included. Thirty-six were in the MCIs group and the remaining 38 patients were in the HC group. **Table 4** shows the results from passing obtained features to the kernel-based multiclass SVM classifier. As can be seen from **Table 4**, our proposed method to combine all four modalities of a biomarker for distinguishing between HC and MCIs achieved good results compared to single modality biomarkers. For this classification problem, our proposed method had achieved 95.24% of AUC, and 95.65% of accuracy with a Cohen's kappa of 0.90. Therefore, we can say that for all classification groups our proposed method has achieved a high level of performance while compared to single modality of biomarkers, ranging from 1 to 5%, and our proposed method has also achieved a high level of agreement between each other for all six classification groups while compared with single modality-based methods. For AD vs. MCIs, AD vs. MCIc, HC vs. MCIs, and HC vs. MCIc groups, CSF individual biomarkers performed very well-compared to other individual modality of biomarkers, and the CSF achieved AUC for these groups are 94.17, 89.58, 94.05, and 92.5%.

TABLE 4 | Classification results for AD vs. HC, MCIs vs. MCIc, AD vs. MCIs, AD vs. MCIc, HC vs. MCIc, and HC vs. MCIs groups.

Groups	Features	Classifier	Performance measure						
			AUC	ACC	SEN	SPEC	PRE	F1-score	Cohen's kappa
AD vs. HC	APOE genotype	SVM	90.83	88.96	90.91	89.46	86.92	87.33	0.79
	CSF		91.54	91.3	88.48	91.67	90.91	93.15	0.82
	sMRI		93.33	92.5	100	89.74	88.47	92.86	0.85
	FDG-PET		92.5	92.56	89.74	90	93.62	91.63	0.84
	Combined		**98.33**	**98.42**	**100**	**96.47**	**97.89**	**98.42**	**0.93**
MCIs vs. MCIc	APOE genotype	SVM	91.21	92	86.67	**100**	**100**	**92.86**	0.83
	CSF		87.73	88	85.71	90.91	92.31	88.89	0.75
	sMRI		86.54	85.43	84.55	83.92	86.96	81.82	0.69
	FDG-PET		90.38	89	100	85	76.92	86.96	0.76
	Combined		**93.59**	**94.86**	**100**	88.71	89.62	91.67	**0.86**
AD vs. MCIs	APOE genotype	SVM	90	89.96	100	82.73	84	88.89	0.75
	CSF		94.17	93.33	91.3	**100**	86.67	92.86	0.86
	sMRI		88.33	87.67	82.61	86.49	73.33	84.62	0.73
	FDG-PET		89.17	90	89.96	91.73	89.96	88.89	0.75
	Combined		**96.83**	**96.65**	**100**	91.67	**93.33**	**96.55**	**0.91**
AD vs. MCIc	APOE genotype	SVM	88.89	88.46	77.78	**94.12**	87.2	82.35	0.71
	CSF		89.58	86.39	86.92	90	87.5	88.67	0.73
	sMRI		84.52	80.36	80.77	81.82	80	78.26	0.69
	FDG-PET		84.03	80.77	66.67	88.24	75	70.59	0.65
	Combined		**94.64**	**92.26**	**91.67**	92.86	**91.67**	**91.67**	**0.84**
HC vs. MCIc	APOE genotype	SVM	87.5	87.12	82.64	87.5	86.67	92.33	0.73
	CSF		94.05	92.31	91.67	90.44	92.26	95.22	0.83
	sMRI		89.58	88.46	90.91	86.67	83.33	86.96	0.76
	FDG-PET		91.07	87.5	88.46	100	82.35	85.71	0.76
	Combined		**96.43**	**94.13**	**94.75**	**100**	**100**	**96.72**	**0.88**
HC vs. MCIs	APOE genotype	SVM	90.83	87.08	86.96	**92.86**	86.67	89.66	0.72
	CSF		92.5	90.47	100	72.73	80	88.89	0.73
	sMRI		91.27	90.16	98.26	86.67	90.91	92	0.71
	FDG-PET		89.68	87.3	92.31	80	85.71	88.89	0.73
	Combined		**95.24**	**95.65**	**100**	88.89	**93.33**	**96.55**	**0.90**

Figure 5 shows Cohen's kappa statistics score for six classification problems, AD vs. HC, MCIs vs. MCIc, AD vs. MCIs, AD vs. MCIc, HC vs. MCIs, and HC vs. MCIc. From this graph, we can see that our proposed method has achieved a good level of agreement between different classification groups.

Here, **Figure 6** shows the AUC curve for AD vs. HC, MCIs vs. MCIc, AD vs. MCIs, AD vs. MCIc, HC vs. MCIs, and HC vs. MCIc. Total AUC-ROC curve is a single index for measuring the performance of a test. The larger the AUC, the better is the overall performance of the diagnostic test to correctly pick up diseased and non-diseased subjects. For AD vs. HC, our proposed model achieved 98.33% AUC, showing that our proposed model performed well when distinguishing positive and negative values. For MCIs vs. MCIc, our proposed model correctly distinguished converted patients from stable patients with an AUC of 93.59%, which is a great achievement for this complex group. Likewise, for AD vs. MCIs, AD vs. MCIc, HC vs. MCIs, and HC vs. MCIc, our proposed model achieved AUCs of 96.83, 94.64, 95.24, and 96.43%. Overall, for all classification methods, our proposed model performed well and its probabilities for the positive classes are well-separated from those of the negative classes.

DISCUSSION

In this experiment, we proposed a novel technique to fuse data from multiple modalities for the classification of AD from different groups, using a kernel-based multiclass SVM method. In addition, earlier studies aimed only for AD vs. HC classification groups. In this paper, we studied six binary classification problem, AD vs. HC, MCIs vs. MCIc, AD vs. MCIs, AD vs. MCIc, HC vs. MCIs, and HC vs. MCIc. More importantly, we combined not only sMRI and FDG-PET images but also their CSF (biochemical) and APOE (genetic) genotype values. Our experiment result shows that each modality (sMRI, FDG-PET, CSF, and APOE) is indispensable in achieving good combination and good classification accuracy.

Some studies (Zhang et al., 2011, 2012; Young et al., 2013) have used a small number of features extracted from automatic or manual segmentation processes for the classification of AD from different groups. Their proposed model has achieved good performance for AD vs. HC; however, for MCIc vs. MCIs, the performance of their proposed model is poor.

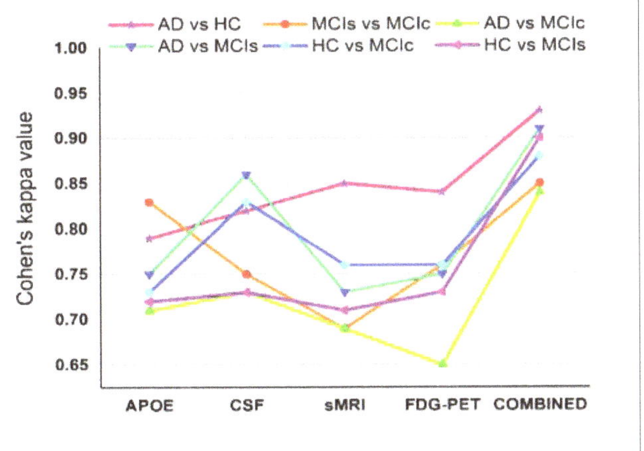

FIGURE 5 | Cohen's kappa score for AD vs. HC, MCIs vs. MCIc, AD vs. MCIc, AD vs. MCIs, HC vs. MCIs, and HC vs. MCIc (each experiment obtained kappa value is shown by different solid color lines). This Cohen's kappa plot shows that combined features outperform the single modality features in all experiments.

Therefore, in our study, we tried to extract as many ROI from two imaging modalities using the 2-mm Brainnetome template image. To the best of our knowledge, this is the first experiment where 246 ROI was extracted from all 158 subjects and all features were used in the classification of AD and MCI subjects.

Furthermore, we later fused features from these two imaging modalities with three CSF and two APOE genotype features offered by the ADNI website for the distinction of AD from different groups using early fusion technique. Moreover, we use a more advanced segmented template image for feature extraction from both imaging modalities with the NiftyReg registration toolbox, compared to other studies (Walhovd et al., 2010; Davatzikos et al., 2011; Zhang et al., 2011; Beheshti et al., 2017; Li et al., 2017; Long et al., 2017). As we can see that from **Table 4**, single modality biomarkers (sMRI and APOE genotype) achieved a good performance for AD vs. HC and MCIs vs. MCIc (using all 246 extracted features and as well as with two APOE genotype feature from each subject) groups, when compared with the obtained outputs reported before (Zhang et al., 2011; Young et al., 2013). Likewise, from same **Table 4**, we can see that CSF individual modality of biomarkers has outperformed other individual biomarkers with 94.17, 89.58, 94.05, 92.5% of AUC for AD vs. MCIs, AD vs. MCIc, HC vs. MCIc, and HC vs. MCIs. Moreover, a lot of studies have shown that different modalities of biomarkers contain complementary

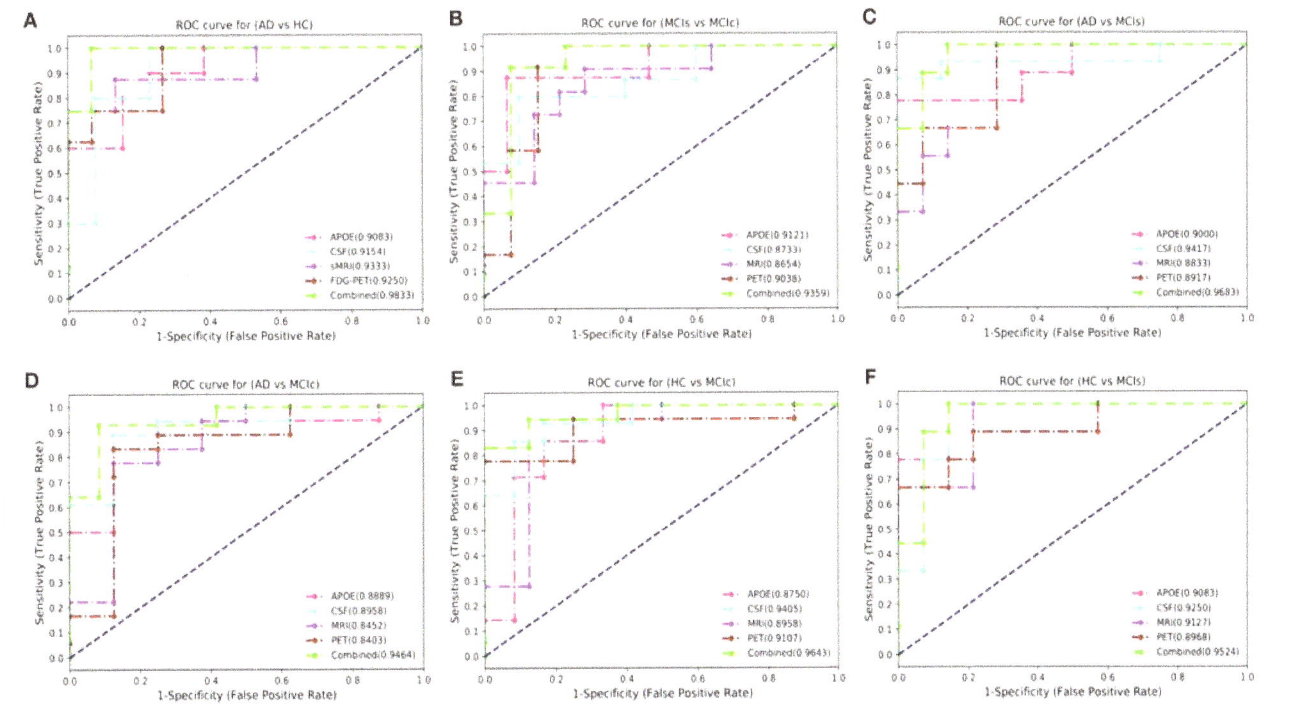

FIGURE 6 | Comparison of the ROC-AUC curve corresponding with the best performance of combined fusion method in each experiment is displayed by the green dashed lines. We also compare these ROC-AUC curves with those of single modality features. This comparison shows that combined features outperform the single modality features in all experiments, which can be seen from above figure **(A)** AD vs. HC, **(B)** MCIs vs. MCIc, **(C)** AD vs. MCIs, **(D)** AD vs. MCIc, **(E)** HC vs. MCIc, and **(F)** HC vs. MCIs.

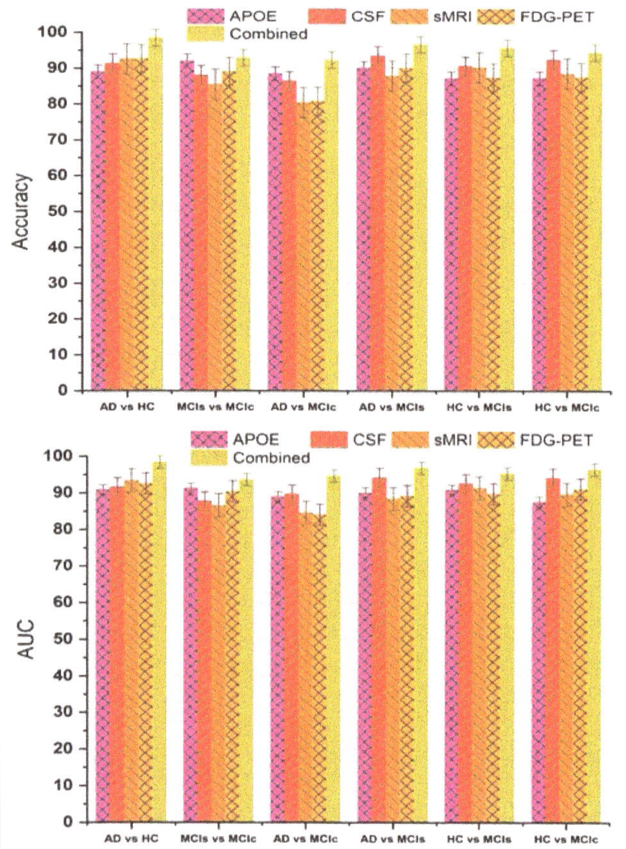

FIGURE 7 | Comparison of single modality results with multi-modality classification result based on obtained accuracy and AUC score. From above figure we can see that in every group combined feature (or multimodal method) has outperformed the single modality results.

information for the discrimination of AD and MCI subjects. Here, we quantitatively measure the discrimination agreement between any two different classification groups using the kappa index. For combined features (for AD vs. HC, AD vs. MCIs, and AD vs. MCIc), the obtained level of agreement between each group is 0.93, 0.91, and 0.84, respectively. Likewise, for HC vs. MCIs and HC vs. MCIc, the obtained level of agreement between each group are 0.90 and 0.88. Moreover, for MCIs vs. MCIc group the obtained level of agreement between each other is the 0.86, respectively. These all scores are achieved using a 10-fold stratified CV method on combined dataset. These results indicate that the combined feature (for AD vs. HC) group has the highest level of agreement between each other while compared to other groups and as well as while compared to the individual performance of each modality.

Recently, many studies have been published using a single modality of biomarkers (Chetelat et al., 2007; Fjell et al., 2010; Chen and Ishwaran, 2012; Beheshti et al., 2016; Jha et al., 2017; Lama et al., 2017; Long et al., 2017), including sMRI, FDG-PET, CSF, and APOE. Most of these studies used biomarkers from the sMRI, because it is practically difficult to get biomarkers from all modalities for the same patients due to the various reasons, including the availability of imaging equipment, cost, lack of patient consent, and patient death in longitudinal studies. Previously proposed models using a single modality have achieved good performance for AD vs. HC classification, where for MCIs vs. MCIc their classification accuracy is very low compared to our proposed multimodal technique. Here, we have performed an experiment to assess the classification performance using features from every single modality independently, as well as with the combination of multimodal biomarkers. A kernel-based multiclass SVM classifier was utilized, and the comparison of the obtained single modality results with the multimodal classification results are shown in **Figure 7**. In terms of accuracy and AUC, the classification performance using features from CSF is generally better than those using genetic and imaging features, which highlights the importance of Aβ plaques as biomarkers in the classification of AD, while in comparison to the performance with multimodal biomarkers, its performance is slightly lower. In addition, we can see that for the MCIs vs. MCIc comparison, each modality of biomarker has performed well. Different methods were used to evaluate the classification of AD using multimodal data. First, we combine all high-dimensional features from four modalities into a single feature vector for classification of AD and MCI subjects. After that, all features were normalized (to have a zero mean ± unit standard deviation) before using them in the classification process. This combined multimodal method provides a straightforward method of using multimodal data. Subsequently, we passed these features to the kernel-based multiclass SVM classifier for classification purposes with a 10-fold stratified CV strategy as described above, and obtained results are shown in **Table 4** and **Figure 7**. As we can see in **Table 4**, our early fusion combination method consistently outperforms the performance of individual modality of biomarkers.

Recently, several studies have investigated neuroimaging techniques for the early detection of AD, with the main focus on MCI subjects, who may or may not convert to AD, and separating patients with AD from healthy controls using multimodal data. However, it is difficult to make direct comparisons with these state-of-the-art methods since a majority of the studies have used different validation methods and datasets, which both crucially influence the classification problem. The first study by Zhang et al. (2012) obtained an accuracy of 76.8% (sensitivity and specificity of 79 and 68%) for the classification of converters and stable MCI subjects within 24 months.

These results were achieved using a multi-kernel SVM on a longitudinal ADNI dataset. Another study (Young et al., 2013) used a Gaussian process method for classification of MCIs vs. MCIc using several modalities. They reported an accuracy of 69.9% and AUC of 79.5%. Another study by Suk et al. (2014) used shared features from two imaging modalities, MRI and PET, using a combination of hierarchical and deep Boltzmann machines for a deep learning process; their proposed method achieved 74.66% accuracy and 95.23% AUC when comparing MCI-C vs. MCI-NC. In another study (Cheng et al., 2015), the authors introduced domain transfer learning using multimodal data (i.e., MRI, CSF, and PET) with an accuracy

TABLE 5 | Classification performance for the proposed method compared with published state-of-the art methods for differentiating between MCIs vs. MCIc.

Method	Modality	Subjects	AUC	ACC	SEN	SPEC
Zhang et al. (2012)	Longitudinal (MRI + PET)	88	76.8	78.4	79	68
Young et al. (2013)	MRI + PET + APOE	143	79.5	69.9	78.7	65.6
Suk et al. (2014)	PET + MRI	204	74.66	75.92	48.04	**95.23**
Cheng et al. (2015)	MRI + PET + CSF	99	84.8	79.4	84.5	72.7
Moradi et al. (2015)	MRI + AGE + Cognitive measure	264	90.20	81.72	86.65	73.64
Beheshti et al. (2017)	MRI	136	75.08	75	76.92	73.23
Liu et al. (2017)	MRI + PET	234	80.8	73.5	76.19	70.37
Long et al. (2017)	MRI (AMYG)	227	93.2	88.99	86.32	90.91
Proposed method	MRI + PET + CSF + APOE genotype	82	**93.59**	**94.86**	**100**	88.71

of 79.4% for MCIs vs. MCIc with an AUC of 84.8%. In another study (Moradi et al., 2015), the authors employed a VBM analysis of gray matter as a feature, combining age and cognitive measures. They reported an AUC of 90.20% with 81.72% accuracy comparing MCIc vs. MCIs sample. Another study (Beheshti et al., 2017), used feature ranking and a genetic algorithm (GA) for selection of optimal features for the classifier. Their method achieved an accuracy of 75%, sensitivity of 76.92%, specificity of 73.23%, and AUC of 75.08% for pMCI vs. sMCI. Liu et al. (2017) proposed combining two imaging modalities using independent component analysis and the Cox model for prediction of MCI progression. They achieved 80.8% AUC with 73.5% accuracy in comparisons of MCIc vs. MCIs. Recently, another author (Long et al., 2017) used Free surfer software to segment 3-T T1 images into many different parts and later used a multi-dimensional scaling method for feature selection before sending the selected features to the classifier. Their proposed method achieved an AUC of 93.2%, accuracy of 88.88%, sensitivity of 86.32, and specificity of 90.91% when differentiating sMCI from pMCI using only specific amygdala features. As shown in **Table 5**, the performance of the proposed system was highly competitive in performance terms when compared to the other systems reported in the literature for MCIs vs. MCIc classification.

CONCLUSION

In this study, we have proposed a novel method that shows how to extract 246 ROI from two imaging modalities, PET and sMRI, using a Brainnetome template image and then combined these features obtained from imaging with CSF and APOE genotype features from the same subjects. In the proposed method, we used a random tree embedding method to transform obtained features to a higher dimensional state and later we used a truncated SVD dimensionality reduction method to select only the important features, which increased the classification accuracy using kernel-based multiclass SVM classifier. The obtained experimental results prove that a combination of biomarkers from all four modalities is a reliable technique for the early prediction of AD or prediction of MCI conversion, especially with regards to high-dimensional data pattern recognition. In addition, our proposed method achieved 94.86% accuracy with 93.59% AUC and a Cohen's kappa index of 0.86 when distinguishing between MCIs vs. MCIc subjects. The performance of the proposed computer-aided system was measured using 158 subjects from the ADNI dataset with a 10-fold stratified cross-validation technique. The experimental results show that the performance of the proposed approach can compete strongly with other state-of-the-art techniques using biomarkers from all four modalities mentioned in the literature.

In future, we plan to combine demographic information of the studied subjects as features with the proposed model for the classification of AD and we will also carry out an investigation of the multimodal multiclass classification of AD using AV-45 and DTI modality of biomarkers.

AUTHOR CONTRIBUTIONS

YG and RL designed the study, collected the original imagining data from ADNI home page, and wrote the manuscript. RL and G-RK managed and analyzed the imaging data. All authors contributed to and have approved the final manuscript.

FUNDING

This work was supported by the National Research Foundation of Korea (NRF) grant funded by the Korea government (MSIT) (No. NRF-2019R1A4A1029769, NRF-2019R1F1A1060166).

ACKNOWLEDGMENTS

Data collection and sharing for this project was funded by the Alzheimer's Disease Neuroimaging Initiative (ADNI) (National Institutes of Health Grant U01 AG024904) and DOD ADNI (Department of Defense award number W81XWH-12-2-0012). As such, the investigators within the ADNI contributed to the design and implementation of ADNI and/or provided data but did not participate in analysis or writing of this report. A complete listing of ADNI investigators can be found at: http://adni.loni.usc.edu/wp-content/uploads/how_to_apply/ADNI_Acknowledgement_List.pdf. ADNI was funded by the National Institute on Aging, the National Institute of Biomedical Imaging and Bioengineering, and through generous contributions from the following: AbbVie, Alzheimer's Association; Alzheimer's Drug Discovery Foundation; Araclon Biotech; BioClinica, Inc.; Biogen; Bristol-Myers Squibb Company; CereSpir, Inc.; Cogstate; Eisai Inc.; Elan Pharmaceuticals, Inc.; Eli Lilly and Company; EuroImmun; F. Hoffmann-La Roche Ltd and its affiliated company Genentech, Inc.; Fujirebio; GE Healthcare; IXICO Ltd.; Janssen Alzheimer Immunotherapy Research & Development, LLC.; Johnson & Johnson Pharmaceutical Research & Development LLC.; Lumosity; Lundbeck; Merck & Co., Inc.; Meso Scale Diagnostics, LLC.; NeuroRx Research; Neurotrack Technologies; Novartis Pharmaceuticals Corporation; Pfizer Inc.; Piramal Imaging; Servier; Takeda Pharmaceutical Company; and Transition Therapeutics. The Canadian Institutes of Health Research is providing funds to support ADNI clinical sites in Canada. Private sector contributions are facilitated by the Foundation for the National Institutes of Health (www.fnih.org). The grantee organization is the Northern California Institute for Research and Education, and the study is coordinated by the Alzheimer's Therapeutic Research Institute at the University of Southern California. ADNI data are disseminated by the Laboratory for Neuro Imaging at the University of Southern California.

REFERENCES

Ahmed, R. M., Paterson, R. W., Warren, J. D., Zetterberg, H., O'Brien, J. T., Fox, N. C., et al. (2014). Biomarkers in dementia: clinical utility and new directions. *J. Neurol. Neurosurg. Psychiatry* 85, 1426–1434. doi: 10.1136/jnnp-2014-307662

Alzheimer's Disease Neuroimaging Initiative, Liu, Y., Tan, L., Wang, H.-F., Liu, Y., Hao, X.-K., et al. (2016). Multiple effect of apoe genotype on clinical and neuroimaging biomarkers across Alzheimer's Disease Spectrum. *Mol. Neurobiol.* 53, 4539–4547. doi: 10.1007/s12035-015-9388-7

Andreasen, N., Vanmechelen, E., Van de Voorde, A., Davidsson, P., Hesse, C., Tarvonen, S., et al. (1998). Cerebrospinal fluid tau protein as a biochemical marker for Alzheimer's disease: a community based follow up study. *J. Neurol. Neurosurg. Psychiatry* 64, 298–305. doi: 10.1136/jnnp.64.3.298

Anoop, A., Singh, P. K., Jacob, R. S., and Maji, S. K. (2010). CSF biomarkers for Alzheimer's disease diagnosis. *Int. J. Alzheimers Dis.* 2010, 1–12. doi: 10.4061/2010/606802

Ashburner, J., and Friston, K. J. (2000). Voxel-based morphometry—The methods. *NeuroImage* 11, 805–821. doi: 10.1006/nimg.2000.0582

Bain, L. J., Jedrziewski, K., Morrison-Bogorad, M., Albert, M., Cotman, C., Hendrie, H., et al. (2008). Healthy brain aging: a meeting report from the Sylvan M. Cohen Annual Retreat of the University of Pennsylvania Institute on Aging. *Alzheimers Dement.* 4, 443–446. doi: 10.1016/j.jalz.2008.08.006

Beheshti, I., Demirel, H., Farokhian, F., Yang, C., and Matsuda, H. (2016). Structural MRI-based detection of Alzheimer's disease using feature ranking and classification error. *Comput. Methods Programs Biomed.* 137, 177–193. doi: 10.1016/j.cmpb.2016.09.019

Beheshti, I., Demirel, H., and Matsuda, H. (2017). Classification of Alzheimer's disease and prediction of mild cognitive impairment-to-Alzheimer's conversion from structural magnetic resource imaging using feature ranking and a genetic algorithm. *Comput. Biol. Med.* 83, 109–119. doi: 10.1016/j.compbiomed.2017.02.011

Blennow, K. (2004). Cerebrospinal fluid protein biomarkers for Alzheimer's disease. *NeuroRx* 1, 213–225. doi: 10.1602/neurorx.1.2.213

Bouts, M. J. R. J., Möller, C., Hafkemeijer, A., van Swieten, J. C., Dopper, E., van der Flier, W. M., et al. (2018). Single subject classification of Alzheimer's disease and behavioral variant frontotemporal dementia using anatomical, diffusion tensor, and resting-state functional magnetic resonance imaging. *J. Alzheimers Dis.* 62, 1827–1839. doi: 10.3233/JAD-170893

Braak, H., and Braak, E. (1995). Staging of alzheimer's disease-related neurofibrillary changes. *Neurobiol. Aging* 16, 271–278. doi: 10.1016/0197-4580(95)00021-6

Braak, H., Braak, E., Bohl, J., and Bratzke, H. (1998). "Evolution of Alzheimer's disease related cortical lesions," in *Alzheimer's Disease — From Basic Research to Clinical Applications*, eds H.-J. Gertz, and Th. Arendt (Vienna: Springer Vienna), 97–106. doi: 10.1007/978-3-7091-7508-8_9

Brainerd, C. J., Reyna, V. F., Petersen, R. C., Smith, G. E., and Taub, E. S. (2011). Is the apolipoprotein e genotype a biomarker for mild cognitive impairment? Findings from a nationally representative study. *Neuropsychology* 25, 679–689. doi: 10.1037/a0024483

Bron, E. E., Smits, M., Papma, J. M., Steketee, R. M. E., Meijboom, R., de Groot, M., et al. (2017). Multiparametric computer-aided differential diagnosis of Alzheimer's disease and frontotemporal dementia using structural and advanced MRI. *Eur. Radiol.* 27, 3372–3382. doi: 10.1007/s00330-016-4691-x

Brown, G. (2016). "Ensemble learning," in *Encyclopedia of Machine Learning and Data Mining*, eds C. Sammut and G. I. Webb (Boston, MA: Springer). doi: 10.1007/978-1-4899-7502-7

Chang, C.-C., and Lin, C.-J. (2011). LIBSVM: a library for support vector machines. *ACM Trans. Intelligent Syst. Technol.* 2, 1–27. doi: 10.1145/1961189.1961199

Chen, X., and Ishwaran, H. (2012). Random forests for genomic data analysis. *Genomics* 99, 323–329. doi: 10.1016/j.ygeno.2012.04.003

Cheng, B., Liu, M., Zhang, D., Munsell, B. C., and Shen, D. (2015). Domain transfer learning for MCI conversion prediction. *IEEE Trans. Biomed. Eng.* 62, 1805–1817. doi: 10.1109/TBME.2015.2404809

Chetelat, G., Desgranges, B., Landeau, B., Mezenge, F., Poline, J. B., de la Sayette, V., et al. (2007). Direct voxel-based comparison between grey matter hypometabolism and atrophy in Alzheimer's disease. *Brain* 131, 60–71. doi: 10.1093/brain/awm288

Chiam, J. T. W., Dobson, R. J. B., Kiddle, S. J., and Sattlecker, M. (2014). Are blood-based protein biomarkers for Alzheimer's disease also involved in other brain disorders? A systematic review. *J. Alzheimers Dis.* 43, 303–314. doi: 10.3233/JAD-140816

Collij, L. E., Heeman, F., Kuijer, J. P. A., Ossenkoppele, R., Benedictus, M. R., Möller, C., et al. (2016). Application of machine learning to arterial spin labeling in mild cognitive impairment and Alzheimer disease. *Radiology* 281, 865–875. doi: 10.1148/radiol.2016152703

Cortes, C., and Vapnik, V. (1995). Support-vector networks. *Mach. Learn.* 20, 273–297. doi: 10.1007/BF00994018

Cui, Y., Liu, B., Luo, S., Zhen, X., Fan, M., Liu, T., et al. (2011). Identification of conversion from mild cognitive impairment to Alzheimer's disease using multivariate predictors. *PLoS ONE* 6:e21896. doi: 10.1371/journal.pone.0021896

Cuingnet, R., Gerardin, E., Tessieras, J., Auzias, G., Lehéricy, S., Habert, M.-O., et al. (2011). Automatic classification of patients with Alzheimer's disease from structural MRI: a comparison of ten methods using the ADNI database. *Neuroimage* 56, 766–781. doi: 10.1016/j.neuroimage.2010.06.013

Davatzikos, C., Bhatt, P., Shaw, L. M., Batmanghelich, K. N., and Trojanowski, J. Q. (2011). Prediction of MCI to AD conversion, via MRI, CSF biomarkers, and pattern classification. *Neurobiol. Aging* 32, 2322.e19–2322.e27. doi: 10.1016/j.neurobiolaging.2010.05.023

Davatzikos, C., Fan, Y., Wu, X., Shen, D., and Resnick, S. M. (2008). Detection of prodromal Alzheimer's disease via pattern classification of magnetic resonance imaging. *Neurobiol. Aging* 29, 514–523. doi: 10.1016/j.neurobiolaging.2006.11.010

De Leon, M. J., Mosconi, L., Blennow, K., Desanti, S., Zinkowski, R., Mehta, P. D., et al. (2007). Imaging and CSF studies in the preclinical diagnosis of Alzheimer's disease. *Ann. N. Y. Acad. Sci.* 1097, 114–145. doi: 10.1196/annals.1379.012

Dickerson, B. (2013). Biomarker-based prediction of progression in MCI: comparison of AD signature and hippocampal volume with spinal fluid amyloid-β and tau. *Front. Aging Neurosci.* 5:55. doi: 10.3389/fnagi.2013.00055

Dixon, R. A., DeCarlo, C. A., MacDonald, S. W. S., Vergote, D., Jhamandas, J., and Westaway, D. (2014). APOE and COMT polymorphisms are complementary biomarkers of status, stability, and transitions in normal aging and early mild cognitive impairment. *Front. Aging Neurosci.* 6:236. doi: 10.3389/fnagi.2014.00236

Elwood, R. W. (1991). The Wechsler memory scale revised: psychometric characteristics and clinical application. *Neuropsychol. Rev.* 2, 179–201. doi: 10.1007/BF01109053

Fan, L., Li, H., Zhuo, J., Zhang, Y., Wang, J., Chen, L., et al. (2016). The human brainnetome atlas: a new brain atlas based on connectional architecture. *Cereb. Cortex* 26, 3508–3526. doi: 10.1093/cercor/bhw157

Fan, Y., Resnick, S. M., Wu, X., and Davatzikos, C. (2008). Structural and functional biomarkers of prodromal Alzheimer's disease: a high-dimensional pattern classification study. *Neuroimage* 41, 277–285. doi: 10.1016/j.neuroimage.2008.02.043

Fjell, A. M., Walhovd, K. B., Fennema-Notestine, C., McEvoy, L. K., Hagler, D. J., Holland, D., et al. (2010). CSF biomarkers in prediction of cerebral and clinical change in mild cognitive impairment and Alzheimer's disease. *J. Neurosci.* 30, 2088–2101. doi: 10.1523/JNEUROSCI.3785-09.2010

Förster, S., Yousefi, B. H., Wester, H.-J., Klupp, E., Rominger, A., Förstl, H., et al. (2012). Quantitative longitudinal interrelationships between brain metabolism and amyloid deposition during a 2-year follow-up in patients with early Alzheimer's disease. *Eur. J. Nucl. Med. Mol. Imaging* 39, 1927–1936. doi: 10.1007/s00259-012-2230-9

Foster, N. L., Heidebrink, J. L., Clark, C. M., Jagust, W. J., Arnold, S. E., Barbas, N. R., et al. (2007). FDG-PET improves accuracy in distinguishing frontotemporal dementia and Alzheimer's disease. *Brain* 130, 2616–2635. doi: 10.1093/brain/awm177

Frölich, L., Peters, O., Lewczuk, P., Gruber, O., Teipel, S. J., Gertz, H. J., et al. (2017). Incremental value of biomarker combinations to predict progression of mild cognitive impairment to Alzheimer's dementia. *Alzheimers Res. Ther.* 9:84. doi: 10.1186/s13195-017-0301-7

Gatz, M., Reynolds, C. A., Fratiglioni, L., Johansson, B., Mortimer, J. A., Berg, S., et al. (2006). Role of genes and environments for explaining Alzheimer disease. *Arch. Gen. Psychiatry* 63, 168–174. doi: 10.1001/archpsyc.63.2.168

Geurts, P., Ernst, D., and Wehenkel, L. (2006). Extremely randomized trees. *Mach. Learn.* 63, 3–42. doi: 10.1007/s10994-006-6226-1

Greiner, M., Pfeiffer, D., and Smith, R. D. (2000). Principles and practical application of the receiver-operating characteristic analysis for diagnostic tests. *Prev. Vet. Med.* 45, 23–41. doi: 10.1016/S0167-5877(00)00115-X

Gupta, Y., Lee, K. H., Choi, K. Y., Lee, J. J., Kim, B. C., and Kwon, G.-R. (2019). Alzheimer's disease diagnosis based on cortical and subcortical features. *J. Healthc. Eng.* 2019, 1–13. doi: 10.1155/2019/2492719

Heister, D., Brewer, J. B., Magda, S., Blennow, K., McEvoy, L. K., and For the Alzheimer's Disease Neuroimaging Initiative (2011). Predicting MCI outcome with clinically available MRI and CSF biomarkers. *Neurology* 77, 1619–1628. doi: 10.1212/WNL.0b013e3182343314

Jack, C. R., Bennett, D. A., Blennow, K., Carrillo, M. C., Dunn, B., Haeberlein, S. B., et al. (2018). NIA-AA research framework: toward a biological definition of Alzheimer's disease. *Alzheimers Dement.* 14, 535–562. doi: 10.1016/j.jalz.2018.02.018

Jack, C. R., Bennett, D. A., Blennow, K., Carrillo, M. C., Feldman, H. H., Frisoni, G. B., et al. (2016). A/T/N: an unbiased descriptive classification scheme for Alzheimer disease biomarkers. *Neurology* 87, 539–547. doi: 10.1212/WNL.0000000000002923

Jack, C. R., Knopman, D. S., Jagust, W. J., Shaw, L. M., Aisen, P. S., Weiner, M. W., et al. (2010). Hypothetical model of dynamic biomarkers of the Alzheimer's pathological cascade. *Lancet Neurol.* 9, 119–128. doi: 10.1016/S1474-4422(09)70299-6

Jha, D., Kim, J.-I., and Kwon, G.-R. (2017). Diagnosis of Alzheimer's disease using dual-tree complex wavelet transform, PCA, and feed-forward neural network. *J. Healthc. Eng.* 2017, 1–13. doi: 10.1155/2017/9060124

Lama, R. K., Gwak, J., Park, J.-S., and Lee, S.-W. (2017). Diagnosis of Alzheimer's disease based on structural MRI images using a regularized extreme learning machine and PCA features. *J. Healthc. Eng.* 2017, 1–11. doi: 10.1155/2017/5485080

Li, Q., Wu, X., Xu, L., Chen, K., Yao, L., and Li, R. (2017). Multi-modal discriminative dictionary learning for Alzheimer's disease and mild cognitive impairment. *Comput. Methods Programs Biomed.* 150, 1–8. doi: 10.1016/j.cmpb.2017.07.003

Li, X., Morgan, P. S., Ashburner, J., Smith, J., and Rorden, C. (2016). The first step for neuroimaging data analysis: DICOM to NIfTI conversion. *J. Neurosci. Methods* 264, 47–56. doi: 10.1016/j.jneumeth.2016.03.001

Li, Y., Rinne, J. O., Mosconi, L., Pirraglia, E., Rusinek, H., DeSanti, S., et al. (2008). Regional analysis of FDG and PIB-PET images in normal aging, mild cognitive impairment, and Alzheimer's disease. *Eur. J. Nucl. Med. Mol. Imaging* 35, 2169–2181. doi: 10.1007/s00259-008-0833-y

Liu, K., Chen, K., Yao, L., and Guo, X. (2017). Prediction of mild cognitive impairment conversion using a combination of independent component analysis and the Cox model. *Front. Hum. Neurosci.* 11:33. doi: 10.3389/fnhum.2017.00033

Long, X., Chen, L., Jiang, C., and Zhang, L. (2017). Prediction and classification of Alzheimer disease based on quantification of MRI deformation. *PLoS ONE* 12:e0173372. doi: 10.1371/journal.pone.0173372

Luciano, M., Gow, A. J., Harris, S. E., Hayward, C., Allerhand, M., Starr, J. M., et al. (2009). Cognitive ability at age 11 and 70 years, information processing speed, and APOE variation: the Lothian Birth Cohort 1936 study. *Psychol. Aging* 24, 129–138. doi: 10.1037/a0014780

Madevska-Bogdanova, A., Nikolik, D., and Curfs, L. (2004). Probabilistic SVM outputs for pattern recognition using analytical geometry. *Neurocomputing* 62, 293–303. doi: 10.1016/j.neucom.2003.03.002

Minoshima, S., Giordani, B., Berent, S., Frey, K. A., Foster, N. L., and Kuhl, D. E. (1997). Metabolic reduction in the posterior cingulate cortex in very early Alzheimer's disease. *Ann. Neurol.* 42, 85–94. doi: 10.1002/ana.410420114

Modat, M., Ridgway, G. R., Taylor, Z. A., Lehmann, M., Barnes, J., Hawkes, D. J., et al. (2010). Fast free-form deformation using graphics processing units. *Comput. Methods Programs Biomed.* 98, 278–284. doi: 10.1016/j.cmpb.2009.09.002

Moosmann, F., Nowak, E., and Jurie, F. (2008). Randomized Clustering Forests for Image Classification. *IEEE Trans. Pattern Anal. Mach. Intell.* 30, 1632–1646. doi: 10.1109/TPAMI.2007.70822

Moradi, E., Pepe, A., Gaser, C., Huttunen, H., and Tohka, J. (2015). Machine learning framework for early MRI-based Alzheimer's conversion prediction in MCI subjects. *NeuroImage* 104, 398–412. doi: 10.1016/j.neuroimage.2014.10.002

Morris, J. C. (1993). The Clinical Dementia Rating (CDR): current version and scoring rules. *Neurology* 43, 2412–2412. doi: 10.1212/WNL.43.11.2412-a

Nozadi, S. H., Kadoury, S., The Alzheimer's Disease Neuroimaging Initiative (2018). Classification of Alzheimer's and MCI patients from semantically parcelled PET images: a comparison between AV45 and FDG-PET. *Int. J. Biomed. Imaging* 2018, 1–13. doi: 10.1155/2018/1247430

Pedregosa, F., Varoquaux, G., Gramfort, A., Michel, V., Thirion, B., Grisel, O., et al. (2011). Scikit-learn: machine learning in python. *J. Mach. Learn. Res.* 12, 2825–2830.

Ritter, K., Schumacher, J., Weygandt, M., Buchert, R., Allefeld, C., and Haynes, J.-D. (2015). Multimodal prediction of conversion to Alzheimer's disease based on incomplete biomarkers. *Alzheimers Dement.* 1, 206–215. doi: 10.1016/j.dadm.2015.01.006

Salvatore, C., Cerasa, A., Battista, P., Gilardi, M. C., Quattrone, A., and Castiglioni, I. (2015). Magnetic resonance imaging biomarkers for the early diagnosis of Alzheimer's disease: a machine learning approach. *Front. Neurosci.* 9:307. doi: 10.3389/fnins.2015.00307

Samper-González, J., Burgos, N., Bottani, S., Fontanella, S., Lu, P., Marcoux, A., et al. (2018). Reproducible evaluation of classification methods in Alzheimer's disease: framework and application to MRI and PET data. *Neuroimage* 183, 504–521. doi: 10.1016/j.neuroimage.2018.08.042

Sapkota, S., Bäckman, L., and Dixon, R. A. (2017). Executive function performance and change in aging is predicted by apolipoprotein E, intensified by catechol-O-methyltransferase and brain-derived neurotrophic factor, and moderated by age and lifestyle. *Neurobiol. Aging* 52, 81–89. doi: 10.1016/j.neurobiolaging.2016.12.022

Schouten, T. M., Koini, M., de Vos, F., Seiler, S., van der Grond, J., Lechner, A., et al. (2016). Combining anatomical, diffusion, and resting state functional magnetic resonance imaging for individual classification of mild and moderate Alzheimer's disease. *NeuroImage* 11, 46–51. doi: 10.1016/j.nicl.2016.01.002

Shaffer, J. L., Petrella, J. R., Sheldon, F. C., Choudhury, K. R., Calhoun, V. D., Coleman, R. E., et al. (2013). Predicting cognitive decline in subjects at risk for Alzheimer disease by using combined cerebrospinal fluid, MR imaging, and PET biomarkers. *Radiology* 266, 583–591. doi: 10.1148/radiol.12120010

Shaw, L. M., Vanderstichele, H., Knapik-Czajka, M., Clark, C. M., Aisen, P. S., Petersen, R. C., et al. (2009). Cerebrospinal fluid biomarker signature in Alzheimer's disease neuroimaging initiative subjects. *Ann. Neurol.* 65, 403–413. doi: 10.1002/ana.21610

Spampinato, M. V., Rumboldt, Z., Hosker, R. J., Mintzer, J. E., and Alzheimer's Disease Neuroimaging Initiative (2011). Apolipoprotein E and gray matter volume loss in patients with mild cognitive impairment and Alzheimer disease. *Radiology* 258, 843–852. doi: 10.1148/radiol.10100307

Suk, H.-I., Lee, S.-W., and Shen, D. (2014). Hierarchical feature representation and multimodal fusion with deep learning for AD/MCI diagnosis. *Neuroimage* 101, 569–582. doi: 10.1016/j.neuroimage.2014.06.077

Tustison, N. J., Avants, B. B., Cook, P. A., Zheng, Y., Egan, A., Yushkevich, P. A., et al. (2010). N4ITK: improved N3 bias correction. *IEEE Trans. Med. Imaging* 29, 1310–1320. doi: 10.1109/TMI.2010.2046908

Vemuri, P., Wiste, H. J., Weigand, S. D., Shaw, L. M., Trojanowski, J. Q., Weiner, M. W., et al. (2009). MRI and CSF biomarkers in normal, MCI, and AD subjects: diagnostic discrimination and cognitive correlations. *Neurology* 73, 287–293. doi: 10.1212/WNL.0b013e3181af79e5

Walhovd, K. B., Fjell, A. M., Brewer, J., McEvoy, L. K., Fennema-Notestine, C., Hagler, D. J., et al. (2010). Combining MR imaging, positron-emission tomography, and CSF biomarkers in the diagnosis and prognosis of Alzheimer disease. *Am. J. Neuroradiol.* 31, 347–354. doi: 10.3174/ajnr.A1809

Young, J., Modat, M., Cardoso, M. J., Mendelson, A., Cash, D., and Ourselin, S. (2013). Accurate multimodal probabilistic prediction of conversion to Alzheimer's disease in patients with mild cognitive impairment. *Neuroimage.* 2, 735–745. doi: 10.1016/j.nicl.2013.05.004

Zetterberg, H., and Burnham, S. C. (2019). Blood-based molecular biomarkers for Alzheimer's disease. *Mol. Brain* 12:26. doi: 10.1186/s13041-019-0448-1

Zhang, D., Shen, D., and Alzheimer's Disease Neuroimaging Initiative (2012). Predicting future clinical changes of MCI patients using longitudinal and multimodal biomarkers. *PLoS ONE* 7:e33182. doi: 10.1371/journal.pone.0033182

Zhang, D., Wang, Y., Zhou, L., Yuan, H., and Shen, D. (2011). Multimodal classification of Alzheimer's disease and mild cognitive impairment. *Neuroimage* 55, 856–867. doi: 10.1016/j.neuroimage.2011.01.008

6

Alcoholism Identification Based on an AlexNet Transfer Learning Model

Shui-Hua Wang [1,2,3†]*, Shipeng Xie* [4†]*, Xianqing Chen* [5†]*, David S. Guttery* [3†]*,*
Chaosheng Tang [1*]*, Junding Sun* [1*] *and Yu-Dong Zhang* [1,3,6*†]

[1] *School of Computer Science and Technology, Henan Polytechnic University, Jiaozuo, China,* [2] *School of Architecture Building and Civil Engineering, Loughborough University, Loughborough, United Kingdom,* [3] *Department of Informatics, University of Leicester, Leicester, United Kingdom,* [4] *College of Telecommunications and Information Engineering, Nanjing University of Posts and Telecommunications, Nanjing, China,* [5] *Department of Electrical Engineering, College of Engineering, Zhejiang Normal University, Jinhua, China,* [6] *Guangxi Key Laboratory of Manufacturing System and Advanced Manufacturing Technology, Guilin, China*

***Correspondence:**
Chaosheng Tang
tcs@hpu.edu.cn
Junding Sun
sunjd@hpu.edu.cn
Yu-Dong Zhang
yudongzhang@ieee.org

[†] *These authors have contributed equally to this work*

Aim: This paper proposes a novel alcoholism identification approach that can assist radiologists in patient diagnosis.

Method: AlexNet was used as the basic transfer learning model. The global learning rate was small, at 10^{-4}, and the iteration epoch number was at 10. The learning rate factor of replaced layers was 10 times larger than that of the transferred layers. We tested five different replacement configurations of transfer learning.

Results: The experiment shows that the best performance was achieved by replacing the final fully connected layer. Our method yielded a sensitivity of 97.44%$\pm$ 1.15%, a specificity of 97.41 $\pm$ 1.51%, a precision of 97.34 $\pm$ 1.49%, an accuracy of 97.42 $\pm$ 0.95%, and an F1 score of 97.37 $\pm$ 0.97% on the test set.

Conclusion: This method can assist radiologists in their routine alcoholism screening of brain magnetic resonance images.

Keywords: alcoholism, transfer learning, AlexNet, data augmentation, convolutional neural network, dropout, local response normalization, magnetic resonance imaging

INTRODUCTION

Alcoholism (1) was previously composed of two types: alcohol abuse and alcohol dependence. According to current terminology, alcoholism differs from "harmful drinking" (2), which is an occasional pattern of drinking that contributes to increasing levels of alcohol-related ill-health. Today, it is defined depending on more than one of the following conditions: alcohol is strongly desired, usage results in social problems, drinking large amounts over a long time period, difficulty in reducing alcohol consumption, and usage resulting in non-fulfillment of everyday responsibilities.

Alcoholism affects all parts of the body, but it particularly affects the brain. The size of gray matter and white matter of alcoholism subjects are less than age-matched controls (3), and this shrinkage can be observed using magnetic resonance imaging (MRI). However, neuroradiological diagnosis using MR images is a laborious process, and it is difficult to detect minor alterations in the brain of alcoholic patient. Therefore, development of a computer vision-based automatic smart alcoholism identification program is highly desirable to assist doctors in making a diagnosis.

Within the last decade, studies have developed several promising alcoholism detection methods. Hou (4) put forward a novel algorithm called predator-prey adaptive-inertia chaotic particle swarm optimization (PAC-PSO), and applied it to identify alcoholism in MR brain images. Lima (5) proposed to use Haar wavelet transform (HWT) to extract features from brain images, and the authors used HWT to detect alcoholic patients. Macdonald (6) developed a logistic regression (LR) system. Qian (7) employed the cat swarm optimization (CSO) and obtained excellent results in the diagnosis of alcoholism. Han (8) used wavelet Renyi entropy (WRE) to generate a new biomarker; whereas Chen (9) used a support vector machine, which was trained using a genetic algorithm (SVM-GA) approach. Jenitta and Ravindran (10) proposed a local mesh vector co-occurrence pattern (LMCoP) feature for assisting diagnosis.

Recently, deep learning has attracted attention in many computer vision fields, e.g., synthesizing visual speech (11), liver cancer detection (12), brain abnormality detection (13), etc. As a result, studies are now focused on using deep learning techniques for alcoholism detection. Compared to manual feature extraction methods (14–18), deep learning can "learn" the features of alcoholism. For example, Lv (19) established a deep convolutional neural network (CNN) containing seven layers. Their experiments found that their model obtained promising results, and the stochastic pooling provided better performance than max pooling and average pooling. Moreover, Sangaiah (20) developed a ten-layer deep artificial neural network (i.e., three fully-connected layers and seven conv layers), which integrated advanced techniques, such as dropout and batch normalization, into their neural network.

Transfer learning (TL) is a new pattern recognition problem-solver (21–23). TL attempts to transfer knowledge learned using one or more source tasks (e.g., ImageNet dataset) and uses it to improve learning in a related target task (24). In perspective of realistic implementation, the advantages of TL compared to plain deep learning are: (i) TL uses a pretrained model as a starting point; (ii) fine-tuning a pretrained model is usually easier and faster than training a randomly-initialized deep neural network.

The contribution of this paper is that we may be the first to apply transfer learning in this field of alcoholism identification. We used AlexNet as the basic transfer learning model and tested different transfer configurations. Further, the experiments showed that the performance (sensitivity, specificity, precision, accuracy, and F1 score) of our model is >97%, which is superior to state-of-the-art approaches. We also validated the effectiveness of using data augmentation which further improves the performance of our model.

DATA PREPROCESSING

Datasets

This study was approved by the ethical committee of Henan Polytechnic University. Three hundred seventy-nine slices were obtained in which there are 188 alcoholic brain images and 191 non-alcoholic brain images. We divided the dataset into three parts: a training set containing 80 alcoholic brain images and 80 non-alcoholic brain images; A validation set containing 30 alcoholic brain images and 30 non-alcoholic brain images; a test set containing 78 alcoholic brain images and 81 non-alcoholic brain images. The division is shown in **Table 1**.

TABLE 1 | Dataset division into training, validation, and test sets.

	Alcoholic	Non-alcoholic	Total
Training	80	80	160
Validation	30	30	60
Test	78	81	159
Total	188	191	379

TABLE 2 | Data augmentation.

	Alcoholic	Non-alcoholic	Total
Original Image	80	80	160
DA_I: Noise Injection	2,400	2,400	4,800
DA_II: Scaling	2,400	2,400	4,800
DA_III: Random Translation	2,400	2,400	4,800
DA_IV: Image Rotation	2,400	2,400	4,800
DA_V: Gamma Correction	2,400	2,400	4,800
Horizontal-flipped Image	80	80	160
DA_I: Noise Injection	2,400	2,400	4,800
DA_II: Scaling	2,400	2,400	4,800
DA_III: Random Translation	2,400	2,400	4,800
DA_IV: Image Rotation	2,400	2,400	4,800
DA_V: Gamma Correction	2,400	2,400	4,800
New Training Data	24,160	24,160	48,320

Data Augmentation

To improve the performance of deep learning, data augmentation (DA) (25) was introduced. This was done because our deep neural network model has many parameters, so we needed to show that our model contains a proportional amount of sample images to achieve optimal performance. For each original image, we generated a horizontally flipped image. Then, for both original and horizontal-flipped images, we applied the following five DA techniques: (i) noise injection, (ii) scaling, (iii) random translation, (iv) image rotation, and (v) gamma correction. Each of those methods produced 30 new images.

Gaussian noise with zero-mean and variance of 0.01 was applied to every image. Scaling was used with a scaling factor of 0.7–1.3, with an increase of 0.02. Random translation was utilized with a random shift within [−40 40] pixels. Image rotation with rotation angle varies from -30° to 30° and a step of 2° was employed. Gamma correction with gamma value varies from 0.4 to 1.6 with a step of 0.04 was utilized.

The DA result is shown in **Table 2**. Each image generated $(1+30*5)*2 = 302$ images including itself. After DA, the training set had 24,160 alcoholism brain images and 24,160 healthy brain images. Altogether, the new training set consisted of a balanced $160*320 = 48,320$ samples.

METHODOLOGY

Fundamentals of Transfer Learning

The core knowledge of transfer learning (TL) is shown in **Figure 1**. The core is to use a relatively complex and successful pre-trained model, trained from a large data source, e.g.,

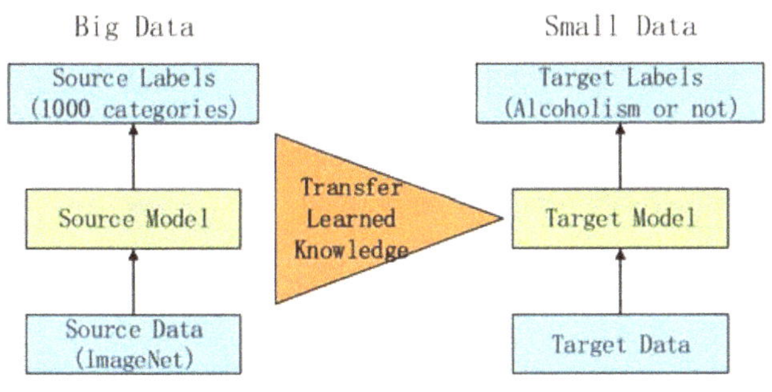

FIGURE 1 | Idea of transfer learning.

ImageNet, which is the large visual database developed for visual object recognition research (26). It contains more than 14,000,000 hand-annotated images and at least one million images are provided with bounding boxes. ImageNet contains more than 20,000 categories (27). Usually, pretrained models are trained on a subset of ImageNet with 1,000 categories. Then we "transferred" the learnt knowledge to the relatively simplified tasks (e.g., classifying alcoholism and non-alcoholism in this study) with a small amount of private data.

Two attributes are important to help the transfer (28): (i) The success of the pretrained model can promote the exclusion of user intervention with the boring hyper-parameter tuning of new tasks; (ii) The early layers in pretrained models can be determined as feature extractors that help to extract low-level features, such as edges, tints, shades, and textures.

Traditional TL only retrains the new layers (29). In this study, we initially used the pretrained model, and then re-trained the whole structure of the neural network. Importantly, the global learning rate is fixed, and the transferred layers will have a low factor, while newly-added layers will have a high factor.

AlexNet

AlexNet competed in the ImageNet challenge (30) in 2012, achieved a top-5 error of only 15.3%, more than 10.8% better than the result of the runner-up that used the shallow neural network. Original AlexNet was performed on two graphical processing units (GPUs). Nowadays, researchers tend to use only one GPU to implement AlexNet. **Figure 2** illustrates the structure of AlexNet. This study only counts layers associated with learnable weights. Hence, AlexNet contains five conv layers (CL) and three fully-connected layers (FCL), totaling eight layers.

The details of learnable weights and biases of AlexNet are shown in **Table 3**. The total weights and biases of AlexNet are 60,954,656 + 10,568 = 60,965,224. In Matlab, the variable is stored in single-float type, taking four bytes for each variable. Hence, in total we needed to allocate 233 MB.

Common Layers in AlexNet

Compared to traditional neural networks, there are several advanced techniques used in AlexNet. First, CLs contain a set of learnable filters. For example, the user has a 3D input with a size of $P_W \times P_H \times D$, a 3D filter with a size of $Q_W \times Q_H \times D$. As a consequence, the size of the output activation map is $S_W \times S_H$. The value of S_W and S_H can be obtained by

$$S_W = 1 + \frac{P_W - Q_W + 2\beta}{\mu} \tag{1}$$

$$S_H = 1 + \frac{P_H - Q_H + 2\beta}{\mu} \tag{2}$$

where μ is the stride size and β represents the margin. Commonly, there may be T filters. One filter will generate one 2D feature map, and T filters will yield an activation map with a size of $S_W \times S_H \times T$. An illustration of convolutional procedure is shown in **Figure 3**. The "feature learning" in the filters here, can be regarded as a replacement of the "feature extraction" in traditional machine learning.

Second, the rectified linear unit (ReLU) function was employed to replace the traditional sigmoid function $S(x)$ in terms of the activation function (31). The reason is because the sigmoid function may come across a gradient vanishing problem in deep neural network models.

$$S(x) = \frac{1}{1 + \exp(-x)} \tag{3}$$

Therefore, the ReLU was proposed and defined as follows:

$$\mathrm{Re\,LU}(x) = \max(0, x) \tag{4}$$

The gradient of ReLU is one at all times, when the input is larger than or equal to zero. Scholars have proven that the convergence speed of deep neural networks, with ReLU as the activation function, is 6x quicker than traditional activation functions. Therefore, the new ReLU function greatly accelerates the training procedure.

Third, a pooling operation is implemented with two advantages: (i) It can reduce the size of the feature map, and thus reduce the computation burden. (ii) It ensures that the representation becomes invariant to the small translation of the input. Map pooling (MP) is a common technique that chooses the maximum value among a 2 × 2 region of interest. **Figure 4** shows a toy example of MP, with a stride of 2 and kernel size of 2.

The fourth improvement is the "local response normalization (LRN)." Krizhevsky et al. (26) proposed the LRNs in order to aid generalization. Suppose that a_i represents a neuron computed by applying kernel i and ReLU non-linearity, then the response-normalized neuron b_i will be expressed as:

$$b_i = \frac{a_i}{\left(m + \alpha \sum_{s=\max(0,i-z/2)}^{\min(Z-1,i+z/2)} a_s^2\right)^{\beta}} \tag{5}$$

where z is the window channel size, controlling the number of channels used for normalization of each element, and Z is the gross number of kernels in that layer. Hyperparameters are set as: $\beta = 0.75$, $\alpha = 10^{-4}$, $m = 1$, and $z = 5$.

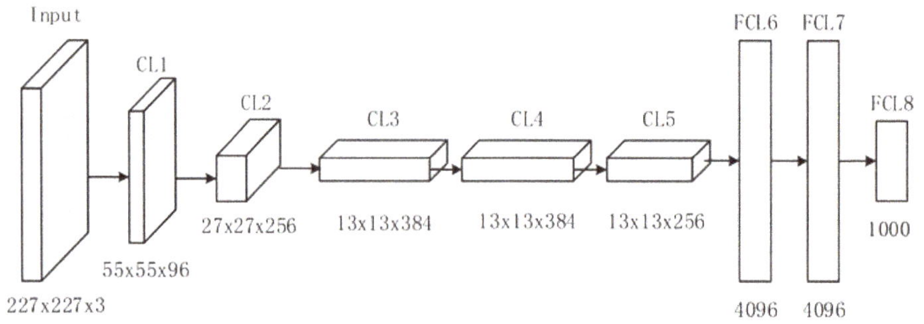

FIGURE 2 | Structure of AlexNet (5 CLs and 3 FCLs).

TABLE 3 | Learnable layers in AlexNet.

Name	Weights	Biases
CL1	11*11*3*96 = 34,848	1*1*96 = 96
CL2	5*5*48*256 = 307,200	1*1*256 = 256
CL3	3*3*256*384 = 884,736	1*1*384 = 384
CL4	3*3*192*384 = 663,552	1*1*384 = 384
CL5	3*3*192*256 = 442,368	1*1*256 = 256
FCL6	4096*9216 = 37,748,736	4096*1 = 4,096
FCL7	4096*4096 = 16,777,216	4096*1 = 4,096
FCL8	1000*4096 = 4,096,000	1000*1 = 1,000
CL Subtotal	2,332,704	1,376
FCL Subtotal	58,621,952	9,192
Total	60,954,656	10,568

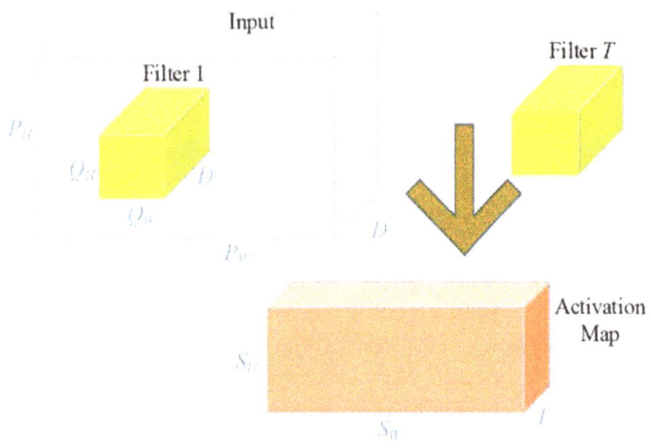

FIGURE 3 | Illustration of convolution operation.

Fifth, the fully connected layers (FCLs) have connections to all activations in the previous layer, so they can be modeled as multiplying the input by a weight matrix and then adds a bias vector. The last fully-connected layer includes the equal number of artificial neurons as the number of total classes *C*. Therefore, each neuron in the last FCL represents the score of that cognate class, as shown in **Figure 5**.

Sixth, the softmax layer (SL), utilizes the multiclass generalization of logistic regression (32), also known as softmax function. SL is commonly connected after the final FCL. From the perspective of the activation function, the sigmoid/ReLU function works on a single input single output mode, while the SL serves as a multiple input multiple output mode, as shown in **Figure 6**. A toy example can be imagined. Suppose we have a four input at the final SL layer with values of (1–4), then after a softmax layer, we have an output of [0.032, 0.087, 0.236, 0.643].

Suppose that $T(f)$ symbolizes the prior class probability of class f, and $T(h|f)$ means the conditional probability of sample h given class f. Then we can conclude that the likelihood of sample h belonging to class f is

$$T(f\,|h) = \frac{T(h\,|f) \times T(f)}{\sum_{i=1}^{F} T(h\,|i) \times T(i)} \tag{6}$$

Here F stands for the whole number of classes. Let Ω_f equals

$$\Omega_f = \ln\left[T(h,f) \times T(f)\right] \tag{7}$$

Afterwards, we get

$$T(f\,|h) = \frac{\exp\left(\Omega_f(h)\right)}{\sum_{i=1}^{F} \exp\left(\Omega_i(h)\right)} \tag{8}$$

Finally, a dropout technique is used, since training a big neural network is too expensive. Dropout freezes neurons at random with a dropout probability (P_D) of 0.5. During training phase, those dropped out neurons are not engaged in both a forward and backward pass. During the test phase, all neurons are used but with outputs multiplied by P_D of 0.5 (33).

It can be regarded as taking a geometric mean of predictive distributions, generated by exponentially-many small-size dropout neural networks. **Figure 7A** shows a plain neural network with numbers of neurons at each layer as (2, 4, 8, 10),

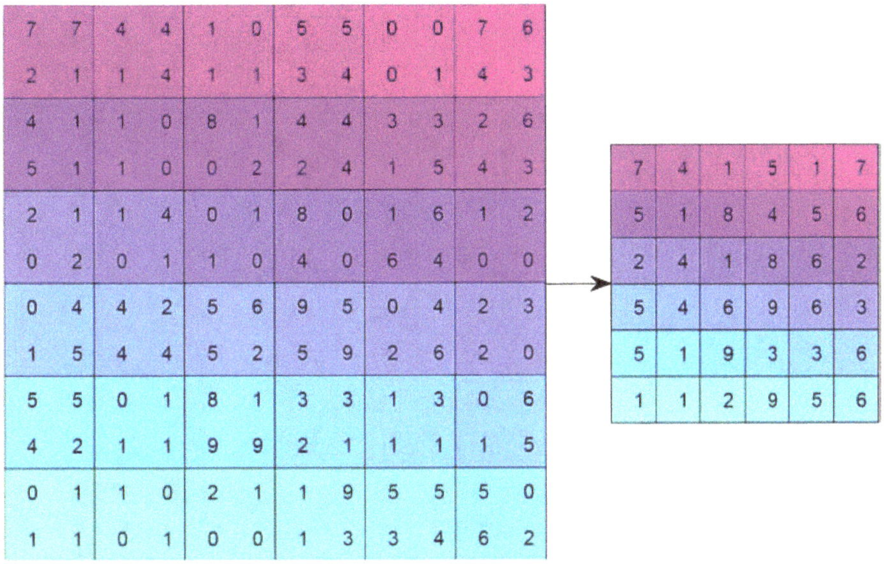

FIGURE 4 | Example of max pooling (stride = 2, kernels size = 2).

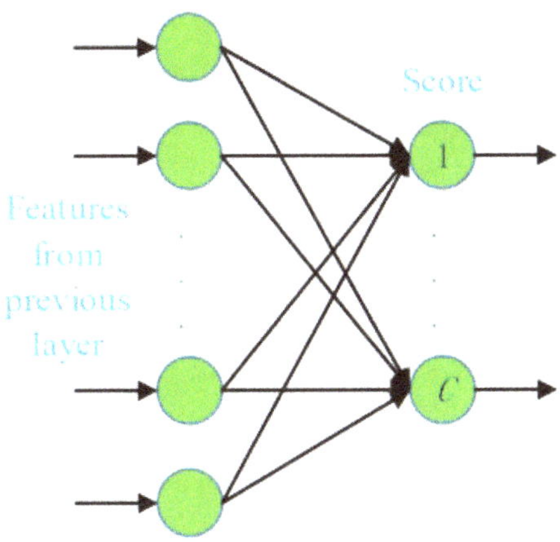

FIGURE 5 | Structure of last fully-connected layer (*C* stands for the number of total classes).

and **Figure 7B** shows the corresponding dropout neural network with P_D of 0.5, where only (1, 2, 4, 5) neurons remain active at each layer.

Transfer AlexNet to Alcoholism Identification

First, we needed to modify the structure. The last FCL was revised, since the original FCLs were developed to classify 1,000 categories. Twenty randomly selected classes were listed as: scale, barber chair, lorikeet, miniature poodle, Maltese dog, tabby, beer bottle, desktop computer, bow tie, trombone, crash helmet, cucumber, mailbox, pomegranate, Appenzeller, muzzle, snow leopard, mountain bike, padlock, diamondback. We observed that none of them are related to the brain image. Hence, we could not directly apply AlexNet as the feature extractor. Therefore, fine-tuning was necessary.

Since the length of output neurons in orthodox AlexNet (1000) is not equal to the number of classes in our task (2), we needed to revise the corresponding softmax layer and classification layer. The revision is shown in **Table 4**. In our transfer learning scheme, we used a new randomly-initialized fully connected layer with two neurons, a softmax layer, and a new classification layer with only two classes (alcoholism and non-alcoholism).

Next, we set the training options. Three subtleties were checked before training. First, the whole training epoch should be small for a transfer learning. In this study, we set the number of training epochs to 10. Second, the global learning rate was set to a small value of 10^{-4} to slow learning down, since the early parts of this neural network were pre-trained. Third, the learning rate of new layers were 10 times that of the transferred layer, since the transferred layers with pre-trained weights/biases and new layers were with random-initialized weights/biases.

Third, we varied the numbers of transferred layers and tested different settings. The AlexNet consists of five conv layers (CL1, CL2, CL3, CL4, and CL5) and three fully-connected layers (FCL6, FL7, FL8). As a result, we tested five different transfer learning settings as shown in **Figure 8** in total, in all experiments. For example, here Setting A means that the layers from the first layer to layer A are transferred directly with learning rate as $10^{-4} \times 1 = 10^{-4}$. The late layers from layer A to the last layer are randomly initialized with a learning rate of $10^{-4} \times 10 = 10^{-3}$.

Implementation and Measure

We ran the experiment many times. Each time, the training-validation-test division was set at random again. The training procedure stopped when either the algorithm reached maximum

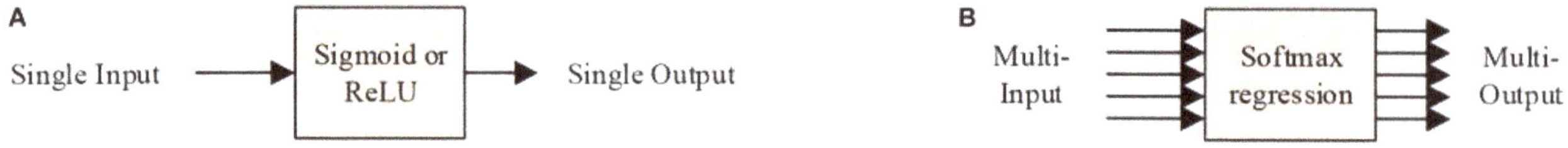

FIGURE 6 | Two modes of activation function. **(A)** Single input single output mode. **(B)** Multiple input multiple output mode.

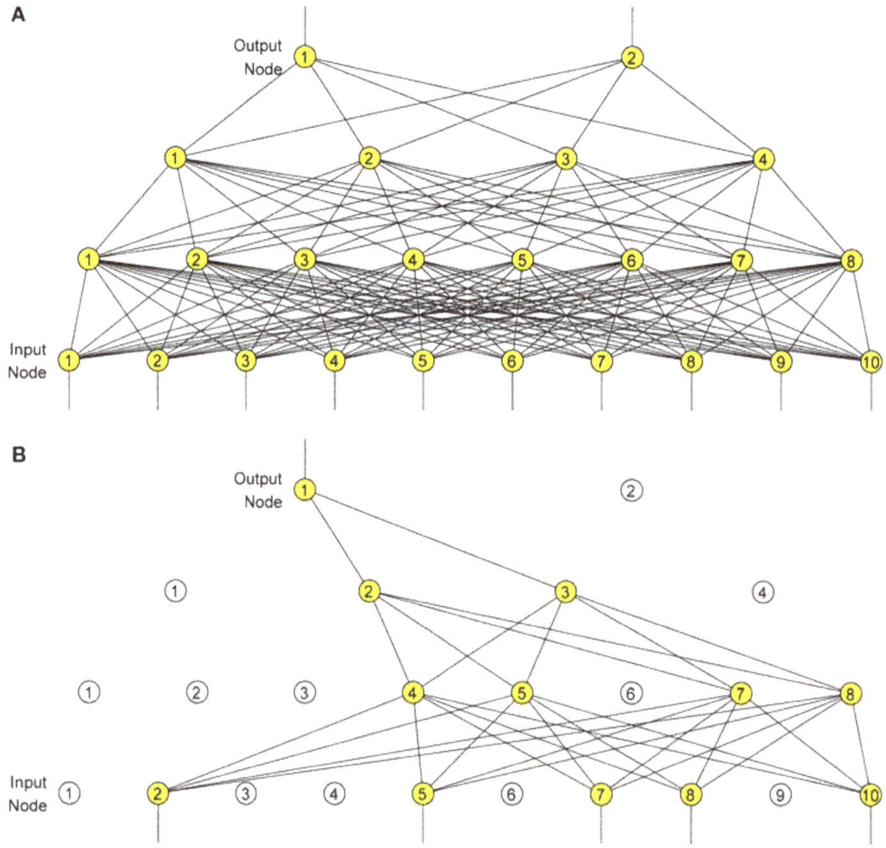

FIGURE 7 | Dropout neural network. **(A)** Before dropout. **(B)** After dropout.

TABLE 4 | Revision of Last three layers of AlexNet.

Layer	Original	Replaced
23	FCL (1000) with pre-trained weights and biases	FCL (2) with random initialization
24	Softmax Layer	Softmax Layer
25	Classification Layer (1,000 classes)	Classification Layer (two classes: alcoholism and non-alcoholism)

epoch, or the performance of validation decreased over a preset training epoch. We repeatedly tuned the hyperparameters and found those optimal hyper-parameters based on a validation set. After the hyperparameters were fixed, we ran the final model on the test set for 10 runs. The test set confusion matrix across all runs was recorded, and the following five measures were calculated: sensitivity (SEN), specificity (SPC), precision (PRC), accuracy (ACC), and F1 score. Assume TP, TN, FP, and FN stands for true positive, true negative, false positive, and false negative, respectively, all five measures were defined as:

$$SEN = \frac{TP}{TP + FN} \tag{9}$$

$$SPC = \frac{TN}{TN + FP} \tag{10}$$

$$PRC = \frac{TP}{TP + FP} \tag{11}$$

$$ACC = \frac{TP + TN}{TP + TN + FP + FN} \tag{12}$$

F_1 considers both the precision and the sensitivity to computer the score (34). That means, the measure of the "F1 score" is

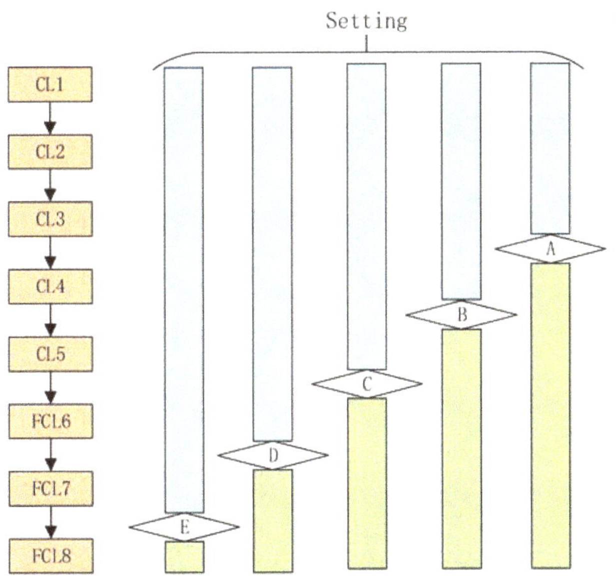

FIGURE 8 | Five different settings A-E (Setting A stands for the layers from first layer till layer A are transferred layers, and the remaining layers are replaced layers).

the harmonic mean of the previous two measures: precision and sensitivity.

$$F_1 = \left(\frac{SEN^{-1} + PRC^{-1}}{2} \right)^{-1} \tag{13}$$

Using simple mathematical knowledge, we can obtain:

$$\begin{aligned} F_1 &= 2/\left(\frac{TP+FN}{TP} + \frac{TP+FP}{TP} \right) \\ &= 2/\left(\frac{2TP+FP+FN}{TP} \right) \\ &= \frac{2 \times TP}{2 \times TP+FP+FN} \end{aligned} \tag{14}$$

Then, the average and standard deviation (SD) of all five measures of 10 runs of the test set were calculated and used for comparison. For ease of understanding, a pseudocode of our experiment is listed below in **Table 5**. The first block is to split the dataset into non-test and test sets. In the second block, the non-test set was split into training and validation randomly. The performance of the retrained AlexNet model was recorded and used to select the optimal transfer learning setting S*. In the final block, the performance on the test set via the retrained AlexNet using setting S* was recorded and outputted.

TABLE 5 | Pseudocode of our experiment.

```
[NonTest, Test]=split(Dataset);

for S = [A, B, C, D, E]
   for i = 1:10
      [train(i), valid(i)] = split(NonTest),
      Model(S, i) = TrainNetwork(AlexNet, train(i), valid(i), Setting = S),
      PerfValid(S, i) = Predict(Model(S, i), valid(i)),
   end
   PerfValid(S) = mean(PerfValid(S, i)),
End
S* = argmax[Performance(S)],
for i = 1:10
   [train(i), valid(i)] = split(NonTest),
   Model(S*, i) = TrainNetwork(AlexNet, train(i), valid(i), Setting = S*),
   PerfTest(S*, i) = predict(Model(S*, i), Test),
End
PerfTest(S*) = mean(PerfTest(S*, i)),
Output PerfTest(S*),
```

RESULTS

Data Augmentation Results

Figure 9 shows the horizontally flipped image. Here, vertical flipping was not carried out because it can be seen as a combination of horizontal flipping with 180-degree rotation.

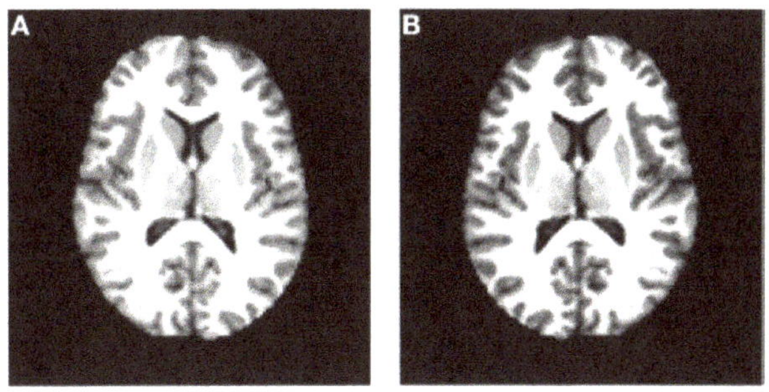

FIGURE 9 | Data augmentation by horizontal flipping. **(A)** Original image. **(B)** Flipped image.

Figure 10 shows the data augmentation results of five different techniques: (a) noise injection; (b) scaling; (c) random translation; (d) image rotation; (e) Gamma correction. Due to the page limit, the data augmentation results on the flipped image are not shown.

Comparison of Setting of TL

In this experiment, we compared five different TL settings on the validation set. The results of Setting A are shown in **Table 6**, where the last row shows the mean and standard deviation value. The results of Setting E are shown in **Table 7**. Due to page limit, we only show the final results of Setting B, C, and D in **Table 8**.

Here, it can be seen from **Table 8** that Setting E, i.e., replacing the FCL8, achieves the greatest performance among all five settings with respect to all measures. The reason may be (i) we expanded a relatively small dataset to a large training set using data augmentation; and (ii) the dissimilarity of our data and the original 1,000-category dataset. The first fact ensures that retraining avoids overfitting; and the latter fact

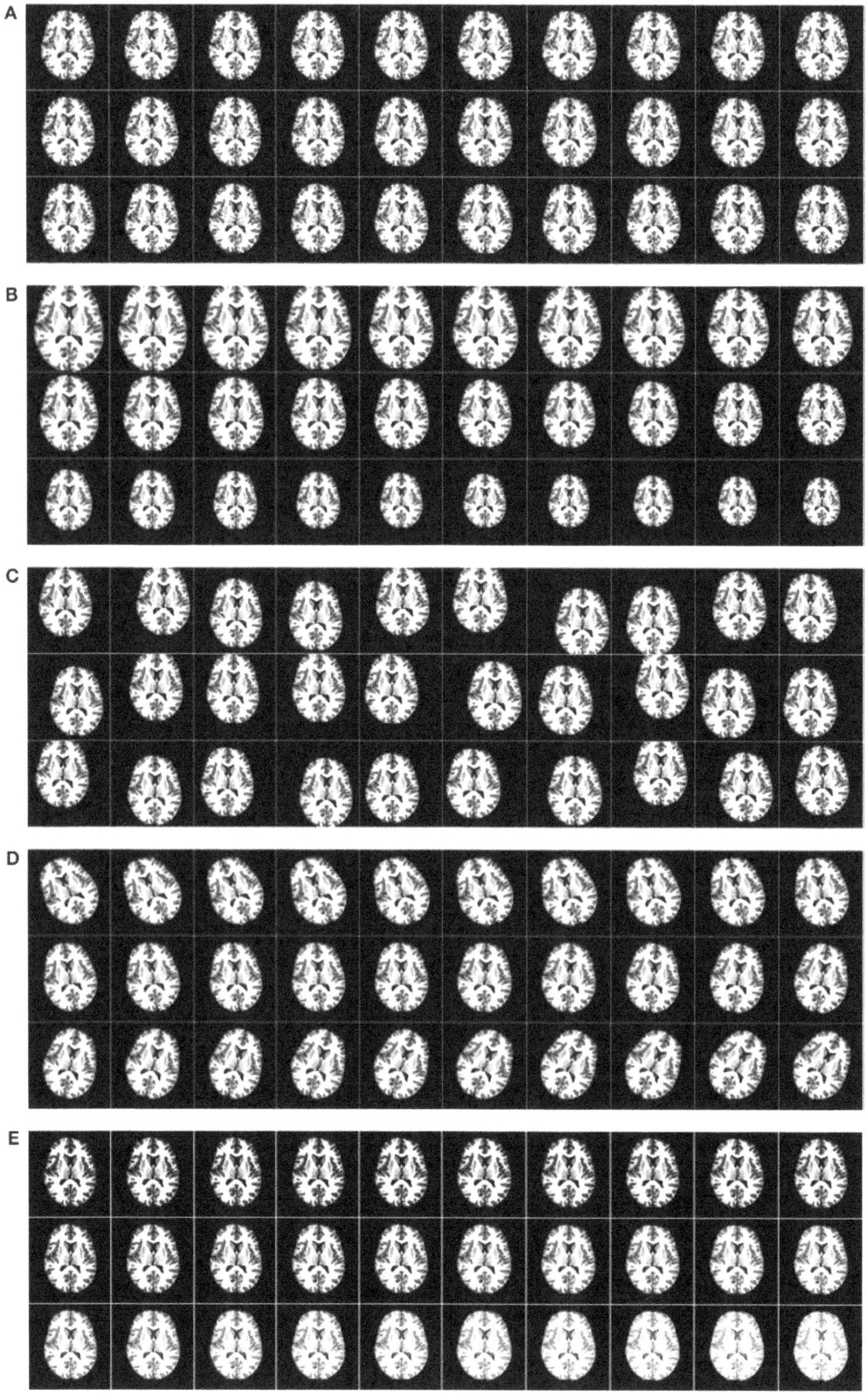

FIGURE 10 | Five augmentation techniques of the original image. **(A)** Noise injection. **(B)** Scaling. **(C)** Random translation. **(D)** Image rotation. **(E)** Gamma correction.

TABLE 6 | Ten runs of validation performance of transfer learning using Setting A.

Run	SEN	SPC	PRC	ACC	F1
1	96.67	93.33	93.54	95.00	95.05
2	100.00	100.00	100.00	100.00	100.00
3	90.00	100.00	100.00	95.00	94.70
4	96.67	90.00	90.63	93.33	93.55
5	90.00	96.67	96.43	93.33	93.10
6	96.67	96.67	96.67	96.67	96.67
7	96.67	96.67	96.88	96.67	96.66
8	96.67	100.00	100.00	98.33	98.28
9	100.00	90.00	90.99	95.00	95.26
10	96.67	93.33	93.54	95.00	95.05
Mean ± *SD*	96.00 ± 3.27	95.67 ± 3.67	95.87 ± 3.40	95.83 ± 2.01	95.83 ± 2.00

TABLE 7 | Ten runs of validation performance of transfer learning using Setting E.

Run	SEN	SPC	PRC	ACC	F1
1	93.33	100.00	100.00	96.67	96.55
2	100.00	96.67	96.88	98.33	98.39
3	100.00	100.00	100.00	100.00	100.00
4	100.00	100.00	100.00	100.00	100.00
5	93.33	93.33	93.33	93.33	93.33
6	96.67	100.00	100.00	98.33	98.28
7	100.00	100.00	100.00	100.00	100.00
8	96.67	93.33	93.54	95.00	95.05
9	96.67	93.33	93.54	95.00	95.05
10	100.00	100.00	100.00	100.00	100.00
Mean ± *SD*	97.67 ± 2.60	97.67 ± 3.00	97.73 ± 2.93	97.67 ± 2.38	97.67 ± 2.37

TABLE 8 | Comparison of different setting.

Setting	SEN	SPC	PRC	ACC	F1
A	96.00 ± 3.27	95.67 ± 3.67	95.87 ± 3.40	95.83 ± 2.01	95.83 ± 2.00
B	96.33 ± 3.79	96.00 ± 2.49	96.12 ± 2.43	96.17 ± 2.36	96.15 ± 2.43
C	96.33 ± 3.48	96.33 ± 3.14	96.49 ± 2.94	96.33 ± 2.08	96.33 ± 2.11
D	97.00 ± 3.79	97.00 ± 2.77	97.06 ± 2.70	97.00 ± 2.56	96.98 ± 2.62
E	**97.67 ± 2.60**	**97.67 ± 3.00**	**97.73 ± 2.93**	**97.67 ± 2.38**	**97.67 ± 2.37**

Bold means the best.

suggests that it is more practical to put most of the layers initialized with weights from a pretrained model, than freezing those layers. For clarity, we plotted the error bar and show it in **Figure 11**.

Analysis of Optimized TL Setting

The structure of the optimal transfer learning model (Setting E) is listed in **Table 9**. Compared to the traditional AlexNet model, the weights and biases of FCL8 were reduced from 4,096,000 to 8,192, and from 1,000 to 2, respectively. The main reason is that we only had two categories in our classification task. Thus, the whole weight of the deep neural network reduced slightly from 60,954,656 to 56,866,848.

Nevertheless, we can observe that FCL6 and FCL7 still constitutes too many weights and biases. For example, FCL6 occupied 37,748,736/56,866,848 = 66.38% of the total weights in this optimal model, and FCL7 occupied 16,777,216/56,866,848 = 29.50% of the total weights. Additionally, the FCL subtotal comprised 95.90% of the total weights. This is the main limitation of our method. To solve it, we need to replace the fully connected layers with 1 × 1 conv layers. Another solution is to choose small-size transfer learning models, such as SqueezeNet, ResNet, GoogleNet, etc.

Effect of Data Augmentation

This experiment compared the performance of runs with data augmentation against runs without data augmentation

(DA). Configuration of transfer learning was set to Setting E. All the other parameters and network structures were the same as the previous experiments. The performance of the 10 runs without using DA are shown in **Table 10**. The results in terms of all measures are equal to or slightly above 95%.

The comparison of using DA against not using DA is shown in **Table 11**. We can discern that DA indeed enhances the classification performance. The reason is that having a large dataset is crucial for good performance. The alcoholism image dataset is commonly of small size, and its size can be augmented to the order of tens of thousands (48,320 in this study). AlexNet can make full use of all its parameters with a big dataset. Without using DA, overfitting is likely to occur in the transferred model.

Results of Proposed Method

In this experiment, we chose Setting E (replace the final block) as shown in **Figure 8**. Here, the retrained neural network was tested on the test set. The results over all 10 runs on the test set are listed in **Table 12** with details of sensitivity, specificity, precision, accuracy, and the F1 score of each run. Setting E yielded a sensitivity of 97.44 ± 1.15%, a specificity of 97.41 ± 1.51%, a precision of 97.34 ± 1.49%, an accuracy of 97.42 ± 0.95%, and an F1 score of 97.37% ± 0.97%. Comparing **Table 12** with **Table 7**, we can see that the mean value of test performance is slightly worse than that of the validation performance, but the standard deviation of the test performance is much smaller than that of the validation performance.

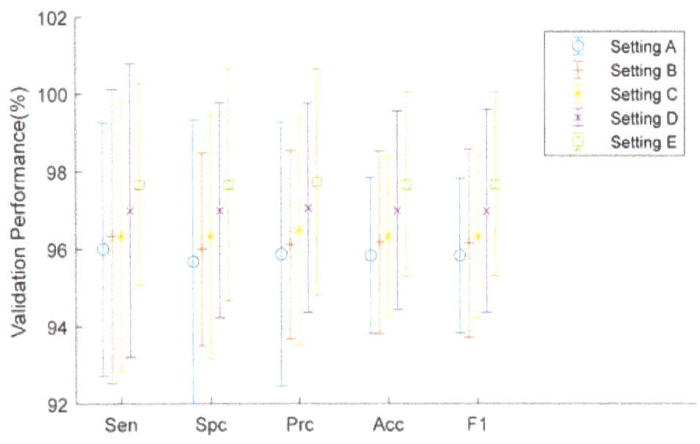

FIGURE 11 | Error bar of five TL settings.

Comparison to Alcoholism Identification Approaches

This proposed transfer learning approach was compared with seven state-of-the-art approaches: PAC-PSO (4), HWT (5), LR (6), CSO (7), WRE (8), SVM-GA (9), and LMCoP (10). The comparison results are shown in **Table 13**. The cognate bar plot is shown in **Figure 12**. We can observe that our AlexNet transfer learning model has more than 3% improvement compared to the next best approach.

The reason is that this proposed model did not need to find features manually; nevertheless, it only used a learned feature from a pretrained model as initialization, and utilized the enhanced training set to fine-tune those learned features. This has two advantages: First, the development is quite fast, which can be reduced to <1 day. Second, the features can be fine-tuned to be more appropriate to this alcoholism classification task than other manually-designated features.

The bioinspired-algorithm may help retraining our AlexNet model. Particle swarm optimization (PSO) (35–37) and other methods will be tested. Cloud computing (38) in particular can be integrated into our method, to help diagnosis of remote patients.

TABLE 9 | Learnable layers in optimal transfer learning model.

Name	Weights	Weights (%)	Biases	Biases (%)
CL1 (Ours)	11*11*3*96 = 34,848	0.06	1*1*96 = 96	1.00
CL2 (Ours)	5*5*48*256 = 307,200	0.54	1*1*256 = 256	2.68
CL3 (Ours)	3*3*256*384 = 884,736	1.56	1*1*384 = 384	4.01
CL4 (Ours)	3*3*192*384 = 663,552	1.17	1*1*384 = 384	4.01
CL5 (Ours)	3*3*192*256 = 442,368	0.78	1*1*256 = 256	2.68
FCL6 (Ours)	4096*9216 = 37,748,736	66.38	4096*1 = 4,096	42.80
FCL7 (Ours)	4096*4096 = 16,777,216	29.50	4096*1 = 4,096	42.80
FCL8 (AlexNet)	1000*4096 = 4,096,000		1000*1 = 1,000	
FCL8 (Ours)	2*4096 = 8,192	0.01	2*1 = 2	0.02
CL Subtotal (AlexNet)	2,332,704		1,376	
CL Subtotal (Ours)	2,332,704	4.10	1,376	14.38
FCL Subtotal (AlexNet)	58,621,952		9,192	
FCL Subtotal (Ours)	54,534,144	95.90	8,194	85.62
Total (AlexNet)	60,954,656		10,568	
Total (Ours)	56,866,848	100	9,570	100

TABLE 10 | Ten runs without using data augmentation (Setting E).

Run	SEN	SPC	PRC	ACC	F1
1	83.33	96.67	96.15	90.00	89.29
2	96.67	93.33	93.54	95.00	95.05
3	96.67	93.33	93.54	95.00	95.05
4	96.67	90.00	90.78	93.33	93.54
5	96.67	100.00	100.00	98.33	98.28
6	96.67	96.67	96.67	96.67	96.67
7	96.67	93.33	93.54	95.00	95.05
8	93.33	100.00	100.00	96.67	96.55
9	93.33	96.67	96.67	95.00	94.94
10	100.00	93.33	93.75	96.67	96.77
Mean ± *SD*	95.00 ± 4.28	95.33 ± 3.06	95.46 ± 2.84	95.17 ± 2.17	95.12 ± 2.32

TABLE 11 | Effect of using data augmentation technique.

DA	SEN	SPC	PRC	ACC	F1
Not use DA	95.00 ± 4.28	95.33 ± 3.06	95.46 ± 2.84	95.17 ± 2.17	95.12 ± 2.32
Use DA (ours)	97.67 ± 2.60	97.67 ± 3.00	97.73 ± 2.93	97.67 ± 2.38	97.67 ± 2.37

TABLE 12 | Ten runs of proposed method on the test set (Setting E).

Run	SEN	SPC	PRC	ACC	F1
1	97.44	96.31	96.22	96.86	96.82
2	98.72	93.81	93.93	96.23	96.25
3	94.87	96.31	96.09	95.61	95.47
4	97.44	98.75	98.72	98.11	98.07
5	98.72	98.75	98.72	98.73	98.72
6	98.72	97.53	97.47	98.11	98.09
7	97.44	98.78	98.72	98.12	98.07
8	97.44	98.75	98.75	98.12	98.05
9	96.15	97.53	97.40	96.84	96.74
10	97.44	97.53	97.44	97.48	97.44
Mean ± *SD*	97.44 ± 1.15	97.41 ± 1.51	97.34 ± 1.49	97.42 ± 0.95	97.37 ± 0.97

TABLE 13 | Comparison with state-of-the-art approaches.

Approach	SEN	SPC	PRC	ACC	F1
PAC-PSO (4)	90.67	91.33	91.28	91.00	90.97
HWT (5)	81.71	81.43	81.48	81.57	81.60
LR (6)	84.00	84.86	84.73	84.43	84.36
CSO (7)	91.84	92.40	91.92	92.13	91.88
WRE (8)	93.60	93.72	93.35	93.66	93.47
SVM-GA (9)	88.42	88.93	88.27	88.68	88.34
LMCoP (10)	89.04	90.00	89.35	89.53	89.19
AlexNet (Ours)	97.44	97.41	97.34	97.42	97.37

CONCLUSIONS

In this study, we proposed an AlexNet-based transfer learning method and applied it to the alcoholism identification task. This paper may be the first paper using transfer learning in the field of alcoholism identification. The results showed that this proposed approach achieved promising results with a sensitivity of 97.44 ± 1.15%, a specificity of 97.41 ± 1.51%, a precision of 97.34 ± 1.49%, an accuracy of 97.42 ± 0.95%, and an F1 score of 97.37 ± 0.97.

Future studies may include the following points: (i) other deeper transfer learning models, such as ResNet, DenseNet, GoogleNet, SqueezeNet, etc. should be tested; (ii) other data augmentation techniques should be attempted. Currently our dataset is small, so data augmentation may have a distinct effect on improving the performance; (iii) how to set the learning rate factor of each individual layer in the whole neural network, remains a challenge and needs to be solved; (iv) this method is ready to run on a larger dataset and can assist radiologists in their routine screening of brain MR images.

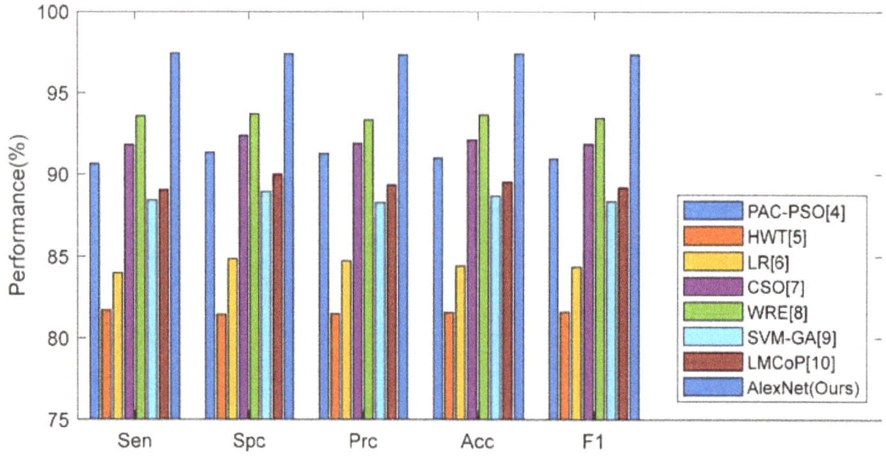

FIGURE 12 | Bar plot of comparison of eight algorithms.

AUTHOR CONTRIBUTIONS

S-HW and Y-DZ conceived the study. SX and XC designed the model. CT, JS, and DG analyzed the data. S-HW, XC, and Y-DZ acquired the preprocessed data. SX and CT wrote the draft. S-HW, CT, JS, and Y-DZ interpreted the results. DG provided English revision of this paper. All authors provided critical revision and consent for this submission.

FUNDING

The authors are grateful for the financial support of the Zhejiang Provincial Natural Science Foundation of China (LY17F010003, Y18F010018), the National key research and development plan (2017YFB1103202), the Open Fund of Guangxi Key Laboratory of Manufacturing System and Advanced Manufacturing Technology (17-259-05-011K), the Natural Science Foundation of China (61602250, U1711263, U1811264), and the Henan Key Research and Development Project (182102310629).

REFERENCES

Khaderi SA. Alcohol and alcoholism introduction. *Clinics in Liver Disease.* (2019) 23:1–2. doi: 10.1016/j.cld.2018.09.009

Bilevicius E, Single A, Rapinda KK, Bristow LA, Keough MT. Frequent solitary drinking mediates the associations between negative affect and harmful drinking in emerging adults. *Addict Behav.* (2018) 87:115–21. doi: 10.1016/j.addbeh.2018.06.026

González-Reimers E, Romero-Acevedo L, Espelosín-Ortega E, Martín-González MC, Quintero-Platt G, Abreu-González P, et al. Soluble klotho and brain atrophy in alcoholism. *Alcohol and Alcohol.* (2018) 53:503–10. doi: 10.1093/alcalc/agy037

Hou XX. Alcoholism detection by medical robots based on Hu moment invariants and predator-prey adaptive-inertia chaotic particle swarm optimization. *Comput Electric Eng.* (2017) 63:126–38. doi: 10.1016/j.compeleceng.2017.04.009

Lima D. Alcoholism detection in magnetic resonance imaging by Haar wavelet transform and back propagation neural network. *AIP Conf Proc.* (2018) 1955: 040012. doi: 10.1063/1.5033676

Macdonald F. Alcoholism detection via wavelet energy and logistic regression. *Adv Intell Syst Res.* (2018) 148:164–8. doi: 10.2991/icitme-18. 2018.33

Qian P. Cat Swarm Optimization applied to alcohol use disorder identification. *Multimedia Tools Appl.* (2018) 77:22875–96. doi: 10.1007/s11042-018-6003-8

Han L, Identification of Alcoholism based on wavelet Renyi entropy and three-segment encoded Jaya algorithm. *Complexity.* (2018) 2018:3198184. doi: 10.1155/2018/3198184

Chen, Y. Alcoholism detection by wavelet entropy and support vector machine trained by genetic algorithm. In: *27th IEEE International Conference on Robot and Human Interactive Communication (ROMAN).* Nanjing: IEEE. (2018). p. 770–5.

Jenitta A, Samson Ravindran R. Image retrieval based on local mesh vector co-occurrence pattern for medical diagnosis from MRI brain images. *J Med Syst.* (2017) 41:157. doi: 10.1007/s10916-017-0799-z

Thangthai A, Milner B, Taylor S. Synthesising visual speech using dynamic visemes and deep learning architectures. *Comput Speech Lang.* (2019) 55:101–19. doi: 10.1016/j.csl.2018.11.003

Das A, Acharya UR, Panda SS, Sabut S. Deep learning based liver cancer detection using watershed transform and Gaussian mixture model techniques. *Cogn Syst Res.* (2019) 54:165–75. doi: 10.1016/j.cogsys.2018.12.009

Talo M, Baloglu UB, Yildirim Ö, Acharya UR. Application of deep transfer learning for automated brain abnormality classification using MR images. *Cogn Syst Res.* (2019) 54:176–88.

Zeng N, Zhang H, Liu W, Liang J, Alsaadi FA. A switching delayed PSO optimized extreme learning machine for short-term load forecasting. *Neurocomputing.* (2017) 240:175–82. doi: 10.1016/j.neucom.2017.01.090

Zeng N, Zhang H, Li Y, Liang J, Dobaie AM. Denoising and deblurring gold immunochromatographic strip images via gradient projection algorithms. *Neurocomputing.* (2017) 247:165–72. doi: 10.1016/j.neucom.2017.03.056

Zeng N, Wang Z, Zhang H, Liu W, Alsaadi FE. Deep belief networks for quantitative analysis of a gold immunochromatographic strip. *Cogn Comput.* (2016) 8:684–92. doi: 10.1007/s12559-016-9404-x

Zeng N, Wang Z, Zhang H. Inferring nonlinear lateral flow immunoassay state-space models via an unscented Kalman filter. *Sci China Inform Sci.* (2016) 59:112204. doi: 10.1007/s11432-016-0280-9

Zeng N, Wang Z, Zineddin B, Li Y, Du M, Xiao L. et al. Image-based quantitative analysis of gold immunochromatographic strip via cellular neural network approach. *IEEE Trans Med Imaging.* (2014) 33:1129–36. doi: 10.1109/TMI.2014.2305394

Wang SH, Lv YD, Sui Y, Liu S, Wang SJ, Zhang YD. Alcoholism detection by data augmentation and convolutional neural network with stochastic pooling. *J Med Syst.* (2018) 42:2. doi: 10.1007/s10916-01 7-0845-x

Sangaiah AK. Alcoholism identification via convolutional neural network based on parametric ReLU, dropout, and batch normalization. *Neural Comput Appl.* (2019). doi: 10.1007/s00521-018-3924-0

Fahimi F, Zhang Z, Goh WB, Lee TS, Ang KK, Guan C. Inter-subject transfer learning with an end-to-end deep convolutional neural network for EEG-based BCI. *J Neural Eng.* (2019) 16:026007. doi: 10.1088/174 1-2552/aaf3f6

Comert Z, Kocamaz AF. Fetal hypoxia detection based on deep convolutional neural network with transfer learning approach. In: *Software Engineering and Algorithms in Intelligent Systems.* Silhavy R, editor. Cham: Springer International Publishing Ag (2019) p. 239–48.

Hussain M, Bird JJ, Faria DR. A study on CNN transfer learning for image classification. In: *Advances in Computational Intelligence Systems.* Lotfi A, Bouchachia H, Gegov A, Langensiepen C, McGinnity M, editors. Cham: Springer International Publishing Ag (2019) p. 191–202.

Soudani A, Barhoumi W. An image-based segmentation recommender using crowdsourcing and transfer learning for skin lesion extraction. *Exp Syst Appl.* (2019) 118:400–10. doi: 10.1016/j.eswa.2018.10.029

Ouchi T, Tabuse M. Effectiveness of data augmentation in automatic summarization system. In: Sugisaka M, Jia Y, Ito T, Lee JJ, editors. *International Conference on Artificial Life and Robotics (ICAROB).* Oita: Alife Robotics Co., Ltd. (2019). p. 177–80.

Krizhevsky A, Sutskever I, Hinton GE. ImageNet classification with deep convolutional neural networks. *Commun ACM.* (2017) 60:84–90. doi: 10.1145/3065386

Mishkin D, Sergievskiy N, Matas J. Systematic evaluation of convolution neural network advances on the Imagenet. *Comput Vis Image Understand.* (2017) 161:11–19. doi: 10.1016/j.cviu.2017.05.007

Serra E, Sharma A, Joaristi M, Korzh O. Unknown landscape identification with CNN transfer learning. In: *IEEE/ACM International Conference on Advances in Social Networks Analysis and Mining.* Barcelona: IEEE (2018). p. 813–20.

Kanuri SN, Navali SP, Ranganath SR, Pujari NV. Multi neural network model for product recognition and labelling. In: *7th International Conference on Computing, Communications and Informatics (ICACCI).* Bangalore: IEEE (2018) p. 1837–42.

Deng J, Dong W, Socher R, Li LJ. ImageNet: a large-scale hierarchical image database. In: *2009 IEEE Conference on Computer Vision and Pattern Recognition.* Miami, FL (2009). p. 248–55.

Godin F, Degrave J, Dambre J, De Neve W. Dual Rectified Linear Units (DReLUs): a replacement for tanh activation functions in quasi-recurrent neural networks. *Patt Recogn Lett.* (2018) 116:8–14. doi: 10.1016/j.patrec.2018.09.006

Tuske Z, Tahir MA, Schluter R, Ney H. Integrating gaussian mixtures into deep neural networks: softmax layer with hidden variables. In *International Conference on Acoustics, Speech, and Signal Processing.* Brisbane, QLD: IEEE (2015). p. 4285–9.

Poernomo A, Kang DK. Biased dropout and crossmap dropout: learning towards effective dropout regularization in convolutional neural network. *Neural Netw.* (2018) 104:60–7. doi: 10.1016/j.neunet.2018.03.016

AlBeladi AA, Muqaibel AH. Evaluating compressive sensing algorithms in through-the-wall radar via F1-score. *Int J Signal Imaging Syst Eng.* (2018) 11:164–71. doi: 10.1504/IJSISE.2018.093268

Zeng NY, Wang Z, Zhang H, Alsaadi FE. A novel switching delayed PSO algorithm for estimating unknown parameters of lateral flow immunoassay. *Cogn Comput.* (2016) 8:143–52. doi: 10.1007/s12559-016-9396-6

Zeng N, Zhang H, Chen Y, Chen B, Liu Y. Path planning for intelligent robot based on switching local evolutionary PSO algorithm. *Assembly Autom.* (2016) 36:120–6. doi: 10.1108/AA-10-2015-079

Zeng NY, You Y, Xie L, Zhang H, Ye L, Hong W, et al. A new imaged-based quantitative reader for the gold immunochromatographic assay. *Optik.* (2018) 152:92–9. doi: 10.1016/j.ijleo.2017.09.109

Aldossary M, Djemame K, Alzamil I, Kostopoulos A, Dimakis A, Agiatzidou E. Energy-aware cost prediction and pricing of virtual machines in cloud computing environments. *Fut Gen Comput Syst.* (2019) 93:442–59. doi: 10.1016/j.future.2018.10.027

7

Deep Learning Based Attenuation Correction of PET/MRI in Pediatric Brain Tumor Patients: Evaluation in a Clinical Setting

*Claes Nøhr Ladefoged, Lisbeth Marner, Amalie Hindsholm, Ian Law, Liselotte Højgaard and Flemming Littrup Andersen**

Department of Clinical Physiology, Nuclear Medicine and PET, Rigshospitalet, Copenhagen, Denmark

Correspondence:
Flemming Littrup Andersen
flemming.andersen@regionh.dk

Aim: Positron emission tomography (PET) imaging is a useful tool for assisting in correct differentiation of tumor progression from reactive changes. O-(2-18F-fluoroethyl)-L-tyrosine (FET)-PET in combination with MRI can add valuable information for clinical decision making. Acquiring FET-PET/MRI simultaneously allows for a one-stop-shop that limits the need for a second sedation or anesthesia as with PET and MRI in sequence. PET/MRI is challenged by lack of a direct measure of photon attenuation. Accepted solutions for attenuation correction (AC) might not be applicable to pediatrics. The aim of this study was to evaluate the use of the subject-specific MR-derived AC method RESOLUTE, modified to a pediatric cohort, against the performance of an MR-AC technique based on deep learning in a pediatric brain tumor cohort.

Methods: The modifications to RESOLUTE and the implementation of a deep learning method were performed using 79 pediatric patient examinations. We analyzed the 36 of these with active brain tumor area above 1 mL. We measured background (B), tumor mean and maximal activity (T_{MEAN}, T_{MAX}), biological tumor volume (BTV), and calculated the clinical metrics T_{MEAN}/B and T_{MAX}/B.

Results: Overall, we found both RESOLUTE and our DeepUTE methodologies to accurately reproduce the CT-AC clinical metrics. Regardless of age, both methods were able to obtain AC maps similar to the CT-AC, albeit with DeepUTE producing the most similar based on both quantitative metrics and visual inspection. In the patient-by-patient analysis DeepUTE was the only technique with all patients inside the predefined acceptable clinical limits. It also had a higher precision with relative %-difference to the reference CT-AC (T_{MAX}/B mean: −0.1%, CI: [−0.8%, 0.5%], $p = 0.54$) compared to RESOLUTE (T_{MAX}/B mean: 0.3%, CI: [−0.6%, 1.2%], $p = 0.67$) and DIXON-AC (T_{MAX}/B mean: 5.9%, CI: [4.5%, 7.4%], $p < 0.0001$).

Conclusion: Overall, we found DeepUTE to be the AC method that most robustly reproduced the CT-AC clinical metrics *per se*, closely followed by RESOLUTE modified to pediatric cohorts. The added accuracy due to better noise handling of DeepUTE, ease of use, as well as the improved runtime makes DeepUTE the method of choice for PET/MRI attenuation correction.

Keywords: pediatric, deep learning, PET/MRI, attenuation correction, brain tumors, bone density, RESOLUTE

INTRODUCTION

Positron emission tomography/Magnetic Resonance Imaging with the combination of MRI and radiolabeled amino acid analog tracers such as O-(2-18F-fluoroethyl)-L-tyrosine (FET) PET offer complimentary information when imaging cerebral brain tumors (Watanabe et al., 1992; Buchmann et al., 2016), especially when estimating the true tumor extent both in low- and high-grade gliomas (Kracht et al., 2004; Vander Borght et al., 2006). The combined information from the two modalities can help to discriminate post-operative changes or radiation damage from true tumor relapse presenting with a contrast-enhanced region (Mullins et al., 2005; Vander Borght et al., 2006; Galldiks et al., 2015a,b). The experience with FET-PET in pediatric and adolescent patients is limited, but it has been shown that FET-PET can add valuable information for clinical decision making (Dunkl et al., 2015). For pediatric patients, there is a clear advantage of acquiring FET-PET simultaneously with conventional MRI, as it offers a one-stop-shop examination, limiting the need for a second sedation or anesthesia as with PET and MRI in sequence, as well as improves co-registration (Henriksen et al., 2016). The advantage of a simultaneous PET/MRI comes with the challenge of accurate attenuation correction (AC) in order for the FET-PET images to be quantitatively correct (Vander Borght et al., 2006).

The initial shortcomings of the vendor-provided AC have been solved for examinations of adult brains without abnormal anatomy to a clinically acceptable precision (Ladefoged et al., 2016), whereas MR-based brain AC methods targeted toward pediatric subjects are scarce. Traditional atlas-based methods are likely to fail, since they are based on a database of adult subjects with normal anatomy (Spick et al., 2016). A database of pediatric age-matched subjects (Bezrukov et al., 2015) is difficult to obtain and might not be sufficient to model anatomical deformations following surgical intervention. An obvious alternative, the MR-based segmentation methods, is often challenged by the fact that traditional MR sequences are not able to distinguish bone and air due to the short relaxation time in bone. However, with special sequences such as ultra-short echo time (UTE) and zero echo time (ZTE), cortical bone can have a high signal despite its very short spin-spin relaxation time (Robson et al., 2003). Unfortunately, the use of these sequences is often hampered by incorrect representation of tissues at air/tissue interfaces (Ladefoged et al., 2015; Sekine et al., 2016) that needs to be specially addressed if a bias is to be avoided. We have recently introduced a PET/MRI-AC method, RESOLUTE (Ladefoged et al., 2015), that makes use of UTE images to calculate an attenuation map with continuous bone representation, and overcomes the air/tissue interface challenges by using anatomical regional masks defined on an aligned template in MNI space. Within these masks, possible bias from the bone surrogate signal is limited. We have shown that RESOLUTE led to the same clinical diagnosis as the reference CT-AC in a challenging cohort consisting of adult post-surgical brain tumor patients with severe anatomical deformations (Ladefoged et al., 2017). A prerequisite for successful application of RESOLUTE to pediatric cohorts is that these masks should be defined on pediatric templates.

Recently, deep learning using convolutional neural networks have demonstrated that they are able to handle complex signals, including noise, while maintaining a high level of accuracy (Han, 2017; Liu et al., 2017; Gong et al., 2018; Leynes et al., 2018). Using this technique, it could therefore be possible to limit the air/tissue interface noise without regional masks, thereby avoiding the need for any registration, as well as benefitting from the improved inference speed usually associated with deep learning. Several techniques using deep learning for MR-AC have been proposed (Han, 2017; Liu et al., 2017; Gong et al., 2018; Leynes et al., 2018), but none have been evaluated on a challenging cohort such as pediatrics.

The aim of this study was to modify the original RESOLUTE method to a pediatric cohort, and implement an MR-AC technique based on deep learning, that takes the UTE images as input and returns an attenuation map without any registration steps or need for regional masks. In a pediatric brain tumor cohort, we evaluated the attenuated FET-PET images of the modified RESOLUTE method, the proposed deep learning method and the vendor-provided DIXON-AC method using CT-AC as reference standard, with the methods evaluated regionally, as well as with metrics used clinically for diagnosis and follow-up examinations.

MATERIALS AND METHODS

Patients

We included children with suspected brain tumor examined with FET-PET using our PET/MRI system (Siemens Biograph mMR, Siemens Healthcare, Erlangen, Germany) (Delso et al., 2011) between February 2015 and October 2017, and 86 FET-PET examinations in total were identified of children under the age of 14. Seven examinations were removed due to missing or corrupt data, resulting in 79 scans used to develop the method (average age: 8 years, min: 2 months, maximum 14 years). For evaluation of the four AC-methods, we included patients with an active tumor area above 1 mL. Patients were part of a larger study of FET-PET/MRI in primary CNS tumors in children and adolescents approved by the regional ethical committee (ID: H-6-2014-095) and registered at clinicaltrials.gov (NCT03402425) and their parents gave written informed consent for participation.

Acquisition of CT

A reference low-dose CT image (120 kVp, 36 mAs, 74 slices, 0.6 mm × 0.6 mm × 3 mm voxels) of the head using a whole-body PET/CT system was used (Biograph TruePoint 40 and 64, Siemens Healthcare) (Jakoby et al., 2009). The CT images were acquired either on the same day as the PET/MRI examination, or at a previous PET/MRI+CT examination with no brain altering surgery in-between. The longest time for any patient between PET/MRI and low dose CT was 8 month.

Acquisition of MRI

The scan protocol included two vendor-provided AC methods: a two-point DIXON-VIBE AC sequence with repetition time (TR) 2,300 ms, echo time 1 (TE1) 1.23 ms, echo time 2 (TE2) 2.46 ms, flip angle 10°, coronal orientation, 19 s acquisition time, voxel size of 2.6 mm × 2.6 mm × 3.12 mm, and a UTE AC sequence with TR/TE1/TE2 = 11.94/0.07/2.46 ms, a flip angle of 10°, axial orientation, 100 s acquisition time, software version VB20P, field of view (FOV) of 300 mm^2, reconstructed on 192 × 192 × 192 matrices (1.6 mm × 1.6 mm × 1.6 mm voxels).

Acquisition of FET-PET

Patients were positioned head first with their arms down on the fully integrated PET/MRI system. Data were acquired for 40 min immediately following injection of 3 MBq/kg (86 ± 37) MBq FET (Langen et al., 2006) over a single bed position of 25.8 cm covering the head and neck. For the purpose of this study, the summed PET data 20–40 min after injection from the PET/MRI acquisition were reconstructed offline (E7tools, Siemens Medical Solutions, Knoxville, TN, United States) using 3D Ordinary Poisson-Ordered Subset Expectation Maximization (OP-OSEM) with 4 iterations, 21 subsets, zoom 2.5 and 5 mm Gaussian post-filtering on 344 × 344 matrices (0.8 × 0.8 × 2 mm^3 voxels) in line with the clinical protocol used at our institution. For all images, default random, scatter and dead time correction were applied.

Attenuation Correction Methods

Four methods for AC were applied to the data. First, the CT image was co-registered to the UTE TE2 image, and was used as our gold standard AC reference following conversion of Hounsfield Units as implemented on the Siemens PET/CT system. Second, vendor-provided MR-based attenuation map were derived using the DIXON VIBE sequence (Martinez-Möller et al., 2009). Third, our recently proposed AC method, RESOLUTE, was updated to process the pediatric cohort on two areas: (1) the regional masks were re-drawn on pediatric templates in MNI space (Fonov et al., 2011) spanning the ages: 0–2 m, <1 year, 1–2, 2–4, 4–8, 8–11, and 11–14 years, and (2) the R_2^*-CT bone mapping was calculated for the pediatric patients by the use of a sigmoid fit rather than a polynomial (Juttukonda et al., 2015). RESOLUTE was derived for each pediatric patient, where we used 2-fold cross validation to ensure that the mapping was not performed on the same patients used to recalibrate the mapping. Lastly, we implemented an MR-AC method based on deep learning convolutional neural networks, denoted DeepUTE. The network was based on a modified version of the U-net architecture (Ronneberger et al., 2015; Çiçek et al., 2016), where the max pool operations were replaced with convolutions with stride 2 (Springenberg et al., 2014), and each convolution, initialized using He normal initializer (He et al., 2015), is followed by a batch normalization, a rectified linear unit (ReLU) activation function, and a dropout layer with increasing fraction from 0.1–0.3 in the encoding part, and vice versa in the decoding part of the network (**Supplementary Figure 1**). The network takes as input 3D volumes consisting of 16 neighboring slices for each of the three UTE images, the echo images and the derived R_2*-map (16 slices × 192 voxels × 192 voxels × 3 channels), and outputs the corresponding CT slices (16 slices × 192 voxels × 192 voxels × 1 channel). We used the HU-converted co-registered CT image as our target. We trained the 3D-network in Keras (Chollet, 2015) with TensorFlow backend (Abadi et al., 2016) using the Adam optimizer (learning rate = 10^{-4}) (Kingma and Ba, 2014), mean-squared-error as loss function, batch size of 2 for 100 epochs. The 35 million parameters that were determined during the training process took 2 days on a Titan V (NVIDIA Corporation, Santa Clara, CA, United States) graphics processing unit. From our cohort of 79 scans, we did a 4-fold cross validation, effectively training 4 networks on approximately 60 scans and evaluation on the remaining. During testing, we predicted the 3D pseudo-CT volumes around each slice, and computed the average voxel value for each of the overlapping volumes.

Since the CT coverage were usually less than the PET/MRI coverage, we added the DIXON-AC attenuation map outside the CT field-of-view. This was also done for the subsequently generated RESOLUTE and DeepUTE attenuation maps to allow for a fair comparison to the reference.

Image Processing and Analysis

Image processing and analysis were performed similar to our previous analysis of adult post-operative brain tumor FET-PET patients (Ladefoged et al., 2017). First, a background (B) region of interest was delineated in healthy appearing gray and white matter at a level above the insula in the contralateral hemisphere to the tumor. The biological tumor volume (BTV) of FET-PET was measured using a 3D auto-contour using Mirada XD software (Mirada Medical, Oxford, United Kingdom) defining tumor tissue at a threshold above 1.6 of the mean standardized uptake value (SUV) in the background ROI (Floeth et al., 2005) for each AC method separately. Extratumoral areas with high FET uptake, e.g., vascular structures, pineal body and skin, were identified on either the T1w or FET-PET image and removed from evaluation. The delineation was performed by a nuclear medicine specialist experienced in pediatric neurooncology (LM).

We assessed the different AC methods ability to produce accurate FET-PET images on a patient-by-patient basis using the most commonly semi-quantitative clinical metrics in the diagnostic workflow. We measured the biological tumor volume (BTV), mean (T_{MEAN}) and max (T_{MAX}), and the ratios T_{MEAN}/B and T_{MAX}/B were calculated. For the BTV we analyzed the tumor contours relative to the CT-AC reference using the Jaccard similarity metric, and a measurement of shape deviations. The calculated ratios were compared to the ratios calculated with the reference CT-AC. These metrics are commonly used as a criterion to identify active tumor tissue from reactive changes. As described previously (Ladefoged et al., 2017), we defined acceptance criteria of < ± 0.05 and 0.1 or 5% for the T_{MEAN}/B and T_{MAX}/B ratios, respectively, and ± 2mL or 10% for the BTV. These were based on differences in clinical practice that may be considered clinically relevant in identifying biologically active tumor tissue or treatment related change in activity (Piroth et al., 2011). The mix of both an absolute and relative cut-off reflects that larger absolute change is acceptable in large or very active tumors. For each clinical metric we calculated the mean difference, 95% confidence intervals (CI) and limits of agreement on the log-transformed data, as the data was found to have log normal distribution. Exponentiation was applied to these results to express the differences as ratios on the original scale and report them as percentage differences. We corrected for repeated measurements from the repeated examinations (Bland and Altman, 1999).

RESULTS

A total of 28 patients met the inclusion criteria of 1 mL active tumor area, 6 of which had one or more follow up examination, resulting in a total of 36 examinations used for evaluation (**Supplementary Table 1**). Both RESOLUTE and DeepUTE were able to derive attenuation maps for all pediatric patients regardless of the age. Ten of the 28 patients (35%) had titanium implants present. Overall, DeepUTE had improved accuracy over RESOLUTE: the Jaccard index was 0.57/0.62 in air, 0.74/0.79 in soft tissue and 0.53/0.70 in bone tissue for RESOLUTE/DeepUTE, respectively. The improved accuracy was also apparent in a direct visual comparison of the estimation of regional attenuation values in the nasal cavities, the skull base and the mastoid processes, and can be appreciated in **Figure 1**, where two patients with challenging anatomy are shown for RESOLUTE-AC, DeepUTE-AC and CT-AC, and the relative difference PET image in **Supplementary Figure 2**. Another example of a typical patient is given in **Figure 2**. There was also a significant improvement in AC runtime with values of 4 s for DeepUTE and ~3 min for of RESOLUTE, which although small, improves the overall imaging workflow.

Across all pediatric patients, the Jaccard index of the tumor delineation was 0.73 ± 0.20 for DIXON-AC, 0.90 ± 0.07 for RESOLUTE and 0.92 ± 0.07 for DeepUTE. The tumor configuration did not change for any of the patients when using RESOLUTE or DeepUTE compared to CT-AC but for DIXON-AC this was found in 4 examinations (mean difference: 1.6 mL), and was completely missed for an additional examination (BTV with CT-AC: 2 mL).

The comparison of the clinical metrics can be seen in **Figure 3**, together with the defined acceptable limits. Across all metrics, using DeepUTE, none of the patients were outside the acceptable limits, whereas two patients fall short of the T_{MAX}/B limit and a single patient in the T_{MEAN}/B limit when using RESOLUTE. In these patients, the largest difference was T_{MAX}/B overestimation

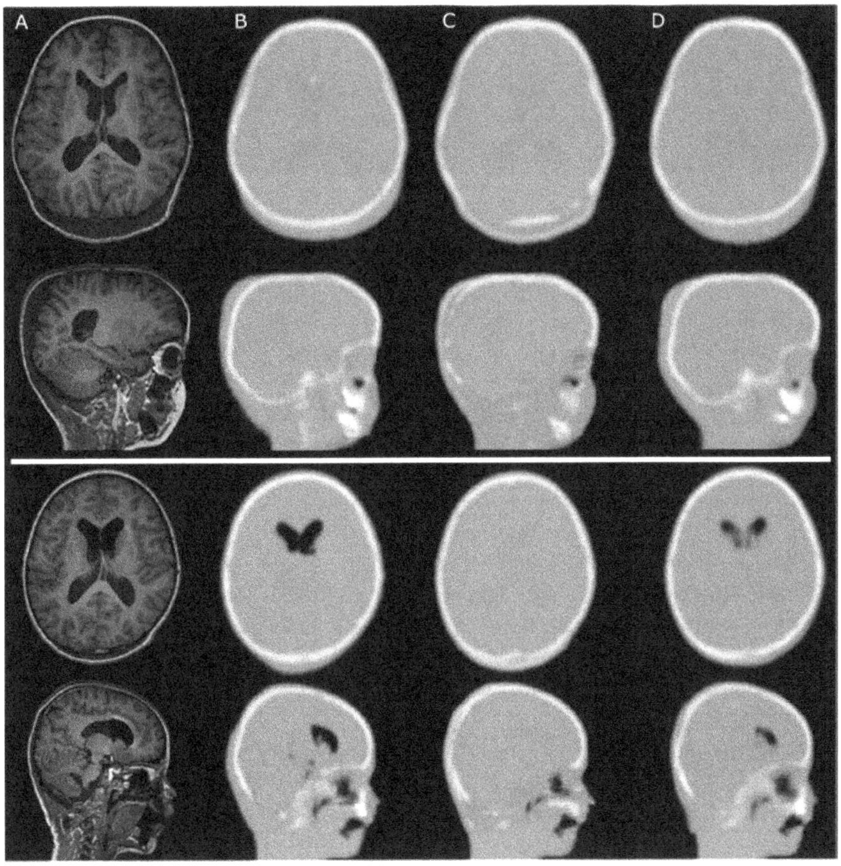

FIGURE 1 | Sample cases for two pediatric patients with irregular anatomy. **(A)** show the T1w MPRAGE, **(B)** CT-AC, **(C)** RESOLUTE-AC, and **(D)** DeepUTE-AC. The top rows show a 5-year-old patient with post-operative subcutaneous soft tissue swelling in the occipital region. RESOLUTE erroneously fills in a dual layer bone layer on both sides of the swelling, along skin and bone. The bottom rows show a 6-year-old patient with air pockets anteriorly in the lateral ventricles that appeared after surgical intervention, and are not imaged in RESOLUTE. Also in this case RESOLUTE crafts a dual layered skull in the occipital region. For both patients, RESOLUTE is challenged in the definition of facial and skull base attenuation value. DeepUTE captures the morphology more confidently.

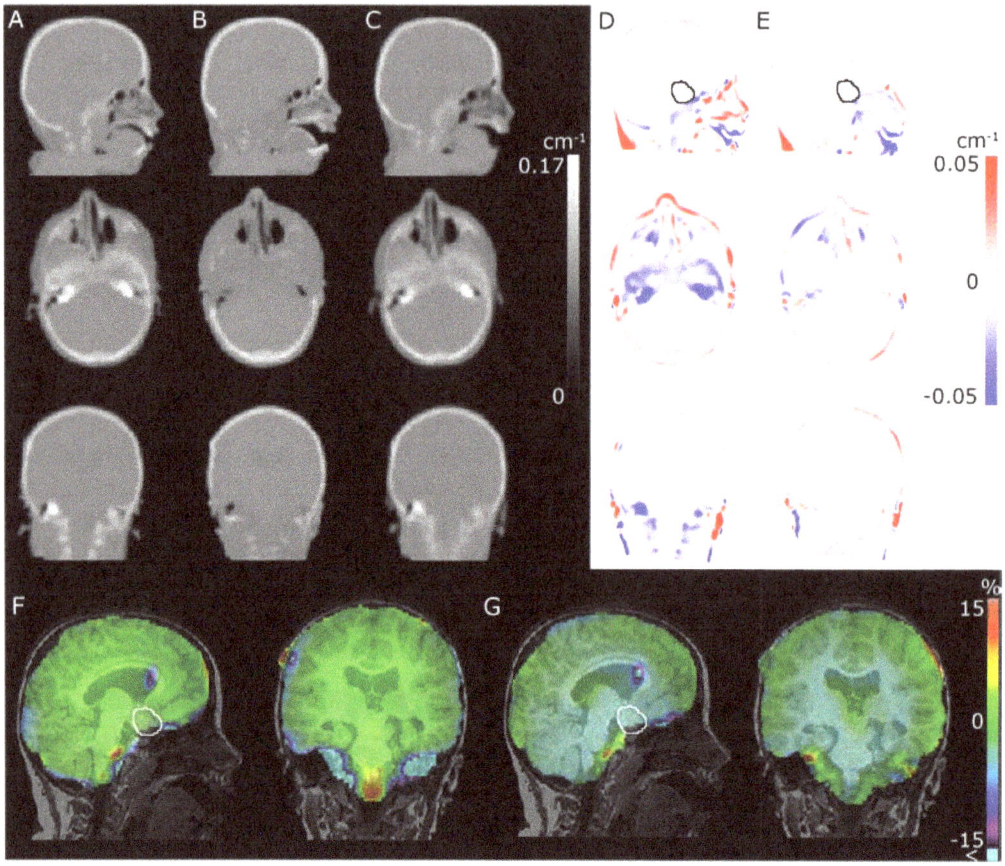

FIGURE 2 | Comparison of CT **(A)**, RESOLUTE **(B)**, and DeepUTE **(C)** attenuation maps in the sagittal, axial and coronal orientation, respectively. **(D,E)** shows **(B,C)** subtracted **(A)**, respectively, and **(F,G)** shows the resulting relative difference in the PET images between RESOLUTE and DeepUTE relative to CT-AC, respectively. The improved accuracy in the nasal cavities, the skull base and the mastoid processes, leads to a clear reduction of the errors in the surrounding regions, e.g., in the medulla. It also appears that, for this patient, a small underestimation of the densities within the brain in DeepUTE leads to a small underestimation globally within the brain. The tumor delineation is show on the sagittal view in **(D–G)**.

of 0.13 a.u. due to overestimated bone area in the skull base. In comparison, DIXON-AC gave a T_{MAX}/B difference over the acceptable limit in 23/36 (64%) examinations, and 13/36 (36%) examinations had changes to BTV over the acceptable limit.

The relative %-difference in the diagnostic measures was similar between RESOLUTE and DeepUTE, again with DeepUTE with the reduced error and variation (**Table 1**). BTV measured using DeepUTE was underestimated by 2% on average (95% CI: −5 to 1%) compared to −1% (95% CI: −5 to 4%) with RESOLUTE. None of the metrics had statistically significant differences compared to the reference CT-AC. In comparison, DIXON-AC had statistically significant differences in all three clinical metrics ($p < 0.001$).

DISCUSSION

Magnetic resonance imaging is the method of choice to diagnose brain tumor patients, but FET-PET can add valuable information for clinical decision making (Dunkl et al., 2015). Examining pediatric and adolescent patients on a hybrid PET/MRI can be preferred over PET/CT to reduce the number of examinations, which is especially relevant when anesthesia is required, and is important for both child and parents. A prerequisite for a confident clinical evaluation of the cohort with PET/MRI is an accurate AC. The skull shape, density, thickness, and composition change considerably during development in childhood especially the first three years after which the sutures and fontanelles gradually calcify and close (Li et al., 2015). Especially the rapid growth of skull thickness and bone density will highly influence attenuation leading to errors in atlas-based methods that cannot account for the thin, low-density infant cranium.

In designing the clinical study, we were acutely aware of these unresolved AC issues and choose to include a separate low-dose CT acquisition. This could be performed safely in all children, although it involved moving sensitive patients to a different scanner for additional radiation exposure and, for some children, extending anesthesia. This additional stress on the patients was regarded ethically acceptable so that future use of hybrid PET/MRI in pediatric brain tumors, which could be one of the most important applications, could be performed with the best possible assessment of risk to the patient caused by

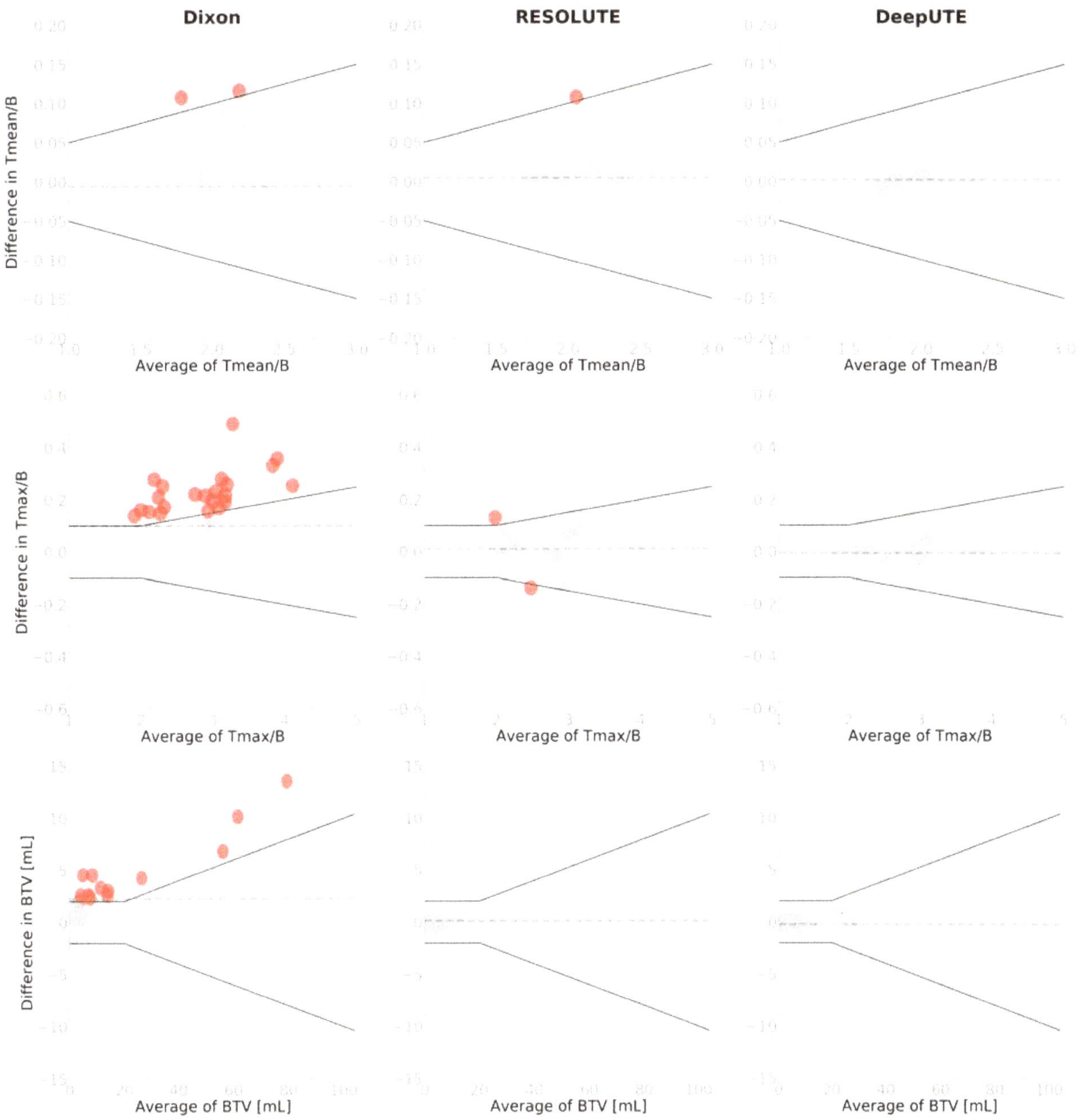

FIGURE 3 | Bland-Altman plot of T_{MEAN}/B (top), T_{MAX}/B (middle) and BTV (bottom) for the two AC-methods RESOLUTE and DeepUTE against the reference standard CT-AC. The black lines indicate the acceptance criteria of T_{MEAN}/B of ± 0.05 or 5%, T_{MAX}/B of ± 0.1 or 5%, and BTV of ± 2mL or 10%, respectively. Points that exceed the criteria have been colored. The age of the children exceeding the threshold using RESOLUTE are 7, 7, and 11 years, respectively. Note the difference on the axes. The dashed gray line indicates the mean value.

quantitative inaccuracies using accepted standard metrics within the field.

We modified the already thoroughly evaluated RESOLUTE method to be applied on pediatric patients, as well as introduced an MR-AC method based on a deep learning convolutional neural network, and also included DIXON-AC. The novelty of DeepUTE does not lie in the chosen type of architecture, but rather in the data that went into training the model. This manuscript is, to the best of our knowledge, the first of its kind to train a deep learning network for MR-AC purposes on a pediatric cohort of this size. The included patients in the evaluated cohort are well suited to test the method's ability to adapt to anatomy changes across different ages.

Pediatric patients are a challenging cohort to examine due to motion, often leading to sedation or anesthesia of the patients. The patients included in this study had, as expected, a larger amount of noise in the MR images than adult patients, leading to increased amount of noise in the bone surrogate signal. The

TABLE 1 | Summary of the relative %-difference* to the reference CT-AC of each clinical metric for the MR-AC methods.

Measured parameter values	Mean % difference			95% lower limits of agreement	95% upper limits of agreement
	Mean	95% CI	*p*		
DIXON-AC					
T_{MEAN}/B	2.2	1.5 to 2.8	< 0.001**	−1.6	6.0
T_{MAX}/B	5.9	4.5 to 7.4	< 0.001**	−2.2	14.7
BTV	32	21 to 45	< 0.001**	−22	124
RESOLUTE					
T_{MEAN}/B	0.2	−0.3 to 0.7	0.38	−2.6	3.1
T_{MAX}/B	0.3	−0.6 to 1.2	0.54	−4.9	5.8
BTV	−1	−5 to 4	0.77	−21	25
DeepUTE					
T_{MEAN}/B	−0.1	−0.2 to 0.5	0.38	−1.7	2.0
T_{MAX}/B	−0.1	−0.8 to 0.5	0.67	−3.7	3.6
BTV	−2	−5 to 1	0.15	−19	17

**Exponentiation was applied to results from analysis on log scale, and results were expressed as percentages. **Indicates a statistical significant ($p < 0.05$) found by a paired t-test. CI = 95% confidence interval for mean difference. BTV is measured in mL. A single examination without BTV with DIXON-AC was left out of this analysis.*

strength of the DeepUTE method is that it is able to robustly handle this noise, which the deep learning methods are known for. An example of the improved noise handling is evident in **Figure 1**, where DeepUTE better models both the thin bone and noise at the posterior part of the head.

Titanium alloy clamps, that were present in 33% of the patients to fix the craniotomy, showed up as small signal voids in the MR images with a size similar to the implants seen on CT. Visual reading showed that both RESOLUTE and DeepUTE filled the signal void with a density similar to dense bone, similar to what has previously been observed (Ladefoged et al., 2017). This meant that a valid attenuation map without artifacts could be calculated in all scans using RESOLUTE and DeepUTE.

Overall, we found both RESOLUTE and our DeepUTE methodology to accurately reproduce the CT-AC clinical metrics with similar accuracy as was seen for RESOLUTE when evaluating adult FET-PET brain tumor patients (Ladefoged et al., 2017). Regardless of age, both methods were able to obtain AC maps similar to the CT-AC, albeit with DeepUTE producing the most similar based on both quantitative metrics and visual inspection. In the patient-by-patient analysis, all patients were inside the predefined acceptable clinical limits with DeepUTE, where three patients (7–11 years old) were outside the limits in the T_{MAX}/B or T_{MEAN}/B metrics when using RESOLUTE (**Figure 3**). A similar result was obtained with RESOLUTE for the adult FET-PET brain tumor patients (Ladefoged et al., 2017) where 5/68 studies exceeded the predefined limit. The errors from RESOLUTE were due to an overestimation of bone density in known "problem" areas near the skull base, but none of the errors impacted the clinical reading of the images. In comparison, the same patients obtained with DeepUTE-AC had a higher precision in the skull base, leading to more accurate measurements. The confidence interval was narrower when using DeepUTE compared to RESOLUTE (**Table 1**). This indicates that there is a smaller variation of the errors in DeepUTE compared to RESOLUTE.

The processing in RESOLUTE was the same for all patients, except for the combination of the segmented tissue maps within regional masks, as these are different depending on the patient age. In DeepUTE, the same method was applied regardless of patient age. Further dividing the training patients into smaller groups depending on age might further reduce the variance, but requires more data, as training a deep learning network with too few patients leads to overfitting. We did not apply transfer learning in this study, as it has been shown that training a deep learning network using less than 30 patients is feasible (Han, 2017; Liu et al., 2017; Gong et al., 2018; Kläser et al., 2018; Leynes et al., 2018). However, using transfer learning, e.g., from a larger adult cohort might further improve the results presented here, as the low-level information are to be expected similar between the cohorts.

In software version VB20P on the Siemens mMR, two vendor-provided solutions for AC is available – DIXON-AC and UTE-AC, that both have been used in the published pediatric neuro-oncology PET/MRI literature (Garibotto et al., 2013; Preuss et al., 2014; Fraioli et al., 2015), however, encompassing only 6 and 12 patients, respectively. This small patient sample may reflect hesitation from the clinical community to use PET/MRI routinely in this difficult patient group because of the well-documented systematic underperformance of particularly DIXON-AC (Andersen et al., 2014; Ladefoged et al., 2017), which is also apparent from our study. DIXON-AC was the only vendor-provided method capable of producing attenuation maps for the full pediatric cohort. In four patients, UTE-AC was not able to produce an attenuation map of patients, aged 0–2 years, which is why we chose to exclude UTE-AC from the comparison.

In this study, we only had 6 patients with repeat examinations. We found that the change of T_{MEAN}/B, T_{MAX}/B and BTV between two examinations with RESOLUTE or DeepUTE were in congruence with the change when measured with CT-AC, as none of the differences were outside the acceptable limit. A larger number of repeat examinations should confirm this.

Limitations

We did not have pediatric data available after the software upgrade to VE11P, which adds a model-based AC method (Paulus et al., 2015; Koesters et al., 2016), but we speculate that the method would be unsuccessful for the younger pediatric cohort since the method was developed for adults.

Both RESOLUTE and DeepUTE are based on the UTE sequence, so while we expect DeepUTE to be directly transferable to any Siemens mMR, which is the case for RESOLUTE, neither method is able to produce attenuation maps from PET/MRI data from other vendors. The fundamental idea behind DeepUTE is not limited to UTE data, and retraining the network on other MR sequences such as the T1w MPRAGE or ZTE could allow for a multi-vendor method. However, it would require a large pediatric dataset across several vendors to confirm this.

Although, the limits of agreement using RESOLUTE and DeepUTE are encouragingly narrow (**Table 1**), the number of patients in each age category is still small. Thus, we cannot rule out artifacts caused by other combinations of anatomy and pathology.

CONCLUSION

The present study performed on FET-PET/MRI examinations of pediatric patients revealed that both RESOLUTE and our deep learning method DeepUTE are able to robustly produce attenuation maps similar to the reference CT-AC. The clinical metrics were within acceptable limits of the reference CT-AC, making either method suitable for imaging of pediatric brain tumor patients - a cohort that is especially challenging for atlas-based methods. For clinical use of any MR-AC map, however, we recommend visually inspection for artifacts with particular attention to areas close to the skull base, anatomically distorted tissue and metal implants. The added accuracy due to better noise handling of DeepUTE, ease of use without the need for regional masks, as well as the improved runtime makes DeepUTE the method of choice for PET/MRI AC. Further refinement of the deep learning method with age-specific data input is likely to improve the performance.

AUTHOR CONTRIBUTIONS

CL designed the method, did the data analysis, and prepared the manuscript. LM and IL designed the method, aided in data analysis, and revised and approved the manuscript. AH, FA, and LH aided in data acquisition, and revised and approved the manuscript.

FUNDING

The generous support by The Danish Childhood Cancer Foundation is highly appreciated (2014-34, 2015-48).

ACKNOWLEDGMENTS

We highly appreciate the scanner assistance of technologists Karin Stahr and Marianne Federspiel, and of radiographers Jákup Martin Poulsen and Nadia Azizi. The John and Birthe Meyer Foundation is thanked for their generous donation of the Siemens mMR hybrid PET/MR system at Copenhagen University Hospital Rigshospitalet.

REFERENCES

Abadi, M., Barham, P., Chen, J., Chen, Z., Davis, A., Dean, J., et al. (2016). "TensorFlow: a system for large-scale machine learning," in *Proceedings of the Twelth USENIX Symposium on Operating Systems Design and Implementation*, Savannah, GA, 265–283.

Andersen, F. L., Ladefoged, C. N., Beyer, T., Keller, S. H., Hansen, A. E., Højgaard, L., et al. (2014). Combined PET/MR imaging in neurology: MR-based attenuation correction implies a strong spatial bias when ignoring bone. *Neuroimage* 84, 206–216. doi: 10.1016/j.neuroimage.2013.08.042

Bezrukov, I., Schmidt, H., Gatidis, S., Schwenzer, N., and Pichler, B. J. (2015). Quantitative evaluation of segmentation- and atlas-based attenuation correction for PET/MR on pediatric patients. *J. Nucl. Med.* 56, 1067–1075. doi: 10.2967/jnumed.114.149476

Bland, J. M., and Altman, D. G. (1999). Measuring agreement in method comparison studies. *Stat. Methods Med. Res.* 8, 135–160. doi: 10.1177/096228029900800204

Buchmann, N., Klasner, B., Gempt, J., Bauer, J. S., Pyka, T., Delbridge, C., et al. (2016). (18)F-fluoroethyl-l-thyrosine positron emission tomography to delineate tumor residuals after glioblastoma resection: a comparison with standard postoperative magnetic resonance imaging. *World Neurosurg.* 89, 420–426. doi: 10.1016/j.wneu.2016.02.032

Çiçek, Ö, Abdulkadir, A., Lienkamp, S. S., Brox, T., and Ronneberger, O. (2016). "3D U-Net: learning dense volumetric segmentation from sparse annotation," in *Proceedings of the International Conference on Medical Image Computing and Computer-Assisted Intervention*, (Berlin: Springer International Publishing), 424–432. doi: 10.1007/978-3-319-46723-8_49

Chollet, F. (2015). *Keras*. Available at: https://github.com/fchollet/keras

Delso, G., Fürst, S., Jakoby, B., Ladebeck, R., Ganter, C., Nekolla, S. G., et al. (2011). Performance measurements of the Siemens mMR integrated whole-body PET/MR scanner. *J. Nucl. Med.* 52, 1914–1922. doi: 10.2967/jnumed.111.092726

Dunkl, V., Cleff, C., Stoffels, G., Judov, N., Sarikaya-Seiwert, S., Law, I., et al. (2015). The usefulness of dynamic O-(2-[18F]fluoroethyl)-L-tyrosine-PET in the clinical evaluation of brain tumors in children and adolescents. *J. Nucl. Med.* 56, 88–92. doi: 10.2967/jnumed.114.148734

Floeth, F. W., Pauleit, D., Wittsack, H. J., Langen, K. J., Reifenberger, G., Hamacher, K., et al. (2005). Multimodal metabolic imaging of cerebral gliomas: positron emission tomography with [18F]fluoroethyl-L-tyrosine and magnetic resonance spectroscopy. *J. Neurosurg.* 102, 318–327. doi: 10.3171/jns.2005.102.2.0318

Fonov, V., Evans, A. C., Botteron, K., Almli, C. R., McKinstry, R. C., Collins, D. L., et al. (2011). Unbiased average age-appropriate atlases for pediatric studies. *Neuroimage* 54, 313–327. doi: 10.1016/j.neuroimage.2010.07.033

Fraioli, F., Shankar, A., Hargrave, D., Hyare, H., Gaze, M. N., Groves, A. M., et al. (2015). 18F-fluoroethylcholine (18F-Cho) PET/MRI functional parameters in pediatric astrocytic brain tumors. *Clin. Nucl. Med.* 40, e40–e45. doi: 10.1097/RLU.0000000000000556

Galldiks, N., Dunkl, V., Stoffels, G., Hutterer, M., Rapp, M., Sabel, M., et al. (2015a). Diagnosis of pseudoprogression in patients with glioblastoma using O-(2-[18F]fluoroethyl)-L-tyrosine PET. *Eur. J. Nucl. Med. Mol. Imaging* 42, 685–695. doi: 10.1007/s00259-014-2959-4

Galldiks, N., Stoffels, G., Filss, C., Rapp, M., Blau, T., Tscherpel, C., et al. (2015b). The use of dynamic O-(2-18F-fluoroethyl)-l-tyrosine PET in the diagnosis of patients with progressive and recurrent glioma. *Neuro Oncol.* 17, 1293–1300. doi: 10.1093/neuonc/nov088

Garibotto, V., Heinzer, S., Vulliemoz, S., Guignard, R., Wissmeyer, M., Seeck, M., et al. (2013). Clinical applications of hybrid PET/MRI in neuroimaging. *Clin. Nucl. Med.* 38, e13–e18. doi: 10.1097/RLU.0b013e3182638ea6

Gong, K., Yang, J., Kim, K., El, Fakhri G, Seo, Y., and Li, Q. (2018). Attenuation correction for brain PET imaging using deep neural network based on dixon and ZTE MR images. *Phys. Med. Biol.* 63:125011. doi: 10.1088/1361-6560/aac763

Han, X. (2017). MR-based synthetic CT generation using a deep convolutional neural network method. *Med. Phys.* 44, 1408–1419. doi: 10.1002/mp.12155

He, K., Zhang, X., Ren, S., and Sun, J. (2015). "Delving deep into rectifiers: Surpassing human-level performance on imagenet classification," in *Proceedings of the IEEE International Conference on Computer Vision*, Nice, 1026–1034. doi: 10.1109/ICCV.2015.123

Henriksen, O. M., Marner, L., and Law, I. (2016). Clinical PET/MR imaging in dementia and neuro-oncology. *PET Clin.* 11, 441–452. doi: 10.1016/j.cpet.2016.05.003

Jakoby, B. W., Bercier, Y., Watson, C. C., Bendriem, B., and Townsend, D. W. (2009). Performance characteristics of a new LSO PET/CT scanner with extended axial field-of-view and PSF reconstruction. *IEEE Trans. Nucl. Sci.* 56, 633–639. doi: 10.1109/TNS.2009.2015764

Juttukonda, M. R., Mersereau, B. G., Chen, Y., Su, Y., Rubin, B. G., Benzinger, T. L. S., et al. (2015). MR-based attenuation correction for PET/MRI neurological studies with continuous-valued attenuation coefficients for bone through a conversion from R2* to CT-Hounsfield units. *Neuroimage* 112, 160–168. doi: 10.1016/j.neuroimage.2015.03.009

Kingma, D. P., and Ba, J. (2014). Adam: a method for stochastic optimization. *arXiv* [Preprint]. arXiv:1412.6980

Kläser, K., Markiewicz, P., Ranzini, M., Li, W., Modat, M., Hutton, B. F., et al. (2018). *International Workshop on Simulation and Synthesis in Medical Imaging*. Cham: Springer, 61–70.

Koesters, T., Friedman, K. P., Fenchel, M., Zhan, Y., Hermosillo, G., Babb, J., et al. (2016). Dixon sequence with superimposed model-based bone compartment provides highly accurate PET/MR attenuation correction of the brain. *J. Nucl. Med.* 57, 918–924. doi: 10.2967/jnumed.115.166967

Kracht, L. W., Miletic, H., Busch, S., Jacobs, A. H., Voges, J., Hoevels, M., et al. (2004). Delineation of brain tumor extent with [11C]L-methionine positron emission tomography: local comparison with stereotactic histopathology. *Clin. Cancer Res.* 10, 7163–7170. doi: 10.1158/1078-0432.CCR-04-0262

Ladefoged, C. N., Andersen, F. L., Kjær, A., Højgaard, L., and Law, I. (2017). RESOLUTE PET/MRI attenuation correction for O-(2-18F-fluoroethyl)-L-tyrosine (FET) in brain tumor patients with metal implants. *Front. Neurosci.* 11:453. doi: 10.3389/fnins.2017.00453

Ladefoged, C. N., Benoit, D., Law, I., Holm, S., Kjær, A., Højgaard, L., et al. (2015). Region specific optimization of continuous linear attenuation coefficients based on UTE (RESOLUTE): application to PET/MR brain imaging. *Phys. Med. Biol.* 60, 8047–8065. doi: 10.1088/0031-9155/60/20/8047

Ladefoged, C. N., Law, I., Anazodo, U., St. Lawrence, K., Izquierdo-Garcia, D., Catana, C., et al. (2016). A multi-centre evaluation of eleven clinically feasible brain PET/MRI attenuation correction techniques using a large cohort of patients. *Neuroimage* 147, 346–359. doi: 10.1016/j.neuroimage.2016.12.010

Langen, K. J., Hamacher, K., Weckesser, M., Floeth, F., Stoffels, G., Bauer, D., et al. (2006). O-(2-[18F]fluoroethyl)-l-tyrosine: uptake mechanisms and clinical applications. *Nucl. Med. Biol.* 33, 287–294. doi: 10.1016/j.nucmedbio.2006.01.002

Leynes, A. P., Yang, J., Wiesinger, F., Kaushik, S. S., Shanbhag, D. D., Seo, Y., et al. (2018). Zero-echo-time and dixon deep pseudo-CT (ZeDD CT): direct generation of pseudo-CT images for pelvic PET/MRI attenuation correction using deep convolutional neural networks with multiparametric MRI. *J. Nucl. Med.* 59, 852–858. doi: 10.2967/jnumed.117.198051

Li, Z., Park, B. K., Liu, W., Zhang, J., Reed, M. P., Rupp, J. D., et al. (2015). A statistical skull geometry model for children 0-3 years old. *PLoS One* 10:e0127322. doi: 10.1371/journal.pone.0127322

Liu, F., Jang, H., Kijowski, R., Bradshaw, T., and McMillan, A. B. (2017). Deep learning MR imaging–based attenuation correction for PET/MR imaging. *Radiology* 286, 676–684. doi: 10.1148/radiol.2017170700

Martinez-Möller, A., Souvatzoglou, M., Delso, G., Bundschuh, R. A., Chefd'hotel, C., Ziegler, S. I., et al. (2009). Tissue classification as a potential approach for attenuation correction in whole-body PET/MRI: evaluation with PET/CT data. *J. Nucl. Med.* 50, 520–526. doi: 10.2967/jnumed.108.054726

Mullins, M. E., Barest, G. D., Schaefer, P. W., Hochberg, F. H., Gonzalez, R. G., and Lev, M. H. (2005). Radiation necrosis versus glioma recurrence: conventional MR imaging clues to diagnosis. *AJNR Am. J. Neuroradiol.* 26, 1967–1972.

Paulus, D. H., Quick, H. H., Geppert, C., Fenchel, M., Hermosillo, G., Faul, D., et al. (2015). Whole-body PET/MR imaging: quantitative evaluation of a novel model-based MR attenuation correction method including bone. *J. Nucl. Med.* 56, 1061–1066. doi: 10.2967/jnumed.115.156000

Piroth, M. D., Pinkawa, M., Holy, R., Klotz, J., Nussen, S., Stoffels, G., et al. (2011). Prognostic value of early [18F]fluoroethyltyrosine positron emission tomography after radiochemotherapy in glioblastoma multiforme. *Int. J. Radiat. Oncol.* 80, 176–184. doi: 10.1016/j.ijrobp.2010.01.055

Preuss, M., Werner, P., Barthel, H., Nestler, U., Christiansen, H., Hirsch, F. W., et al. (2014). Integrated PET/MRI for planning navigated biopsies in pediatric brain tumors. *Child's Nerv. Syst.* 30, 1399–1403. doi: 10.1007/s00381-014-2412-9

Robson, M. D., Gatehouse, P. D., Bydder, M., and Bydder, G. M. (2003). Magnetic resonance: an introduction to ultrashort TE (UTE) imaging. *J. Comput. Assist. Tomogr.* 27, 825–846. doi: 10.1097/00004728-200311000-00001

Ronneberger, O., Fischer, P., and Brox, T. (2015). U-Net: convolutional networks for biomedical image segmentation. *Med Image Comput. Comput. Interv.* 9351, 234–241. doi: 10.1007/978-3-319-24574-4_28

Sekine, T., Voert, E. E. G. W., Warnock, G., Buck, A., Huellner, M., Veit-haibach, P., et al. (2016). Clinical evaluation of zero-echo-time attenuation correction for brain 18F-FDG PET/MRI: comparison with atlas attenuation correction. *J. Nucl. Med.* 57, 1927–1932. doi: 10.2967/jnumed.116.175398

Spick, C., Herrmann, K., and Czernin, J. (2016). PET/CT and PET/mri perform equally well in cancer: evidence from studies on more Than 2,300 patients. *J. Nucl. Med.* 57, 420–431. doi: 10.2967/jnumed.115.158808

Springenberg, J. T., Dosovitskiy, A., Brox, T., and Riedmiller, M. (2014). Striving for simplicity: the all convolutional net. *arXiv* [Preprint]. arXiv:1412.6806

Vander Borght, T., Asenbaum, S., Bartenstein, P., Halldin, C., Kapucu, O., Van Laere, K., et al. (2006). EANM procedure guidelines for brain tumour imaging using labelled amino acid analogues. *Eur. J. Nucl. Med. Mol. Imaging* 33, 1374–1380. doi: 10.1007/s00259-006-0206-3

Watanabe, M., Tanaka, R., and Takeda, N. (1992). Magnetic resonance imaging and histopathology of cerebral gliomas. *Neuroradiology* 34, 463–469. doi: 10.1007/BF00598951

8

Diagnosis of Brain Diseases via Multi-Scale Time-Series Model

Zehua Zhang[1], *Junhai Xu*[2], *Jijun Tang*[1,3], *Quan Zou*[4*] *and Fei Guo*[1*]

[1] School of Computer Science and Technology, College of Intelligence and Computing, Tianjin University, Tianjin, China, [2] School of Artificial Intelligence, College of Intelligence and Computing, Tianjin University, Tianjin, China, [3] Department of Computer Science and Engineering, University of South Carolina, Columbia, SC, United States, [4] Institute of Fundamental and Frontier Sciences, University of Electronic Science and Technology of China, Chengdu, China

***Correspondence:**
Quan Zou
zouquan@nclab.net
Fei Guo
fguo@tju.edu.cn

The functional magnetic resonance imaging (fMRI) data and brain network analysis have been widely applied to automated diagnosis of neural diseases or brain diseases. The fMRI time series data not only contains specific numerical information, but also involves rich dynamic temporal information, those previous graph theory approaches focus on local topology structure and lose contextual information and global fluctuation information. Here, we propose a novel multi-scale functional connectivity for identifying the brain disease via fMRI data. We calculate the discrete probability distribution of co-activity between different brain regions with various intervals. Also, we consider nonsynchronous information under different time dimensions, for analyzing the contextual information in the fMRI data. Therefore, our proposed method can be applied to more disease diagnosis and other fMRI data, particularly automated diagnosis of neural diseases or brain diseases. Finally, we adopt Support Vector Machine (SVM) on our proposed time-series features, which can be applied to do the brain disease classification and even deal with all time-series data. Experimental results verify the effectiveness of our proposed method compared with other outstanding approaches on Alzheimer's Disease Neuroimaging Initiative (ADNI) dataset and Major Depressive Disorder (MDD) dataset. Therefore, we provide an efficient system via a novel perspective to study brain networks.

Keywords: functional magnetic resonance imaging, multi-scale time-series, Alzheimer's disease, major depressive disorder, functional connection

1. INTRODUCTION

The functional Magnetic Resonance Imaging (fMRI) technique provides an opportunity to quantify functional integration via measuring the correlation between intrinsic Blood-Oxygen-Level-Dependent (BOLD) signal fluctuations of distributed brain regions at rest. The BOLD signal is sensitive to spontaneous neural activity within brain regions, thus it can be used as an efficient and noninvasive way for investigating neurological disorders at the whole-brain level. Functional connectivity (FC), defined as the temporal correlation of BOLD signals in different brain regions, can exhibit how structurally segregated and functionally specialized brain regions interact with each other. Therefore, the brain network analysis using fMRI data will provide great advantages to automated diagnosis of neural diseases or brain diseases.

Some researchers model the FC information as a specific network by using graph theoretic techniques. Differences between normal and disrupted FC networks caused by pathological attacks provide important biomarkers to understand pathological underpinnings, in terms of the topological structure and connection strength. The network analysis has been becoming an increasingly useful tool for understanding the cerebral working mechanism and mining sensitive biomarkers for neural or mental diseases. Zeng et al. (2018) propose a new switching delayed particle swarm optimization (SDPSO) algorithm is proposed to optimize the SVM parameters. Using graph theories, the brain network analysis provides an effective solution to concisely quantify the connectivity properties of brain networks, where each node denotes a particular anatomical element or a brain region, and each edge represents the relationship between a pair of nodes, such as anatomical, functional or effective connections (Friston, 2011). The anatomical connection typically corresponds to white matter tracts between many pairs of brain regions. The functional connection corresponds to magnitudes of temporal correlations in activity and occurs between some pairs of anatomically unconnected regions, which may reflect linear or nonlinear interactions, as well as interactions within different time scales (Zhou et al., 2009). The effective connection represents direct or indirect causal influences of one region on another region, which may be estimated from observed perturbations whether synchronous or asynchronous (Friston et al., 2003). As a brain network analysis approach, the graph theory offers two important advantages (Tijms et al., 2013). One is that it provides quantitative measurement, which can preserve the connectivity information in the network and thus reflect the segregated and integrated nature of local brain activity. The other is that, it provides a general framework for comparing heterogeneous graphs constructed by different types of data, such as anatomical and functional data.

However, these graph theory approaches have many drawbacks that must be overcome. First, the graph theory has many limitations, on the one hand, common graph theory features such as edge weights, path lengths and clustering coefficients (Rubinov and Sporns, 2010; Chen et al., 2011) usually focus on local topology structure and lose their global topology characteristics (Sanz-Arigita et al., 2010; Jie et al., 2018); on the other hand, each node in the brain networks is uniquely corresponding to a specific brain region, mostly ignoring the label information of each node (Jie et al., 2018). Second. the functional connectivity is more sensitive to local information rather than the global topology, but some recent studies (Hutchison et al., 2013; Leonardi et al., 2013; Zeng et al., 2013, 2014; Allen et al., 2014) indicate that the FC network contains rich dynamic temporal information. To be more concrete, for each brain region, a sliding window approach is performed to generate a set of BOLD subseries on schizophrenia disease diagnosis (Damaraju et al., 2014) and others (Chen et al., 2016; Wee et al., 2016). Third, the raw functional data is underutilized, building brain network from raw data may lose the temporal or context information. For example, Pearson's Correlation Coefficient (PCC) is the simplest and most commonly scheme in functional connectivity estimation, which is the covariance of the two variables divided by the product of their standard deviations. Clearly, according to the mathematical definition, the PCC value is context-independent or order-independent in time series, not considering nonsynchronous information under different time dimensions.

In view of the above, the fMRI time series not only contains specific numerical information, but also involves contextual information and global fluctuation information. In this paper, we propose a novel time-series model based on Jensen-Shannon divergence for identifying the brain disease via fMRI data, and the flow chart is shown in **Figure 1**. First, we calculate the discrete probability distribution of co-activity between different brain regions with various intervals in multi-scale time series data. Second, the contextual information is taken into account in analyzing the correlation and causality among the fMRI data. Third, we design a novel method based on time-series to measure the similarity between two object co-activity intensity of brain functional connectivity. Finally, we adopt Support Vector Machine (SVM) on our proposed time-series features, which can be applied to do the brain disease classification and even deal with all time-series data. Experimental results verify the effectiveness of our proposed method compared with other outstanding approaches on Alzheimer's Disease Neuroimaging Initiative (ADNI) dataset and Major Depressive Disorder (MDD) dataset. The rest of this paper is organized as follows. We start by a brief review of dataset and pre-processing. Then, we formulate the problem and present our proposed method. Finally, experimental results are reported, followed by the conclusion of this work.

2. MATERIALS AND METHODS

In this section, we introduce the flow of our method. First, we preprocessed the original data, removed the noise from the original data, and segmented the fMRI image data through the brain region template. Next, we extract information or features from the perspective of functional connection between brain regions. To overcome the shortcoming of traditional Pearson Correlation Coefficient (PCC) methods, we propose a novel framework for feature extraction of brain functional connection. Then, through feature selection, we use the classification model for predicting brain disease. Finally, we discuss parameter settings in the model.

2.1. Dataset

We carry out experiments on two different datasets. One is a public Alzheimer's Disease Neuroimaging Initiative database (Jack et al., 2010), and another one is a volunteer experiment of Major Depressive Disorder (Geng et al., 2018). In the data pre-processing, we deal with the raw data by a widely used software package (SPM12), and then divide one brain into 116 brain regions.

2.1.1. ADNI

In Alzheimer's Disease Neuroimaging Initiative database, we emply a total of 169 subjects, including 87 Alzheimer's patients (49 females and 38 males) and 82 normal controls (46 females and 36 males). We download the ADNI data from website http://adni.loni.usc.edu/.

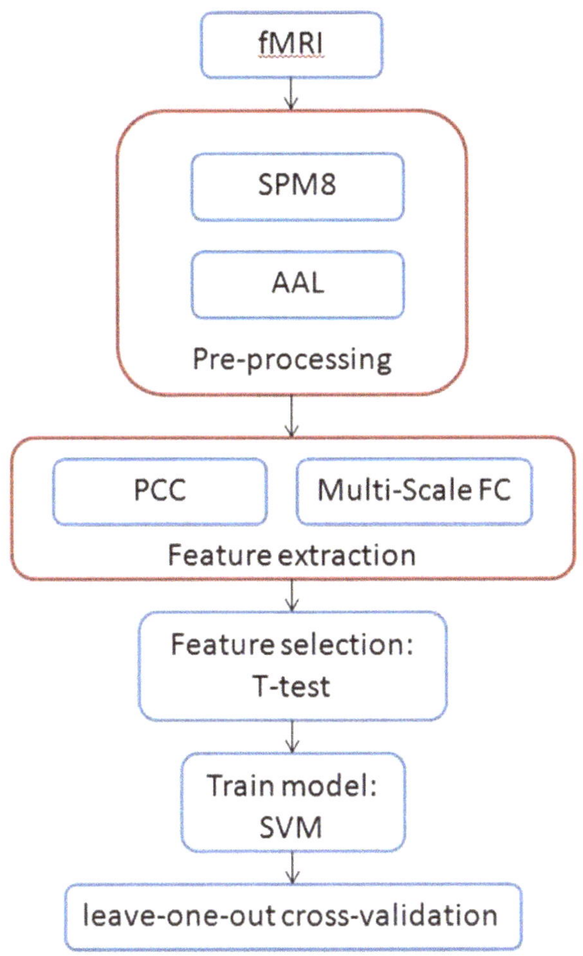

FIGURE 1 | The framework of our proposed multi-scale time-series model for brain diseases diagnosis.

2.1.2. MDD

In volunteer experiment, we use a total of 60 subjects, including 31 volunteers with Major Depressive Disorder (MDD) (22 females and 8 males, aged 60.5 ± 11.2 years, range 25 − 65 years) and 29 healthy volunteers (18 females and 11 males, aged 50.1 ± 10.6 years, range 25 − 65 years). Those major depressive disorder subjects without comorbidity had a minimum duration of illness more than 3 months. Each participant provided written informed consent and the study was conducted in accordance with the local Ethics Committee.

2.2. Pre-processing

We perform image pre-processing for the fMRI data using a standard pipeline, carried out via the statistical parametric mapping (SPM12, www.fil.ion.ucl.ac.uk/spm/software/spm12/) software package on Matlab. The data pre-processing procedure includes slice timing, realign, segment, normalization and band-pass filtered. For more detailed data pre-processing procedure, please refer to website.

The whole brain of each subject in fMRI space is parcellated into 116 brain regions of interest (ROI) according to the Automated Anatomical Labeling (AAL) template. This atlas divided the brain into 78 cortical regions, 26 cerebellar regions and 12 subcortical regions according to anatomy, details in literature (Tzourio-Mazoyer et al., 2002). For each of the 116 ROIs, the mean time series was calculated by averaging the Blood-Oxygen-Level-Dependent (BOLD) signals among all voxels within the specifically ROI. There exist many similar templates such as Brainnetome template (Fan et al., 2016) and Harvard-Oxford template.

2.3. Feature Extraction

After pre-processing, how to excavate the location and cause of lesions is the focus of our research and attention. The most common method is to calculate the correlation between two brain regions through Pearson Correlation Coefficient (PCC), and analyze lesions by observing the changes of correlation. However, the PCC value is context-independent or order-independent, that is not considering nonsynchronous information at different time intervals. Here, we first give a basic introduction to PCC, and then elaborate on our approach.

2.3.1. Pearson Correlation Coefficient

Pearson's correlation coefficient (PCC) is the simplest and most commonly scheme in functional connectivity estimation. For any two brain regions, the coordination degree of blood-oxygen-level dependent fluctuation is calculated as the functional connection strength between these two brain regions. Typically, in the case of the AAL template, this step extracts the 6,670-dimensional features. Mathematical definition is the covariance of the two variables divided by the product of their standard deviations, as follows:

$$PCC_{X,Y} = \frac{\mathrm{E}[(X-\mu_X)(Y-\mu_Y)]}{\sigma_X \sigma_Y} \tag{1}$$

Clearly, according to the formula, the value of the Pearson's correlation coefficient is context-independent or order-independent in time series, which it only limits alignment at the same time, so information about the time dimension or context is missing.

2.3.2. Multi-Scale Functional Connectivity of Brain Regions

We extract the discrete probability distribution of co-activity in time series data. First, we use the function $\phi(\cdot)$ to evaluate temporal dynamic property of the time series data. In addition, we convert $\phi(\cdot)$ to $g(\cdot)$, defined as follows:

$$\phi(t^{k_1}_{i_1,j_1}, t^{k_2}_{i_2,j_2}) = g(f_\varphi(t^{k_1}_{i_1,j_1}), f_\varphi(t^{k_2}_{i_2,j_2})) \tag{2}$$

where $f(\cdot)$ represents a mapping function that makes use of prior knowledge in order to map the original time series into another specific form, $g(\cdot)$ represents the function to evaluate temporal information after the mapping operation.

We utilize the prior knowledge in order to map the original multivariate time series data into another specific form, such as a mapping of numeric, state and character. The mapping function is defined as follows:

$$\begin{aligned} f_\varphi(A_k) &= f_\varphi\{T_1^k, T_2^k, \cdots, T_i^k, \cdots, T_N^k\} \\ &= \{f_\varphi(T_1^k), f_\varphi(T_2^k), \cdots, f_\varphi(T_N^k)\} \end{aligned} \quad (3)$$

where A_k denotes the original time series data, and φ denotes the prior knowledge.

In the multivariate time series data A_k, the correlation value between T_i^k and T_j^k is defined as follows:

$$C_{\phi(\cdot)}^k(i,j) = \sum_{m=1}^{M} \phi(t_{i,m}^k, t_{j,m}^k) \quad (4)$$

In addition, the correlation value between T_i^k and T_j^k in interval $I_t = [r_t, s_t]$ is defined as follows:

$$C_{\phi(\cdot)}^k(i,j,I_t) = \sum_{m=1}^{M} \sum_{l=r_t}^{s_t} \phi(t_{i,m}^k, t_{j,m+l}^k) \quad (5)$$

Notably, it is obvious that $C_{\phi(\cdot)}^k(i,j,I_t) \neq C_{\phi(\cdot)}^k(j,i,I_t)$.

Generally, we explore the correlation of time series data in multiple intervals. Let $C_{\phi(\cdot)}^k \in \mathcal{R}^{N\times N\times T}$ denotes the multi-scale weighted correlation coefficient in multivariate time series data A_k. Here, $C_{\phi(\cdot)}^k$ is a 3-order tensor, N is the number of time series data, T is the number of intervals.

Next, we transform the tensor $C_{\phi(\cdot)}^k$ into a discrete probability distribution $P_{\phi(\cdot)}^k$ for analyzing co-activity in multi-scale time series data, as follows:

$$P_{\phi(\cdot)}^k = \{p_{\phi(\cdot)}^k(i,j,I_t) | i,j \in [1,N], I_t \in I\} \quad (6)$$

where $p_{\phi(\cdot)}^k(i,j,I_t)$ represents the proportion of correlation value between i-th time series data and j-th time series data based on function $\phi(\cdot)$ in interval I_t, defined as follows:

$$p_{\phi(\cdot)}^k(i,j,I_t) = \frac{C_{\phi(\cdot)}^k(i,j,I_t)}{\sum_{i=1}^{N}\sum_{j=1}^{N}\sum_{t=1}^{T} C_{\phi(\cdot)}^k(i,j,I_t)} \quad (7)$$

2.4. Classification Model for Predicting Brain Disease

In disease prediction, the number of samples is limited, but the feature dimension is usually large, so we need to both compress the feature space to improve the accuracy and analyze the etiology with more meaningful features. We use t-test for feature selection, and then we use Support Vector Machine (SVM) as the learning model, which is described in detail as follows.

2.4.1. Feature Selection

We use the two-sample t-test as the feature selection method. We assume that one feature of positive and negative samples is subject to the distribution of the same mean, and we set the significance parameter $p = 0.05$.

2.4.2. Support Vector Machine

We adopt Support Vector Machine (SVM) technique developed by Cortes and Vapnik (1995) for solve the binary classification problem. Also, various kinds of binary classification model can be applied in many other biomedical prediction problems (Guo et al., 2014, 2015, 2016; Ding et al., 2016a,b, 2017a,b; Liu et al., 2016; Zeng et al., 2016; Shen et al., 2017a,b; Xuan et al., 2017; Pan et al., 2018). The decision function is shown as follows:

$$\gamma(A_k) = sign\{\sum_{i=1}^{K} \alpha_i y_i \cdot \mathcal{K}(A_k, A_i) + b\} \quad (8)$$

where $\mathcal{K}(A_k, A_i)$ represents our proposed novel time-series kernel function, and α_i is calculated as follows:

$$\begin{aligned} \text{Maximize} \quad & \sum_{i=1}^{K} \alpha_i - \frac{1}{2}\sum_{i=1}^{K}\sum_{j=1}^{K} \alpha_i\alpha_j \cdot y_i y_j \cdot \mathcal{K}(A_i, A_j) \\ \text{s.t.} \quad & 0 \le \alpha_i \le C \\ & \sum_{i=1}^{K} \alpha_i y_i = 0 \end{aligned} \quad (9)$$

where C is a regularization parameter that controls the tradeoff between margin and misclassification error.

2.5. Model Parameter

In practice, we make more detailed discussion for parameters in our method. We discuss some prior knowledge and assumptions in our problem of Alzheimer's disease and Major Depression Disorder diagnosis, and some details need to be clarified. The time series data not only carry specific numerical information, but also include contextual and fluctuation trend information.

Here, due to the BOLD imaging principle, we pay more attention to the time points of high activity state, that is, time points with high values in time series. We define a dynamic or soft threshold to distinguish whether a time point is active or not, that is, converting a numeric sequence into a state sequence or 0/1 sequence.

For all active time points in one set of time series, we count the number of time points of simultaneous responses in other sets of time series. Moreover, we analyze the co-active between two sets of time series in asynchronous. As we get more details with asynchronous analysis, we'll get more essential information. In the experiments, it is also proved by the higher classification accuracy.

2.5.1. Time Series Mapping

We adopt a empirical rule to indicate the dynamic threshold, called three-sigma method (WalterA, 1986). This method converts a numeric sequence into a state sequence, the dynamic threshold represented as follows:

$$th(T_i^k) = \mu(T_i^k) + \eta \cdot \sigma(T_i^k) \tag{10}$$

where

$$\mu(T_i^k) = \frac{\sum_{m=1}^{M} t_{i,m}^k}{|T_i^k|} \tag{11}$$

and

$$\sigma(T_i^k) = \frac{\sum_{m=1}^{M} (t_{i,m}^k - \mu(T_i^k))^2}{|T_i^k| - 1} \tag{12}$$

In a multivariate time series A_k, we calculate a corresponding dynamic threshold $th(T_i^k)$ for each set of time series T_i^k. Then, for a set of time series T_i^k, we convert a numeric sequence into a 0/1 sequence according to mapping function $f(\cdot)$, as follows:

$$f(t_{i,m}^k) = \begin{cases} 1, & t_{i,m}^k \geq th(T_i^k) \\ 0, & \text{else} \end{cases} \tag{13}$$

The magnitude of η indicates the sensitivity of our method to the active state. In our experiment, η is set to 1.

2.5.2. Correlation Function ϕ

The correlation function represents the relationship between a couple of time points in time series. In disease diagnosis, we only focus on co-activity, that is, both brain region i in time point m and brain region j in time point n are in active states. To be more concrete, $t_{i,m}^k$ and $t_{j,n}^k$ are greater than the threshold $th(T_i^k)$ and $th(T_j^k)$, respectively.

$$g(f(t_{i,m}^k), f(t_{j,n}^k)) = \begin{cases} 1, & f(t_{i,m}^k) = f(t_{j,n}^k) = 1 \\ 0, & \text{else} \end{cases} \tag{14}$$

Corresponding to Formula 2 above, $\phi(\cdot)$ in our experiment is:

$$\phi(t_{i,m}^k, t_{j,n}^k) = \begin{cases} 1, & t_{i,m}^k \geq th(T_i^k) \;\&\; t_{j,n}^k \geq th(T_j^k) \\ 0, & \text{else} \end{cases} \tag{15}$$

2.5.3. Interval Set *I*

For a collection of multiple intervals I, we extract local information by the element of interval, that is, greater element, more detailed information. Easy to be over-fit and sparse; if the element of interval is little, we may lose some key information. Also, for a interval $I_t \in I$, if I_t is close to zero, it means that two time points that we're interested in are very close; if I_t is far from zero, it indicates that we extract long-distance asynchronous information.

In our experiments, the interval collection I is set to $\{[0,0], [1,1], [2,2], [3,12]\}$. Here, $[0,0]$ represents information for synchronization, $[1,1]$ and $[2,2]$ represent short-distance correlation for asynchronism, $[3,12]$ represents a loose interval for asynchronism. Empirically, it is sensitive to close interval of zero and loose for long distances.

3. RESULTS

Our experiment consists of three parts. To proof the effectiveness of our approach, we perform on automated diagnoses of Alzheimer's disease and Major Depressive Disorder, respectively. We evaluate the classification performance using the leave-one-out cross-validation (LOOCV). And also, we adopt Accuracy, Sensitivity, Specificity and AUC as evaluation standards. First, we compare the results of the traditional PCC method and our feature extraction method in the two data sets of AD and MDD. Then, we compare the effects of different classifiers. Finally, we compare our approach with some recent research works.

3.1. Comparison of Different Features

Here, we compare the performance of traditional PCC method and our feature extraction method to analyze fMRI data. In addition to feature extraction, we use the same experimental steps and parameters, including preprocessing, feature selection and classifier. The results are shown in **Table 1**.

On Alzheimer's disease and major depressive disorder database, we compare our method to traditional PCC method, and classification results are summarized in **Table 1**. The information extracted by our multi-scale functional connection (Multi-Scale FC) method is used for predicting brain disease, which is obviously higher than the traditional PCC method. On Alzheimer's disease dataset, our method achieves best specificity of 0.9268. Moreover, by combining PCC and our method, we achieve better results, with ACC of 0.8935 and AUC of 0.8748. On MDD dataset, our method also achieve the best results, but the difference is that PCC and multi-scale functional connection are actually lower when combined. The experimental results indicate that our approach is more effective than traditional PCC or graph theory feature-based methods. Combining different methods will yield better results, but there is also a risk of over-fitting.

3.2. Comparison of Different Classifiers

In this part, we use the feature extraction model in the previous step to compare the performance of different classifiers. Specifically, we compare three classifiers: random forest (RF), logistic regression (LR) and support vector machine (SVM). The results are shown in **Table 2**.

TABLE 1 | Comparison of different features.

Method	Data set	Accuracy	Sensitivity	Specificity	AUC
PCC	AD	0.5858	0.5747	0.5976	0.5612
Multi-Scale FC	AD	0.8876	0.8506	0.9268	0.8562
Multi-Scale FC + PCC	AD	0.8935	0.8850	0.9024	0.8748
PCC	MDD	0.6167	0.6129	0.6207	0.6514
Multi-Scale FC	MDD	0.9000	0.8710	0.9310	0.9295
Multi-Scale FC + PCC	MDD	0.8667	0.8065	0.9310	0.8961

TABLE 2 | Comparison of different classifiers.

Method	Data set	Accuracy	Sensitivity	Specificity	AUC
LR	AD	0.8579	0.7931	0.9268	0.8347
RF	AD	0.8343	0.8276	0.8415	0.8284
SVM	AD	0.8935	0.8850	0.9024	0.8748
LR	MDD	0.8333	0.8387	0.8276	0.8684
RF	MDD	0.8833	0.9032	0.8621	0.8921
SVM	MDD	0.8667	0.8065	0.9310	0.8961

TABLE 3 | Comparison of different existing methods on ADNI.

Method	Accuracy	Sensitivity	Specificity	AUC
Baseline	0.5858	0.5747	0.5976	0.5612
FON	0.8580	0.8161	0.9024	0.8195
Shortest-path	0.7396	0.8161	0.6585	0.6938
WL-edge	0.6272	0.6437	0.6098	0.6084
WL-subtree	0.7811	0.7816	0.7805	0.7645
WL-Shortestpath	0.6095	0.5977	0.6220	0.5735
SKL	0.8462	0.8046	0.8902	0.8166
Our method	0.8876	0.8506	0.9268	0.8562

In this part, we use our proposed multi-scale functional connection method to extract features, and compare the results of different classifiers. Comparing these three classifiers, SVM can achieve the highest AUC in both AD dataset and MDD dataset, the best ACC can also be obtained on the AD data set, which is generally a stable classifier. In addition, RF can obtain the best ACC on the MDD dataset, and LR can obtain the best Spe on the AD dataset. Overall, all three classifiers can achieve good accuracy, indicating that the information extracted by our method is effective and stable.

3.3. Comparison of Different Existing Methods

We compare our proposed method to recent outstanding studies. Baseline represents the traditional graph theory feature-based method. Moreover, the state-of-the-art methods represent three major groups of graph kernels on edge, subtree and shortest-path, respectively. These graph kernel belong to the Weisfeiler-Lehman graph kernel framework (Shervashidze et al., 2011), denoted as WL-edge, WL-subtree and WL-shortestpath, respectively. In addition, in the Alzheimer's disease diagnosis, we also compare with the graph kernel method with shortest-path (Shortest-path) (Borgwardt and Kriegel, 2006), the sliding window method (FON: 70-length sliding window with 1-step) (Chen et al., 2016) and the sub-network kernel method (SKL) (Jie et al., 2018). In the Major Depressive Disorder classification problem, we compare to the method of Geng et al. (2018).

On Alzheimer's Disease Neuroimaging Initiative database, we compare our method to seven existing methods, and classification results are summarized in **Table 3**. Our method achieves best accuracy of 0.8876 and best AUC of 0.8562.

TABLE 4 | Comparison of different existing methods on MDD.

Method	Accuracy	Sensitivity	Specificity	AUC
Baseline	0.6167	0.6129	0.6207	0.6514
Shortest-path	0.7833	0.8065	0.7586	0.8135
Xu et al.	0.8667	0.8710	0.8621	0.9103
Our Method	0.9000	0.8710	0.9310	0.9295

However, the accuracy values for Baseline, FON, Shortest-path, WL-edge, WL-subtree, WL-Shortestpath and SKL are 0.5858, 0.8580, 0.7396, 0.6272, 0.7811, and 0.6095, respectively. Also, the AUC values for these seven methods are 0.5612, 0.8195, 0.6938, 0.6084, 0.7645, and 0.5735, respectively. Comparing to these methods, our method achieves accuracy improvement of 0.0296 and AUC improvement of 0.0367, respectively. The experimental results indicate that our approach is far better than traditional graph theory feature-based methods, and slightly better than the state-of-the-art graph kernel-based methods.

On the volunteer experiments of Major Depressive Disorder, we compare our method to three existing methods, and classification results are summarized in **Table 4**. Our method achieves best accuracy of 0.9000 and best AUC of 0.9295. However, the accuracy values for Baseline, Shortest-path and method of Xu et al. are 0.6167, 0.7833, and 0.8667, respectively. Also, the AUC values for these three methods are 0.6514, 0.8135, and 0.9103, respectively. Comparing to these methods, our method achieves accuracy improvement of 0.0333 and AUC improvement of 0.0192, respectively. The experimental results indicate that our approach is far better than traditional graph methods, and slightly better than the current outstanding methods.

4. CONCLUSIONS

The fMRI time series data not only contains specific numerical information, but also involves rich dynamic temporal information. However, those previous graph theory approaches focus on local topology structure and lose contextual information and global fluctuation information. Here, we propose a novel multi-scale functional connectivity for identifying the brain disease via fMRI data. We calculate the discrete probability distribution of co-activity between different brain regions with various intervals. Also, we consider nonsynchronous information under different time dimensions, for analyzing the contextual information in the fMRI data. Therefore, our proposed method can be applied to more disease diagnosis and other fMRI data, particularly automated diagnosis of neural diseases or brain diseases. Experimental results verify the effectiveness of our proposed method, so we provide an efficient system via a novel perspective to study brain networks.In the future, parallel computing (Zou et al., 2017), computational intelligence (Xu et al., 2017; Zou et al., 2017) and neural networks (Song et al., 2018; Xu et al., 2018) can be considered with the growing of dataset.

AUTHOR CONTRIBUTIONS

FG and QZ conceived and designed the experiments. ZZ and JX performed the experiments and analyzed the data. FG and ZZ wrote the paper. FG and JT supervised the experiments and reviewed the manuscript.

FUNDING

This work is supported by a grant from the National Science Foundation of China (NSFC 61772362) and the Tianjin Research Program of Application Foundation and Advanced Technology (16JCQNJC00200), and National Key R&D Program of China (2018YFC0910405, 2017YFC0908400).

REFERENCES

Allen, E. A., Damaraju, E., Plis, S. M., Erhardt, E. B., Eichele, T., and Calhoun, V. D. (2014). Tracking whole-brain connectivity dynamics in the resting state. *Cereb. Cortex* 24, 663–676. doi: 10.1093/cercor/bhs352

Borgwardt, K. M., and Kriegel, H. P. (2006). "Shortest-path kernels on graphs," in *IEEE International Conference on Data Mining* (Houston, TX), 74–81. doi: 10.1109/ICDM.2005.132

Chen, G., Ward, B. D., Xie, C., Li, W., Wu, Z., Jones, J. L., et al. (2011). Classification of alzheimer disease, mild cognitive impairment, and normal cognitive status with large-scale network analysis based on resting-state functional MR imaging. *Int. J. Med. Radiol.* 259, 213–221. doi: 10.1148/radiol.10100734

Chen, X., Zhang, H., Gao, Y., Wee, C. Y., Li, G., and Shen, D. (2016). High-order resting-state functional connectivity network for MCI classification. *Hum. Brain Mapp.* 37, 3282–3296. doi: 10.1002/hbm.23240

Cortes, C., and Vapnik, V. (1995). Support-vector networks. *Mach. Learn.* 20, 273–297. doi: 10.1007/BF00994018

Damaraju, E., Allen, E. A., Belger, A., Ford, J. M., Mcewen, S., Mathalon, D. H., et al. (2014). Dynamic functional connectivity analysis reveals transient states of dysconnectivity in schizophrenia. *Neuroimage Clin.* 5, 298–308. doi: 10.1016/j.nicl.2014.07.003

Ding, Y., Tang, J., and Guo, F. (2016a). Identification of protein-protein interactions via a novel matrix-based sequence representation model with amino acid contact information. *Int. J. Mol. Sci.* 17:1623. doi: 10.3390/ijms17101623

Ding, Y., Tang, J., and Guo, F. (2016b). Predicting protein-protein interactions via multivariate mutual information of protein sequences. *BMC Bioinformatics* 17:398. doi: 10.1186/s12859-016-1253-9

Ding, Y., Tang, J., and Guo, F. (2017a). Identification of drug-target interactions via multiple information integration. *Inform. Sci.* 418–419, 546–560. doi: 10.1016/j.ins.2017.08.045

Ding, Y., Tang, J., and Guo, F. (2017b). Identification of protein-ligand binding sites by sequence information and ensemble classifier. *J. Chem. Inform. Model.* 57, 3149–3161. doi: 10.1021/acs.jcim.7b00307

Fan, L., Li, H., Zhuo, J., Yu, Z., Wang, J., Chen, L., et al. (2016). The human brainnetome atlas: a new brain atlas based on connectional architecture. *Cereb. Cortex* 26, 3508–3526. doi: 10.1093/cercor/bhw157

Friston, K. J. (2011). Functional and effective connectivity in neuroimaging: a synthesis. *Brain Connect* 1, 13–36. doi: 10.1089/brain.2011.0008

Friston, K. J., Harrison, L., and Penny, W. (2003). Dynamic causal modelling. *Neuroimage* 19, 1273–1302. doi: 10.1016/S1053-8119(03)00202-7

Geng, X., Xu, J., Liu, B., and Shi, Y. (2018). Multivariate classification of major depressive disorder using the effective connectivity and functional connectivity. *Front. Neurosci.* 12:38. doi: 10.3389/fnins.2018.00038

Guo, F., Ding, Y., Li, S. C., Shen, C., and Wang, L. (2016). Protein-protein interface prediction based on hexagon structure similarity. *Comput. Biol. Chem.* 63, 83–88. doi: 10.1016/j.compbiolchem.2016.02.008

Guo, F., Ding, Y., Li, Z., and Tang, J. (2015). Identification of protein-protein interactions by detecting correlated mutation at the interface. *J. Chem. Inform. Model.* 55, 2042–2049. doi: 10.1021/acs.jcim.5b00320

Guo, F., Li, S. C., Du, P., and Wang, L. (2014). Probabilistic models for capturing more physicochemical properties on protein-protein interface. *J. Chem. Inform. Model.* 54, 1798–1809. doi: 10.1021/ci5002372

Hutchison, R. M., Womelsdorf, T., Allen, E. A., Bandettini, P. A., Calhoun, V. D., Corbetta, M., et al. (2013). Dynamic functional connectivity: promise, issues, and interpretations. *Neuroimage* 80, 360–378. doi: 10.1016/j.neuroimage.2013.05.079

Jack, C. R., Bernstein, M. A., Fox, N. C., Thompson, P., Alexander, G., Harvey, D., et al. (2010). The Alzheimer's disease neuroimaging initiative (ADNI): MRI methods. *J. Magn. Reson. Imaging* 27, 685–691. doi: 10.1002/jmri.21049

Jie, B., Liu, M., Zhang, D., and Shen, D. (2018). Sub-network kernels for measuring similarity of brain connectivity networks in disease diagnosis. *IEEE Trans. Image Process.* 27, 2340–2353. doi: 10.1109/TIP.2018.2799706

Leonardi, N., Richiardi, J., Gschwind, M., Simioni, S., Annoni, J. M., Schluep, M., et al. (2013). Principal components of functional connectivity: a new approach to study dynamic brain connectivity during rest. *Neuroimage* 83, 937–950. doi: 10.1016/j.neuroimage.2013.07.019

Liu, Y., Zeng, X., He, Z., and Zou, Q. (2016). Inferring microrna-disease associations by random walk on a heterogeneous network with multiple data sources. *IEEE/ACM Trans. Comput. Biol. Bioinformatics* 14, 905–915. doi: 10.1109/TCBB.2016.2550432

Pan, G., Jiang, L., Tang, J., and Guo, F. (2018). A novel computational method for detecting dna methylation sites with dna sequence information and physicochemical properties. *Int. J. Mol. Sci.* 19:E511. doi: 10.3390/ijms19020511

Rubinov, M., and Sporns, O. (2010). Complex network measures of brain connectivity: uses and interpretations. *Neuroimage* 52, 1059–1069. doi: 10.1016/j.neuroimage.2009.10.003

Sanz-Arigita, E. J., Schoonheim, M. M., Damoiseaux, J. S., Rombouts, S. A. R. B., Maris, E., Barkhof, F., et al. (2010). Loss of 'small-world' networks in Alzheimer's disease: graph analysis of fmri resting-state functional connectivity. *PLoS ONE* 5:e13788. doi: 10.1371/journal.pone.0013788

Shen, C., Ding, Y., Tang, J., Song, J., and Guo, F. (2017a). Identification of dna-protein binding sites through multi-scale local average blocks on sequence information. *Molecules* 22:2079. doi: 10.3390/molecules22122079

Shen, C., Ding, Y., Tang, J., Xu, X., and Guo, F. (2017b). An ameliorated prediction of drug-target interactions based on multi-scale discrete wavelet transform and network features. *Int. J. Mol. Sci.* 18:1781. doi: 10.3390/ijms18081781

Shervashidze, N., Schweitzer, P., Leeuwen, E. J. V., Mehlhorn, K., and Borgwardt, K. M. (2011). Weisfeiler-lehman graph kernels. *J. Mach. Learn. Res.* 12, 2539–2561. doi: 10.1016/j.websem.2011.06.001

Song, T., Liu, X., and Zeng, X. (2018). Asynchronous spiking neural p systems with anti-spikes. *IEEE Trans. Nanobiosci.* 16, 888–895. doi: 10.1007/s11063-014-9378-1

Tijms, B. M., Wink, A. M., De, H. W., Wm, V. D. F., Stam, C. J., Scheltens, P., et al. (2013). Alzheimer's disease: connecting findings from graph theoretical studies of brain networks. *Neurobiol. Aging* 34, 2023–2036. doi: 10.1016/j.neurobiolaging.2013.02.020

Tzourio-Mazoyer, N., Landeau, B., Papathanassiou, D., Crivello, F., Etard, O., Delcroix, N., et al. (2002). Automated anatomical labeling of activations in spm using a macroscopic anatomical parcellation of the mni mri single-subject brain. *Neuroimage* 15, 273–289. doi: 10.1006/nimg.2001.0978

WalterA (1986). *Statistical Method From the Viewpoint of Quality Control.* New York, NY: Dover.

Wee, C. Y., Yang, S., Yap, P. T., and Shen, D. (2016). Sparse temporally dynamic resting-state functional connectivity networks for early mci identification. *Brain Imaging Behav.* 10, 342–356. doi: 10.1007/s11682-015-9408-2

Xu, H., Zeng, W., Zeng, X., and Yen, G. G. (2018). An evolutionary algorithm based on minkowski distance for many-objective optimization. *IEEE Trans. Cybern.* 1–12. Available online at: https://ieeexplore.ieee.org/document/8423202

Xu, H., Zeng, W., Zhang, D., and Zeng, X. (2017). MOEA/HD: a multiobjective evolutionary algorithm based on hierarchical decomposition. *IEEE Trans. Cybern.* 49, 517–526. doi: 10.1109/TCYB.2017.2779450

Xuan, Z., Quan, Z., Rodruguez-Paton, A., and Zeng, X. (2017). Meta-path methods for prioritizing candidate disease mirnas. *IEEE/ACM Trans. Comput. Biol. Bioinformatics* 16, 283–291. doi: 10.1109/TCBB.2017.2776280

Zeng, N., Qiu, H., Wang, Z., Liu, W., Zhang, H., and Li, Y. (2018). A new switching-delayed-pso-based optimized SVM algorithm for diagnosis of alzheimer's disease. *Neurocomputing* 320, 195–202. doi: 10.1016/j.neucom.2018.09.001

Zeng, N., Wang, Z., Li, Y., Du, M., Cao, J., and Liu, X. (2013). Time series modeling of nano-gold immunochromatographic assay via expectation maximization algorithm. *IEEE Trans. Biomed. Eng.* 60, 3418–3424. doi: 10.1109/TBME.2013.2260160

Zeng, N., Wang, Z., Zineddin, B., Li, Y., Du, M., Xiao, L., et al. (2014). Image-based quantitative analysis of gold immunochromatographic strip via cellular neural network approach. *IEEE Trans. Med. Imaging* 33, 1129–1136. doi: 10.1109/TMI.2014.2305394

Zeng, X., Liao, Y., Liu, Y., and Zou, Q. (2016). Prediction and validation of disease genes using hetesim scores. *IEEE/ACM Trans. Comput. Biol. Bioinformatics* 14, 687–695. doi: 10.1109/TCBB.2016.2520947

Zhou, D., Thompson, W. K., and Siegle, G. (2009). Matlab toolbox for functional connectivity. *Neuroimage* 47, 1590–1607. doi: 10.1016/j.neuroimage.2009.05.089

Zou, Q., Wan, S., Zeng, X., and Ma, Z. S. (2017). Reconstructing evolutionary trees in parallel for massive sequences. *BMC Syst. Biol.* 11(Suppl. 6):100. doi: 10.1186/s12918-017-0476-3

9

A Fully Automatic Framework for Parkinson's Disease Diagnosis by Multi-Modality Images

Jiahang Xu[1,2], *Fangyang Jiao*[3], *Yechong Huang*[1], *Xinzhe Luo*[1], *Qian Xu*[4], *Ling Li*[5], *Xueling Liu*[6], *Chuantao Zuo*[5], *Ping Wu*[5]* *and Xiahai Zhuang*[1,2]*

[1] School of Data Science, Fudan University, Shanghai, China, [2] Fudan-Xinzailing Joint Research Center for Big Data, Fudan University, Shanghai, China, [3] Department of Nuclear Medicine, Daping Hospital, Army Medical University, Chongqing, China, [4] Department of Nuclear Medicine, North Huashan Hospital, Fudan University, Shanghai, China, [5] PET Center, Huashan Hospital, Fudan University, Shanghai, China, [6] Department of Radiology, Huashan Hospital, Fudan University, Shanghai, China

***Correspondence:**
Xiahai Zhuang
zxh@fudan.edu.cn
Ping Wu
wupingpet@fudan.edu.cn*

Background: Parkinson's disease (PD) is a prevalent long-term neurodegenerative disease. Though the criteria of PD diagnosis are relatively well defined, current diagnostic procedures using medical images are labor-intensive and expertise-demanding. Hence, highly integrated automatic diagnostic algorithms are desirable.

Methods: In this work, we propose an end-to-end multi-modality diagnostic framework, including segmentation, registration, feature extraction and machine learning, to analyze the features of striatum for PD diagnosis. Multi-modality images, including T1-weighted MRI and ^{11}C-CFT PET, are integrated into the proposed framework. The reliability of this method is validated on a dataset with the paired images from 49 PD subjects and 18 Normal (NL) subjects.

Results: We obtained a promising diagnostic accuracy in the PD/NL classification task. Meanwhile, several comparative experiments were conducted to validate the performance of the proposed framework.

Conclusion: We demonstrated that (1) the automatic segmentation provides accurate results for the diagnostic framework, (2) the method combining multi-modality images generates a better prediction accuracy than the method with single-modality PET images, and (3) the volume of the striatum is proved to be irrelevant to PD diagnosis.

Keywords: Parkinson's disease, multi-modality, image classification, U-Net, striatum

INTRODUCTION

Parkinson's disease (PD) is the second-most prevalent long-term neurodegenerative disease characterized by bradykinesia, rigidity and rest tremor (Postuma et al., 2015). At present, PD is responsible for about 346,000 deaths per year and is thus one of the major concerns of neuroscience community (Roth et al., 2018). The diagnosis of PD mainly refers to the Movement Disorder Society Clinical Diagnostic Criteria for Parkinson's disease (MDS-PD Criteria) (Postuma et al., 2015). According to the MDS-PD criteria, the motor symptoms of PD are linked with the loss of dopaminergic neurons, which mainly affects the anatomical regions of the striatum (SARs). Therefore, SARs, which include the caudate nucleus, the putamen and the pallidum, are commonly explored (Strafella et al., 2017).

Functional neuroimaging of the presynaptic dopaminergic system is highlighted according to the MDS-PD criteria (Liu et al., 2018). Positron-emission tomography (PET) is one of the neuroimaging modalities that indicate the regional activity of the tissues. Accordingly, PET tracers are developed to observe the activity of the dopamine transporter (DAT) in early stage of PD, such as ^{11}C-CFT, which is a biomarker of the presynaptic dopaminergic system with high sensitivity (Kazumata et al., 1998; Ilgin et al., 1999; Wang et al., 2013). However, due to the low resolution of the PET images, the anatomical and structural information related to the brain that PET can provide is limited. Therefore, the structural neuroimaging methods, such as T1-weighted magnetic resonance imaging (T1-MRI), are introduced to assist the multi-modality diagnosis of PD (Ibarretxe-Bilbao et al., 2011). Bu et al. (2018) worked on the subtypes of multiple system atrophy (MSA) utilizing T1-MRI and ^{11}C-CFT PET. Huang et al. (2019) combined these two modalities with ^{18}F-FDG PET and analyzed Rapid Eye Movement (REM) Sleep Behavior Disorder research. In both of their studies, T1-MR images were registered to PET images to identify the region of interest (ROIs) in the PET images.

Recently, researchers attempt to improve the accuracy in diagnostic methods with the help of machine learning algorithms, for example, the support vector machine (SVM) has been widely used. Long et al. (2012) used SVM to distinguish early PD patients from NL subjects utilizing resting-state functional MRI, and obtained an accuracy of 86.96%. Haller et al. (2012) used SVM and reached an accuracy of 97% when classifying PD from other atypical forms of Parkinsonism by combining Diffusion Tensor Imaging (DTI) and ^{123}I ioflupane Single-Photon Emission Computed Tomography (SPECT). These works combining multi-modality imaging have proved the reliability of artificial intelligence (AI)-assisted PD diagnosis, while few works are reported including ^{11}C-CFT PET, to the best of our knowledge.

In this work, we proposed an end-to-end multi-modality diagnostic framework for PD combining T1-MR and ^{11}C-CFT PET images. In the framework, MR images were segmented by a U-Net (Ronneberger et al., 2015; Wong et al., 2018). The resulting segmentation was then used to locate the SARs of the PET images by registration. Finally, features extracted from these SARs were used to diagnose PD. Our main contributions include:

(1) We have shown that the automatic segmentation provides accurate results for the proposed diagnostic framework of PD.
(2) We have shown that MR images provide important information to obtain the SAR information in the PET images.
(3) We have demonstrated that the *volume* feature of the striatum is irrelevant to PD diagnosis.

METHODOLOGY

The proposed framework is shown in **Figure 1**. It contains three major steps: (1) segmentation, (2) registration, and (3) feature extraction and prediction. In the first two steps, MRI-assisted PET segmentation is performed by MRI segmentation and MRI-PET registration, and in the subsequent step, only information of PET images is considered for PD diagnosis.

Striatum Segmentation via Deep Neural Network

To obtain the fine structure of the brain tissues, a 3D deep neural network, i.e., U-Net (Ronneberger et al., 2015; Wong et al., 2018), is implemented to segment the striatum in the MR images. The obtained segmentation is used as a reference for SAR localization and extraction in the subsequent procedures.

Figure 2 shows the network architecture for the segmentation, which outputs a mask indicating the segmented labels of the input image. The network further incorporates the idea of deep supervision introduced by Mehta and Sivaswamy (2017) for faster training convergence. Specifically, the network comprises encoding and decoding paths. The encoding path captures contextual information by residual blocks and max-pooling operations at different resolutions, while the decoding path sequentially recovers the spatial resolution and object boundaries. Besides, skip connections between the upsampled feature maps in the decoder and the corresponding feature maps in the encoder are employed for the combination of local and contextual information. Moreover, the deep supervision scheme is adopted to allow more direct backpropagation to the hidden layers for faster convergence. A final $1 \times 1 \times 1$ convolution layer with a softmax function produces the segmentation probabilities. Gaussian blurring and dropout operations are adopted to avoid overfitting. A loss function is defined to handle the relatively small anatomical structures of labels for accurate segmentation, i.e.,

$$L = w_D L_{Dice} + w_C L_{Cross}, \tag{1}$$

where, w_D and w_C denote the weights of L_{Dice} and L_{Cross}, respectively; L_{Dice} denotes the Dice-related loss, and L_{Cross} denotes the cross-entropy. They are respectively, given by

$$L_{Dice} = E_i\left[\left(-\ln Dice_i\right)^{\gamma}\right], \tag{2}$$

with

$$Dice_i = \frac{2\left(\sum_x \delta_{il}(x) \cdot p_i(x)\right)}{\sum_x \left(\delta_{il}(x) + p_i(x)\right)}, \tag{3}$$

and

$$L_{Cross} = E_x\left[-\ln p_l(x)\right]. \tag{4}$$

In Eq. (3), $\delta_{il}(x)$ is the Kronecker delta, which equals to 1 if the segmentation label $i(x)$ equals to the ground-truth label $l(x)$ at the voxel position x, and 0 otherwise; $p_i(x)$ is the probability of voxel x being labeled as i. In our implementations, we chose $w_D = 0.8$, $w_C = 0.2$ and $\gamma = 0.3$ for the loss function and pretrained the model using an Adam optimizer with a learning rate of 1×10^{-3} for 10 epochs (Kingma and Ba, 2014). Due to the computational limitations, an ROI of MR images with a size of $96 \times 96 \times 96$ voxels was cropped, which contains the whole structure of SARs.

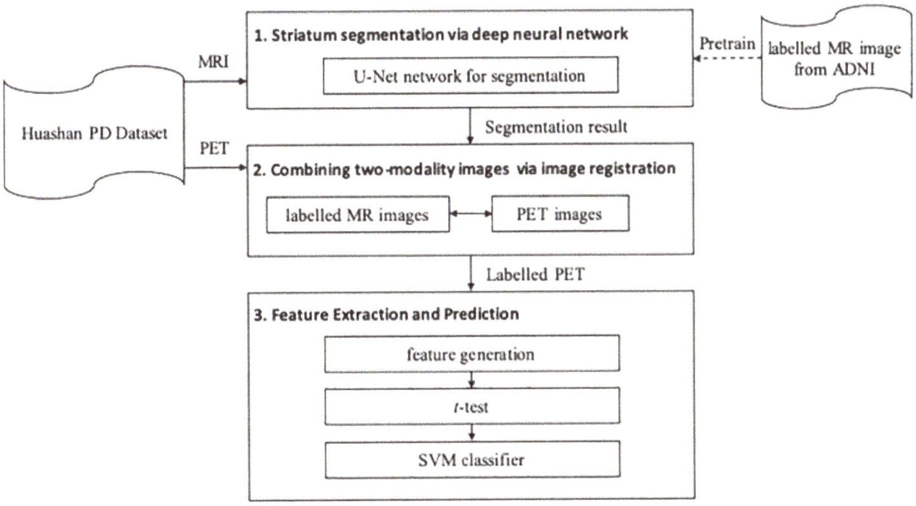

FIGURE 1 | The architecture of the proposed framework.

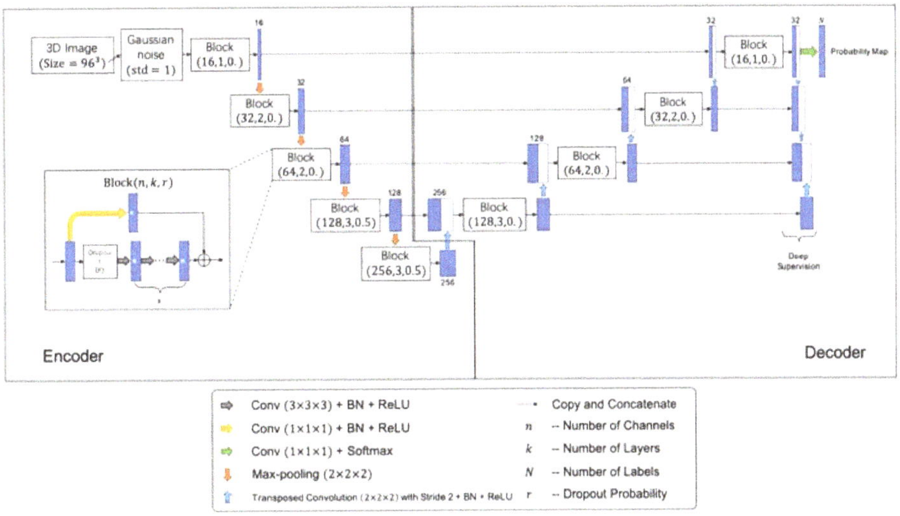

FIGURE 2 | The proposed segmentation network architecture. Each block is represented by (n, k, r), where n, k, and r denote number of channels, number of layers, and the dropout probability, respectively.

We employ T1-MR brain images from the Alzheimer's Disease Neuroimaging Initiative (ADNI[1]) database for pretraining, for the size of the clinical data used in this work is far from being enough for the U-Net training. Note that the information related to AD or other modality data is not used in this study, namely we solely employ the 1859 brain T1-MR images to assist the U-Net training. The ADNI MR images are segmented by the multi-atlas label propagation with the expectation-maximization (MALP-EM[2]) framework (Ledig et al., 2015). The manual segmentation of the caudate nucleus, the putamen and the pallidum are chosen to be the gold standards in the pretraining stage.

[1]adni.loni.usc.edu

[2]https://biomedia.doc.ic.ac.uk/software/malp-em/

Combining Two-Modality Images via Image Registration

We propose to combine two-modality images for the automatic diagnosis of PD, where T1-MRI provides the morphological information of SARs, and ^{11}C-CFT offers pathological information related to PD. The extraction of the SAR information from the MR images is achieved by the DNN segmentation method, as described in Section "Striatum Segmentation via Deep Neural Network." With this information, one can extract the shape or substructure features from each of anatomical regions. For the combination of the two-modality images, we propose to use image registration, which propagates the anatomical and structural information of SARs in the MRI to the PET.

The registration in the multi-modality diagnostic framework is achieved via the zxhproj[3] platform (Zhuang et al., 2011). Firstly, the image with prior label information is registered to the target PET image. The resulting transformation is then used to propagate the prior label information to the PET, which results in the automatic localization of the SARs for the target PET image. Since the MRI and PET images are from the same subject at the same acquisition session, we propose to use a rigid registration. By registration, the caudate nucleus, the putamen and the pallidum, as well as the parieto-occipital regions are labeled.

For comparisons, we propose a single-modality diagnostic framework using solely PET images. To achieve the fully automated diagnosis, we propose to achieve the anatomical information in the PET images via the same registration method used for the multi-modality scheme. In this scenario, the image with prior label information is defined using a pre-labeled PET template, and the registration between the template and the target PET is achieve via an affine registration following a pre-rigid registration.

Feature Extraction and Prediction

To extract adequate features from the SARs, the caudate nucleus and the putamen are further divided into three substructures using a k-means algorithm (Ng et al., 2006). After clustering, statistics of image intensity are calculated to represent the feature information in each region, including *maximum*, *minimum*, *median*, *1st* and *3rd quantile*, and *mean* of PET intensity. Several studies characterize radioactive uptake by the striatal-to-occipital ratio (SOR), as the parieto-occipital region is widely considered of lacking CFT uptake (Ma et al., 2002; Carbon et al., 2004; Huang et al., 2007). In this work, the SOR, which is defined as *(striatum-occipital)/occipital*, is calculated with each kind of intensity value. Meanwhile, the *volumes* of the six anatomical SARs are included into the feature set. In all, 90 features are generated (for a list of specific features, see **Supplementary Table S1**).

After feature extraction, a t-test is performed to analyze the significance of each feature. Setting significance level $\alpha = 0.01$, features with a p-value less than 0.01 are considered as being statistically significant. Only significant features would be regarded as the arguments of the machine learning models.

Consequently, the SVM classifier is trained to classify the subjects (Haller et al., 2012; Long et al., 2012). Furthermore, to estimate the generalization ability and stability of the method, the leave-n-out cross-validation strategy is employed to evaluate the performance of the models. In addition, we implement the random forest algorithm to calculate the importance of the features (Gray et al., 2013).

EXPERIMENTS

The following parts in this section are organized as follows. Section "Data Acquisition" describes the data used in this work; Section "Evaluation of Automatic Striatum Segmentation" validates the reliability of the automatic segmentation method; Section "Advantages of Multi-Modality Images" investigates the advantages of combining multi-modality images; and Section "Efficacy of Volume Features" explores the efficacy of the volume features of SARs for the diagnostic of PD.

Data Acquisition

Data used in this study was collected from the Department of Neurology, Huashan Hospital, Fudan University. It contains paired ^{11}C-CFT PET and T1-MR images of PD patients and healthy participants. MR images were acquired by a 3.0-T MR scanner (DiscoveryTM MR750, GE Healthcare, Milwaukee, WI, United States). Each MR image was visually inspected to rule out motion artifacts (Bu et al., 2018; Huang et al., 2019). PET images were acquired by a Siemens Biograph 64 PET/CT scanner (Siemens, Munich, Germany) in three-dimensional (3D) mode. A CT transmission scan was first performed for attenuation correction. Static emission data were acquired 60 min after the intravenous injection of 370 MBq of ^{11}C-CFT and lasted for 15 min. All subjects were scanned in a supine position with a dimly lighted and noise-free surrounding (Bu et al., 2018; Huang et al., 2019). The synchronous MRI data were acquired using a T1-weighted 3D inversion recovery spoiled gradient recalled acquisition (IR-SPGR) with the following parameters: TE/TR = 2.8/6.6 ms, inversion time = 400 ms, flip angle = 15°, matrix = 256 × 256 × 170, field-of-view = 24 cm, and slice thickness = 1 mm. MR and PET images acquisition for each subject had a time interval of no more than 3 months.

Forty-nine patients with PD and 18 age-matched normal control (NL) subjects were recruited. All subjects were screened and clinically examined by a senior investigator of movement disorders before entering the study and were followed up for at least 1 year. The diagnosis of PD was made referring to the MDS-PD Criteria. The Unified Parkinson's Disease Rating Scale (UPDRS) and Hoehn and Yahr scale (HY) were assessed after the cessation of oral anti-parkinsonian medications (if used) for at least 12 h. The following exclusion criteria were used for the NL subjects' recruitment: (1) being tested positive by the REM Sleep Behavior Disorder Single-Question Screen (Postuma et al., 2012), (2) a history of neurological or psychiatric illness, (3) a prior exposure to neuroleptic agents or drugs, (4) an abnormal neurological examination. The data are summarized in **Table 1**. In this study, gender proportion differences between groups could be ignored, as previous studies have shown no significant difference in DAT bindings between genders (Eshuis et al., 2009). The research was approved by the Ethics Committee of Huashan

TABLE 1 | Summary for the studied dataset.

Subject	HY	Count	Gender (M/F)	Age	UPDRS
NL	0	18	4/14	64.1 ± 6.7	–
PD	1	15	10/5	61.2 ± 7.6	14.3 ± 5.1
	2	26	16/10	62.0 ± 7.9	21.6 ± 7.5
	3	8	4/4	58.8 ± 5.9	34.6 ± 7.4

For gender, the expression means Male/Female, and for age and Unified Parkinson's Disease Rating Scale, the expression means mean ± standard deviation.

[3]http://www.sdspeople.fudan.edu.cn/zhuangxiahai/0/zxhproj/

TABLE 2 | Average DSCs of the segmentation of each anatomy.

	Right caudate	Left caudate	Right pallidum	Left pallidum	Right putamen	Left putamen
DSCs	88.5 ± 6.3%	90.1 ± 7.2%	89.3 ± 11.4%	86.9 ± 13.0%	92.2 ± 5.0%	91.4 ± 5.5%

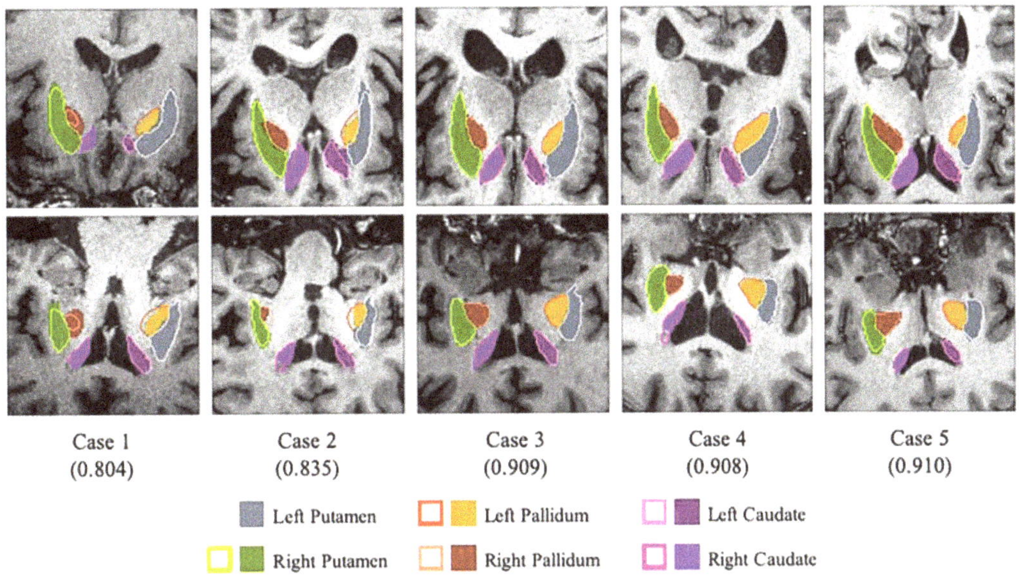

FIGURE 3 | Visualization of the segmentation results with slices of the axial view (top row) and the coronal view (bottom row). Case 1 and case 2 are two worst segmentation results, and case 3, case 4 and case 5 are three median results. Values in the parentheses refer to the corresponding dice similarity coefficients. As for the legends, the colored contours represent the automatic segmentation boundaries while the colored blocks are the corresponding ground truth masks.

Hospital. All subjects or legally responsible relatives signed written informed consent in accordance with the Declaration of Helsinki before the study.

After data acquisition, both sides of the caudate nucleus, the putamen and the pallidum of each MR image were manually labeled by an experienced clinician from the Department of Neurology, Huashan Hospital. To ensure the qualities of the segmentation results, boundaries of these anatomical structures were double-checked by another clinician from the same department.

Evaluation of Automatic Striatum Segmentation

To test the performance of the segmentation network, three-fold cross-validation was performed. The whole dataset was split into three disjoint parts, and the model was fine-tuned for 5 epochs on the union of every two disjoint subsets. **Table 2** illustrates the average Dice Similarity Coefficient (DSC) of each anatomical region, and **Figure 3** provides a visualization of the segmentation results of five example cases. One can find that the left pallidum (colored goldenrod in **Figure 3**) is worst segmented with the maximal standard deviation while the right putamen (colored olive drab in **Figure 3**) is best segmented with the minimal standard deviation.

Figure 4 shows the average accuracy (ACC) and the number of wrong predictions with leave-n-out cross-validation of the different segmentation methods, i.e., automatically and manually. Both accuracies reached 100% when $n = 1$, and the accuracies and the numbers of wrong predictions of the two experiments result in no significant difference in a pairwise t-test (p-value = 0.1017). Furthermore, when training classifiers using features of manually segmented images and testing it using features of automatically segmented images, we still obtained 100% accuracy. All results indicate that the automatic segmentation provides accurate results for the proposed diagnostic framework of PD.

Advantages of Multi-Modality Images

To evaluate the influence of multi-modality images, the single-modality method using solely PET images was compared. In the multi-modality scheme, the MR images provides accurate anatomical and structural SAR information of the subject. By contrast, in the single-modality method this information is achieved by registering the PET images to a pre-labeled Automated Anatomical Labeling (AAL) PET template. We conducted the rest of the pipeline in the same way for the two methods.

Figure 5 shows the results of the comparative experiments with leave-n-out cross-validation. The results demonstrate that with the assistance of MR images, the performance of the multi-modality group is better than the single-modality PET group in the PD/NL task. When $n = 1$, the accuracy of the multi-modality

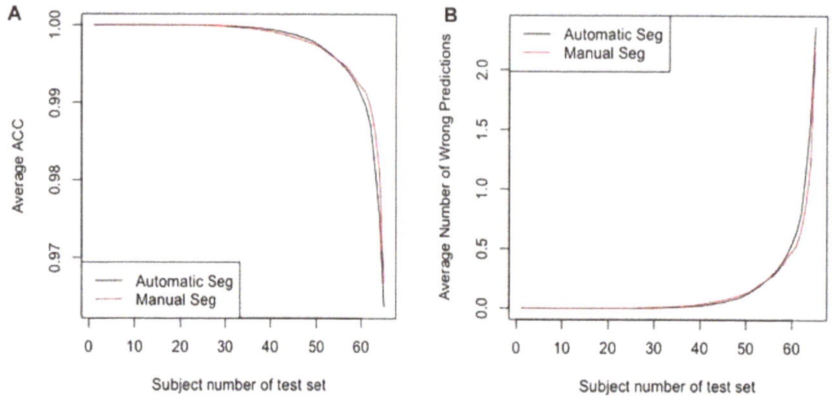

FIGURE 4 | The results for the leave-*n*-out cross-validation of the classification with automatic segmentation and manual segmentation. Panel **(A)** presents the average ACC, and panel **(B)** presents the average number of wrong predictions. The horizontal axes in the two panels represent subjects numbers of the test set, i.e., the *n* in the leave-*n*-out cross-validation.

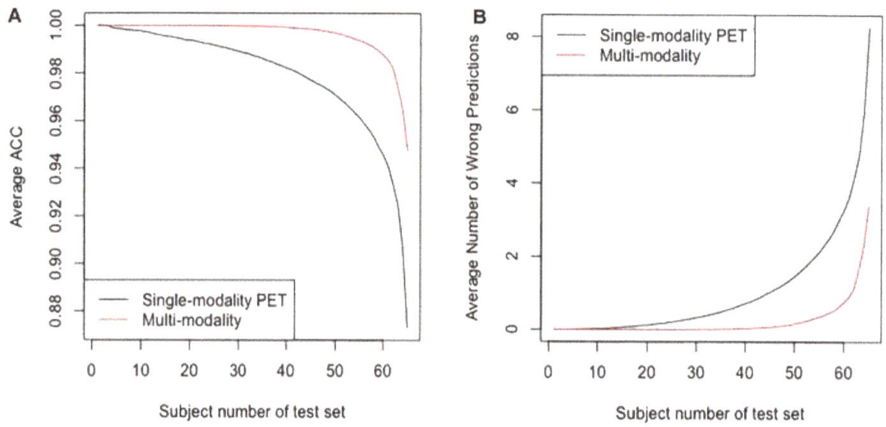

FIGURE 5 | The results for the leave-*n*-out cross-validation of the classification by the multi-modality diagnostic method and the single-modality method. Panel **(A)** presents the average ACC, and panel **(B)** presents the average number of wrong predictions. The horizontal axes in the two panels represent subjects numbers of the test set, i.e., the *n* in the leave-*n*-out cross-validation.

TABLE 3 | Feature importance of groups with/without *volume*.

Feature	Group with *Volume*	Group without *Volume*
mean	0.2030	0.2006
median	0.2024	0.1965
3rd quantile	0.1961	0.1946
1st quantile	0.1825	0.1835
maximum	0.1443	0.1497
minimum	0.0715	0.0751
volume	0.0002	–

The importance values were calculated by the random forest algorithm.

TABLE 4 | Feature importance of groups with manual segmentation results and automatic segmentation results.

Feature	Manual segmentation	Automatic segmentation
mean	0.2064	0.2031
median	0.2010	0.2025
3rd quantile	0.2008	0.1962
1st quantile	0.1654	0.1825
maximum	0.1660	0.1443
minimum	0.0605	0.0716

The importance values were calculated by the random forest algorithm.

group reached 100% in the PD/NL task, while the accuracy of the single-modality PET group was 98.51%.

To test the uniformity of the classifiers based on the different groups, we also trained the classifier using features of multi-modality images and tested it using features of single-modality PET, and the accuracy dropped to 88.05%, with 8 subjects misclassified.

Efficacy of Volume Features

In the feature extraction step, *t*-tests were performed to evaluate the significances of all feature, and results indicated that the features of the *volume* are not statistically significant with $\alpha = 0.01$ (see **Supplementary Table S1** for more details). To further evaluate the effects of the *volume* of SARs, we compared the importance of different features based on groups with and without *volume*, as **Table 3** shows. One can see that the importance values of the two groups are similar. Hence, the effect of *volume* to the model is negligible. Note that the *volume* is calculated based on the original MR images without downsampling.

DISCUSSION AND CONCLUSION

In this work, we proposed a fully automatic framework for PD diagnosis. This method utilized two modalities, i.e., ^{11}C-CFT PET and T1-MR imaging, performed MRI-assisted PET segmentation, selected features and employed SVM to give the predictions. To validate the performance of the framework, we applied the proposed method on the clinical data from Huashan Hospital.

One of the major differences between the proposed method and the traditional methods is that the SARs are located according to the labels of the automatic segmentation by U-Net. To evaluate the performance of the U-Net, we calculated the DSCs between automatic and manual segmentation. In addition, we compared the proposed pipeline, whose SARs were located according to the automatic segmentation, to the method whose SARs were manually segmented. The leave-*n*-out experiment shows the two methods performed comparably,

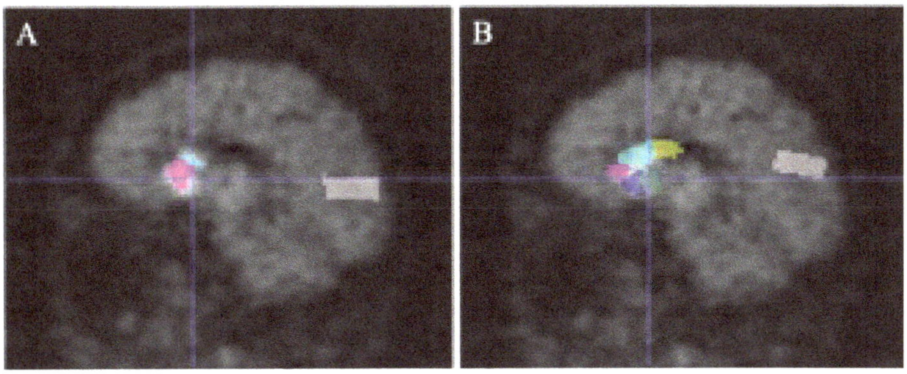

FIGURE 6 | The comparison of gold standard and wrongly placed SARs of the wrongly predicted subject. Panel **(A)** shows the segmentation result in gold standard, and panel **(B)** shows the segmentation in the wrongly predicted subject. Images are in sagittal plane and have the same cursor position.

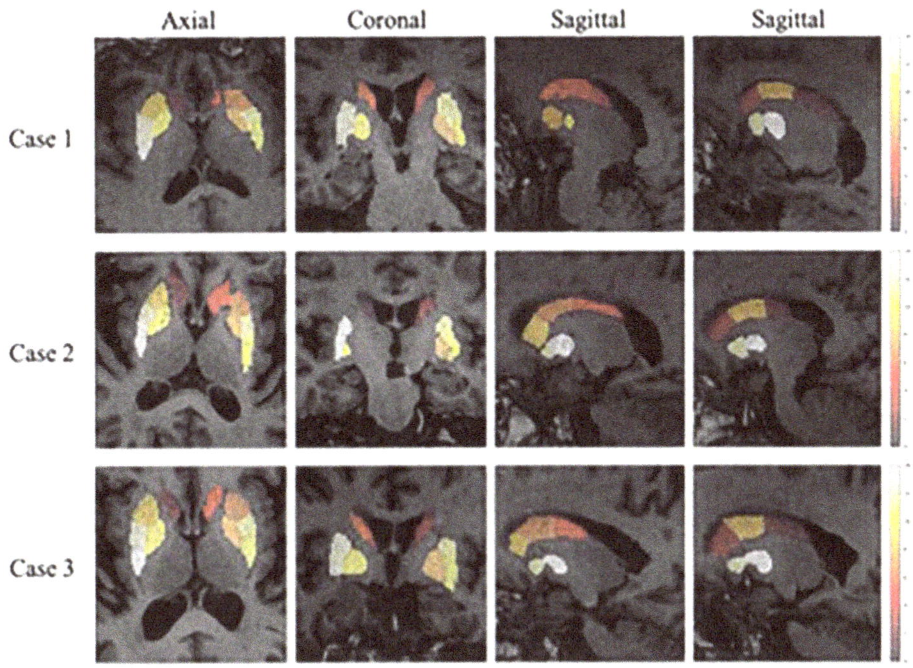

FIGURE 7 | The importance of the SARs in the proposed framework. One axial slice, one coronal slice and two sagittal slices (right and left side of the regions, respectively) of three subjects are chosen to show the importance of the SARs.

indicating that the automatic segmentation could provide accurate results for the proposed diagnostic framework of PD. Further investigation of the feature importance of the two groups is illustrated in **Table 4**. It indicates that the *minimum* has lower importance than the first five features. Given that the striatum region has a higher uptake value compared with its adjacent areas, voxels with minimal intensity value are more likely to appear on the edge of the SARs. Therefore, the inaccurate delineation of the anatomical boundary as a potential result of the automatic segmentation could not cause a significant decline in the performance of the overall diagnostic framework.

An alternative way to locate SARs for subsequent feature extraction is to apply a pre-labeled PET template by registration. In Section "Advantages of Multi-Modality Images," AAL PET template was used as the PET template, and was registered to PET images for the localization of SARs. Experiments show that the diagnostic capability of this single-modality PET group is worse than the proposed multi-modality framework. Though the single-modality PET approach gives a favorable prediction, the multi-modality approach performs better. This is because the localization of the SARs occupies a significant place in the diagnostic framework, and the additional structural information from MR images can better locate SARs. **Figure 6** demonstrates that the single-modality PET approach might be affected by the erroneous delineation of the SARs. The error could be attributed to the ignored inter-subject variations in brain structures when defining SARs from a PET template.

To test the uniformity of the classifiers based on different segmentation approaches, we trained classifiers using features of manually segmented multi-modality images, and tested it using features of other methods. When testing with features of multi-modality automatic segmentation method, we still obtained 100% accuracy, indicating that the features of manual and automatic segmentation are highly consistent. However, testing with the single-modality method resulted in an accuracy of 88.05%. The lower accuracy might be explained by the lack of adequate extracted features due to the falsely located SARs. Hence, compared with the multi-modality group, single-modality PET group naturally needs more feature engineering and better-designed algorithms.

In the feature extraction, features of *volume* were rejected according to the *t*-test. This could be the reason why the volume of SARs does not change significantly with the progression of PD, as concluded from the literature (Ibarretxe-Bilbao et al., 2011). **Figure 7** shows the heatmaps of feature distribution on the SARs, displaying the influence of each subregion for the classification in the PD/NL task. The difference of influence is expressed by the color scale. One can find that the most relevant region influencing the separation of PD/NL is localized in the middle and rear of the putamen, then the pallidum, and the caudate nucleus reveals the least significance on this task.

Several future studies could be completed explored based on the current pipeline. Firstly, the classifiers can be trained with Parkinsonian disorders (PDS) dataset to classify PD and atypical PDS, such as MSA and Progressive Supranuclear Palsy (PSP), which has important clinical values but is with great challenges. Secondly, this framework only contains medical imaging information currently, while other aspects of information, such as age, gender, motor ratings and other biomarkers are not included, which may further improve the diagnostic accuracy. Future research could be undertaken to incorporate additional multimodal data for better disease prediction. Finally, the sample size of subjects in this work is relatively small, and a bigger dataset is expected to validate our experiment results and improve the performance of the framework.

To conclude, we proposed a fully automatic framework combining the two modalities for PD diagnosis. This framework obtained a promising diagnostic accuracy in the PD/NL task. In addition, this work also emphasized the high value of the ^{11}C-CFT PET in the PD diagnosis.

ETHICS STATEMENT

All data were collected from Department of Neurology, Huashan Hospital, Fudan University, and the study was approved by the Ethics Committee of Huashan Hospital. All subjects or a legally responsible relative were given written informed consent before the study.

AUTHOR CONTRIBUTIONS

XZ is the principle investigator of this work, designed the experiments, and supervised and revised the manuscript. PW co-investigated the research and revised the manuscript. CZ co-investigated the research. JX led the implementation and experiments and wrote the manuscript. YH co-led the work and wrote the manuscript. XiL provided support to the work of coding, experiments, and manuscript writing. FJ, QX, and LL collected the data. XuL collected the data and segmented the striatum of the subjects.

FUNDING

This work was funded by the Science and Technology Commission of Shanghai Municipality Grant (17JC1401600), and the National Natural Science Foundation of China (NSFC) Grant (61971142). Collection of the PD data was supported by the National Natural Science Foundation of China (81671239 and 81361120393).

ACKNOWLEDGMENTS

We thank Lei Li and Yuncheng Zhou, whose dedicated comments helped us to modify the organization of the manuscript and improve its quality.

REFERENCES

Bu, L., Liu, F. T., Jiang, C. F., Guo, S. S., Yu, H., Zuo, C. T., et al. (2018). Patterns of dopamine transporter imaging in subtypes of multiple system atrophy. *Acta Neurol. Scand.* 138, 170–176. doi: 10.1111/ane.12932

Carbon, M., Ma, Y., Barnes, A., Dhawan, V., Chaly, T., Ghilardi, M. F., et al. (2004). Caudate nucleus: influence of dopaminergic input on sequence learning and brain activation in Parkinsonism. *Neuroimage* 21, 1497–1507. doi: 10.1016/j.neuroimage.2003.12.014

Eshuis, S. A., Jager, P. L., Maguire, R. P., Jonkman, S., Dierckx, R. A., and Leenders, K. L. (2009). Direct comparison of FP-CIT SPECT and F-DOPA PET in patients with Parkinson's disease and healthy controls. *Eur. J. Nucl. Med. Mol. Imaging* 36, 454. doi: 10.1007/s00259-008-0989-5

Gray, K. R., Aljabar, P., Heckemann, R. A., Hammers, A., Rueckert, D., and Alzheimer's Disease Neuroimaging Initiative, (2013). Random forest-based similarity measures for multi-modal classification of Alzheimer's disease. *Neuroimage* 65, 167–175. doi: 10.1016/j.neuroimage.2012.09.065

Haller, S., Badoud, S., Nguyen, D., Garibotto, V., Lovblad, K. O., and Burkhard, P. R. (2012). Individual detection of patients with Parkinson disease using support vector machine analysis of diffusion tensor imaging data: initial results. *Am. J. Neuroradiol.* 33, 2123–2128. doi: 10.3174/ajnr.A3126

Huang, C., Tang, C., Feigin, A., Lesser, M., Ma, Y., Pourfar, M., et al. (2007). Changes in network activity with the progression of Parkinson's disease. *Brain* 130, 1834–1846. doi: 10.1093/brain/awm086

Huang, Z. M., Li, L., Xu, Q., Xu, Q., Ge, J., Li, M., et al. (2019). Correlations between dopaminergic dysfunction and abnormal metabolic network activity in REM sleep behavior disorder. *J. Cereb. Blood Flow Metab.* doi: 10.1177/0271678X19828916 [Epub ahead of print].

Ibarretxe-Bilbao, N., Junque, C., Marti, M. J., and Tolosa, E. (2011). Brain structural MRI correlates of cognitive dysfunctions in Parkinson's disease. *J. Neurol. Sci.* 310, 70–74. doi: 10.1016/j.jns.2011.07.054

Ilgin, N., Zubieta, J., Reich, S. G., Dannals, R. F., Ravert, H. T., and Frost, J. J. (1999). PET imaging of the dopamine transporter in progressive supranuclear palsy and Parkinson's disease. *Neurology* 52, 1221–1226.

Kazumata, K., Dhawan, V., Chaly, T., Antonini, A., Margouleff, C., Belakhlef, A., et al. (1998). Dopamine transporter imaging with fluorine-18-FPCIT and PET. *J. Nucl. Med.* 39, 1521.

Kingma, D. P., and Ba, J. (2014). Adam: a method for Stochastic optimization. *arXiv*

Ledig, C., Heckemann, R. A., Hammers, A., Lopez, J. C., Newcombe, V. F. J., Makropoulos, A., et al. (2015). Robust whole-brain segmentation: application to traumatic brain injury. *Med. Image Anal.* 21, 40–58. doi: 10.1016/j.media.2014.12.003

Liu, F. T., Ge, J., Wu, J. J., Wu, P., Ma, Y., Zuo, C. T., et al. (2018). Clinical, dopaminergic, and metabolic correlations in Parkinson disease: a dual-tracer PET study. *Clin. Nucl. Med.* 43, 562–571. doi: 10.1097/RLU.0000000000002148

Long, D., Wang, J., Xuan, M., Gu, Q., Xu, X., Kong, D., et al. (2012). Automatic classification of early Parkinson's disease with multi-modal MR imaging. *PLoS One* 7:e47714. doi: 10.1371/journal.pone.0047714

Ma, Y., Dhawan, V., Mentis, M., Chaly, T., Spetsieris, P. G., and Eidelberg, D. (2002). Parametric mapping of [18F] FPCIT binding in early stage Parkinson's disease: a PET study. *Synapse* 45, 125–133. doi: 10.1002/syn.10090

Mehta, R., and Sivaswamy, J. (2017). "M-net: a convolutional neural network for deep brain structure segmentation," in *Proceedings of the 2017 IEEE 14th International Symposium on Biomedical Imaging (ISBI 2017)*, (Melbourne, VIC: IEEE), 437–440.

Ng, H. P., Ong, S. H., Foong, K. W. C., and Nowinski, W. L. (2006). "Medical image segmentation using k-means clustering and improved watershed algorithm," in *Proceedings of the 2006 IEEE Southwest Symposium on Image Analysis and Interpretation*, (Denver, CO: IEEE), 61–65.

Postuma, R. B., Arnulf, I., Hogl, B., Iranzo, A., Miyamoto, T., Dauvilliers, Y., et al. (2012). A single-question screen for rapid eye movement sleep behavior disorder: a multicenter validation study. *Mov. Disord.* 27, 913–916. doi: 10.1002/mds.25037

Postuma, R. B., Berg, D., Stern, M., Poewe, W., Olanow, C. W., Oertel, W., et al. (2015). MDS clinical diagnostic criteria for Parkinson's disease. *Mov. Disord.* 30, 1591–1601. doi: 10.1002/mds.26424

Ronneberger, O., Fischer, P., and Brox, T. (2015). *U-Net: Convolutional networks for biomedical image segmentation[C]//International Conference on Medical image computing and computer-assisted intervention.* Cham: Springer, 234–241.

Roth, G. A., Abate, D., Abate, K. H., Abay, S. M., Abbafati, C., Abbasi, N., et al. (2018). Global, regional, and national age-sex-specific mortality for 282 causes of death in 195 countries and territories, 1980-2017: a systematic analysis for the Global Burden of Disease Study 2017. *Lancet* 392, 1736–1788. doi: 10.1016/S0140-6736(18)32203-7

Strafella, A. P., Bohnen, N. I., Perlmutter, J. S., Eidelberg, D., Pavese, N., Van Eimeren, T., et al. (2017). Molecular imaging to track Parkinson's disease and atypical parkinsonisms: new imaging frontiers. *Mov. Disord.* 32, 181–192. doi: 10.1002/mds.26907

Wang, J., Hoekstra, J. G., Zuo, C., Cook, T. J., and Zhang, J. (2013). Biomarkers of Parkinson's disease: current status and future perspectives. *Drug Discov. Today* 18, 155–162. doi: 10.1016/j.drudis.2012.09.001

Wong, K. C. L., Moradi, M., Tang, H., and Syeda-Mahmood, T. (2018). *3D segmentation with exponential logarithmic loss for highly unbalanced object sizes[C]//International Conference on Medical Image Computing and Computer-Assisted Intervention.* Cham: Springer, 612–619.

Zhuang, X., Arridge, S., Hawkes, D. J., and Ourselin, S. (2011). A nonrigid registration framework using spatially encoded mutual information and free-form deformations. *IEEE Trans. Med. Imaging* 30, 1819–1828. doi: 10.1109/TMI.2011.2150240

10

Analysis of Progression Toward Alzheimer's Disease Based on Evolutionary Weighted Random Support Vector Machine Cluster

Xia-an Bi[1], Qian Xu[1], Xianhao Luo[2], Qi Sun[1] and Zhigang Wang[1]*

[1] *College of Information Science and Engineering, Hunan Normal University, Changsha, China,* [2] *College of Mathematics and Statistics, Hunan Normal University, Changsha, China*

***Correspondence:**
Xia-an Bi
bixiaan@hnu.edu.cn

Alzheimer's disease (AD) could be described into following four stages: healthy control (HC), early mild cognitive impairment (EMCI), late MCI (LMCI) and AD dementia. The discriminations between different stages of AD are considerably important issues for future pre-dementia treatment. However, it is still challenging to identify LMCI from EMCI because of the subtle changes in imaging which are not noticeable. In addition, there were relatively few studies to make inferences about the brain dynamic changes in the cognitive progression from EMCI to LMCI to AD. Inspired by the above problems, we proposed an advanced approach of evolutionary weighted random support vector machine cluster (EWRSVMC). Where the predictions of numerous weighted SVM classifiers are aggregated for improving the generalization performance. We validated our method in multiple binary classifications using Alzheimer's Disease Neuroimaging Initiative dataset. As a result, the encouraging accuracy of 90% for EMCI/LMCI and 88.89% for LMCI/AD were achieved respectively, demonstrating the excellent discriminating ability. Furthermore, disease-related brain regions underlying the AD progression could be found out on the basis of the amount of discriminative information. The findings of this study provide considerable insight into the neurophysiological mechanisms in AD development.

Keywords: Alzheimer's disease progression, functional connectivity, classification, disease-related brain regions, evolutionary weighted random support vector machine cluster

INTRODUCTION

Alzheimer's disease (AD) is a devastating neuro-cognitive disorder of the human brain (Keren-Shaul et al., 2017; Kodis et al., 2018), which is characterized by the progressive loss of cognition and memory in elderly adults (Roy et al., 2016). Along with the aging of global population, the number of individuals suffering from AD will increase (Novak et al., 2017). It is predicted that there will be more than 100 million elderly people worldwide affected by AD by 2050 (Cortes-Canteli et al., 2015; Branca and Oddo, 2017). Therefore, the identification of AD and particularly its transitional phase, namely mild cognitive impairment (MCI), have received increasingly growing attentions in recent years (Cui et al., 2018). The individuals diagnosed with MCI could be further subdivided into the early MCI (EMCI) and late MCI (LMCI) (Lee et al., 2017) and the distinguishing criterions for EMCI and LMCI have been previously depicted in Alzheimer's Disease Neuroimaging Initiative (ADNI) cohort (Nuttall et al., 2016). At present, there is still no therapy to prevent or reverse the AD pathological process (Forster et al., 2017). It is hence important to develop a new approach that could identify different stages of AD to enhance the understanding of AD pathophysiological progression, which is helpful to the preclinical AD studies.

A great deal of neuroimaging techniques could be utilized to image human brain function and structure, e.g., diffusion tensor imaging (DTI), magnetic resonance spectroscopy (MRS), electroencephalogram (EEG), functional magnetic resonance imaging (fMRI), and so on (Busato et al., 2016; Thanh Vu et al., 2017). Due to the advantages of high temporal and spatial resolutions, fMRI especially resting-state fMRI have gained increasingly growing popularities in the investigation of the whole-brain neural connectivity recently (Goense et al., 2016). As an advanced brain imaging technology, resting-state fMRI has shown a great potential in providing comprehensive information to achieve a high level of identification of the neurological diseases (Phillips, 2012; Rosa et al., 2015). Accordingly, the application of non-invasive resting-state fMRI is highly advantageous to unfold the complexity of brain connectivity network and examine the brain dynamic changes from EMCI to LMCI to AD.

Machine learning (ML) technologies were extensively used in automatic pattern recognition based on imaging data (dos Santos Siqueira et al., 2014; Moradi et al., 2015; Wang et al., 2018; Zeng et al., 2018). In existing literature, there has been a widespread interest to utilize ML methods to classify different stages of AD. Nozadi et al. (2018) employed a random forest (RF) algorithm based on the whole-brain approach to achieve the accuracies of 72.5 and 81.7% for 164 EMCI versus 189 LMCI and 189 LMCI versus 99 AD respectively. Goryawala et al. (2015) reported the accuracies of 73.6 and 90.1% for 114 EMCI versus 91 LMCI and 91 LMCI versus 55 AD using the linear discriminant analysis (LDA). Jie et al. (2018) utilized the multi-kernel SVM and displayed a high accuracy of 78.8% classifying 56 EMCI from 43 LMCI. It is noteworthy that the discrimination between EMCI and LMCI is more challenging in comparison to LMCI and AD.

In order to improve the classification performances especially of EMCI and LMCI, and enhance the understanding of neuropathology in the AD progression, a new method of evolutionary weighted random SVM cluster (EWRSVMC) was presented in this paper to diagnose different stages of AD. The EWRSVMC combined multiple weighted SVM classifiers to make the final decision, which was believed to be considerably stable and robust compared to other individual classifiers such as artificial neural network and decision tree. In addition, the EWRSVMC employed a method of evolution to guide feature selection to explore the optimal feature set for better classification performance. We performed the experiment 1 for EMCI/LMCI classification and the experiment 2 for LMCI/AD classification, yielding high accuracies of 90 and 88.89% respectively using this new framework. Furthermore, the disease-related brain regions were ranked according to the corresponding optimal features' frequencies and the top-ranked brain regions could be found out. On the one hand, several high-frequency brain regions [e.g., superior temporal gyrus (STG.R), insula (INS.L) and middle temporal gyrus (MTG.L)] are presented in the two groups of experiments at the same time, which suggested that these brain regions play crucial roles in the progression of AD. On the other hand, some brain areas displayed high frequencies only in one group of experiment [e.g., superior frontal gyrus (SFGmed.L) and olfactory cortex (OLF.R) in the experiment 1, and parahippocampal gyrus (PHG.L) and posterior cingulate gyrus (PCG.L) in the experiment 2], which facilitated to understand differences in disease progression. These findings are in agreement with the claims of the previous studies on AD (Douaud et al., 2013; Xiang et al., 2013; Zhu et al., 2014) and provide a novel perspective to AD progression's neurophysiological mechanisms.

MATERIALS AND METHODS

Subjects

The neuroimaging data we utilized in this study came from the ADNI cohort[1] (Morris et al., 2014). We collected the resting-state fMRI data of 105 participants, which contained 42 EMCI patients (18 male, average age 72.34 years), 38 LMCI patients (23 male, average age 72.99 years) and 25 AD subjects (12 male, average age 74.59 years). Every participant had clinical dementia rating (CDR) scores and mini-mental state examination (MMSE) scores to ensure that the data was homologous. Chi-squared test was utilized for gender comparisons and two-sample *t*-test was utilized for age, MMSE and CDR comparisons. The detailed demographic information for the patient cohorts was listed in **Table 1**.

All participants were asked to lie still in a Siemens TRIO 3 Tesla machine using the same scanning parameters as follows: 64 × 64 acquisition matrix; flip angle = 80°; echo time (TE) / repetition time (TR) =30/3000 ms; pixel spacing Y/pixel spacing X = 3.3/3.3mm; 140 image volumes; 48 axial slices; 3.313 mm slice thickness with no gap. During the scan, all participants should close eyes but keep awake with thinking of nothings (Liu et al., 2018).

Data Preprocessing

The same image preprocessing for EMCI, LMCI and AD patients was performed by utilizing the Data Processing

[1] http://adni.loni.usc.edu/

TABLE 1 | Demographic information.

Variable (Mean ± SD)	EMCI	LMCI	AD	*P*-value
Male/Female	18/24	23/15	12/13	0.11[a]/0.33[b]
Age	72.34 ± 6.87	72.99 ± 7.79	74.59 ± 7.03	0.69[a]/0.41[b]
MMSE	28.10 ± 1.57	27.11 ± 2.44	21.24 ± 3.44	0.03[a]/0.00[b]
CDR	0.45 ± 0.22	0.54 ± 0.14	0.92 ± 0.31	0.04[a]/0.00[b]

[a] *The P-value of the comparison between the EMCI and LMCI.* [b] *The P-value of the comparison between the LMCI and AD.*

Assistant for Resting State fMRI (DPARSF) toolbox (Dan et al., 2017). Briefly, the data was preprocessed in nine steps: converting the data into NIFTI format; exclusion of the first 10 volumes; slice-timing correction; realignment for head movement compensation; normalization; smoothing (utilizing a Gaussian kernel); removing linear trend; temporal band-pass filtering; 9) regressing out the nuisance signals.

Functional Connectivity Features

The brain is a dynamic system constructed by large-scale complex networks comprised of the connections between different brain regions (Braun et al., 2015). In this paper, we employ a popular automated anatomical labeling template (Rolls et al., 2015) to divide the cerebrum into 90 brain areas (45 for left and right hemisphere respectively). A representative resting-state fMRI signal for each brain region is generated by averaging the time series of voxels within each of 90 brain regions. The Pearson correlation coefficient between the representative signals of each pair of the brain regions is computed and treated as a proxy of functional connectivity (FC) (Noble et al., 2017). As a result, a total of 4005 ($80 \times 90/2$) FCs are obtained for each subject and served as predictor features for the proposed EWRSVMC algorithm, which is considered to be a promising approach.

The Evolutionary Weighted Random SVM Cluster

EWRSVMC Design

Machine learning techniques are widely used for pattern recognition (Zeng et al., 2017), among which the SVM model has received increasing popularities in the analysis of neurological disease based on the high-dimensional imaging data recently. Nevertheless, utilizing the single SVM classifier is too challenging to achieve excellent diagnostic performance due to the noise of brain imaging data. Bi et al. (2018) put forward a random SVM cluster (RSVMC) in which multiple SVM classifiers are combined for a final decision-making, which outperforms an individual SVM classifier. But, it could not be ignored that the diagnostic power of each individual classifier in the ensemble classifier may be greatly differential from others. The previous method of RSVMC ignores the fact that the individual SVM classifier with relatively high training error is likely to perform wrong voting on the new samples, which is likely to degrade the discriminative ability. Accordingly, there still remains room for the improvement with respect to the RSVMC method.

This paper presents a novel algorithm of EWRSVMC with two successive steps, i.e., the construction and evolution of weighted ensemble of SVMs respectively. First, in order to reduce the influence of the weak classifiers on the voting, the classification accuracy of each SVM classifier is calculated using the validation set, which is regarded as a proxy of weight of every SVM classifier. The output of EWRSVMC is a weighted average of the outputs of multiple SVMs, which could further reduce classification error rate. Second, in order to select out the most discriminative features from a large-scale feature vector, the method of evolution is introduced to dynamically eliminate the redundant features for further improving final classification performance. The idea of our proposed architecture is showed in **Figure 1**, where each row and column corresponds to a subject and feature respectively in the left data matrixes.

We suppose $X = \{x_1, ...x_k, ...x_n\} \in R^{N \times d}$ as the connectivity features vectors where N and d are the numbers of all subjects and features. $y_i \in \{+1, -1\}$ is the response class label representing two different states (e.g., EMCL or LMCI). The construction of the weighted random SVM cluster is performed using the following steps:

(1) Stepl: The available dataset X is divided into two data subset, i.e., a "training and validation" set and a test set respectively.
(2) Step2: Then, the training subset and feature subset are respectively obtained by randomly selecting partial samples from above "training and validation" set and partial features from total features to build an individual SVM model.
(3) Step3: The remaining validation subset is utilized for the estimation of diagnostic accuracy W_l of l-th SVM, which is considered as a proxy of weight of the SVM.

$$W_l = \frac{T_l^{correct}}{T_L} \tag{1}$$

where $T_l^{correct}$ denotes the number of validation samples correctly classified by l-th SVM classifier, T_L represents the number of validation samples.
(4) Step4: The step 2 to step 4 are repeated for n times to build a weighted ensemble of n SVM classifiers.

Following the above steps, a weighted ensemble of multiple SVM classifiers could be constructed and then an approach of evolution is applied to the ensemble classifier to guide feature selection.

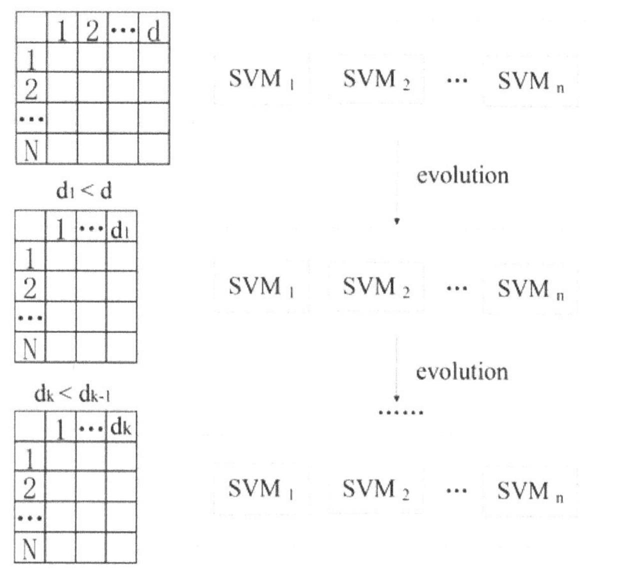

FIGURE 1 | The idea of our proposed EWRSVMC.

Specifically, the SVM classifiers whose classification accuracies are lower than 0.5 are first picked out from the weighted random SVM cluster and considered as weak classifiers. Similarly, the remaining SVM classifiers are regarded as strong classifiers due to the good performance. Then the features selected by these weak classifiers are found out and the weights corresponding to the common features are accumulated. The total weight of each feature in weak classifiers is denoted as Tw_j:

$$Tw_j = \sum_{l=1}^{p} w_{l,j} \tag{2}$$

where p is the number of weak classifiers; $w_{l,j}$ represents the weight of the j-th feature corresponding to l-th weak classifier.

Next, we remove the features whose total weight Tw_j exceeds a certain threshold q, because these features play crucial roles in the weak classifiers and are likely to make few contributions to the excellent performance of the overall system. As a result, we obtain the remaining features with lower total weights in the weak classifiers and all the features determined by the strong classifiers as an evolutionary feature set, leading to the reduced dimensionality of total feature space. Finally, the above-obtained evolutionary feature set is employed to rebuild a weighted random SVM cluster for the further reduction of feature dimensionality. This procedure is repeated iteratively until it reaches the times of evolutions we set. The optimal EWRSVMC with the highest accuracy during the evolution process could be found out and the features determined by this optimal EWRSVMC are considered as the optimal feature set. The feature selection procedure of the EWRSVMC is exhibited in **Figure 2**.

The Evaluation of the EWRSVMC

The EWRSVMC perform a weighted average of the outputs of multiple SVM classifiers, which could predict the class label of each new testing sample. To be specific, a new sample is firstly input into a EWRSVMC system and each individual SVM classifier performs a weighted vote in accordance with its accuracy dealing with the validation samples. Then the weighted voting values belonging to the same predicted label are added up. Lastly, the label having the highest voting value represents new sample's final predicted label.

In this paper, we employ the three metrics, i.e., accuracy, sensitivity and specificity to estimate our proposed EWRSVMC's final performances. The diagnostic accuracy A_c stands for a fraction of correctly identified samples (Schröder et al., 2015):

$$A_c = \frac{TP + TN}{TP + FP + FN + TN} \tag{3}$$

where TP, FP, FN, and TN respectively represents the number of true positives, false positives, false negatives and true negatives.

Sensitivity (S_n) stands for a proportion of actual positive samples which are correctly identified (Mondal and Pai, 2014):

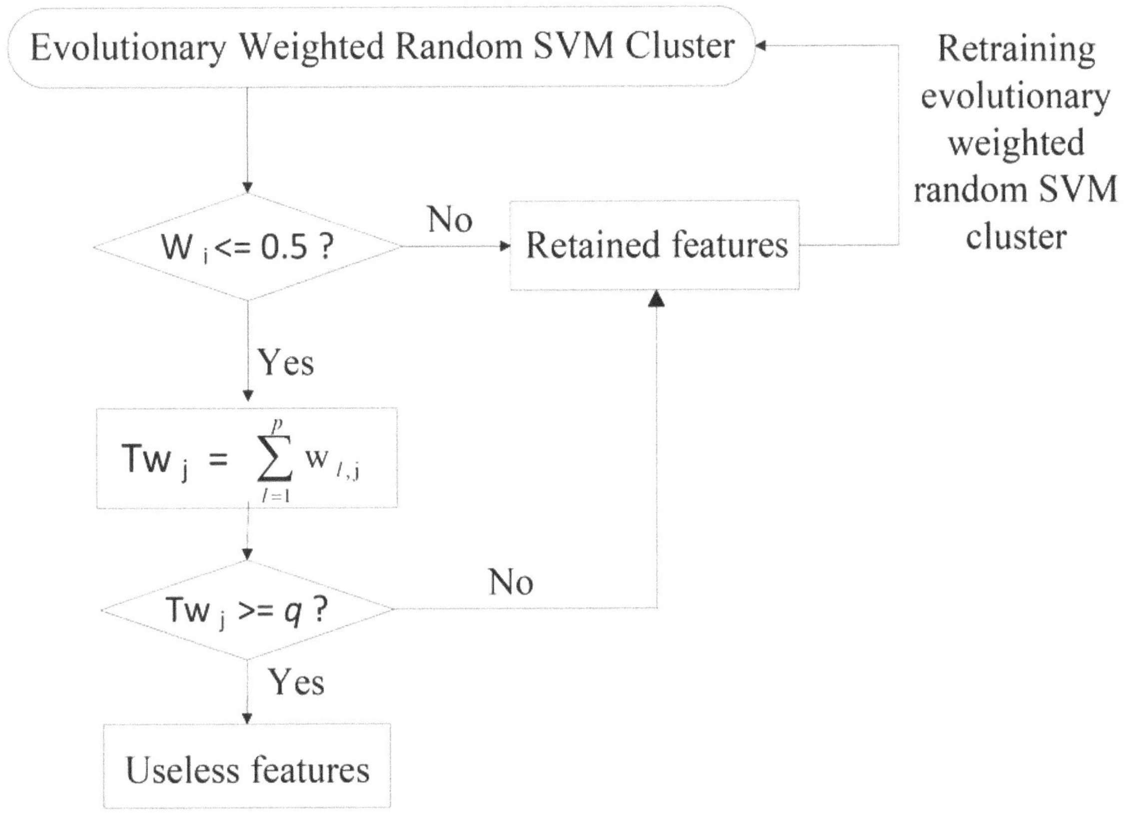

FIGURE 2 | Feature selection procedure of the EWRSVMC.

$$S_n = \frac{TP}{TP + FN} \quad (4)$$

Specificity (S_p) stands for a proportion of actual negative samples which are correctly identified (Kumar and Helenprabha, 2017):

$$S_p = \frac{TN}{TN + FP} \quad (5)$$

The Application of the EWRSVMC

In the current study, we conducted multiple binary classifications, including EMCI vs. LMCI and LMCI vs. AD to confirm the performance of our proposed EWRSVMC using 4005 FCs as the raw features. In addition to optimizing the classification accuracy as with most existing studies, we also paid great attentions to exploring and analyzing the alterations of the brain in patients with different cognitive stages of AD. Accordingly, another sub-procedure for the exploration of the disease-related brain regions using the optimal features set was carried out. First, we detected the brain regions which are relevant to the optimal features in the EWRSVMC with the highest classification accuracy. Then, disease-related brain regions were sorted in a descending mode, which is consistent with their occurrence frequencies. The higher the frequencies are, the greater the abnormal degrees of the brain regions are.

Experiment Design

In this paper, we conducted the experiment 1 for EMCI vs. LMCI classification and the experiment 2 for LMCI vs. AD classification. Each group of experiment could be mainly divided into four parts:

(1) Division of data sets. A 3:1 ratio is set to divide entire resting-state data set into the "training and validation" set for training the EWRSVMC and the test set for examining the generalization ability of the overall system. Furthermore, a 2:1 ratio is set to subdivide the "training and validation" set into the training set for training the SVM classifier and the validation set for obtaining the weight corresponding to the SVM classifier.

(2) Building an ERWSVMC. Firstly, we randomly select $\sqrt{4005} \approx 62$ features from all 4005 features based on the training set to build a radial basis function (RBF) kernel SVM classifier. The kernel bandwidth σ and penalty parameter C for each SVM model are primarily set as 3 and Inf respectively. The number of initial base classifiers is set to 500 to get the weighted ensemble of SVMs. Then, we make the ensemble classifier evolves for 50 times. In each evolution, we find out the features selected by the weak classifiers and remove the features whose total weight Tw_j exceeding the certain threshold $q = 7$. As a result, the EWRSVMCs with different evolution times are obtained.

(3) Finding out the optimal subset of features. We compute the diagnostic accuracies of the EWRSVMCs with different evolution times. The features selected by the optimal EWRSVMC having the lowest diagnostic error rate form the optimal features subset.

(4) Exploring the abnormal brain regions. We seek out the features with high discriminative ability in the optimal EWRSVMC, and then investigate the corresponding disease-related brain regions associated with these features.

RESULTS

The Experiment 1

We investigated the performance of classification between EMCI and LMCI in the experiment 1. According to Section "Experiment Design," we conducted 50 evolutions for the EWRSVMC. Consequently, the EWRSVMC yielded a maximum accuracy of 90% in the 32nd evolution (as shown in **Figure 3**), which suggested that 32 was the optimal times of evolutions. Meanwhile, a sensitivity of 90.9% and a specificity of 88.89% were achieved based on the optimal feature set. The experiment results showed that the novel framework could significantly enhance diagnostic performance for EMCI/LMCI classification in compared with some other existing algorithms.

Feature selection was a crucial stage in our EWRSVMC algorithm classifying LMCI from EMCI and the process was shown in **Figure 4**. On the one hand, the number of removed features increased rapidly and exceeded 100 after two evolutions. Then it became gradually stable and fluctuated around 120. On the other hand, the number of remained features showed a trend of linear decline. There were 248 features left after completing the 32nd evolution, which constituted the optimal feature set and were utilized for subsequent study on the exploration of disease-related brain regions.

By counting the high-frequency FCs, we could detect the most discriminative brain regions which were ranked in the **Table 2**. The brain regions exceeding the frequency of 10 comprise inferior temporal gyrus (ITG.R), temporal pole: middle temporal gyrus (TPOmid.L), temporal pole: superior temporal gyrus (TPOsup.R), middle temporal gyrus (MTG.L) and insula (INS.L). As seen from **Table 2**, some sub-regions of the temporal lobe showed higher frequencies compared to other regions, indicating the temporal lobe made an essential contribution to the evolution from EMCI to LMCI. The locations of brain regions were mapped in **Figure 5** and the size of the red node

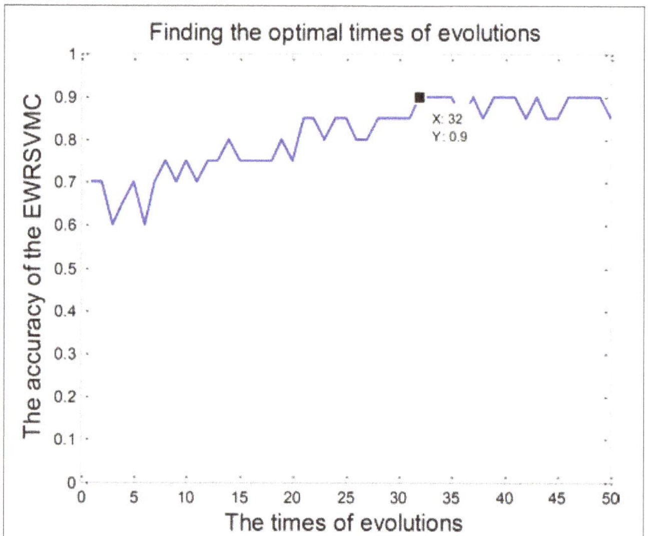

FIGURE 3 | Finding the optimal times of evolutions in the experiment 1.

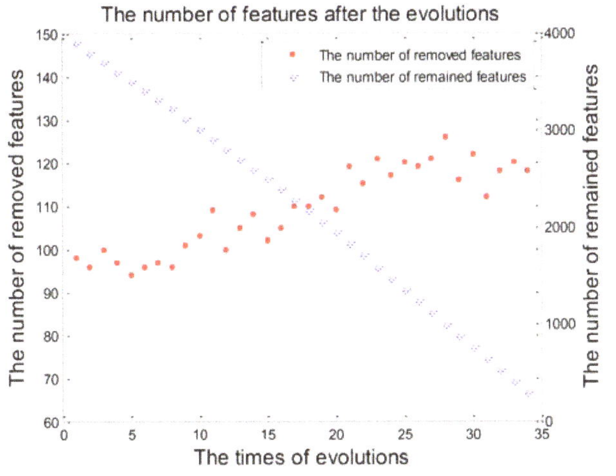

FIGURE 4 | The number of features after each evolution in the experiment 1.

TABLE 2 | The frequencies of the most discriminative brain regions in the experiment 1.

Frequency	Brain region
15	ITG.R
14	TPOmid.L
12	TPOsup.R MTG.L
11	INS.L
10	SFGmed.L PAL.R
9	OLF.R ITG.L

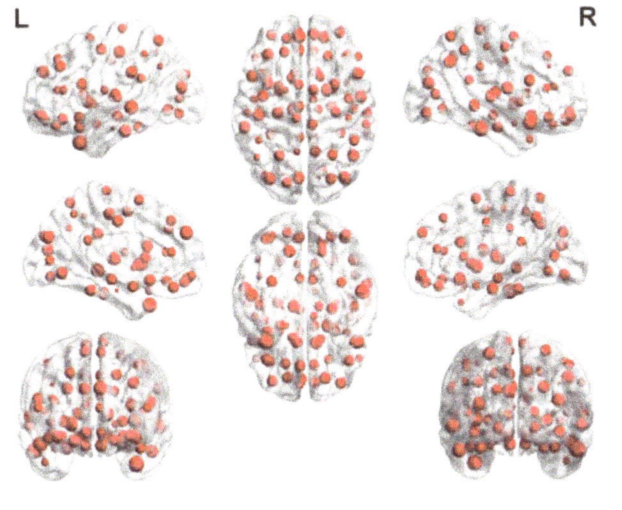

FIGURE 5 | The locations of abnormal brain regions in the experiment 1.

represented the degree of abnormality of the corresponding brain regions.

The Experiment 2

The classification of patients with LMCI and AD was carried out in the experiment 2. Similarly, 50 evolutions were performed and the EWRSVMC reported the highest accuracy of 88.89% in the 34nd evolution (please see **Figure 6**), which indicated that 34 was the optimal times of evolutions in LMCI/AD classification. At the same time, the optimal EWRSVMC achieved 85.71% sensitivity and 90.9% specificity. The encouraging performances demonstrated the potential of our new framework for the diagnosis of AD dementia.

The process of feature selection in LMCI/AD classification was plotted in **Figure 7**. The number of removed features showed an overall upward trend, while the number of remained features exhibited a trend of linear decline. There were 293 features left after finishing the 34th evolution, which formed the optimal feature set for the further analysis of progression from LMCI to AD.

We were able to explore the most discriminative brain regions by counting the high-frequency FCs. The disease-related

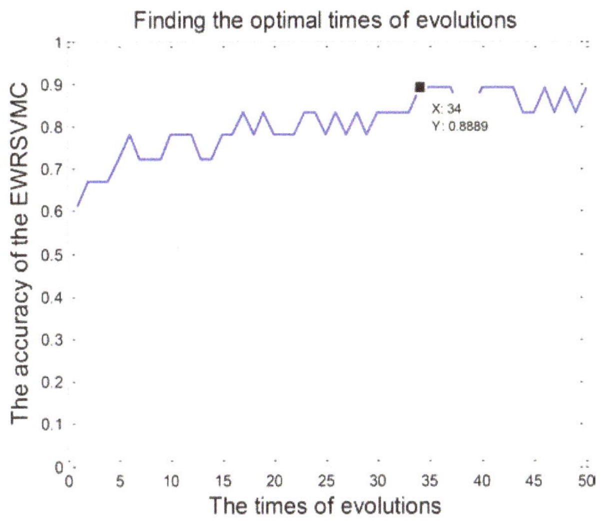

FIGURE 6 | Finding the optimal times of evolutions in the experiment 2.

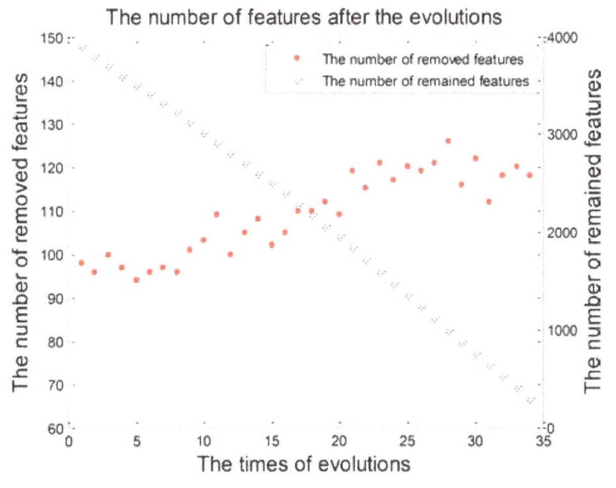

FIGURE 7 | The numbers of features after each evolution in the experiment 2.

brain regions in LMCI/AD classification were ranked in the **Table 3** and the ones exceeding the frequency of 10 were listed as follows: superior temporal gyrus (STG.R), parahippocampal gyrus (PHG.L), middle frontal gyrus, orbital part (ORBmid.R), calcarine fissure and surrounding cortex (CAL.R), insula (INS.L), temporal pole: middle temporal gyrus (TPOmid.R), and posterior cingulate gyrus (PCG.L). Similarly, some subregions of the temporal lobe and insula showed higher frequencies than other brain regions, suggesting the temporal lobe and insula made greater contributions to the evolution of AD. **Figure 8** described the locations of brain regions.

DISCUSSION

Classification Effect

In this paper, we propose an advanced framework of EWRSVMC based on resting-state fMRI data to accurately classify different stages of AD. Resting-state fMRI is an effective tool for exploring the dynamical changes in human brain because of the high temporal and spatial resolutions (Lee M.H. et al., 2016). In addition, to the best of our knowledge, no investigation is available about the EWRSVMC in AD studies using brain imaging data. The EWRSVMC is able to efficiently perform EMCI/LMCI and LMCI/AD classifications with the high accuracies of 90 and 88.89%, sensitivities of 90.9 and 85.71%, specificities of 88.89 and 90.9% respectively. The results of two groups of experiments demonstrate the availability of novel EWRSVMC algorithm for early detection of AD and the potential of resting-state fMRI for identification of the transition from EMCI to LMCI to AD.

TABLE 3 | The frequencies of the most discriminative brain regions in the experiment 2.

Frequency	Brain region
14	STG.R
13	PHG.L
12	ORBmid.R
11	CAL.R INS.L TPOmid.R PCG.L
10	ACG.R FFG.L TPOsup.L MTG.L

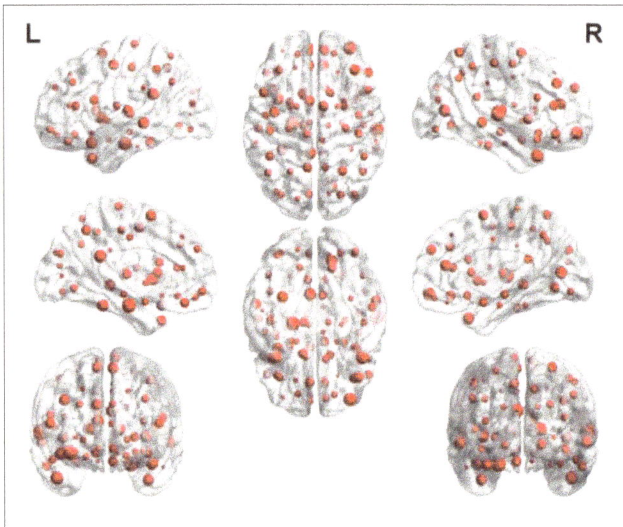

FIGURE 8 | The locations of brain regions in the experiment 2.

The ML techniques have received increasingly growing attentions recently in imaging data (Zeng et al., 2014; Wang et al., 2017), and have been shown to be a reliable method to diagnose different cognitive stages of AD using neuroimaging data. Jiang et al. (2014) achieved a high accuracy around 80% for 56 EMCI versus 44 LMCI combining a sparse learning with the SVM classifier. Prasad et al. (2015) reported the accuracy of 63.4% for 74 EMCI vs. 38 LMCI using the SVM classifier with the feature set of the fiber network measures (FIN) and the flow network measures (FLN). Mahjoub et al. (2018) combined the proposed deep similarity network architectures with the single SVM classifier utilizing the cross-validation method to classify 41 AD from 36 LMCI with a classification accuracy peaking at 77.92%.

The majority of ML methods had the slightly lower classification performances especially classifying EMCI from LMCI because of image noise and small-sample size of data. In addition, a great deal of studies have paid more attention to the classification but rarely explored disease-related brain regions underlying the AD evolution. To address these issues, a new framework of EWRSVMC using the FCs as the raw features was presented in this paper. The output of EWRSVMC is a weighted average of the outputs of SVMs, which could further reduce classification error rate compared to some previous methodologies. Additionally, Due to the high dimensionality of feature space, the complexity of the algorithm is likely to be increased and the performance of model estimation is degraded. Accordingly, a method of evolution is employed to dynamically eliminate the redundant features and the features in the optimal EWRSVMC are regarded as the optimal features. Moreover, disease-related brain regions could be found out by identifying these features with high discriminative ability, which provides new insights in the pathology of AD.

The issue of overfitting is a major concern in the training process of our EWRSMC algorithm and more details about it are discussed here. In order to building an individual SVM classifier in EWRSVMC, the training set was randomly chosen out from the all experimental dataset and 62 FCs was randomly chosen out from total 4005 FCs as input features. Because of the randomness of samples and features, each SVM base classifier is greatly different from others, which could reduce the effects of overfitting. Furthermore, the EWRSVMC shows a good classification performance in the test set, suggesting a low risk of overfitting phenomenon.

In our proposed EWRSVMC, two hyperparameters, namely the penalty parameter C and the kernel bandwidth σ, need to be determined. Initially, we set parameter C and σ to *Inf* and 3 to train the individual RBF-SVM classifier. For comparison, we tested different values for C and σ and found no considerable changes in terms of the classification performances of the EWRSVMC, suggesting that the proposed EWRSVMC is considerably robust and universal.

Analysis of Higher-Frequency Brain Regions

In this part, we mainly discussed about four abnormal brain regions, i.e., temporal lobe, insula, superior frontal gyrus, and parahippocampal gyrus respectively.

The Temporal Lobe

Some subregions of the temporal lobe had relatively greater frequencies in both EMCI/LMCI and LMCI/AD classifications, indicating that the temporal lobe is likely to play a crucial role in AD progression. The temporal lobe is situated beneath the lateral sulcus on both hemispheres of the human cerebrum (Kiernan, 2012), which is known to be associated with visual memory, language comprehension, emotion association and executive function (Riley et al., 2010; Bell et al., 2011).

Several previous studies have reported the abnormal temporal lobe in AD progression. Younes et al. (2014) found that the volume of medial temporal lobe structures were relevant to time of progress from MCI to AD. Davatzikos et al. (2011) observed the positive baseline Spatial Pattern of Abnormalities for Recognition of Early AD in temporal lobe in patients with MCI who progressed to AD dementia. Stein et al. (2010) observed the temporal lobe volume differences in brain MRI scans of AD patients, MCI patients and healthy elderly participants. Douaud et al. (2013) found that the cerebral atrophy in medial temporal lobe was vulnerable to the AD progression. Blasko et al. (2008) reported the changes of medial temporal lobe atrophy (MTA) through the evolution from cognitive health to MCI and to AD in a prospective cohort of subjects aged 75 years. The discovery of abnormal temporal lobe may help to improve the understanding of AD progression.

The Insula

The insula had a relatively higher frequency than other brain regions in both EMCI/LMCI and LMCI/AD classifications as well, indicating that the insula may make a great contribution in the progression of AD. The insula is a crucial hub of the human brain networks and is folded deep in the floor of lateral sulcus (Cauda et al., 2011). It is reported that the human insula is involved in perception, motor control, general cognition and self-awareness (Kang et al., 2011; Chang et al., 2013).

The insula abnormality was reported in numerous previous literatures in AD pathology. Xie et al. (2012) found out the altered functional integration of the insula networks in AD development. Zhu et al. (2014) observed the significantly greater gray matter volume loss in the bilateral insula in the progression of conversion from HC to MCI to AD with a linear trend. Sojkova et al. (2008) reported the longitudinal alterations in regional cerebral blood flow which involved insula and superior temporal regions in AD progression. Hafkemeijer et al. (2012) mentioned that the patients diagnosed with AD exhibited extensive decreases in gray matter volume in insula and temporal lobe. Patel et al. (2013) reported that the default mode network (DMN) regions, e.g., insula and superior temporal gyrus, were significantly affected by AD pathology. The discovery of the insula abnormality may help to illuminate the underlying neuromechanism of AD disorder.

The Superior Frontal Gyrus

The superior frontal gyrus possessed a relatively higher frequency compared to other brain regions in the EMCI/LMCI classification, suggesting that the superior frontal gyrus made an important contribution to the evolution from EMCI to LMCI. The superior frontal gyrus (SFG) is situated at the frontal lobe' superior part and makes up about one third of the prefrontal cortex of the human brain (Li et al., 2013). It has been reported that the superior frontal gyrus is associated with motor functions and cognitive control especially execution within working memory (Chiao et al., 2009; Van den Stock et al., 2011).

We have reviewed a great deal of previous literature about EMCI and LMCI, and found that there were relatively few studies to make inferences about the brain dynamic differences in the cognitive process from EMCI to LMCI. Accordingly, the discovery of abnormal superior frontal gyrus could be clinically helpful for early detection of AD evolution at MCI stage. Lee E.S. et al. (2016) showed the decreased FC in the right superior frontal gurus in patients with LMCI compared with EMCI, which was agreement with our finding.

The Parahippocampal Gyrus

The parahippocampal gyrus obtained a higher frequency in 90 brain regions in the LMCI/AD classification, indicating that the parahippocampal gyrus acted a crucial part in the evolution from LMCI to AD. The parahippocampal gyrus is a part of the limbic system (Enatsu et al., 2015; Arnone et al., 2016), which is involved in the memory encoding and retrieval (Puri et al., 2012; Monti et al., 2018).

Several previous studies have reported the parahippocampal gyrus abnormality in AD pathology. Liang et al. (2014) found out the altered amplitude of low-frequency fluctuations in right parahippocampal gyrus from LMCI and AD. Xiang et al. (2013) reported that AD patients showed less activity than MCI patients in the right parahippocampal gyrus during a visual memory task. Yetkin et al. (2006) mentioned that the AD group had less activation in bilateral parahippocampal gyri than the MCI group in a memory-encoding task. Echávarri et al. (2011) found out the significant differences of volumes of the parahippocampal gyrus between the groups with the following order: AD < aMCI < healthy. The discovery of parahippocampal gyrus abnormality may provide assistant for clinical diagnosis of early AD.

Limitations

The current study is limited by the following two factors. Firstly, we utilized one modality, i.e., RS-fMRI for multiple binary classifications. Nevertheless, there exist other modalities [e.g., cerebrospinal fluid (CSF) and positron emission tomography (PET)] which may also contain commentary information for better classification performance. Secondly, it is crucial to visualize the learned decision process for better understanding the classification approach and gaining clinical insights. However, as with most previous AD classification algorithms, the visualization of the learned decision process in our proposed EWRSVMC is not informative, which is still a limitation which is expected to be addressed in the future.

ETHICS STATEMENT

This study was carried out in accordance with the recommendations of National Institute of Aging-Alzheimer's Association (NIA-AA) workgroup guidelines, Institutional Review Board (IRB). The study was approved by IRB of each participating site, including the Banner Alzheimer's Institute, and was conducted in accordance with Federal Regulations, the Internal Conference on Harmonization (ICH), and Good Clinical Practices (GCP).

AUTHOR CONTRIBUTIONS

X-aB proposed the design of the work and revised it critically for important intellectual content. QX and QS carried out the experiment for the work and drafted part of the work. XL and ZW collected, interpreted the data, and drafted part of the work. All the authors approved the final version to be published and agreed to be accountable for all aspects of the work in ensuring that questions related to the accuracy or integrity of any part of the work are appropriately investigated and resolved.

FUNDING

This work was supported by the National Natural Science Foundation of China (No. 61502167).

REFERENCES

Arnone, D., Job, D., Selvaraj, S., Abe, O., Amico, F., Cheng, Y., et al. (2016). Computational meta-analysis of statistical parametric maps in major depression. *Hum. Brain Mapp.* 37, 1393–1404. doi: 10.1002/hbm.23108

Bell, B., Lin, J. J., Seidenberg, M., and Hermann, B. (2011). The neurobiology of cognitive disorders in temporal lobe epilepsy. *Nat. Rev. Neurol.* 7, 154–164. doi: 10.1038/nrneurol.2011.3

Bi, X.-A., Wang, Y., Shu, Q., Sun, Q., and Xu, Q. (2018). Classification of autism spectrum disorder using random support vector machine cluster. *Front. Genet.* 9:18. doi: 10.3389/fgene.2018.00018

Blasko, I., Jellinger, K., Kemmler, G., Krampla, W., Jungwirth, S., Wichart, I., et al. (2008). Conversion from cognitive health to mild cognitive impairment and Alzheimer's disease: prediction by plasma amyloid beta 42, medial temporal lobe atrophy and homocysteine. *Neurobiol. Aging* 29, 1–11. doi: 10.1016/j.neurobiolaging.2006.09.002

Branca, C., and Oddo, S. (2017). Paving the way for new clinical trials for Alzheimer's Disease. *Biol. Psychiatry* 81, 88–89. doi: 10.1016/j.biopsych.2016.10.016

Braun, U., Schäfer, A., Walter, H., Erk, S., Romanczuk-Seiferth, N., Haddad, L., et al. (2015). Dynamic reconfiguration of frontal brain networks during executive cognition in humans. *Proc. Natl. Acad. Sci. U.S.A.* 112, 11678–11683. doi: 10.1073/pnas.1422487112

Busato, A., Feruglio, P. F., Parnigotto, P. P., Marzola, P., and Sbarbati, A. (2016). In Vivo imaging techniques: a new era for histochemical analysis. *Eur. J. Histochem.* 60:2725. doi: 10.4081/ejh.2016.2725

Cauda, F., D'Agata, F., Sacco, K., Duca, S., Geminiani, G., and Vercelli, A. (2011). Functional connectivity of the insula in the resting brain. *Neuroimage* 55, 8–23. doi: 10.1016/j.neuroimage.2010.11.049

Chang, L. J., Yarkoni, T., Khaw, M. W., and Sanfey, A. G. (2013). Decoding the role of the insula in human cognition: functional parcellation and large-scale reverse inference. *Cereb. Cortex* 23, 739–749. doi: 10.1093/cercor/bhs065

Chiao, J. Y., Harada, T., Komeda, H., Li, Z., Mano, Y., Saito D., et al. (2009). Neural basis of individualistic and collectivistic views of self. *Hum. Brain Mapp.* 30, 2813–2820. doi: 10.1002/hbm.20707

Cortes-Canteli, M., Mattei, L., Richards, A. T., Norris, E. H., and Strickland, S. (2015). Fibrin deposited in the Alzheimer's disease brain promotes neuronal degeneration. *Neurobiol. Aging* 36, 608–617. doi: 10.1016/j.neurobiolaging.2014.10.030

Cui, X., Xiang, J., Guo, H., Yin, G., Zhang, H., Lan, F., et al. (2018). Classification of Alzheimer's Disease, mild cognitive impairment, and normal controls with subnetwork selection and graph kernel principal component analysis based on minimum spanning tree brain functional network. *Front. Computat. Neurosci.* 12:31. doi: 10.3389/fncom.2018.00031

Dan, L., Peiyu, H., Yufeng, Z., Yuting, L., Zhidong, C., Quanquan, G., et al. (2017). Abnormal baseline brain activity in Parkinson's disease with and without REM sleep behavior disorder: a resting-state functional MRI study. *J. Magn. Reson. Imaging* 46, 697–703. doi: 10.1002/jmri.25571

Davatzikos, C., Bhatt, P., Shaw, L. M., Batmanghelich, K. N., and Trojanowski, J. Q. (2011). Prediction of MCI to AD conversion, via MRI, CSF biomarkers, and pattern classification. *Neurobiol. Aging* 32, 2322.e19–2322.e27. doi: 10.1016/j.neurobiolaging.2010.05.023

dos Santos Siqueira, A., Biazoli Junior, C. E., Comfort, W. E., Rohde, L. A., and Sato, J. R. (2014). Abnormal functional resting-state networks in ADHD: graph theory and pattern recognition analysis of fMRI data. *BioMed Res. Int.* 2014:380531. doi: 10.1155/2014/380531

Douaud, G., Refsum, H., de Jager, C. A., Jacoby, R. E., Nichols, T., Smith, S. M., et al. (2013). Preventing Alzheimer's disease-related gray matter atrophy by B-vitamin treatment. *Proc. Natl. Acad. Sci. U.S.A.* 110, 9523–9528. doi: 10.1073/pnas.1301816110

Echávarri, C., Aalten, P., Uylings, H. B., Jacobs, H. I., Visser, P. J., Gronenschild, E. H., et al. (2011). Atrophy in the parahippocampal gyrus as an early biomarker of Alzheimer's disease. *Brain Struct. Funct.* 215, 265–271. doi: 10.1007/s00429-010-0283-8

Enatsu, R., Gonzalez-Martinez, J., Bulacio, J., Kubota, Y., Mosher, J., Burgess, R. C., et al. (2015). Connections of the limbic network: a corticocortical evoked potentials study. *Cortex* 62, 20–33. doi: 10.1016/j.cortex.2014.06.018

Forster, A. B., Abeywickrema, P., Bunda, J., Cox, C. D., Cabalu, T. D., Egbertson, M., et al. (2017). The identification of a novel lead class for phosphodiesterase 2 inhibition by fragment-based drug design. *Bioorgan. Med. Chem. Lett.* 27, 5167–5171. doi: 10.1016/j.bmcl.2017.10.054

Goense, J., Bohraus, Y., and Logothetis, N. K. (2016). fMRI at high spatial resolution: implications for BOLD-Models. *Front. Computat. Neurosci.* 10:66. doi: 10.3389/fncom.2016.00066

Goryawala, M., Zhou, Q., Barker, W., Loewenstein, D. A., Duara, R., and Adjouadi, M. (2015). Inclusion of neuropsychological scores in atrophy models improves diagnostic classification of Alzheimer's disease and Mild Cognitive Impairment. *Intell. Neurosci.* 2015:865265. doi: 10.1155/2015/865265

Hafkemeijer, A., van der Grond, J., and Rombouts, S. A. R. B. (2012). Imaging the default mode network in aging and dementia. *Biochimica Biophysica Acta* 1822, 431–441. doi: 10.1016/j.bbadis.2011.07.008

Jiang, X., Zhang, X., and Zhu, D. (2014). Intrinsic functional component analysis via sparse representation on Alzheimer's disease neuroimaging initiative database. *Brain Connect.* 4, 575–586. doi: 10.1089/brain.2013.0221

Jie, B., Liu, M., and Shen, D. (2018). Integration of temporal and spatial properties of dynamic connectivity networks for automatic diagnosis of brain disease. *Med. Image Anal.* 47, 81–94. doi: 10.1016/j.media.2018.03.013

Kang, Y., Williams, L. E., Clark, M. S., Gray, J. R., and Bargh, J. A. (2011). Physical temperature effects on trust behavior: the role of insula. *Soc. Cogn. Affect. Neurosci.* 6, 507–515. doi: 10.1093/scan/nsq077

Keren-Shaul, H., Spinrad, A., Weiner, A., Matcovitch-Natan, O., Dvir-Szternfeld, R., Ulland, T. K., et al. (2017). A unique microglia type associated with restricting development of Alzheimer's Disease. *Cell* 169, 1276.e17–1290.e17. doi: 10.1016/j.cell.2017.05.018

Kiernan, J. A. (2012). Anatomy of the temporal lobe. *Epilepsy Res. Treat.* 2012:176157. doi: 10.1155/2012/176157

Kodis, E. J., Choi, S., Swanson, E., Ferreira, G., and Bloom, G. S. (2018). N-methyl-D-aspartate receptor–mediated calcium influx connects amyloid-β oligomers to ectopic neuronal cell cycle reentry in Alzheimer's disease. *Alzheimers Dement.* (in press). doi: 10.1016/j.jalz.2018.05.017

Kumar, T. S., and Helenprabha, K. (2017). Top-Hat transform based retinal nerve fiber layer thickness measurement for Alzheimer detection using OCT images. *J. Computat. Theor. Nanosci.* 14, 1499–1505. doi: 10.1166/jctn.2017.6434

Lee, E. S., Yoo, K., Lee, Y.-B., Chung, J., Lim, J.-E., Yoon, B., et al. (2016). Default mode network functional connectivity in early and late mild cognitive impairment: results from the Alzheimer's Disease neuroimaging initiative. *Alzheimer Dis. Assoc. Disord.* 30, 289–296. doi: 10.1097/wad.0000000000000143

Lee, M. H., Miller-Thomas, M. M., Benzinger, T. L., Marcus, D. S., Hacker, C. D., Leuthardt, E. C., et al. (2016). Clinical resting-state fMRI in the preoperative setting: are we ready for prime time? *Top. Magn. Reson. Imaging* 25, 11–18. doi: 10.1097/RMR.0000000000000075

Lee, P., Ryoo, H., Park, J., and Jeong, Y. (2017). Morphological and microstructural changes of the hippocampus in early MCI: a study utilizing the Alzheimer's Disease neuroimaging initiative database. *J. Clin. Neurol.* 13, 144–154. doi: 10.3988/jcn.2017.13.2.144

Li, W., Qin, W., Liu, H., Fan, L., Wang, J., Jiang, T., et al. (2013). Subregions of the human superior frontal gyrus and their connections. *Neuroimage* 78, 46–58. doi: 10.1016/j.neuroimage.2013.04.011

Liang, P., Xiang, J., Liang, H., Qi, Z., Li, K., and Alzheimer's Disease NeuroImaging, Initiative. (2014). Altered amplitude of low-frequency fluctuations in early and late mild cognitive impairment and Alzheimer's disease. *Curr. Alzheimer Res.* 11, 389–398. doi: 10.2174/1567205011666140331225335

Liu, L., Chen, S., Zeng, D., Li, H., Shi, C., and Zhang, L. (2018). Cerebral activation effects of acupuncture at Yanglinquan(GB34) point acquired using resting-state fMRI. *Comput. Med. Imaging Graph.* 67, 55–58. doi: 10.1016/j.compmedimag.2018.04.004

Mahjoub, I., Mahjoub, M. A., and Rekik, I. (2018). Brain multiplexes reveal morphological connectional biomarkers fingerprinting late brain dementia states. *Sci. Rep.* 8:4103. doi: 10.1038/s41598-018-21568-7

Mondal, S., and Pai, P. P. (2014). Chou×s pseudo amino acid composition improves sequence-based antifreeze protein prediction. *J. Theor. Biol.* 356, 30–35. doi: 10.1016/j.jtbi.2014.04.006

Monti, D. A., Tobia, A., Stoner, M., Wintering, N., Matthews, M., Conklin, C. J., et al. (2018). Changes in cerebellar functional connectivity and autonomic regulation in cancer patients treated with the neuro emotional technique for traumatic stress symptoms. *J. Cancer Survivorsh.* 12, 145–153. doi: 10.1007/s11764-017-0653-9

Moradi, E., Pepe, A., Gaser, C., Huttunen, H., and Tohka, J. (2015). Machine learning framework for early MRI-based Alzheimer's conversion prediction in MCI subjects. *Neuroimage* 104, 398–412. doi: 10.1016/j.neuroimage.2014.10.002

Morris, J. K., Vidoni, E. D., Honea, R. A., and Burns, J. M. (2014). Impaired glycemia increases disease progression in mild cognitive impairment. *Neurobiol. Aging* 35, 585–589. doi: 10.1016/j.neurobiolaging.2013.09.033

Noble, S., Scheinost, D., Finn, E. S., Shen, X., Papademetris, X., McEwen, S. C., et al. (2017). Multisite reliability of MR-based functional connectivity. *Neuroimage* 146, 959–970. doi: 10.1016/j.neuroimage.2016.10.020

Novak, P., Schmidt, R., Kontsekova, E., Zilka, N., Kovacech, B., Skrabana, R., et al. (2017). Safety and immunogenicity of the tau vaccine AADvac1 in patients with Alzheimer's disease: a randomised, double-blind, placebo-controlled, phase 1 trial. *Lancet Neurol.* 16, 123–134. doi: 10.1016/S1474-4422(16)30331-3

Nozadi, S. H., Kadoury, S., and The Alzheimer's Disease Neuroimaging Initiative (2018). Classification of Alzheimer's and MCI patients from semantically parcelled PET Images: a comparison between AV45 and FDG-PET. *Int. J. Biomed. Imaging* 2018:1247430. doi: 10.1155/2018/1247430

Nuttall, R., Pasquini, L., Scherr, M., and Sorg, C. (2016). Degradation in intrinsic connectivity networks across the Alzheimer's disease spectrum. *Alzheimer's Dementia* 5, 35–42. doi: 10.1016/j.dadm.2016.11.006

Patel, K. T., Stevens, M. C., Pearlson, G. D., Winkler, A. M., Hawkins, K. A., Skudlarski, P., et al. (2013). Default mode network activity and white matter integrity in healthy middle-aged ApoE4 carriers. *Brain Imaging Behav.* 7, 60–67. doi: 10.1007/s11682-012-9187-y

Phillips, M. L. (2012). Neuroimaging in psychiatry: bringing neuroscience into clinical practice. *Br. J. Psychiatry* 201, 1–3. doi: 10.1192/bjp.bp.112.109587

Prasad, G., Joshi, S. H., Nir, T. M., Toga, A. W., and Thompson, P. M. (2015). Brain connectivity and novel network measures for Alzheimer's disease classification. *Neurobiol. Aging* 36, S121–S131. doi: 10.1016/j.neurobiolaging.2014.04.037

Puri, B. K., Jakeman, P. M., Agour, M., Gunatilake, K. D. R., Fernando, K. A. C., Gurusinghe, A. I., et al. (2012). Regional grey and white matter volumetric changes in myalgic encephalomyelitis (chronic fatigue syndrome): a voxel-based morphometry 3 T MRI study. *Br. J. Radiol.* 85, e270–e273. doi: 10.1259/bjr/93889091

Riley, J. D., Franklin, D. L., and Choi, V. (2010). Altered white matter integrity in temporal lobe epilepsy: association with cognitive and clinical profiles. *Epilepsia* 51, 536–545. doi: 10.1111/j.1528-1167.2009.02508.x

Rolls, E. T., Joliot, M., and Tzourio-Mazoyer, N. (2015). Implementation of a new parcellation of the orbitofrontal cortex in the automated anatomical labeling atlas. *Neuroimage* 122, 1–5. doi: 10.1016/j.neuroimage.2015.07.075

Rosa, M. J., Portugal, L., Hahn, T., Fallgatter, A. J., Garrido, M. I., Shawe-Taylor, J., et al. (2015). Sparse network-based models for patient classification using fMRI. *Neuroimage* 105, 493–506. doi: 10.1016/j.neuroimage.2014.11.021

Roy, D. S., Arons, A., Mitchell, T. I., Pignatelli, M., Ryan, T. J., and Tonegawa, S. (2016). Memory retrieval by activating engram cells in mouse models of early Alzheimer's disease. *Nature* 531, 508–512. doi: 10.1038/nature17172

Schröder, J., Girirajan, S., Papenfuss, A. T., and Medvedev, P. (2015). Improving the power of structural variation detection by augmenting the reference. *PLoS One* 10:e0136771. doi: 10.1371/journal.pone.0136771

Sojkova, J., Beason-Held, L., Zhou, Y., An, Y., Kraut, M. A., Ye, W., et al. (2008). Longitudinal cerebral blood flow and amyloid deposition: an emerging pattern? *J. Nuclear Med.* 49, 1465–1471. doi: 10.2967/jnumed.108.051946

Stein, J. L., Hua, X., Morra, J. H., Lee, S., Hibar, D. P., Ho, A. J., et al. (2010). Genome-wide analysis reveals novel genes influencing temporal lobe structure with relevance to neurodegeneration in Alzheimer's disease. *Neuroimage* 51, 542–554. doi: 10.1016/j.neuroimage.2010.02.068

Thanh Vu, A., Jamison, K., Glasser, M. F., Smith, S. M., Coalson, T., Moeller, S., et al. (2017). Tradeoffs in pushing the spatial resolution of fMRI for the 7T human connectome project. *Neuroimage* 154, 23–32. doi: 10.1016/j.neuroimage.2016.11.049

Van den Stock, J., Tamietto, M., Sorger, B., Pichon, S., Grézes, J., and de Gelder, B. (2011). Cortico-subcortical visual, somatosensory, and motor activations for perceiving dynamic whole-body emotional expressions with and without striate cortex (V1). *Proc. Natl. Acad. Sci. U.S.A.* 108, 16188–16193. doi: 10.1073/pnas.1107214108

Wang, T., Bhuiyan, M. Z. A., Wang, G., Rahman, M. A., Wu, J., and Cao, J. (2018). Big data reduction for a smart city's critical infrastructural health monitoring. *IEEE Commun. Mag.* 56, 128–133. doi: 10.1109/MCOM.2018.1700303

Wang, T., Zeng, J., Lai, Y., Cai, Y., Tian, H., Chen, Y., et al. (2017). Data collection from WSNs to the cloud based on mobile Fog elements. *Fut. Gen. Comput. Syst.* (in press). doi: 10.1016/j.future.2017.07.031

Xiang, J., Guo, H., Cao, R., Liang, H., and Chen, J. (2013). An abnormal resting-state functional brain network indicates progression towards Alzheimer's disease. *Neural Regen. Res.* 8, 2789–2799. doi: 10.3969/j.issn.1673-5374.2013.30.001

Xie, C., Bai, F., Yu, H., Shi, Y., Yuan, Y., Chen, G., et al. (2012). Abnormal insula functional network is associated with episodic memory decline in amnestic mild cognitive impairment. *Neuroimage* 63, 320–327. doi: 10.1016/j.neuroimage.2012.06.062

Yetkin, F. Z., Rosenberg, R. N., Weiner, M. F., Purdy, P. D., and Cullum, C. M. (2006). FMRI of working memory in patients with mild cognitive impairment and probable Alzheimer's disease. *Eur. Radiol.* 16, 193–206. doi: 10.1007/s00330-005-2794-x

Younes, L., Albert, M., and Miller, M. I. (2014). Inferring changepoint times of medial temporal lobe morphometric change in preclinical Alzheimer's disease. *Neuroimage* 5, 178–187. doi: 10.1016/j.nicl.2014.04.009

Zeng, N., Wang, Z., Zineddin, B., Li, Y., Du, M., Xiao, L., et al. (2014). Image-Based quantitative analysis of gold immunochromatographic strip via cellular neural network approach. *IEEE Trans. Med. Imaging* 33, 1129–1136. doi: 10.1109/TMI.2014.2305394

Zeng, N., Zhang, H., Li, Y., Liang, J., and Dobaie, A. M. (2017). Denoising and deblurring gold immunochromatographic strip images via gradient projection algorithms. *Neurocomputing* 247, 165–172. doi: 10.1016/j.neucom.2017.03.056

Zeng, N., Zhang, H., Song, B., Liu, W., Li, Y., and Dobaie, A. M. (2018). Facial expression recognition via learning deep sparse autoencoders. *Neurocomputing* 273, 643–649. doi: 10.1016/j.neucom.2017.08.043

Zhu, X., Suk, H.-I., and Shen, D. (2014). A novel matrix-similarity based loss function for joint regression and classification in AD diagnosis. *Neuroimage* 100, 91–105. doi: 10.1016/j.neuroimage.2014.05.078

11

Low-Rank Based Image Analyses for Pathological MR Image Segmentation and Recovery

Chuanlu Lin, Yi Wang, Tianfu Wang and Dong Ni*

National-Regional Key Technology Engineering Laboratory for Medical Ultrasound, Guangdong Provincial Key Laboratory of Biomedical Measurements and Ultrasound Imaging, Health Science Center, School of Biomedical Engineering, Shenzhen University, Shenzhen, China

Correspondence:
Yi Wang
onewang@szu.edu.cn

The presence of pathologies in magnetic resonance (MR) brain images causes challenges in various image analysis areas, such as registration, atlas construction and atlas-based segmentation. We propose a novel method for the simultaneous recovery and segmentation of pathological MR brain images. Low-rank and sparse decomposition (LSD) approaches have been widely used in this field, decomposing pathological images into (1) low-rank components as recovered images, and (2) sparse components as pathological segmentation. However, conventional LSD approaches often fail to produce recovered images reliably, due to the lack of constraint between low-rank and sparse components. To tackle this problem, we propose a transformed low-rank and structured sparse decomposition (TLS^{2}D) method. The proposed TLS^{2}D integrates the structured sparse constraint, LSD and image alignment into a unified scheme, which is robust for distinguishing pathological regions. Furthermore, the well recovered images can be obtained using TLS^{2}D with the combined structured sparse and computed image saliency as the adaptive sparsity constraint. The efficacy of the proposed method is verified on synthetic and real MR brain tumor images. Experimental results demonstrate that our method can effectively provide satisfactory image recovery and tumor segmentation.

Keywords: MR brain images, image recovery, tumor segmentation, structured sparsity, low-rank, matrix decomposition

1. INTRODUCTION

Automated image computing routines (e.g., segmentation, registration, atlas construction) that can analyze the magnetic resonance (MR) brain tumor scans are of essential importance for improved disease diagnosis, treatment planning and follow-up of individual patients (Iglesias and Sabuncu, 2015; Mai et al., 2015; Menze et al., 2015; Chen et al., 2018). Lately, a wave of deep learning is taking over traditional computer aided diagnosis techniques, by learning abundant multi-level features from large amount of training repository for image representation and analyzing (Litjens et al., 2017; Shen et al., 2017). Various architectures of deep convolutional neural networks have been developed and employed for brain tumor segmentation (Pereira et al., 2016; Havaei et al., 2017; Kamnitsas et al., 2017; Zhao et al., 2018). Despite achieving satisfactory performance, deep learning based approaches require enormous amount of labeled images to train a segmentation model. Collecting and labeling useful training samples may last a lengthy duration thus sometimes is clinically impractical. In addition, the presence of pathologies in MR brain images causes difficulties in most of other image analyses, such as image registration, atlas construction and atlas-based anatomical segmentation. The recovery of pathological regions with normal brain appearances can facilitate subsequent image computing procedures. For example, the recovered images could further be used for atlas construction and specific patient's follow-up (Joshi et al., 2004; Liu et al., 2014; Zheng et al., 2017; Han et al., 2018). However, there is lack of deep learning based methods developed for pathological medical image recovery. In contrast, the low-rank and sparse decomposition (LSD) (Wright et al., 2009; Candès et al., 2011) scheme, learning normal image appearance from unlabeled population data, has been widely employed to decompose pathological MR brain images into recovered normal brain appearances and pathological regions (Liu et al., 2015; Tang et al., 2018).

Although the low-rank and sparse analyses of computational brain tumor segmentation has attracted considerable attention during last decade, it remains several challenges. First, conventional LSD methods have to be computed on a series of aligned images (Otazo et al., 2015; Tang et al., 2018), because the image misalignment causes undesired structure differences that would interfere the representation of sparse component. Thus, the image alignment should be conducted before/during the LSD computation; however, the image alignment itself is a challenging task. Second, specific spatial constraint should be imposed on sparse component to restrict the structured sparsity of the tumor region in the whole image. Third, LSD methods often produce recovered images (i.e., low-rank component) with distorted pathological regions (Liu et al., 2015), due to the lack of effective constraint between low-rank and sparse components. Thus it is essential to adaptively balance the low-rank and sparse components to reliably recover tumor regions meanwhile retaining normal brain regions.

To address aforementioned issues, this paper presents a novel method for the simultaneous recovery and segmentation of pathological MR brain images (see **Figure 1**). Specifically, we propose a transformed low-rank and structured sparse decomposition (TLS^{2}D) method. The proposed TLS^{2}D integrates the structured sparsity constraint, LSD and image alignment into a unified framework, which is robust for extracting pathological regions. Furthermore, the well recovered images can be obtained using TLS^{2}D with the combined structured sparse and computed image saliency as the adaptive sparsity constraint. Experimental results on synthetic and real MR brain tumor images demonstrate that the proposed TLS^{2}D can effectively extract and recover tumor regions.

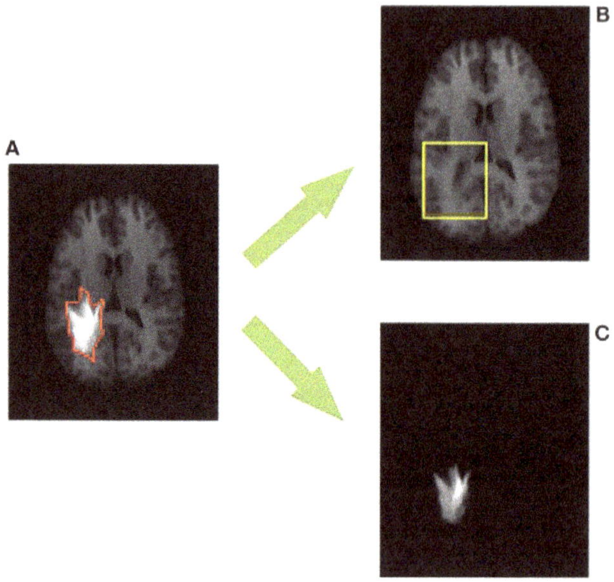

FIGURE 1 | The proposed TLS^{2}D method can decompose **(A)** the MR brain tumor image into **(B)** the recovered MR image with quasi-normal brain appearances, and **(C)** the extracted tumor region. The red contour in **(A)** indicates the manually delineated tumor boundary. The yellow box in **(B)** indicates the reliably recovered region.

2. METHODS

The proposed recovery and segmentation framework is shown in **Figure 2**. Our TLS^{2}D first iteratively aligns all images and decomposes aligned images into low-rank and structured sparse components. Then the structured sparse components are combined with the computed saliency maps to generate tumor probability maps as the adaptive sparsity constraint. The final recovery and segmentation is obtained by imposing the adaptive sparsity constraint on the TLS^{2}D.

The following subsections present a brief review of classical LSD, the details of our method and elaborate the novel TLS^{2}D.

2.1. Review of Low-Rank and Sparse Decomposition (LSD)

Suppose we are given n previously aligned MR brain images $A_1, A_2, ..., A_n \in \mathbb{R}^{w \times h}$, where w and h denotes width and height of the image, respectively. We can vectorize each image matrix A_n to form the column of $A = [vec(A_1), vec(A_2), ..., vec(A_n)] \in \mathbb{R}^{m \times n}$, where $m = w \times h$.

The conventional LSD method decomposes A into a low-rank matrix L and a sparse matrix S, where L indicates the linearly correlated normal images, and S represents sparse tumor regions. The decomposition can be solved by the following convex optimization:

$$\min_{L,S} \|L\|_* + \lambda \|S\|_1 \quad s.t.\ A = L + S, \tag{1}$$

where $\|L\|_*$ is the nuclear norm of L (i.e., the sum of its singular values), $\|S\|_1$ is the ℓ_1 norm of S, and regularizing parameter λ weights the relationship between low-rank and sparse components. The optimization in Equation (1) can be solved by augmented Lagrangian multiplier (ALM) method (Lin et al., 2010).

To realize practical and reliable recovery and segmentation of pathological MR images, the LSD remains three issues to be addressed: (1) all images shall be aligned in the same spatial domain; (2) S shall be structured sparse to better represent

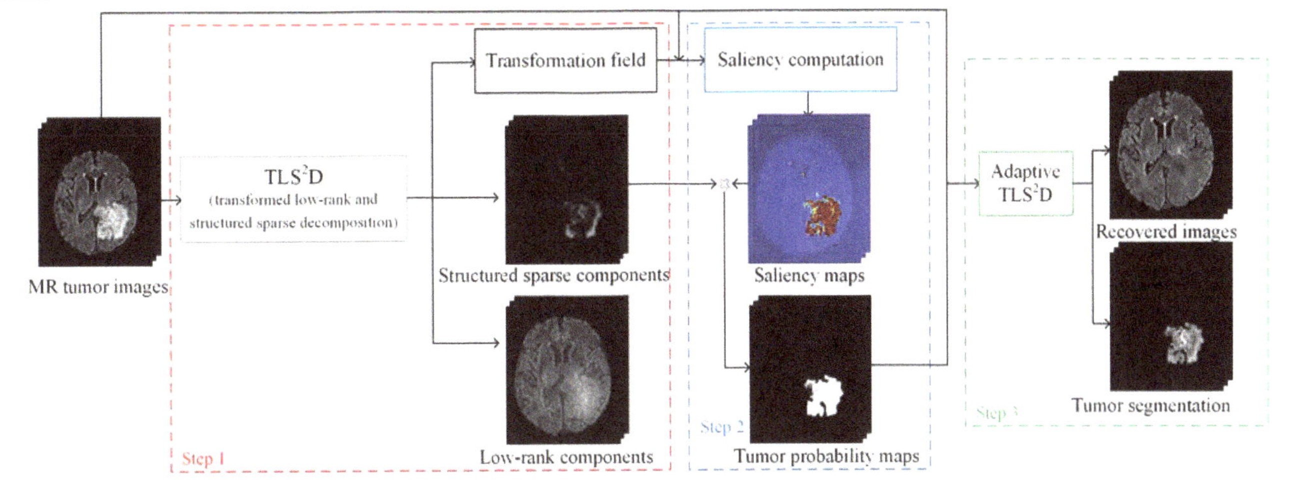

FIGURE 2 | The illustration of the whole recovery and segmentation framework using the proposed transformed low-rank and structured sparse decomposition (TLS^2D) method.

the structured sparsity of the contiguous tumor region in the whole image; (3) as illustrated in **Figure 3**, as the parameter λ becomes smaller, the low-rank images can recover tumor regions more reliably, but also generate more blurred appearances in originally normal regions. Therefore, regularizing parameter λ shall be different regarding to normal and tumor regions, thus to adaptively balance the low-rank and sparse components to reliably recover tumor regions meanwhile retaining normal brain regions.

2.2. Transformed Low-Rank and Structured Sparse Decomposition (TLS^2D)

To tackle the issues in LSD, we propose a transformed low-rank and structured sparse decomposition. Firstly, considering the tumor region usually occupies a contiguous portion of the brain image, thus it is reasonable to model the tumor region using the structured sparsity norm. Inspired by the structured sparsity in Jia et al. (2012), we introduce a structured sparsity norm $\Omega(S)$ to model tumor region, and define low-rank and structured sparse decomposition (LS^2D) as:

$$\min_{L,S} \|L\|_* + \lambda\Omega(S) \quad s.t.\ A = L + S, \tag{2}$$

where

$$\Omega(S) = \sum_{i=1}^{n}\sum_{g\in G} \left\| mat(S_i)_g \right\|_\infty . \tag{3}$$

In Equation (3), $S_i \in \mathbb{R}^m$ is the ith column in S; $mat(S_i) \in \mathbb{R}^{w\times h}$ is the matrix form of S_i. We define 3×3 overlapping-patch groups G in $mat(S_i)$, and $g \in G$ represents each 3×3 group. Each group overlaps 6 pixels with its neighbor group. $\|\cdot\|_\infty$ is the ℓ_∞ norm (i.e., the maximum value in a group g). The structured sparsity norm $\Omega(S)$ in Equation (2) can constrain S to be structured distribution thus better representing tumor region.

During the decomposition, the spatial mismatch between different images may cause undesired sparse noise. To alleviate the spatial mismatch, we perform image alignment in our decomposition procedure (Zheng et al., 2017). The proposed TLS^2D is defined as follows:

$$\min_{L,S,\tau} \|L\|_* + \lambda\Omega(S) \quad s.t.\ A \circ \tau = L + S, \tag{4}$$

where τ denotes a set of n affine transformations $\tau_1, \tau_2, ..., \tau_n$ that warps A to align all images; $A \circ \tau = [vec(A_1 \circ \tau_1), vec(A_2 \circ \tau_2), ..., vec(A_n \circ \tau_n)] \in \mathbb{R}^{m\times n}$.

The optimization of our TLS^2D in Equation (4) is non-convex and difficult to solve directly due to the nonlinearity of the τ. To tackle this issue, we can iteratively linearize about the estimate of τ according to Boyd et al. (2011) and Wang et al. (2018). Specifically, we linearize the constraint by using the local first order Taylor approximation for each image as $A \circ (\tau + \Delta\tau) \approx A \circ \tau + \sum_{i=1}^{n} J_i \Delta\tau_i \epsilon_i \epsilon_i^T$, where $\Delta\tau = [\Delta\tau_1, \Delta\tau_2, ..., \Delta\tau_n] \in \mathbb{R}^{p\times n}$, and each $\Delta\tau_i \in \mathbb{R}^p$ is defined by p parameters of the transformation; $J_i = \frac{\partial}{\partial\zeta} vec(A_i \circ \zeta)|_{\zeta=\tau_i} \in \mathbb{R}^{m\times p}$ is the Jacobian of the image A_i with respect to the transformation τ_i, and $\{\epsilon_i\}$ denotes the standard basis for $\mathbb{R}^n$. Thus, Equation (4) can be relaxed into the following optimization:

$$\min_{L,S,\Delta\tau} \|L\|_* + \lambda\Omega(S) \quad s.t.\ A \circ \tau + \sum_{i=1}^{n} J_i \Delta\tau_i \epsilon_i \epsilon_i^T = L + S. \tag{5}$$

Then the resulting convex programming in Equation (5) can be solved by ALM method (Lin et al., 2010). We formulate the following augmented Lagrangian function:

$$\begin{aligned}\mathcal{L}(L, S, \Delta\tau, Y; \mu) &= \|L\|_* + \lambda\Omega(S) + \langle Y, h(L, S, \Delta\tau)\rangle \\ &\quad + \frac{\mu}{2}\left\|h(L, S, \Delta\tau)\right\|_F^2,\end{aligned} \tag{6}$$

where $h(L, S, \Delta\tau) = A \circ \tau + \sum_{i=1}^{n} J_i \Delta\tau_i \epsilon_i \epsilon_i^T - L - S$; $Y \in \mathbb{R}^{m\times n}$ is the Lagrangian multiplier and μ is a positive hyperparameter;

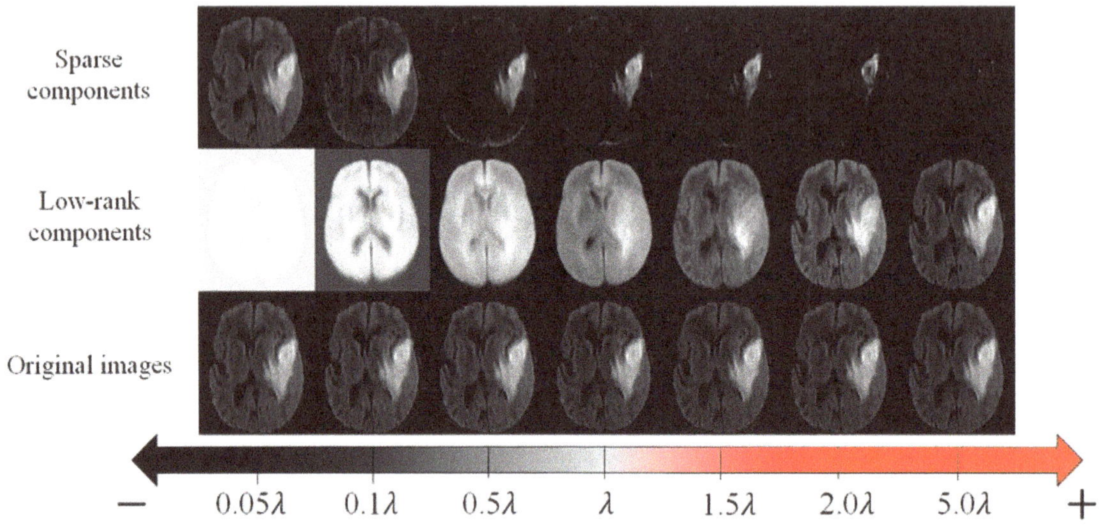

FIGURE 3 | The original MR images **(bottom row)**, and corresponding recovered low-rank components **(middle row)** and sparse components **(top row)** given by conventional LSD method, with different values of regularizing parameter λ.

$\langle \cdot, \cdot \rangle$ denotes the matrix inner product, and $\|\cdot\|_F$ is the Frobenius norm. The ALM algorithm then estimates both the optimal solution and the Lagrange multiplier by iteratively solving the following four subproblems:

$$\begin{aligned} L^{t+1} &= \arg\min_{L} \mathcal{L}(L, S^t, \Delta\tau^t, Y^t; \mu^t), \\ S^{t+1} &= \arg\min_{S} \mathcal{L}(L^{t+1}, S, \Delta\tau^t, Y^t; \mu^t), \\ \Delta\tau^{t+1} &= \arg\min_{\Delta\tau} \mathcal{L}(L^{t+1}, S^{t+1}, \Delta\tau^t, Y^t; \mu^t), \\ Y^{t+1} &= Y^t + \mu^t h(L^{t+1}, S^{t+1}, \Delta\tau^{t+1}), \end{aligned} \tag{7}$$

where superscript t denotes the iteration. In each iteration, the first problem in Equation (7) can be expressed as

$$L^{t+1} = \arg\min_{L} \left\{ \|L\|_* + \frac{\mu^t}{2} \|H_L - L\|_F^2 \right\}, \tag{8}$$

where $H_L = A \circ \tau + \sum_{i=1}^{n} J_i \Delta\tau_i^t \epsilon_i \epsilon_i^T - S^t + Y^t/\mu^t$. The problem in Equation (8) has a simple closed-form solution by soft thresholding operator (Parikh et al., 2014). Suppose the singular value decomposition of H_L is $(U, \Sigma, V) = svd(H_L)$, then $L^{t+1} = U\mathcal{S}_{\frac{1}{\mu^t}}[\Sigma]V^T$, where $\mathcal{S}_{\frac{1}{\mu}}(x) = \{[x - \frac{1}{\mu}]_+ - [-x - \frac{1}{\mu}]_+\}$ is the soft thresholding operator and $[\cdot]_+ = max(\cdot, 0)$.

The second problem in Equation (7) can be rewritten as

$$S^{t+1} = \arg\min_{S} \left\{ \frac{\mu^t}{2} \|H_S - S\|_F^2 + \lambda\Omega(S) \right\}, \tag{9}$$

where $H_S = A \circ \tau + \sum_{i=1}^{n} J_i \Delta\tau_i^t \epsilon_i \epsilon_i^T - L^{t+1} + Y^t/\mu^t$. The problem in Equation (9) is the proximal operator associated with the structured sparsity norm, which can be calculated by solving a quadratic min-cost flow problem (Mairal et al., 2010).

Then given the current estimated L^{t+1} and S^{t+1}, the solution of the third problem in Equation (7) can be calculated as

$$\Delta\tau^{t+1} = \sum_{i=1}^{n} J_i^{\dagger}(L^{t+1} + S^{t+1} - A \circ \tau - Y^t/\mu^t)\epsilon_i\epsilon_i^T, \tag{10}$$

where $J_i^{\dagger}$ denotes the Moore-Penrose pseudoinverse of J_i. We summarize the solver for Equation (4) in Algorithm 1.

2.3. Recovery and Segmentation Framework

In our recovery and segmentation framework, at the first step we employ the proposed TLS^{2}D to align all MR images and meanwhile obtaining low-rank and structured sparse images (see **Figure 2**). The low-rank images at this step blur the tumor region and yet cannot reliably recover the normal image appearances. To address this problem, we propose to leverage the obtained structured sparse component to adjust the regularizing parameter λ in Equation (4) for the adaptive sparsity constraint.

Specifically, we compute the saliency maps of the MR images using (Perazzi et al., 2012). The saliency map indicates the saliency of each pixel to catch the human attention, with value 1 denoting the highest attention and 0 denoting no attention. According to (Perazzi et al., 2012), in order to calculate the saliency of an image, we first abstract this image into perceptually homogeneous elements using (Achanta et al., 2012). We then employ a set of high-dimensional Gaussian filters (Adams et al., 2010) to calculate two contrast measures (i.e., the uniqueness and spatial distribution of elements), and use these two measures to predict the final saliency of each pixel. In pathological MR images, the most salient part shall be the tumor regions. We then obtain the tumor probability map of an image by computing the dot product between its binary structured sparse image and its corresponding saliency map, as shown in **Figure 2**.

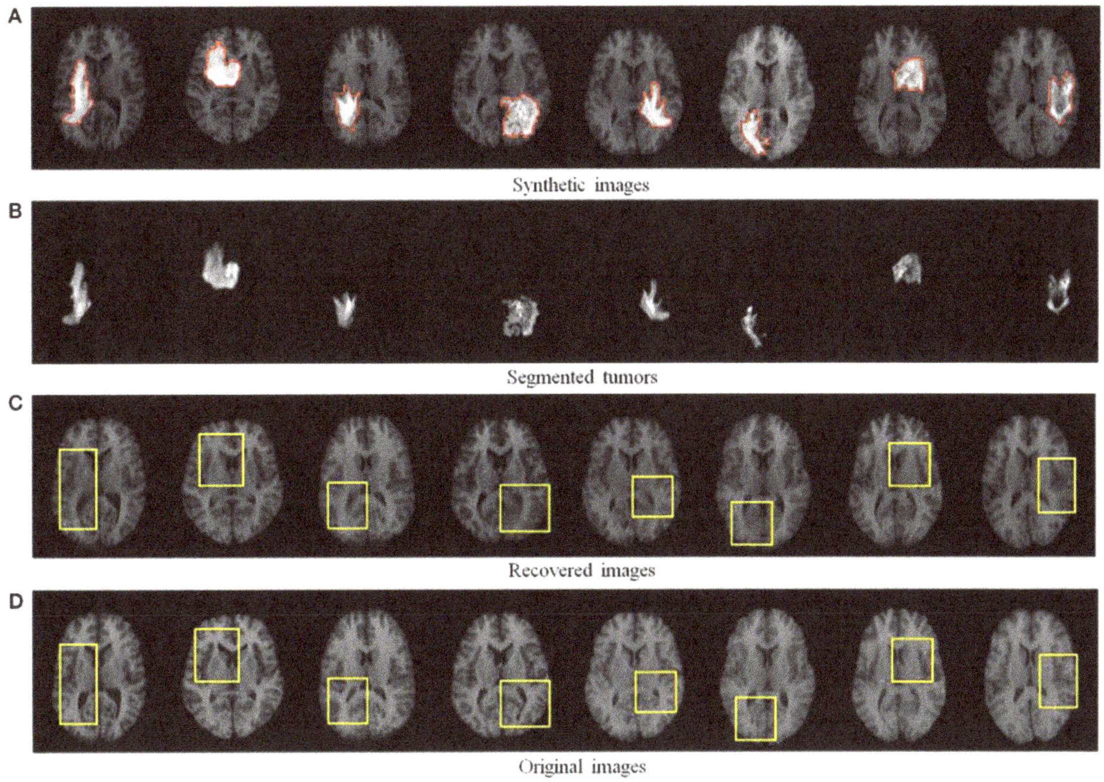

FIGURE 4 | Recovery and segmentation of **(A)** synthetic MR brain tumor images: **(B)** the segmented tumors, **(C)** the recovered images with normal brain appearances, **(D)** the corresponding original MR images from LPBA40 (Shattuck et al., 2008). Yellow boxes illustrate the reliably recovered regions.

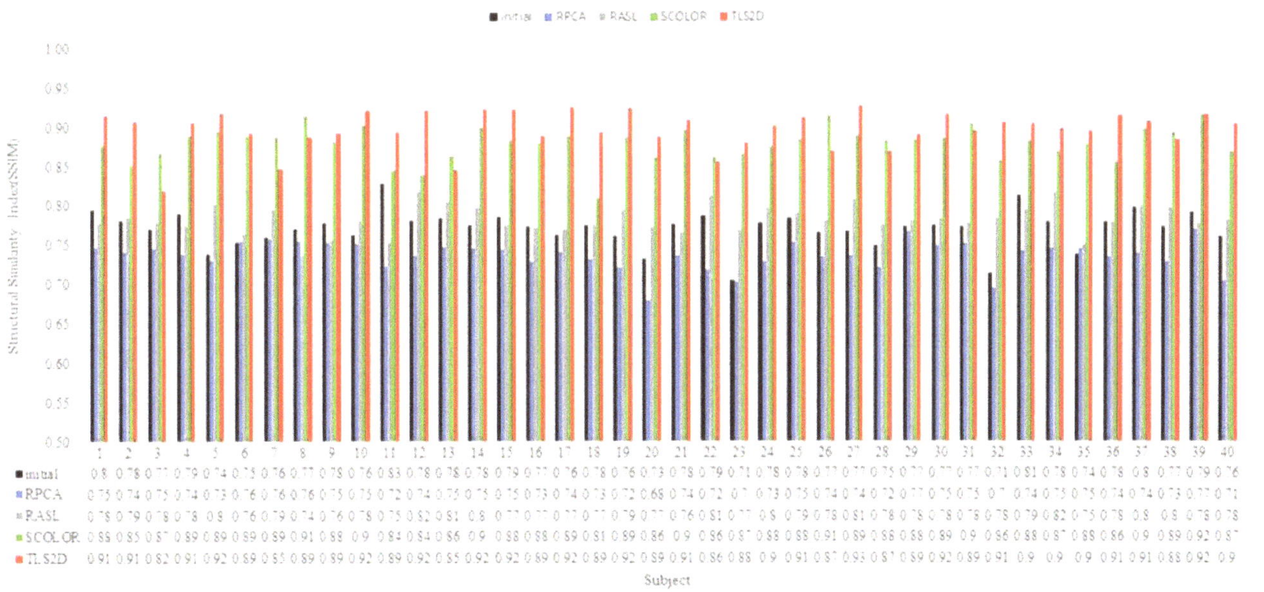

FIGURE 5 | The structural similarity index (SSIM) between each of the original MR images and the corresponding recovered images by different methods. The "Initial" indicates the SSIM between the synthetic tumor images and the corresponding original images.

Algorithm 1: Transformed Low-Rank and Structured Sparse Decomposition (TLS^{2}D)

Input : $A = [vec(A_1), vec(A_2), ..., vec(A_n)] \in \mathbb{R}^{m \times n}$, the regularizing parameter λ, the penalty constant ρ, the tolerance ϵ, and maximal iteration *maxIter*.

Output: Solution $(L, S, \Delta\tau)$ to the problem in Equation (5)

Initialize: $L^0 = S^0 = \mathbf{0} \in \mathbb{R}^{m \times n}$, $Y^0 = A$, $\Delta\tau^0 = \mathbf{0} \in \mathbb{R}^{p \times n}$, $\lambda = \frac{1}{\sqrt{\max(m,n))}}$, $\mu^0 = 1$, $\rho = 1.25$, $\epsilon = 10\text{e}{-7}$, $maxIter = 1000$

while $t \leq maxIter$ **do**

  Update L: $H_L = A \circ \tau + \sum_{i=1}^{n} J_i \Delta\tau_i^t \epsilon_i \epsilon_i^T - S^t + Y^t/\mu^t$;

  $(U, \Sigma, V) = \text{svd}(H_L)$;

  $L^{t+1} = U S_{\frac{1}{\mu^t}}[\Sigma] V^T$.

  Update S: $H_S = A \circ \tau + \sum_{i=1}^{n} J_i \Delta\tau_i^t \epsilon_i \epsilon_i^T - L^{t+1} + Y^t/\mu^t$;

  $S^{t+1} = prox_{\frac{\lambda}{\mu^t}}(H_S)$.

  Update $\Delta\tau$:

  $\Delta\tau^{t+1} = \sum_{i=1}^{n} J_i^{\dagger}(L^{t+1} + S^{t+1} - A \circ \tau - Y^t/\mu^t)\epsilon_i \epsilon_i^T$.

  Update Y: $Y^{t+1} = Y^t + \mu^t h(L^{t+1}, S^{t+1}, \Delta\tau^{t+1})$.

  Update μ: $\mu^{t+1} = \rho\mu^t$.

  if $||h(L^{t+1}, S^{t+1}, \Delta\tau^{t+1})||_2 \leq \epsilon$ **then**

    Converge and break

  end

end

return $L = L^{t+1}$, $S = S^{t+1}$, $\Delta\tau = \Delta\tau^{t+1}$ *and* $Y = Y^{t+1}$

The tumor probability map indicates the probability of each pixel being tumor region. We denote tumor probability map $P = [vec(P_1), vec(P_2), ..., vec(P_n)] \in \mathbb{R}^{m \times n}$.

Finally, we use the tumor probability map to adaptively adjust the regularizing parameter λ in Equation (4). We define the adaptive TLS^{2}D to obtain the final tumor segmentation and well recovered quasi-normal images:

$$\min_{L,S,\tau} ||L||_* + \lambda(\mathbf{1} - P) \odot \Omega(S) \quad s.t.\, A \circ \tau = L + S, \tag{11}$$

where $\mathbf{1} \in \mathbb{R}^{m \times n}$, with each element equals to 1. $\lambda(\mathbf{1} - P)$ is the adaptive regularizing matrix. $\odot$ denotes dot product. In such a way, the sparse constraints for tumor and normal regions are set differently, thus our TLS^{2}D can reliably recover tumor regions meanwhile retaining normal regions.

3. EXPERIMENTS AND RESULTS

The proposed TLS^{2}D method was evaluated on both synthetic and real MR brain tumor images. We also extensively compared our method with state of the art, including Robust Principal Component Analysis (RPCA) (Candès et al., 2011), Robust Alignment by Sparse and Low-rank decomposition (RASL) (Peng et al., 2012), and Spatially COnstraint LOw-Rank (SCOLOR) (Tang et al., 2018). Specifically, the RPCA method is one of the most classical and successful low-rank and sparse decomposition schemes; the RASL method considers spatial mismatch between different images and hence adds image alignment into the low-rank based decomposition procedure; the SCOLOR method imposes spatial constraint on sparse component to restrict its structured sparsity.

TABLE 1 | Dice values of different methods on synthetic and real MR brain tumor images.

Data type	RPCA	RASL	SCOLOR	TLS^{2}D (Ours)
Synthetic tumor images	0.54 ± 0.25	0.62 ± 0.26	0.70 ± 0.26	**0.80 ± 0.28**
Real tumor images	0.46 ± 0.20	0.51 ± 0.20	0.63 ± 0.30	**0.75 ± 0.26**

Best results are highlighted in bold.

The metrics employed to quantitatively evaluate recovery and segmentation performance was structural similarity index (SSIM) (Wang et al., 2004) and Dice index (Chang et al., 2009), respectively. The SSIM index is the most popular metric to evaluate the similarity of two images by using structural information. The SSIM of two images x and y is:

$$SSIM(x, y) = \frac{(2\mu_x\mu_y + c_1)(2\sigma_{xy} + c_2)}{(\mu_x^2 + \mu_y^2 + c_1)(\sigma_x^2 + \sigma_y^2 + c_2)}, \tag{12}$$

where μ_x and μ_y is the average of x and y; σ_x and σ_y is the variance of x and y, respectively; σ_{xy} is the covariance of x and y; c_1 and c_2 are two constants to stabilize the division. The Dice index is used for comparing the similarity of two regions, and can be calculated as:

$$Dice = \frac{2|G \cap T|}{|G| + |T|}, \tag{13}$$

where T and G denotes the segmented tumor region and ground truth, respectively.

3.1. Validation on Synthetic MR Brain Tumor Images

We first quantitatively evaluated the recovery performance of our method on synthetic tumor images. The synthetic MR brain tumor images are based on images from a public dataset LPBA40 (Shattuck et al., 2008). The LPBA40 dataset includes 40 T1-weighted MR normal brain images. Some example normal images from LPBA40 are shown in **Figure 4D**. We generated the synthetic tumor images by fusing tumor regions derived from a real MR tumor image dataset BRATS2018 (Menze et al., 2015) (see **Figure 4A**).

Figure 4 visualizes some recovery and segmentation results obtained by our method. It can be observed that our method can reliably extract the tumor regions, and recover these regions with normal brain appearances. **Figure 5** further illustrates the quantitative SSIM values between the original MR images and the recovered images by different methods. Our TLS^{2}D method consistently achieves the most similar image appearance to the original images from LPBA40. In addition, **Table 1** lists the Dice indices of the segmented tumor regions by different methods. Our TLS^{2}D achieves the best segmentation performance.

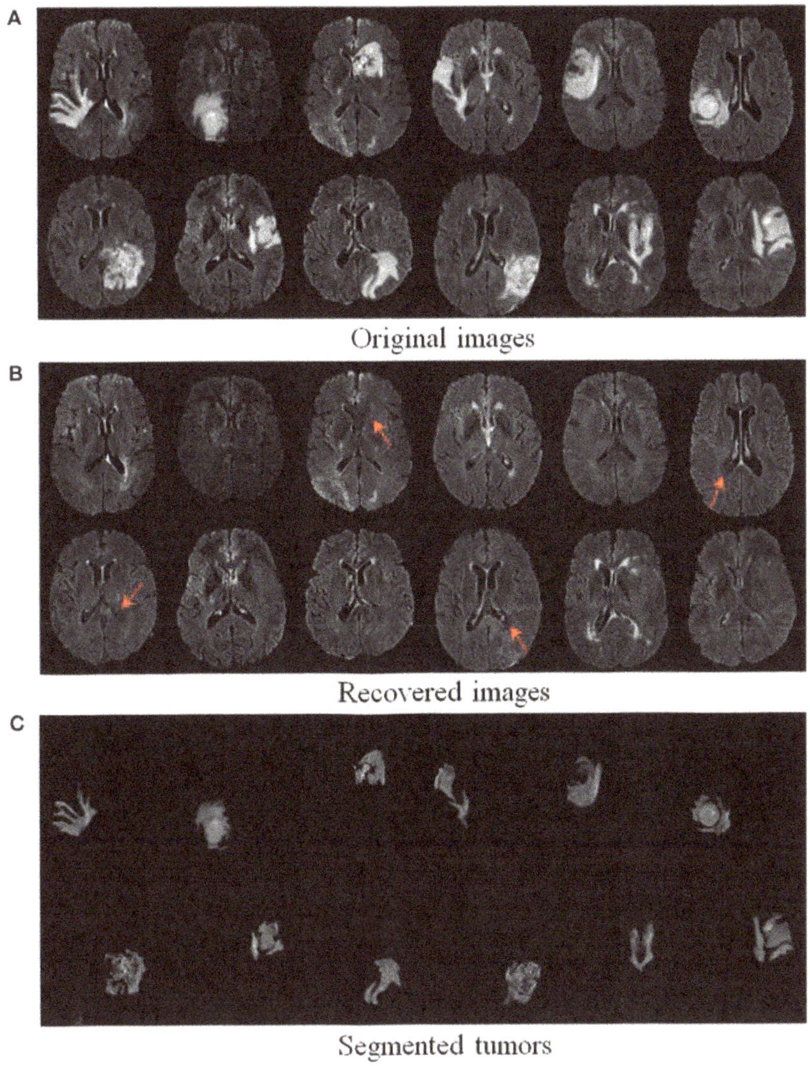

FIGURE 6 | Recovery and segmentation of **(A)** real MR brain tumor images from BRATS2018 (Menze et al., 2015); **(B)** the recovered images with normal brain appearances, **(C)** the tumor segmentation results. Red arrows indicate well recovered brain structures.

3.2. Evaluation on Real MR Brain Tumor Images

We further evaluated the efficacy of our method on 124 real T2-weighted FLAIR MR brain tumor images from the dataset BRATS2018 (Menze et al., 2015). **Table 1** demonstrates that our TLS^{2}D method achieves the best tumor segmentation results. **Figure 6** illustrates some example recovery and segmentation results obtained by our method. It can be seen from **Figure 6** that our method can achieve satisfactory recovery and segmentation performance. The recovered images by our method could infer the plausible brain structures, see red arrows in **Figure 6B**.

3.3. Application to Multi-Atlas Segmentation

The recovery of pathological regions with normal brain appearances is beneficial for other image computing tasks, such as multi-atlas segmentation (MAS). The MAS attempts to register multiple normal brain atlases to a new brain image, thus to map their corresponding anatomical labels to the new brain image for the brain segmentation. Conventional MAS methods may not perform well when images are with tumor regions, because the appearance change induced by these regions cause difficulties in registering multiple atlases to the brain tumor image. We conducted multi-atlas segmentation based on the recovered images to demonstrate the benefit of our method on image recovery.

We used 40 T1-weighted MR images and their corresponding segmentation labels from LPBA40 (Shattuck et al., 2008) to conduct MAS. For each time of MAS, we chose one image to generate synthetic tumor image, and employed the remaining 39 images as multiple atlases. As shown in **Figure 7**, we then used the proposed TLS^{2}D method to obtain the recovered image, and utilized an intensity-based non-rigid registration

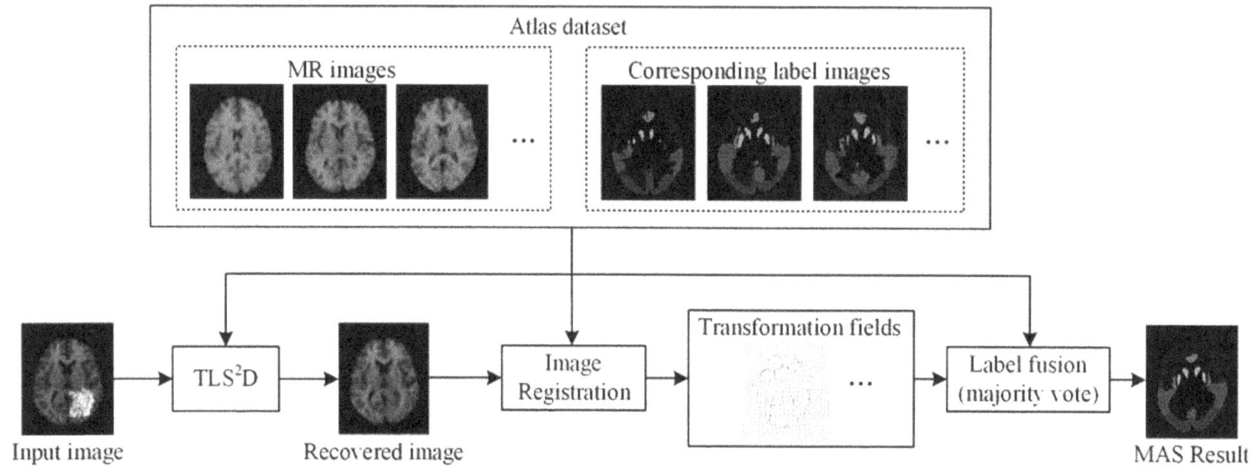

FIGURE 7 | The illustration of the multi-atlas segmentation framework.

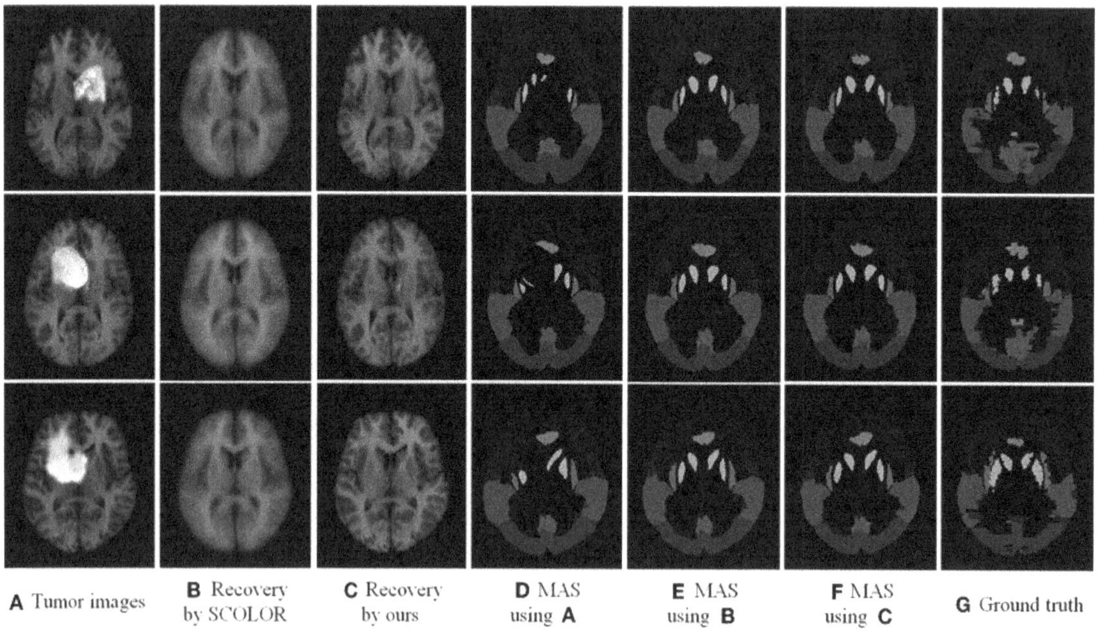

FIGURE 8 | Multi-atlas segmentation results: **(A)** brain tumor images, **(B)** the recovered images by SCOLOR method, **(C)** our recovered images with quasi-normal brain appearances, **(D)** the MAS results by using original tumor images, **(E)** the MAS results by using the recovered images from SCOLOR, **(F)** the MAS results by using our recovered images, and **(G)** the segmentation ground truth.

method (Myronenko and Song, 2010) to map multiple atlases to the recovered image for the brain segmentation via majority vote based label fusion. **Figure 8** shows some MAS results obtained by using the recovered images and original images, respectively. It can be observed that the brain segmentations using our recovered images outperform those using original tumor images, especially in the regions tumor occupied. It also can be observed from **Figure 8** that compared to SCOLOR method, our method can produce much clearer recovered images. **Figure 9** further illustrates the average Dice indices of different brain regions of 40 segmented brain tumor images using MAS+original images, MAS+SCOLOR recovered images and MAS+our recovered images, respectively. The MAS using our recovered images consistently achieve better Dice indices compared to the MAS using original images and recovered images from SCOLOR, which demonstrates our method is potentially useful to improve the MAS when images are with pathological regions.

4. DISCUSSION AND CONCLUSION

In this study, we have proposed a novel low-rank based method, called transformed low-rank and structured sparse

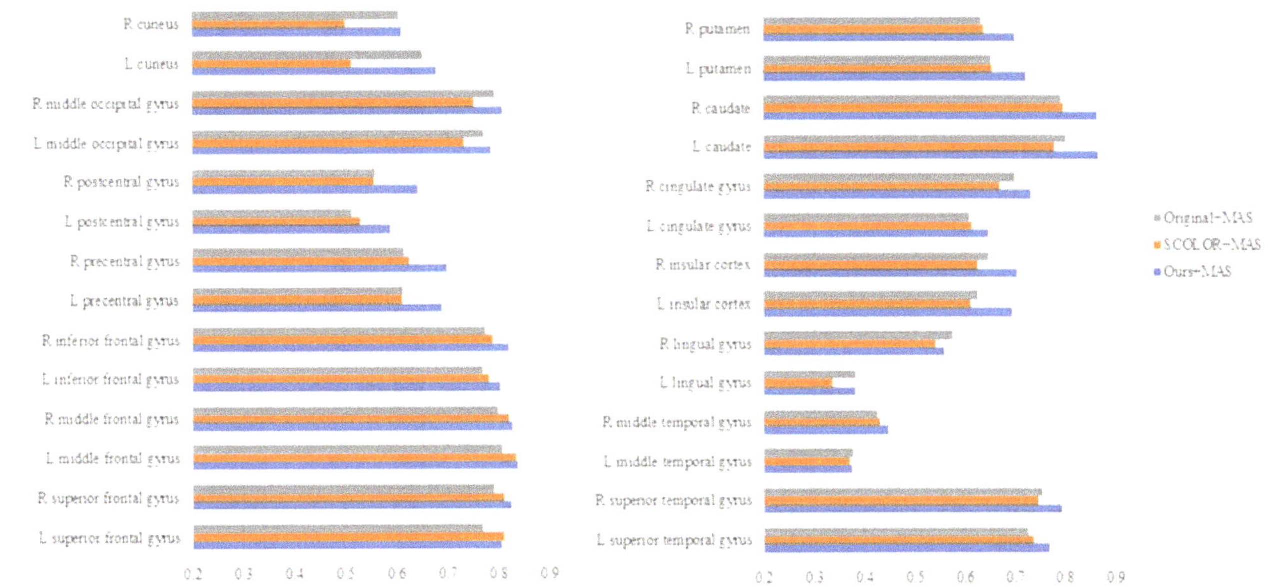

FIGURE 9 | The average Dice indices of different brain regions of 40 segmented brain tumor images using MAS+original images, MAS+SCOLOR recovered images, and MAS+our recovered images, respectively.

decomposition (TLS^{2}D), for the reliable recovery and segmentation of pathological MR brain images. By integrating the structured sparsity, image alignment, and adaptive spatial constraint into a unified matrix decomposition framework, our method is robust for extracting pathological regions, and also is reliable for recovering quasi-normal MR appearances. The recovered image is beneficial for subsequent image computing procedures, such as atlas-based segmentation. We have compared the proposed TLS^{2}D method with several state-of-the-art low-rank based approaches on synthetic and real MR brain images. Regarding these compared methods, the RPCA method is a conventional low-rank and sparse decomposition method; the RASL method embeds image alignment into LSD framework; the SCOLOR method imposes spatial constraint on sparse component. Experimental results show our method consistently outperforms all compared methods, which demonstrates the contribution of the proposed transformed low-rank and structured sparse decomposition with adaptive sparse constraint on simultaneous recovery and segmentation.

Computer aided methods that can assist clinicians to analyze the MR brain tumor scans are of essential significance for improved diagnosis, treatment planning and patients' follow-up. Automated tumor segmentation is the primary research task for analyzing the pathological images, and has been extensively investigated in the literature (Gordillo et al., 2013; Menze et al., 2015; Zhou et al., 2017). However, in addition to tumor segmentation task, the presence of pathologies in MR images poses challenges in other image computing tasks, such as intensity-/feature-based image registration (Sotiras et al., 2013) and atlas-based segmentation of brain structures (Cabezas et al., 2011), due to the structure and appearance changes of pathological brain images. Thus the recovery of pathological regions with normal brain appearances is beneficial for most image computing procedures. To this end, we consider to integrate the registration, segmentation and recovery procedures into a unified decomposition framework. The proposed TLS^{2}D is a generic method for analyzing the MR brain tumor scans. It is worth noting that although our method is able to provide recovered images with quasi-normal brain appearances, the recovered regions may have some artifacts, located in the region around original tumor boundary, as shown in **Figure 8**. This is mainly due to the distinction of sparse constraints between inner boundary (tumor region) and outer boundary (normal region). Even so, compared to the original pathological images, our recovered images are more similar to the normal brain images, thus are more convenient to be used for other image computing tasks, such as multi-atlas segmentation shown in section 3.3.

The tumor region usually occupies a contiguous portion in the MR brain image, thus the distributions of tumor pixels are not pixel-wised sparse but structurally sparse. This motivates us to model the tumor region using the structured sparsity norm. Considering that the structured sparsity norm described in Jia et al. (2012) can effectively encourage sparse component to distribute in structured patterns and also its facility to be implemented in the low-rank and sparse decomposition scheme, we employ this structured sparsity norm (Jia et al., 2012) to model tumor region in this study. Note that the structured sparsity (Jia et al., 2012) could be replaced by sparsity in a different basis (e.g., a wavelet basis), but such sparsity needs to take into account the spatial connection of the sparse pixels.

The tumor segmentation performance of our method still could be improved, especially compared with the state-of-the-art deep learning based segmentation models (Pereira et al., 2016; Havaei et al., 2017). However, these deep learning based methods typically require enormous amount of high-quality labeled images to train a model for medical image segmentation. Although some recent approaches (Mlynarski et al., 2018; Shah et al., 2018) proposed a mixed-supervision scheme, which employed a minority of images with high-quality per-pixel labels and a majority of images with coarse-level annotations (bounding boxes, landmarks or image-level annotations) to train the deep neural networks; preparing annotations such as bounding boxes and landmarks is still laborious. Compared with deep learning based methods, our advantage is that the proposed TLS^{2}D does not require labeled images to train a segmentation model; it extracts tumor regions by analyzing normal MR image appearances from unlabeled population data. What's more, the segmentation results of our method can alleviate the image labeling procedure by the clinicians. Our segmentation results could further be used as label information for the semi-supervised training of deep learning based segmentation models (Papandreou et al., 2015; Bai et al., 2017).

AUTHOR CONTRIBUTIONS

CL, YW, TW, and DN: response for study design; CL: implemented the research and conducted the experiments; CL and YW: conceived the experiments, analyzed the results, and wrote the main manuscript text and prepared the figures. All authors reviewed the manuscript.

ACKNOWLEDGMENTS

The work described in this paper was supported in part by the National Natural Science Foundation of China (No. 61701312), in part by the Natural Science Foundation of Shenzhen University (No. 2018010), and in part by the Shenzhen Peacock Plan under Grant KQTD2016053112051497.

REFERENCES

Achanta, R., Shaji, A., Smith, K., Lucchi, A., Fua, P., Süsstrunk, S., et al. (2012). SLIC superpixels compared to state-of-the-art superpixel methods. *IEEE Trans. Pattern Anal. Mach. Intel.* 34, 2274–2282. doi: 10.1109/TPAMI.2012.120

Adams, A., Baek, J., and Davis, M. A. (2010). Fast highdimensional filtering using the permutohedral lattice. *Computer Graph. Forum.* 29, 753–762. doi: 10.1111/j.1467-8659.2009.01645.x

Bai, W., Oktay, O., Sinclair, M., Suzuki, H., Rajchl, M., Tarroni, G., et al. (2017). "Semi-supervised learning for network-based cardiac MR image segmentation," in *International Conference on Medical Image Computing and Computer-Assisted Intervention (MICCAI)* (Quebec City, QC: Springer), 253–260.

Boyd, S., Parikh, N., Chu, E., Peleato, B., and Eckstein, J. (2011). Distributed optimization and statistical learning via the alternating direction method of multipliers. *Found. Trends Mach. Learn.* 3, 1–122. doi: 10.1561/2200000016

Cabezas, M., Oliver, A., Lladó, X., Freixenet, J., and Cuadra, M. B. (2011). A review of atlas-based segmentation for magnetic resonance brain images. *Comput. Methods Programs Biomed.* 104, e158–e177. doi: 10.1016/j.cmpb.2011.07.015

Candès, E. J., Li, X., Ma, Y., and Wright, J. (2011). Robust principal component analysis? *J. ACM (JACM)* 58, 11. doi: 10.1145/1970392.1970395

Chang, H.-H., Zhuang, A. H., Valentino, D. J., and Chu, W.-C. (2009). Performance measure characterization for evaluating neuroimage segmentation algorithms. *Neuroimage* 47, 122–135. doi: 10.1016/j.neuroimage.2009.03.068

Chen, H., Dou, Q., Yu, L., Qin, J., and Heng, P.-A. (2018). Voxresnet: deep voxelwise residual networks for brain segmentation from 3D MR images. *NeuroImage* 170, 446–455. doi: 10.1016/j.neuroimage.2017.04.041

Gordillo, N., Montseny, E., and Sobrevilla, P. (2013). State of the art survey on MRI brain tumor segmentation. *Magn. Reson. Imaging* 31, 1426–1438. doi: 10.1016/j.mri.2013.05.002

Han, X., Kwitt, R., Aylward, S., Bakas, S., Menze, B., Asturias, A., et al. (2018). Brain extraction from normal and pathological images: a joint PCA/image-reconstruction approach. *NeuroImage* 176, 431–445. doi: 10.1016/j.neuroimage.2018.04.073

Havaei, M., Davy, A., Warde-Farley, D., Biard, A., Courville, A., Bengio, Y., et al. (2017). Brain tumor segmentation with deep neural networks. *Med. Image Anal.* 35, 18–31. doi: 10.1016/j.media.2016.05.004

Iglesias, J. E., and Sabuncu, M. R. (2015). Multi-atlas segmentation of biomedical images: a survey. *Med. Image Anal.* 24, 205–219. doi: 10.1016/j.media.2015.06.012

Jia, K., Chan, T. H., and Ma, Y. (2012). "Robust and practical face recognition via structured sparsity," in *Proceedings of the IEEE European Conference on Computer Vision (ECCV)* (Florence), 331–344.

Joshi, S., Davis, B., Jomier, M., and Gerig, G. (2004). Unbiased diffeomorphic atlas construction for computational anatomy. *Neuroimage* 23, S151–S160. doi: 10.1016/j.neuroimage.2004.07.068

Kamnitsas, K., Ledig, C., Newcombe, V. F., Simpson, J. P., Kane, A. D., Menon, D. K., et al. (2017). Efficient multi-scale 3D cnn with fully connected CRF for accurate brain lesion segmentation. *Med. Image Anal.* 36, 61–78. doi: 10.1016/j.media.2016.10.004

Lin, Z., Chen, M., Wu, L., and Ma, Y. (2010). The augmented lagrange multiplier method for exact recovery of corrupted low-rank matrices. *Eprint Arxiv* 9. doi: 10.1016/j.jsb.2012.10.010

Litjens, G., Kooi, T., Bejnordi, B. E., Setio, A. A. A., Ciompi, F., Ghafoorian, M., et al. (2017). A survey on deep learning in medical image analysis. *Med. Image Anal.* 42, 60–88. doi: 10.1016/j.media.2017.07.005

Liu, X., Niethammer, M., Kwitt, R., McCormick, M., and Aylward, S. (2014). "Low-rank to the rescue–atlas-based analyses in the presence of pathologies," in *International Conference on Medical Image Computing and Computer-Assisted Intervention (MICCAI)* (Cambridge, MA: Springer), 97–104.

Liu, X., Niethammer, M., Kwitt, R., Singh, N., McCormick, M., and Aylward, S. (2015). Low-rank atlas image analyses in the presence of pathologies. *IEEE Trans. Med. Imaging* 34, 2583–2591. doi: 10.1109/TMI.2015.2448556

Mai, J. K., Majtanik, M., and Paxinos, G. (2015). *Atlas of the Human Brain.* Cambridge, MA: Academic Press.

Mairal, J., Jenatton, R., Bach, F. R., and Obozinski, G. R. (2010). "Network flow algorithms for structured sparsity," in *Advances in Neural Information Processing Systems* (Vancouver, BC), 1558–1566.

Menze, B. H., Jakab, A., Bauer, S., Kalpathy-Cramer, J., Farahani, K., Kirby, J., et al. (2015). The multimodal brain tumor image segmentation benchmark (BRATS). *IEEE Trans. Med. Imaging* 34, 1993. doi: 10.1109/TMI.2014.2377694

Mlynarski, P., Delingette, H., Criminisi, A., and Ayache, N. (2018). Deep learning with mixed supervision for brain tumor segmentation. *arXiv* [Preprint] *arXiv:1812.04571.*

Myronenko, A., and Song, X. (2010). Intensity-based image registration by minimizing residual complexity. *IEEE Trans. Med. Imaging* 29, 1882–1891. doi: 10.1109/TMI.2010.2053043

Otazo, R., Candès, E., and Sodickson, D. K. (2015). Low-rank plus sparse matrix decomposition for accelerated dynamic MRI with separation of background and dynamic components. *Magn. Reson. Med.* 73, 1125–1136. doi: 10.1002/mrm.25240

Papandreou, G., Chen, L.-C., Murphy, K. P., and Yuille, A. L. (2015). "Weakly- and semi-supervised learning of a deep convolutional network for semantic image segmentation," in *Proceedings of the IEEE International Conference on Computer Vision (ICCV)* (Santiago), 1742–1750.

Parikh, N., and Boyd, S. (2014). Proximal algorithms. *Found. Trends Optim.* 1, 127–239. doi: 10.1561/2400000003

Peng, Y., Ganesh, A., Wright, J., Xu, W., and Ma, Y. (2012). RASL: robust alignment by sparse and low-rank decomposition for linearly correlated images. *IEEE Trans. Pattern Anal. Mach. Intel.* 34, 2233–2246. doi: 10.1109/TPAMI.2011.282

Perazzi, F., Krähenbühl, P., Pritch, Y., and Hornung, A. (2012). "Saliency filters: Contrast based filtering for salient region detection," in *Proceedings of the IEEE Conference on Computer Vision and Pattern Recognition (CVPR)* (Providence, RI), 733–740.

Pereira, S., Pinto, A., Alves, V., and Silva, C. A. (2016). Brain tumor segmentation using convolutional neural networks in MRI images. *IEEE Trans. Med. Imaging* 35, 1240–1251. doi: 10.1109/TMI.2016.2538465

Shah, M. P., Merchant, S., and Awate, S. P. (2018). "Ms-net: mixed-supervision fully-convolutional networks for full-resolution segmentation," in *International Conference on Medical Image Computing and Computer-Assisted Intervention* (Granada: Springer), 379–387.

Shattuck, D. W., Mirza, M., Adisetiyo, V., Hojatkashani, C., Salamon, G., Narr, K. L., et al. (2008). Construction of a 3D probabilistic atlas of human cortical structures. *NeuroImage* 39, 1064–1080. doi: 10.1016/j.neuroimage.2007.09.031

Shen, D., Wu, G., and Suk, H.-I. (2017). Deep learning in medical image analysis. *Ann. Rev. Biomed. Eng.* 19, 221–248. doi: 10.1146/annurev-bioeng-071516-044442

Sotiras, A., Davatzikos, C., and Paragios, N. (2013). Deformable medical image registration: a survey. *IEEE Trans. Med. Imaging* 32, 1153–1190. doi: 10.1109/TMI.2013.2265603

Tang, Z., Ahmad, S., Yap, P. T., and Shen, D. (2018). Multi-atlas segmentation of MR tumor brain images using low-rank based image recovery. *IEEE Trans. Med. Imaging* 37, 2224–2235. doi: 10.1109/TMI.2018.2824243

Wang, Y., Zheng, Q., and Heng, P. A. (2018). Online robust projective dictionary learning: shape modeling for MR-TRUS registration. *IEEE Trans. Med. Imaging* 37, 1067–1078. doi: 10.1109/TMI.2017.2777870

Wang, Z., Bovik, A. C., Sheikh, H. R., and Simoncelli, E. P. (2004). Image quality assessment: from error visibility to structural similarity. *IEEE Trans. Image Proc.* 13, 600–612. doi: 10.1109/TIP.2003.819861

Wright, J., Ganesh, A., Rao, S., Peng, Y., and Ma, Y. (2009). "Robust principal component analysis: exact recovery of corrupted low-rank matrices via convex optimization," in *Advances in Neural Information Processing Systems*, (Vancouver, BC), 2080–2088.

Zhao, X., Wu, Y., Song, G., Li, Z., Zhang, Y., and Fan, Y. (2018). A deep learning model integrating FCNNs and CRFs for brain tumor segmentation. *Med. Image Anal.* 43, 98–111. doi: 10.1016/j.media.2017.10.002

Zheng, Q., Wang, Y., and Heng, P. A. (2017). "Online robust image alignment via subspace learning from gradient orientations," in *Proceedings of the IEEE Conference on Computer Vision (ICCV)* (Venice), 1771–1780.

Zhou, S. K., Greenspan, H., and Shen, D. (2017). *Deep Learning for Medical Image Analysis*. Cambridge, MA: Academic Press.

12

Brain White Matter Hyperintensity Lesion Characterization in T_2 Fluid-Attenuated Inversion Recovery Magnetic Resonance Images: Shape, Texture and Potential Growth

Chih-Ying Gwo[1*†], *David C. Zhu*[2†] *and Rong Zhang*[3†]

[1] *Department of Information Management, Chien Hsin University of Science and Technology, Zhongli District, Taiwan,* [2] *Department of Radiology and Psychology, and Cognitive Imaging Research Center, Michigan State University, East Lansing, MI, United States,* [3] *Department of Neurology and Neurotherapeutics, Department of Internal Medicine, University of Texas Southwestern Medical Center and Institute for Exercise and Environmental Medicine, Texas Health Presbyterian Hospital Dallas, Dallas, TX, United States*

Correspondence:
Chih-Ying Gwo
ericgwo@uch.edu.tw

†These authors have contributed equally to this work as co-authors

Prior methods in characterizing age-related white matter hyperintensity (WMH) lesions on T_2 fluid-attenuated inversion recovery (FLAIR) magnetic resonance images (MRI) have mainly been limited to understanding the sizes of, and occasionally the locations of WMH lesions. Systematic morphological characterization has been missing. In this work, we proposed innovative methods to fill this knowledge gap. We developed an innovative and proof-of-concept method to characterize and quantify the shape (based on Zernike transformation) and texture (based on fuzzy logic) of WMH lesions. We have also developed a multi-dimension feature vector approach to cluster WMH lesions into distinctive groups based on their shape and then texture features. We then developed an approach to calculate the potential growth index (PGI) of WMH lesions based on the image intensity distributions at the edge of the WMH lesions using a region-growing algorithm. High-quality T_2 FLAIR images containing clearly identifiable WMH lesions with various sizes from six cognitively normal older adults were used in our method development Analyses of Variance (ANOVAs) showed significant differences in PGI among WMH group clusters in terms of either the shape ($P = 1.06 \times 10^{-2}$) or the texture ($P < 1 \times 10^{-20}$) features. In conclusion, we propose a systematic framework on which the shape and texture features of WMH lesions can be quantified and may be used to predict lesion growth in older adults.

Keywords: brain T_2 FLAIR hyperintensity, shape, texture, potential growth, morphology

INTRODUCTION

The presence of white matter hyperintensities (WMH) on T_2 fluid-attenuated inversion recovery (FLAIR) magnetic resonance images (MRI) is common in older adults over 65 years old with a prevalence rate of ~ 60–80% in the general population (De Leeuw et al., 2001; Wen and Sachdev, 2004). WMH lesions are even more extensive in those with vascular or Alzheimer's disease (AD) type of dementia when compared with cognitively normal older adults, suggesting its role in dementia pathogenesis and neurocognitive dysfunction (Bombois et al., 2007; Kloppenborg et al., 2014; Lee et al., 2016). WMH is also frequently observed in patients with multiple sclerosis (MS) (Loizou et al., 2015; Newton et al., 2017). Qualitative and quantitative WMH characterization has been used as a biomarker to assist cerebrovascular and neurodegenerative disease diagnosis and to assess treatment effects (Wardlaw et al., 2013). The pathogenic mechanisms of WMH are not well-understood, and have been attributed to cerebral small vessel disease (CSVD), white matter demyelization, or both, indicating brain white matter lesions (Greenberg, 2006; Wardlaw et al., 2013). Furthermore, periventricular and subcortical deep WMHs may have different pathogenic mechanisms (Schmidt et al., 2011; Poels et al., 2012; Tseng et al., 2013).

The most commonly used methods for WMH quantification in brain aging, vascular, and AD type of dementia are to measure its regional or total volume (i.e., the sum of WMH voxel size) within the whole brain based on image tissue segmentation algorithms (DeCarli et al., 2005; Wardlaw et al., 2013). This method, however, neglects entirely the typological or morphological features of WMH lesions which may have important clinical significance as demonstrated in recent studies in patients with MS (Loizou et al., 2015; Newton et al., 2017).

WMH shape is a basic morphological feature which can be derived from T_2 FLAIR images after tissue segmentation. Shape feature extraction, recognition, and classification can be implemented either in the original or the transformed image space (Khotanzad and Hong, 1990; Mikolajczyk et al., 2003; Carmichael and Hebert, 2004; Tahmasbi et al., 2011). Current shape classification methods include mainly the following: (1) one-dimensional function shape representation (Kauppinen et al., 1995; Yadav et al., 2007; Zhang and Lu), (2) polygonal approximation (ShuiHua and ShuangYuan), (3) spatial interrelation feature (Sebastian et al., 2004; Guru and Nagendraswamy, 2007; Bauckhage and Tsotsos), (4) moments (Mukundan, 2004; Celebi and Aslandogan; Taubin and Cooper), (5) scale-space methods (Zhang and Lu, 2003; Kpalma and Ronsin, 2006), and (6) shape transform domains (Chen and Bui, 1999; Zhang and Lu). These methods for shape classification may be suitable for specific applications in various fields but have major limitations for shape characterization of brain lesions. For example, method (1) is highly sensitive to noise, and inaccurate boundary definition can cause large errors; method (2) can only represent the object appearance but not all shape features; method (3) may be used to describe the general appearance of an object, but is limited by the orientation and size of the object; method (4) contains redundant information in the image feature vectors and thus unique images cannot be reconstructed back; method (5) is limited to the shapes which have shallow concavities/convexities; and method (6) requires the definition of the shape contour starting point derived from other methods. In order to characterize the complex shapes of brain lesions, a technique needs to be invariant to the orientation of a lesion, be resistant to image noise and be able to define a one-to-one relationship between feature vector and shape. In this regard, Zernike transformation can satisfy these criteria (Khotanzad and Hong, 1990). Similar to Fourier analysis, shape features of an object captured on MRI can be represented by the coefficients of shape function of the Zernike polynomial expansion (i.e., Zernike transform), referred to as Zernike moments (ZMs) (Zernike, 1934). In this study, we applied Zernike transformation to extract WMH shape features for pattern recognition and classification in cognitively normal older adults.

Image texture is another morphological feature which can be categorized through modeling (Chen et al., 1989), structure (Chow and Rahman, 2007), transformation (Tsai and Hsiao, 2001), and statistics based methods (Haralick et al., 1973; Iivarinen et al., 1996). Model-based and structure-based methods work best for repeating texture patterns but are not suitable for irregular texture patterns such as those in brain lesion images. The transformation based method works best in identifying sub-regions with known characteristics, but does not work well on unknown and potentially complicated patterns such as those in brain lesion images. Statistical-based methods describe the texture in the distribution of and relationships between gray-level values in an image. These statistics-based methods can normally describe objects better than the structure and transformation based methods because they are invariant to the orientation, the size of an object, and also robust to the noise inside the object (Castellano et al., 2004). Since WMH lesions often have various sizes, orientations, and locations, and are manifested across multiple image slices, a statistics-based method is likely to be the best choice to accommodate these complexities. Therefore, we adopted a statistical method based on fuzzy logic to construct the image intensity histogram of WMH lesions for texture feature extraction.

Finally, we have thought that as a potential imaging biomarker of brain aging and CSVD, the size, shape, and image texture of WMH lesion may change with time (Sachdev et al., 2007; Godin et al., 2011) which may reflect the progression of the underlying pathological process. In this regard, recent studies have shown that the immediate surrounding areas of clearly defined WMH lesions may be at risk for further tissue damage and conversion to lesions (Maillard et al., 2014; Promjunyakul et al., 2016). These areas are classified as WMH penumbras (Maillard et al., 2014). To characterize WMH lesions as well as their penumbras, we developed a seed-based region-growing algorithm to characterize WMH boundaries to explore the potential growth of WMH lesions. We defined this specific WMH boundary characteristic as potential growth index (PGI). To explore whether the shape and texture characterization techniques can potentially be used to predict lesion growth, we assessed whether different shape and texture patterns are related to PGI.

METHODS AND RESULTS

MRI Acquisition

Full-brain 2D T_2 FLAIR images were collected on a Philips Achieva 3T scanner (Philips Healthcare, Best, the Netherlands) with the following parameters: axial, time of echo (TE) = 125 ms, time of repetition (TR) = 11 s, time of inversion (TI) = 2,800 ms, field of view (FOV) = 23 cm × 23 cm, slice thickness = 2.5 mm, number of slices = 64 with no gaps, acquisition matrix size =

352 × 212, and reconstructed matrix size = 512 × 512. All subjects signed informed consent approved by the Institutional Review Boards of the UT Southwestern Medical Center and Texas Health Presbyterian Hospital of Dallas. Six T_2 FLAIR brain image datasets (two male, four female, 75 ± 4 years old and normal cognition), which contained clearly identifiable white matter hyperintensity (WMH) lesions with various sizes, were selected from an healthy aging study we published previously (Tarumi et al., 2014).

T_2 FLAIR Image Segmentation

T_2 FLAIR WMH regions were segmented on each 2D image through the lesion prediction algorithm (LPA) implemented in the Lesion Segmentation Toolbox (LST) version 2.0.12 for Statistical Parametric Mapping (SPM12). In LPA, the algorithm is trained using a logistic regression model on T_2 FLAIR brain images from 53 MS patients with severe lesion patterns. LPA was also validated in other patient populations such as older adults with diabetes (Maldjian et al., 2013). The fitness of a new T_2 FLAIR brain image to this model provides an estimate of lesion probability for each voxel in the image. In this study, we used a threshold of 0.5, as suggested by LST, on the obtained lesion probability maps to identify WMH regions. The segmentation accuracy was further verified through visual inspection. **Figure 1** shows an example of the segmentation.

Lesion Size Distribution

WMH binary masks generated from 2D T_2 FLAIR images (**Figure 1**) were used to obtain WMH size distribution. To minimize artifacts, only those masks with more than 10 connected WMH voxels (voxel size: 0.45 mm × 0.45 mm) on an image were considered probable lesions and were used for further characterization, which resulted in a total of 993 WMH lesions. Fitting each of these lesions within a square, these lesions had a size range of from 6 × 6 to 176 × 176 voxels. The lesion size distributions of six subjects are shown in **Figure 2**. Of note, more than 93% of these lesions are ≤ 60 × 60, and only about 1.5% are ≥ 120 × 120 voxels.

WMH Shape Feature Extraction and Classification in 2D

WMH Shape Feature Extraction Using Zernike Transformation

Zernike transformation has been used extensively in imaging shape feature extraction and pattern recognition (Papakostas et al., 2007; Wee and Paramesran, 2007). The coefficients of Zernike polynomial expansion of an object are referred to as Zernike moments (ZMs) which are used to represent the shape features of analyzed objects. In this study, Zernike polynomials were expressed in polar coordinates defined on a unit disc, which are a complete set of orthogonal basis functions (Papakostas et al., 2007; Wee and Paramesran, 2007). The lower-order ZMs describe global contour and gross shape features, and the higher-order ZMs describe regional and fine topological details of a shape (Gwo and Wei, 2016). Of note, the magnitudes of ZMs are not only rotational invariant but also robust to small perturbations on the contour of a shape image (Teh and Chin, 1988).

For a 2D image object (a WMH lesion image segmented from a T2 FLAIR image in this work), using polar coordinates, the complex Zernike moments of order n with repetition m can be represented as the inner product of a shape function $f(r,\theta)$ with the basis function of Zernike polynomials, $V_{nm}(r,\theta)$, specifically as

$$Z_{nm} = \frac{n+1}{\pi} \int_0^{2\pi} \int_0^1 f(r,\theta)\, V_{nm}^*(r,\theta)\, r dr d\theta, \quad |r| \le 1, \tag{1}$$

where $V_{nm}^*(r,\theta)$ denotes the complex conjugation of $V_{nm}(r,\theta)$. The basis function of Zernike polynomial is given by

$$V_{nm}(r,\theta) = R_{nm}(r)\, e^{im\theta}, \quad i = \sqrt{-1} \tag{2}$$

where the radial polynomial, $R_{nm}(r)$, is defined as follows:

$$R_{nm}(r) = \sum_{k}^{\frac{n-|m|}{2}} (-1)^k \frac{(n-k)!}{k!\left(\frac{n+|m|}{2}-k\right)!\left(\frac{n-|m|}{2}-k\right)!} r^{n-2k} \tag{3}$$

where $0 \le |m| \le n$, $n-|m|$ is an even integer, and $n \ge 0$.

Since the shape features represented by ZMs at orders higher than six are usually too small (small ZM magnitude) to be detected reliably by human eyes (Charman, 2005), the maximum Zernike transformation order was set to five in this study (**Figure 3**). In Zernike transformation, $|V_{n,+m}(r,\theta)| = |V_{n,-m}(r,\theta)|$, and $|Z_{n,+m}| = |Z_{n,-m}|$. The number of distinctive ZM magnitudes for an expansion up to order n is computed as follows:

$$\begin{cases} \left(\frac{n+2}{2}\right)^2 & \text{if ordern is even} \\ \frac{(n+3)(n+1)}{4} & \text{if order n is odd} \end{cases} \tag{4}$$

Shape feature extraction procedures based on Zernike transformation are illustrated in **Figure 4**. In this illustration, we chose three WMH masks, two with a similar shape but different sizes, and one with both different shape and size. To simplify computation complexity, these image masks with different sizes were first scaled to the same size of 60 × 60 voxels so that the ZM magnitudes can be compared on a same scale. Each Z_{nm} was calculated using Equation (1–3). The calculation resulted with 21 ZM complex coefficients with maximum order $n = 5$. Based on the magnitudes of the ZM coefficient, only 12 coefficients were needed to extract shape features since the WMH shape (mask) generated with tissue segmentation is rotational invariant. As shown in the right column of **Figure 4**, the two lesion images (a) and (b) with a similar shape have similar ZMs magnitudes at all 12 coefficients. On the contrary, the ZM magnitudes of WMH lesions with a different shape are different from the other two.

WMH Shape Classification

We then classified the lesion images to different clusters (groups) based on the similarity on shape features. Current common clustering algorithms, such as the K-means clustering algorithm,

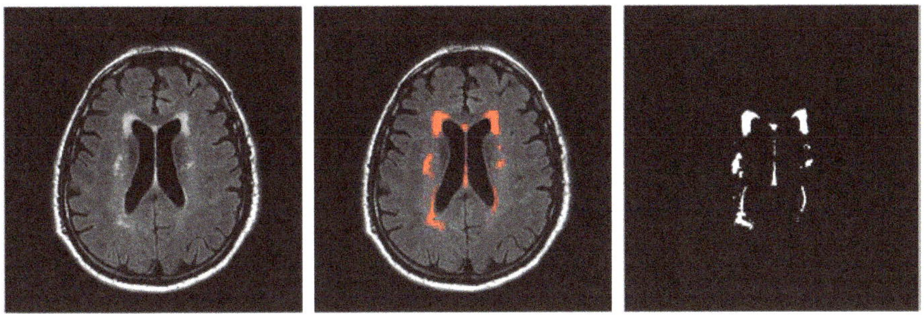

FIGURE 1 | An example T_2 FLAIR image from one subject showing multiple white-matter hyperintensity (WMH) lesions; the results of WMH segmentation using the lesion prediction algorithm (LPA) showing in red, and a WMH binary mask after tissue segmentation, which was used in shape feature extraction.

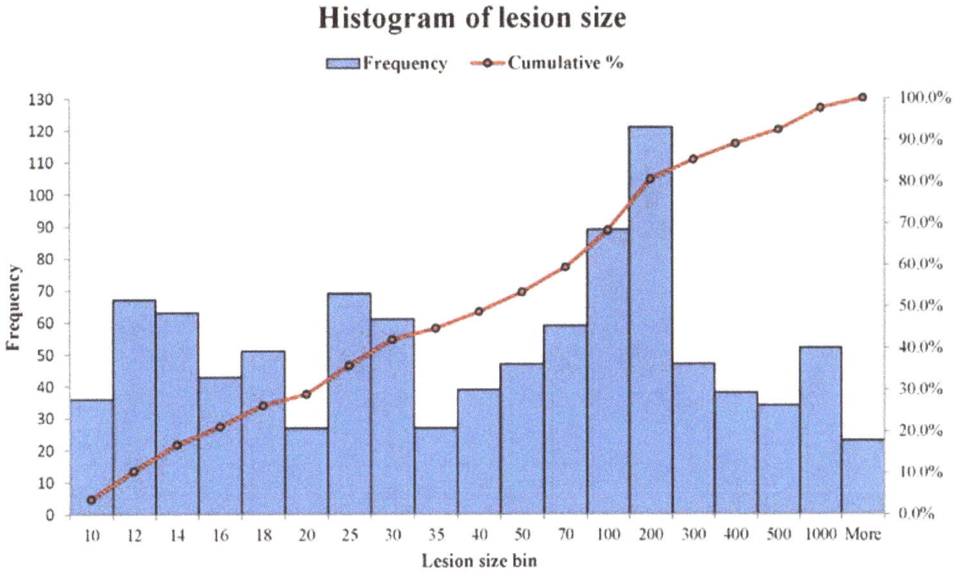

FIGURE 2 | The histograms of WMH lesion size distributions in two representative subjects. The lesion size bin of 50 represents the lesion size range from 40 × 40 to 50 × 50 voxels. The frequency scale (the left vertical axis) is the counts the number of lesion sizes within a lesion size bin. The cumulative percentage of lesion size relative to the total lesion counts is labeled on the right vertical axis.

requires data-specific a priori selection on the number of clusters (Zhao, 2012). For instance, if the number of clusters is too small, the WMH lesion images with noticeable different shapes may be grouped inappropriately into a same cluster. On the other hand, if the number of clusters is too large, lesion images with trivial differences may be assigned into different clusters, confounding potential clinical significance. Finding the appropriate number of clusters using model simulation is one way to resolve this dilemma (Zhao, 2012). However, this procedure has to be carried out for all choices of shape feature dimensions. To simplify the procedures, the estimation of cluster characteristic indices based on sum of within-cluster dispersions [W_k in Equation (5)] or its variants were proposed (Ball and Hall, 1965; Calinski and Harabasz, 1974; Xu, 1997; Tibshirani et al., 2001). For a better understanding of the influences of the classifiable number of clusters and the feature dimensions derived from the Zernike transform on W_k, we plotted W_k as a function of cluster numbers and feature dimensions which are equivalent to the numbers of the distinctive magnitudes of the ZMs (**Figure 5**). The ZMs for WMH shapes from one to 10 orders were calculated to generate 2 to 36 dimensional feature vectors (Equation 4). Euclidean distance was then calculated to assess the similarity between the feature vectors. The K-means clustering algorithm was applied for grouping purpose. W_k was calculated based on the 2 to 20 cluster groups at each feature dimensions. W_k, in general, decreases with the increase of the number of clusters but increases with the increase of the number of feature dimensions (**Figure 5**). For a specified feature dimension, a better grouping result is likely achieved at a lower W_k value by finding a local minimum. However, in some feature dimensions, a local minimum cannot be found even after W_k decreases to nearly constant. For example, when two is selected as the feature dimension, the W_k value remains small even at small number of clusters because two-dimensional feature vectors only represents

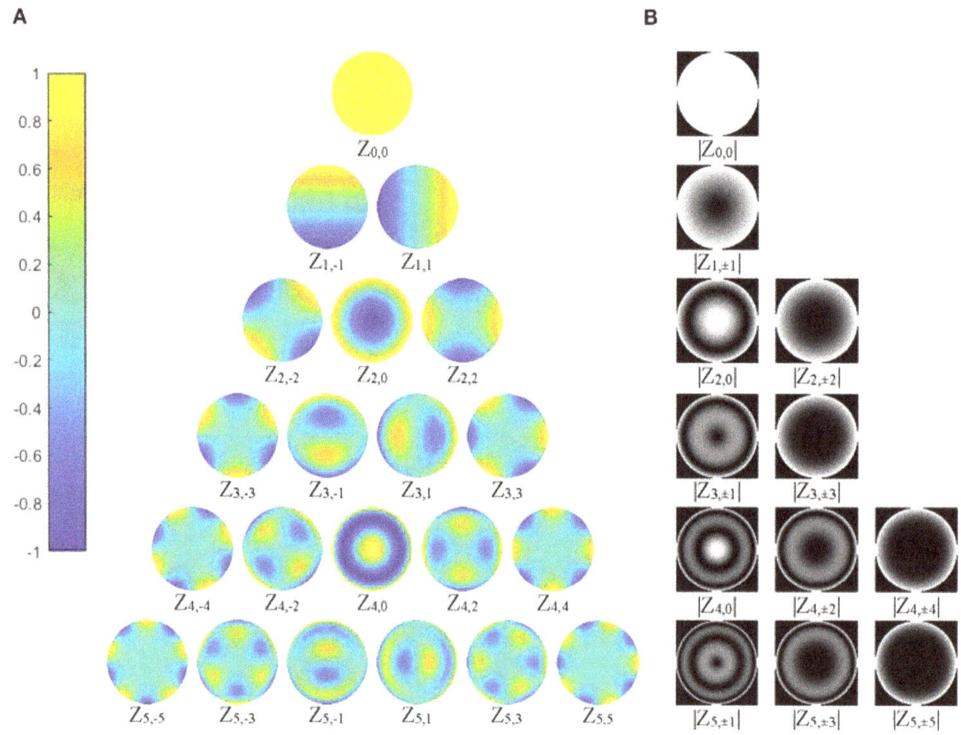

FIGURE 3 | (A) The 21 basis functions of Zernike polynomials, $V_{nm}(r, \theta)$, with order $n \leq 5$, are illustrated. The polynomials have a radial range of [−1, 1] ($|V_{nm}(r, \theta)| \leq 1$), shown by the color bar on the left column; **(B)** 12 distinctive magnitude images, which are rotational invariance, are shown, corresponding to the polynomials in **(A)**.

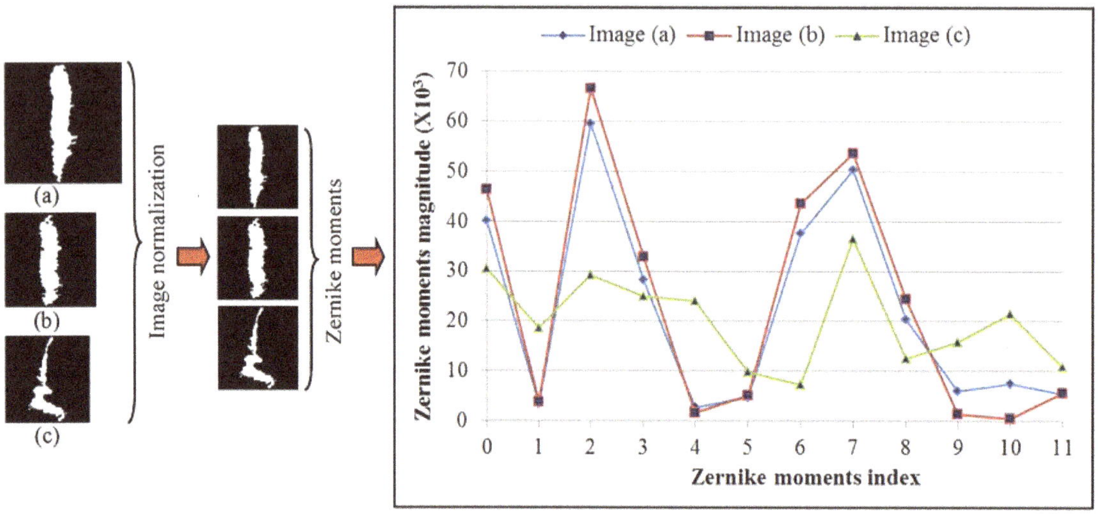

FIGURE 4 | Three representative white mater hyperintensity masks generated after tissue segmentation with different sizes and shape are shown in the left column. The images are normalized to the same size of 60 × 60 voxels shown in the middle column. The magnitudes of 12 Zernike moments coefficients based on ZM orders ≤5 of Zernike polynomial expansion are shown in the right column for comparison.

the gross global contour and thus cannot differentiate shapes with enough details. Therefore, selecting an appropriate feature dimension is also crucial and will be discussed later. Nevertheless, once a feature dimension is selected [which was selected to be 12 in this study based on our exploration of data features (**Figures 4, 5**)], the optimal number of clusters can be determined based on the estimation of cluster characteristics discussed below (Desgraupes, 2013).

The distance between two points in a share feature vector space can be calculated based on Euclidian distance. The overall distance of all points in a cluster to their mean indicates the compactness of a cluster, or within-cluster dispersion. To determine the optimal number of shape clusters for WMH shape classification, we then employed a gap statistics method proposed by Tibshirani et al. (2001). This method estimates the optimal number of clusters by comparing the logarithm of the sum of within-cluster dispersions of a set of clusters to that from the reference datasets created through sampling uniformly at random from the original dataset. The sum of all within-cluster dispersions decreases gradually with the increase of number of clusters but becomes nearly constant at some points as demonstrated in **Figure 5**. This is so called "elbow" phenomenon, which has been used to find the optimal number of clusters (Tibshirani et al., 2001). The algorithm used to estimate the optimal number of WMH shape clusters based on the gap statistic is presented below:

1. Group the shape vectors by varying the number of shape clusters from $k = 1, 2, \ldots, N$ (pre-defined as the maximum to evaluate), and compute the sum of the within-cluster dispersion W_k for each choice k.

$$W_k = \sum_{r=1}^{k} \sum_{x_i \in C_r} (x_i - \bar{x}_r)^2 \quad (5)$$

where x_i is a data point, C_r denotes cluster r, and $\bar{x}_r$ is the vector mean of C_r.

Generate reference datasets (total number $= B$) by sampling uniformly at random from the original dataset within its distribution ranges of all dimensions. Although a better statistically randomness is likely achieved with a large B, the choice of B is bounded by computation demand. For each reference dataset b, we can generate k clusters, and we can calculate the sum of the within-cluster dispersion W_{kb} for each k based on Equation (5) above, where $b = 1, 2, \ldots, B$; $k = 1, 2, \ldots, N$. The gap statistics for each k is calculated as below:

$$Gap\left(k\right) = \frac{1}{B}\sum_{b=1}^{B} \log\left(W_{kb}\right) - \log\left(W_k\right) \quad (6)$$

2. let$l = (1/B) \sum_b \log\left(W_{kb}\right)$, compute the standard deviation

$$sd_k = \left[\frac{1}{B}\sum_{b=1}^{B} \left(\log\left(W_{kb}\right) - l\right)^2\right]^{1/2} \quad (7)$$

Let $s_k = sd_k\sqrt{(1 + 1/B)}$. Choose the optimal number of shape clusters k_{opt} by Equation (8)

$$k_{opt} = \text{smallest } k \text{ such that Gap}\left(k\right) \geq Gap\left(k+1\right) - s_{k+1} \quad (8)$$

In the gap statistic procedure above, N is a pre-selected number of shape clusters such that k_{opt} can be determined in the range of $[1, N]$. B is selected such that the value of sd_k converges. In this study, N and B were set to 20 and 10, respectively.

For the WMH shape datasets in this study, based on the previous discussion and **Figure 5**, the "elbow" phenomenon was sufficiently noticeable when the feature dimension was set to 12. At this feature dimension, only ZM magnitudes corresponding to ZM orders of $n = 0$ to 5 were used in clustering [cf. Equation (4)]. The Gap values were calculated and displayed in **Figure 6**; the optimal number of shape clusters was selected to be six according to Equation (8).

Figure 7 shows the WMH shape classification results using the K-means algorithm based on the cluster number of six and feature dimension of 12. Unique shape difference can be visualized between the six clusters.

WMH Texture Feature and Classification

Texture Feature Extraction

Image texture characterizes the voxel signal intensity distribution patterns in a WMH region. Statistics-based methods quantify the distribution and relationships of voxel signal values in an image region. These methods often provide better discrimination indexes than structure and spectral transformation based methods (Castellano et al., 2004).

WMH lesions often have various sizes, orientations and locations, and manifest across multiple image slices. In this study, the distributions of WMH lesion size measured in the number of voxels are presented in **Figure 8**.

Most lesions are small, with 48.64% of lesions $\leq$40 voxels (8 mm^2 on a slice). Therefore, a robust texture analysis method needs to satisfy three requirements: (1) Texture feature should be independent of lesion orientation and location; (2) texture feature should be able to quantify small lesions, and (3) texture characterization needs to go beyond a single image slice. A statistics-based method for WMH texture feature extraction is described next.

Since WMH lesions manifests across multiple slices, we used the "WMH3D" term to emphasize the 3D perspective. Specifically, if a WMH lesion image in a slice connects directly either above, below, or diagonally to another WMH lesion image in an adjacent slice, we treat these lesion images belonging to the same lesion, called it a "WMH3D" for texture analysis. This treatment also reduces the chance of false positive in lesion identification. To characterize the voxel signal intensity distribution, potential voxel spike noise, which is often seen in images, needs to remove first. This can be accomplished by setting the voxel intensities within the boundaries of above or below three standard deviations of the mean values. To reduce the slice variation in signal intensity, a min-max normalization was applied to a WMH3D to normalize its voxel intensity based on the equation,

$$s\left(x, y, z\right) = \frac{f\left(x, y, z\right) - gMin}{gMax - gMin} \quad (9)$$

where $f\left(x, y, z\right)$ is the intensity of voxel (x, y) at the zth slice and $s \in [0,1]$, $gMax = Max$(voxel intensities of WMH3D) and $gMin = Min$ (voxel intensities of WMH3D).

For feature extraction, the normalized data were quantized into one of the pre-selected bins to create a histogram that

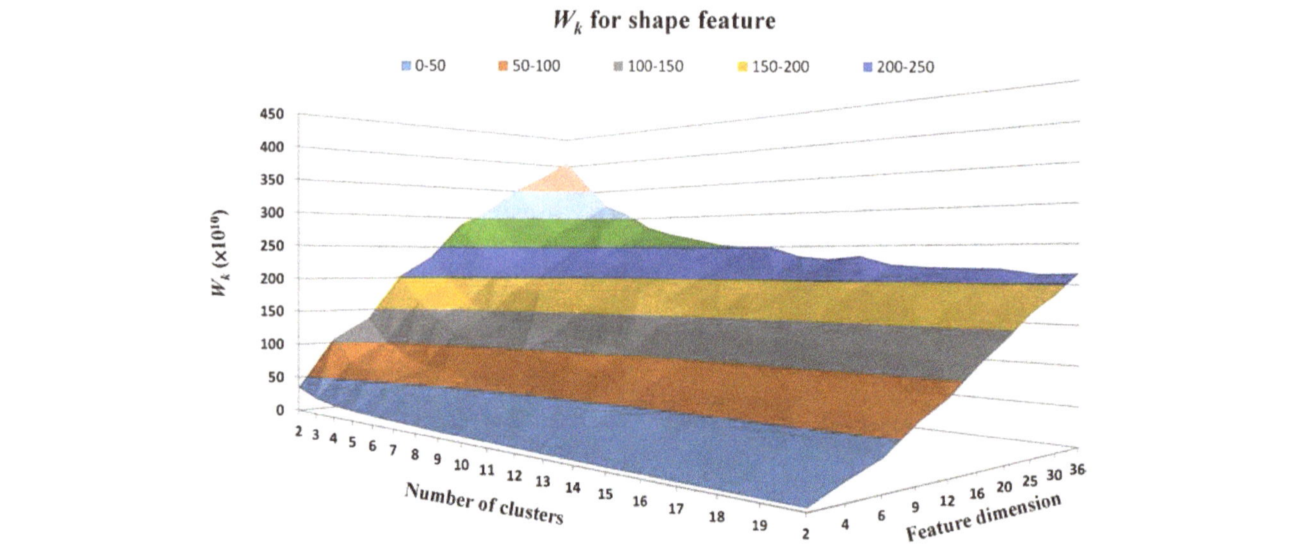

FIGURE 5 | The within-cluster dispersion W_k as a function of the number of shape clusters and feature dimensions. The feature dimensions are the number of distinctive magnitudes of the ZMs. W_k, in general, tends to decrease with the number of clusters but increase with the number of feature dimensions.

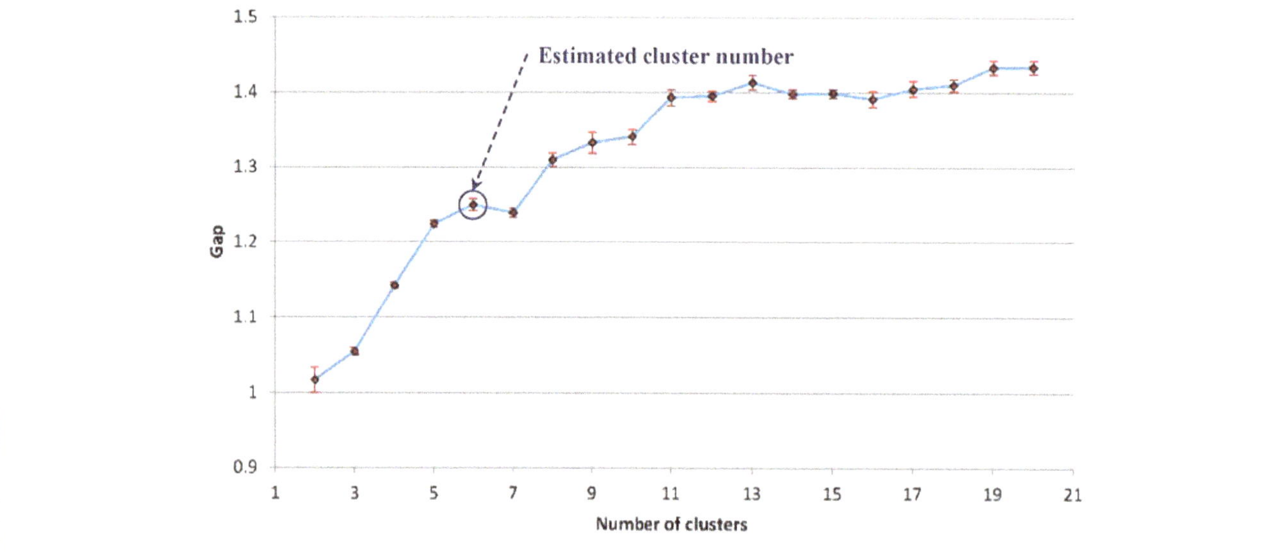

FIGURE 6 | The estimated gap statistic Gap as a function of shape cluster number k (dots and solid curve), error bars are $\pm s_k$.

represents voxel intensity distribution of a WMH3D. To minimize the interference of image noise to the frequency histogram, we propose a fuzzy logic method (Gwo and Wei, 2013) to allocate voxel intensity values to each of the pre-selected bins. Specifically, a normalized voxel intensity s is assigned proportionally two values, called fuzzy values, to the two neighboring bins according its relative positions to the bin centers (**Figure 9**). The fuzzy logic method not only is able to characterize the local image signal intensity distribution of a lesion, but also its global distribution, producing different histogram skewness based on the intensity mean value.

The fuzzy logic functions used for assigning voxels to the frequency histogram are presented in Equation (10). The fuzzy value v[j] at bin j is calculated as:

$$\begin{cases} v[0] = 1 \quad \text{if } s \le \frac{1}{2n} \\ \left.\begin{array}{l} v[j-1] = \frac{2j+1}{2} - s \times n \\ v[j] = s \times n - \frac{2j-1}{2} \end{array}\right\} \text{if } s \le \frac{2j+1}{2n} \\ \left.\begin{array}{l} v[j] = \frac{2j+3}{2} - s \times n \\ v[j+1] = s \times n - \frac{2j+1}{2} \end{array}\right\} \text{if } s > \frac{2j+1}{2n} \\ v[n-1] = 1 \text{ if } s \ge 1 - \frac{1}{2n} \end{cases} \tag{10}$$

Shape type	Number of lesions	The six lesion images closest to the cluster center
1	105	
2	86	
3	176	
4	237	
5	211	
6	178	

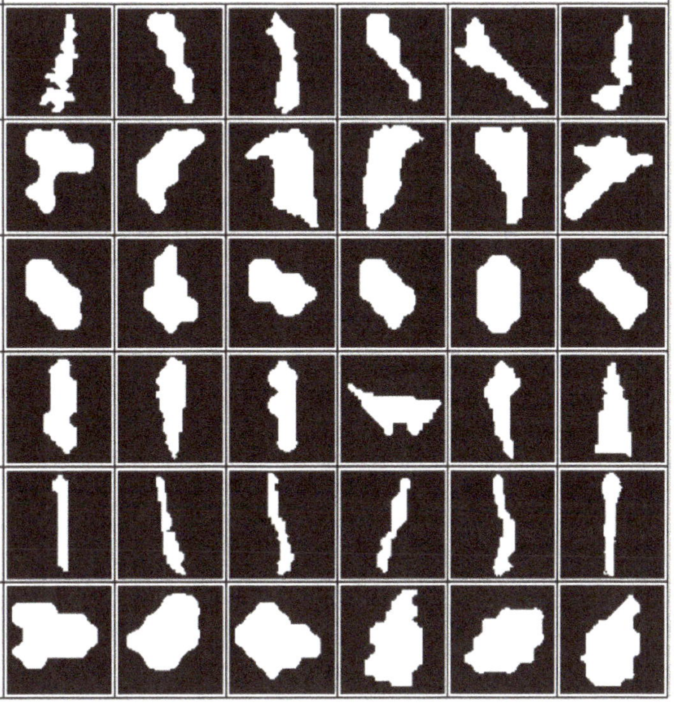

FIGURE 7 | WMH shape classification results using the K-means algorithm based on the cluster number of six and feature dimension of 12. The number of lesion images in each cluster and the six normalized lesion images closest to the cluster mean in each cluster are shown. All lesion images shown in the figure were normalized to the size of 60 × 60 voxels.

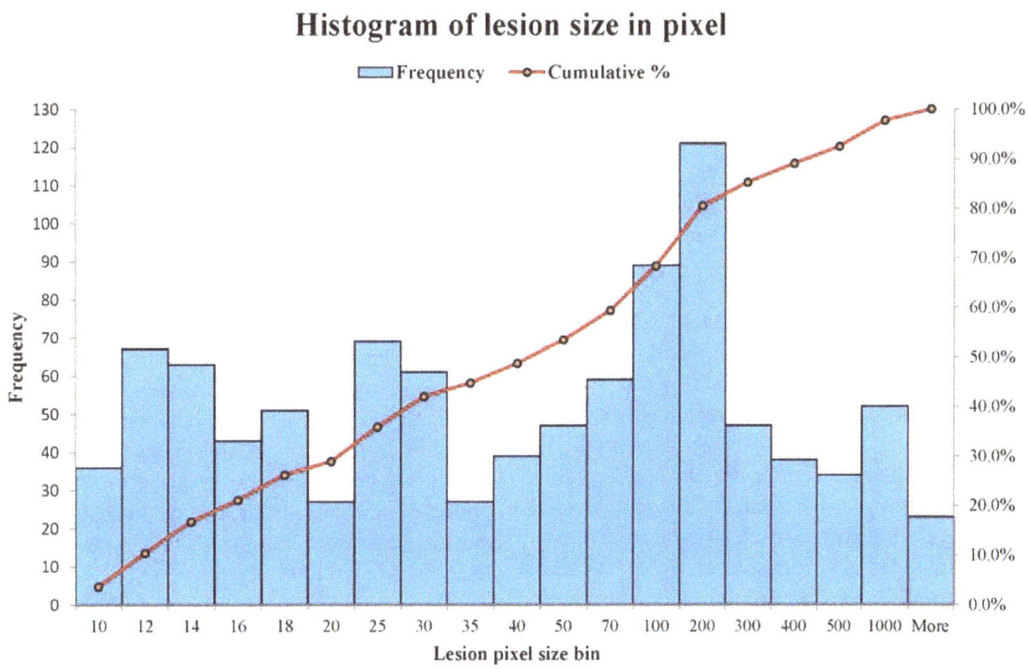

FIGURE 8 | The distributions of WMH lesion size measured in number of voxels from the six subjects. A number shown in a lesion size bin (the horizontal axis) represents a lesion size range. For example, lesion size bin of 50 represents the lesion size range of 40 × 40 to 50 × 50 voxels. Frequency (the vertical axis) counts the number of lesion sizes at the lesion size bins.

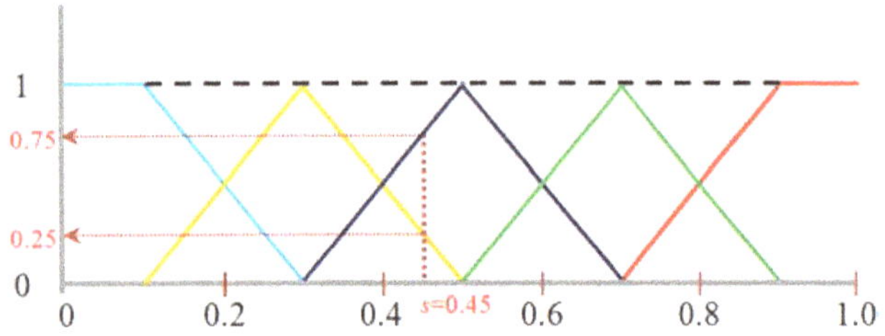

FIGURE 9 | The fuzzy logic functions used for assigning voxels to five bins: bin [0, 0.2] shown in blue, bin [0.2, 0.4] in orange, bin [0.4, 0.6] in black, bin [0.6, 0.8] in green, and bin [0.8, 1.0] in red. A normalized image intensity value is assigned to its two neighboring bins based on these assignments functions. For example, s of 0.45 is assigned to a frequency value of 0.25 to the bin [0.2, 0.4], and 0.75 to the bin [0.4, 0.6] as indicated by the vertical and horizontal dotted lines.

where n = the total number of bins, and j = 0, ..., n-1. To choose a proper number of bins, there are two considerations: (1) When the number of bins increases, the accumulated fuzzy values in some bins become sparse, especially for small size lesions. Sparsity is problematic for any statistical analysis method (Hughes, 1968). The amount of data needed to obtain a reliable statistical result grows exponentially with the number of bins (Hughes, 1968); (2) conversely, if the number of bins is too small, image features may not be differentiated effectively. In this study, to facilitate WMH texture feature classification discussed below, we selected five bins for texture feature extraction.

Since the sizes of WMH lesions vary in a wide range (**Figure 8**), the image intensity frequency distribution histograms need to be further normalized before they can be compared. Herein, each histogram is normalized to have a total accumulative frequency of 1. For example, for a WMH lesion shown in the first row in **Figure 10**, the original distributions of histogram with five bins and 814 voxels would produce a texture feature vector of (266.6, 240.2, 153.9, 125.3, 28.0). To compare with other WMH lesions with different sizes, this vector was divided by 814 to become the normalized distribution of (0.3275, 0.2951, 0.1891, 0.1539, 0.0343).

WMH Texture Feature Classification

Texture feature classification of individual WMH lesion images was conducted using a feature vector clustering method similar to those discussed above in the section of "WMH Shape Classification." Of note, the texture feature vector is based on the histogram presented above using the fuzzy logic method. The influences of different texture feature dimensions (i.e., the number of bins used to construct the intensity histogram) and the numbers of clusters on texture feature classification were explored using the same strategy discussed above for WMH shape feature classification. Based on prior works (Shapiro and Stockman, 2001), Manhattan distance is a more preferred choice over Euclidean distance in accessing the similarity between feature vectors described in histograms. Thus, Manhattan distance was used to assess the similarity between the texture feature vectors in our work. The sum of within-cluster dispersion W_k value was calculated with the cluster number from 2 to 20 and

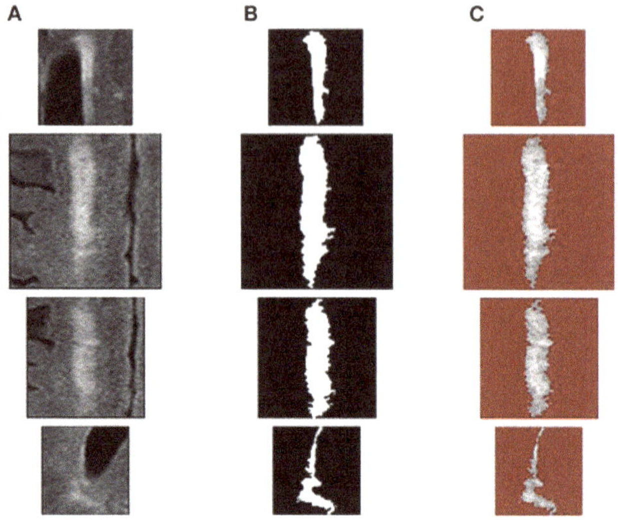

FIGURE 10 | WMH texture feature extraction procedures: **(A)** source WMH lesion images, **(B)** WMH lesion mask images, and **(C)** WMH texture quantized images using fuzzy logic method.

the feature dimensions from 3 to 15. As illustrated in **Figure 11**, W_k tends to decrease with the increase of the cluster numbers. A noticeable "elbow" phenomenon was seen for a wide range of texture feature dimensions from 3 to 15.

The gap statistics discussed above was applied to determine the optimal number of texture feature cluster for pattern recognition based on the K-means algorithm for grouping (Hartigan and Wong, 1979). **Figure 12** shows that five is the optimal number of cluster.

Figure 13 shows the texture classification results, demonstrating five unique clusters.

WMH Potential Growth Index in 2D

We developed a seed-based region-growing algorithm to characterize WMH boundary conditions in order to explore potential growth of WMH lesions (Maillard et al., 2014; Promjunyakul et al., 2016). We hypothesized that the area of potential growth of WMH lesions has similar signal intensity as WMH lesions and is located around the boundary of WMH lesions. With a pre-defined signal intensity threshold, calculated by the extreme values in the WMH3D [Equation (9)], we can use a seed-based region-growing algorithm to find the "potential growth" voxels around the WMH boundary. The region-growing algorithm is initiated by selecting the WMH mask boundary voxels as the growing seeds. At each growing seed voxel, the eight connected neighbor voxels, defined as $A_8(x, y)$ in Equation (11) below, are examined iteratively until no more voxels meet a given criterion in signal intensity.

$$A_8(x,y) = \begin{Bmatrix} (x-1,y-1),(x,y-1),(x+1,y-1),(x-1,y) \\ (x+1,y),(x-1,y+1),(x,y+1),(x+1,y+1) \end{Bmatrix} \quad (11)$$

In the study, the stopping criterion used for iterative seed growing is determined by comparing a neighboring voxel

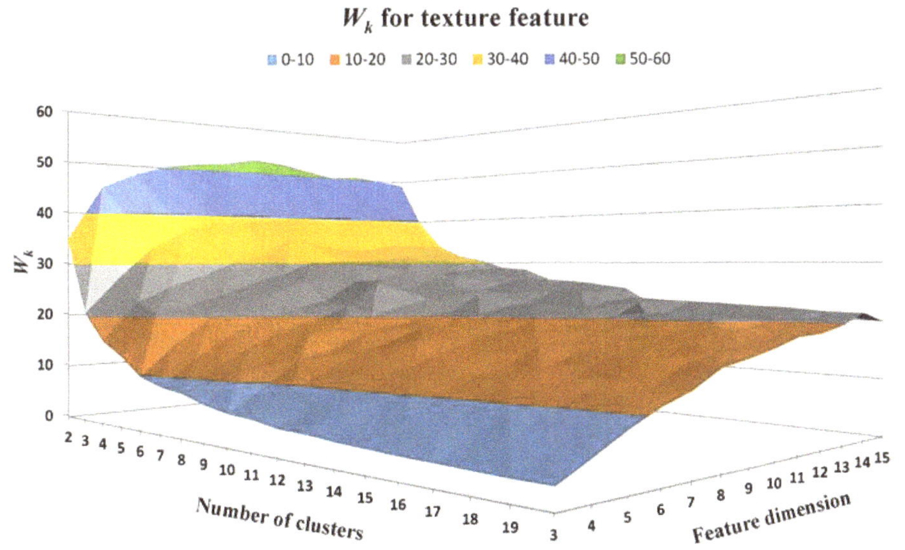

FIGURE 11 | The within-cluster dispersion W_k as the function of the number of texture cluster and feature dimension. Note that a noticeable "elbow" phenomenon presents for a wide range of texture feature dimensions from 3 to 15.

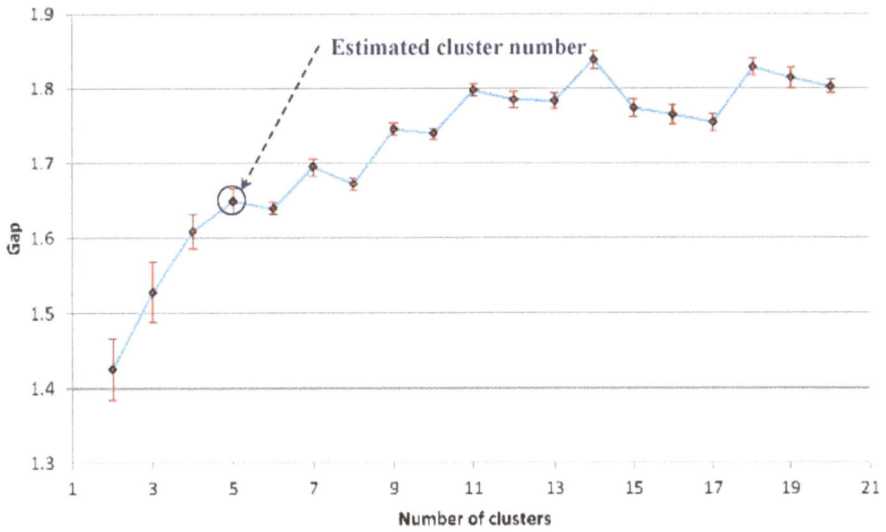

FIGURE 12 | The estimated gap statistic Gap as a function of texture cluster number k (dots and solid curve), error bars are $\pm s_k$.

intensity with the highest and lowest signal intensity, *gMax* and *gMin* of a WMH3D. If the voxel intensity difference from the *gMax* is less than a threshold, as defined below in Equation (12), the corresponding voxel is designated to a growth voxel set, R_g, and assigned to the boundary seed voxel list S_l for further searching. The pseudo-code of the seed-based region-growing algorithm is presented in **Figure 14A**. Note that M_k is the set of voxels in a WMH lesion mask, and $f(p)$ is the signal intensity at neighbor voxel p of a lesion boundary seed voxel, as defined in Equation (11).

$$Threshold = \gamma \times (gMax - gMin) \qquad (12)$$

where γ is the threshold control coefficient. The choice of γ represents the user-defined steepness of the edge around the WMH boundaries. Of note, if the value of γ is too large, the potential growth region would spread around all boundaries of the WMH lesions regardless of lesion shape or texture features. In this study, we chose $\gamma = 1.02$ to demonstrate the presence of potential growth regions of WMH lesions using the seed-based growing algorithm (**Figure 14B**).

After all "potential growth" voxels are found, the potential growth index (PGI) of a WMH lesion can be calculated. To calculate this index, first a set of four-connected voxels [Equation (13)] to a voxel (x, y) on the mask boundary is applied to generate

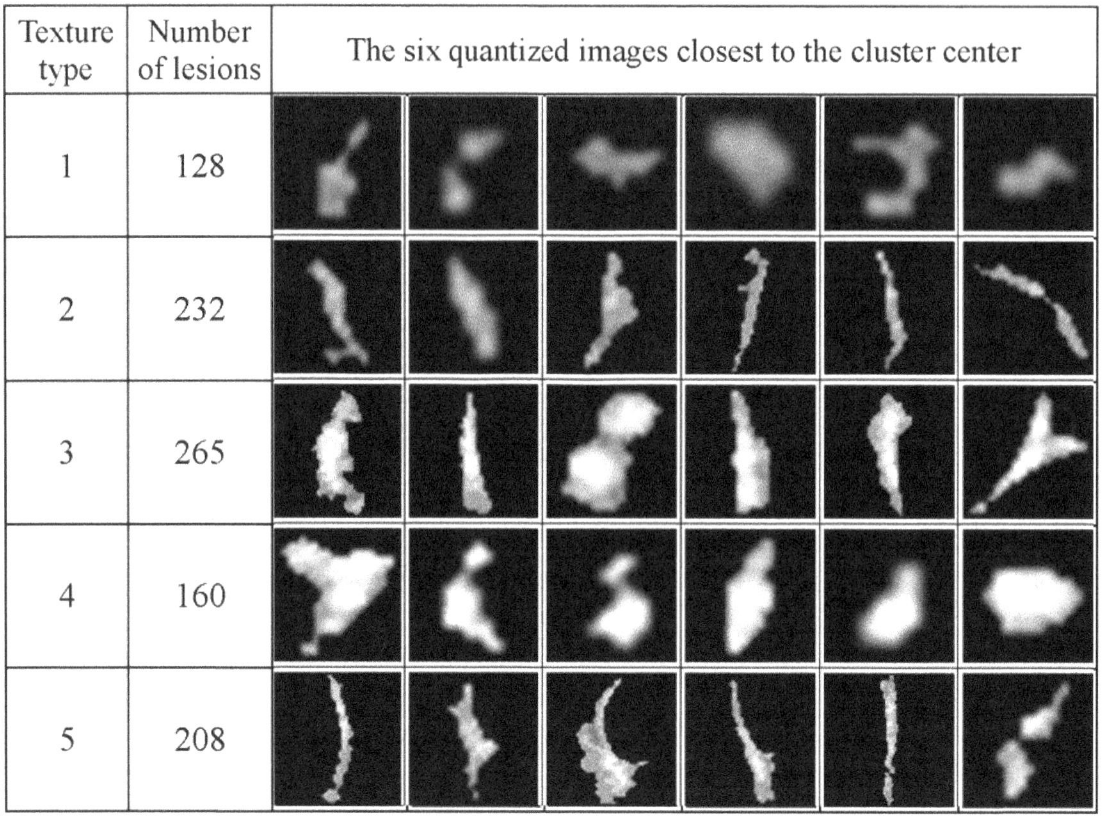

FIGURE 13 | The WMH lesion images from six subjects were classified to five clusters based on their texture features. The six lesion images closest to their cluster means based on the Manhattan distance are shown for each cluster.

successively l layers of apparent masks surrounding the lesion with a layer thickness of one voxel.

$$A_4(x,y) = \begin{Bmatrix} (x,y-1),(x-1,y), \\ (x+1,y),(x,y+1) \end{Bmatrix} \tag{13}$$

The pseudo-code of generating l layers around a WMH lesion growing algorithm is presented in **Figure 14C**. The notations S_l and M_k are the same as in **Figure 14A**. l is the number of layers to be generated and the ith layer voxels are kept in the $E[i]$ list.

These apparent layer masks are used to identify the relative location of a growth voxel. A growth voxel at an outer layers of these masks weights more in its contribution to the potential growth index. Specifically, the weight w_i at i^{th} layer, with total l layers, is given by the following equation:

$$w_i = \frac{i}{\sum_{j=1}^{l} j} \tag{14}$$

Once the number of growth voxels at each layers were calculated, the potential growth index P_g for each WMH lesion is calculated below:

$$P_g = \frac{\sum_{i=1}^{l} GV_i w_i}{V_l} \tag{15}$$

where, GV_i = number of "growth voxels" found at the ith layer, and V_l = the total number of voxels in all l layers for a WMH.

To demonstrate the potential application, all lesion images were evaluated for their potential growth indices with l set to three (**Figure 14D**).

The Relationship Between Potential Growth Index and WMH Shape and Texture Features

The relationship between PGI and WMH Shape and texture features was investigated in the study. The K-means algorithm is the most commonly used clustering algorithm in unsupervised learning due to its simplicity and efficiency (Hung et al., 2005), and thus is appropriate for this proof-of-concept development. However, the initial cluster seeds in K-means algorithm can generate different clustering results. To demonstrate the applicability of the K-means algorithm, we performed 1,000 trials with randomly selected initial cluster seeds from the feature vectors of shape and then texture of the lesions (a total of 993 lesions) to examine the clustering results. For the shape and texture clusters classified as shown in **Figures 7**, **13** above, one-way Analyses of Variance (ANOVAs) were performed to evaluate if there were significant differences in potential growth index generated from each trial among the shape or the texture clusters.

A

```
Initialize: S_l = the boundary voxels of a WMH lesion mask
            R_g = the holder of the growth voxel set to be found
            M_k = the set of voxels in a WMH lesion mask
repeat
   Remove the first voxel q at (x, y) from S_l
   for all voxel p in A_8(x, y), as defined in Eq. (11)
       if p is not in M_k then
           if gMax − f(p) < Threshold then
               Add p into S_l
               Add p into R_gl
               Add p into M_k
until S_l is empty
```

B

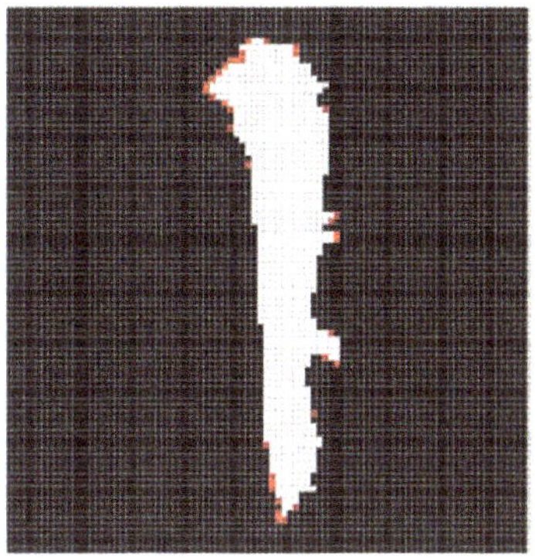

C

```
Initialize: l = the number of layers
            S_l = the boundary voxels of a WMH lesion mask
            E[l] = the holder of the voxel set for l layers
            M_k = the set of voxels in a WMH lesion mask
for all n=1,...,l
    repeat
      Remove the first voxel q at (x, y) from S_l
      for all voxel p in A_4(x, y), as defined in Eq. (13)
          if p is not in M_k then
              Add p into E[n]
              Add p into M_k
    until S_l is empty
    S_l ← E[n]
```

D

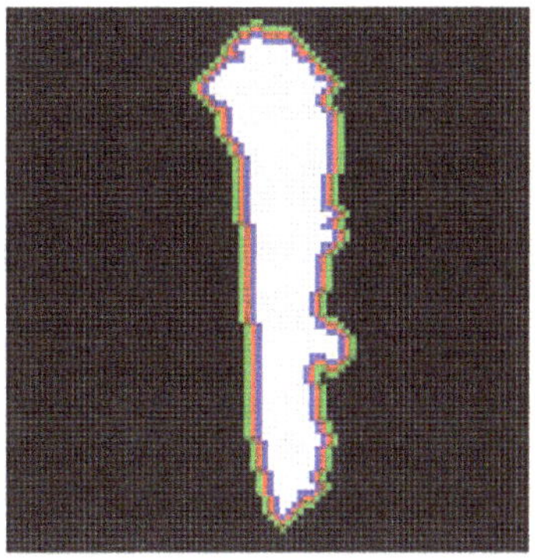

FIGURE 14 | (A) The pseudo-code of seed-based region-growing algorithm of WMH lesions; **(B)** a WMH lesion mask and the potential growth voxels marked in red color which are identified using the seed-based region-growing algorithm. **(C)** The pseudo-code of layer generating algorithm for WMH lesions; **(D)** three one-voxel-thick layers surrounding the WMH lesion, which are used to locate a growth voxel.

Significant growth index differences for all trials were found among both shape ($P = 2.04\times10^{-10}$ to $P = 1.06\times10^{-2}$) and texture ($P < 1\times10^{-40}$ to $P < 1\times10^{-20}$) clusters. **Table 1** shows the most conservative results.

DISCUSSION AND CONCLUSION

In this study, we have developed innovative and proof-of-concept methods to quantitatively characterize the shape (based on Zernike transformation) and texture (based on fuzzy logic) of WMH lesions. A multi-dimension feature vector approach based on these new features was used to cluster WMH lesions into distinctive groups to assess whether these features can potentially be used as image biomarkers. We have also developed an approach to calculate the potential growth index (PGI) of WMH lesions using a region-growing algorithm along the WMH boundaries. From preliminary data analyses of six subjects with a total of 993 lesions, we observed significant differences in PGI among the clustered WMH groups in terms of either the shape or the texture features. These findings, even though only a proof-of-concept, suggest that the shape and texture features of WMH can potentially be used as new imaging biomarkers to predict lesion growth in brain aging, vascular dementia, or AD.

This work demonstrates the feasibility and potential usefulness of our methods. However, there are several limitations, which are beyond the scope of this study to address completely. In WMH lesion segmentation, we adopted the mid-range point of 0.5 of the lesion probability map as the cut-off threshold suggested by the authors of the LST Toolbox. This threshold appears logical for a wide range of populations. However, different thresholds might be suitable for different study populations. Maldjian et al. (2013) suggested to use a 0.25 threshold in their study on older adults with diabetes. The change of segmentation threshold may introduce small change in the quantification of lesion sizes, which is not the focus of

TABLE 1 | Potential growth indices (PGIs) for the classified shape and texture clusters.

SHAPE						
	Cluster 1	**Cluster 2**	**Cluster 3**	**Cluster 4**	**Cluster 5**	**Cluster 6**
Number of images	105	86	176	237	211	178
PGI	0.1535 ± 0.0790	0.1702 ± 0.0818	0.1376 ± 0.1051	0.1399 ± 0.0885	0.1500 ± 0.0700	0.1636 ± 0.1011
	Between-cluster difference: $P = 1.06 \times 10^{-2}$, $F = 3.0070$					
TEXTURE						
	Cluster 1	**Cluster 2**	**Cluster 3**	**Cluster 4**	**Cluster 5**	
Number of images	128	232	265	160	208	
PGI	0.1928 ± 0.1023	0.1863 ± 0.0879	0.1037 ± 0.0683	0.1191 ± 0.0751	0.1656 ± 0.0828	
	Between-cluster difference: $P < 1 \times 10^{-20}$, $F = 48.4009$					

Results presented are the most conservative case from 1,000 trials with randomly selected initial cluster seeds from the feature vectors of the shape and texture of the white matter lesions.

our work. The effects of change of segmentation threshold on characterizations of the WMH shape, texture, and potential growth should be further studied.

In shape feature extraction, all images were proportionally scaled to the same size of 60 × 60 voxels. This scaling procedure resulted in blurring the shape contours of small-size images and losing the contour details of large-size images. This one-size-fit-all scaling treatment can lead to quantification inaccuracy at higher orders of ZM. Nevertheless, we have observed that high ZM orders are not required to represent primary WMH shape features. In this study, we limit the feature characteristics at ZM ≤5. Thus, the scaling factor used in this study should have minimal effects on the shape feature extraction results. When there is a large number of WMH lesions, a more proper procedure in shape analysis can be applied to reduce the influence of this image scaling issue on shape feature extraction. Specifically, WMH lesion images can be first divided into several groups based on the size, and then are scaled appropriately based on their corresponding size groups. Shape feature analyses can then be carried in each size group. It should also be mentioned that image shape feature extraction using the Zernike transform, in theory, is independent of the image sizes to be analyzed (Teague, 1980). The purpose of image scaling in this study was to improve computational efficiency.

In texture analysis, a linear fuzzy logic method was proposed to quantize the distribution of voxel signal intensity in a lesion image. This approach is robust in handling the potential quantization error due to imaging noise (Gwo and Wei, 2013). We have chosen a linear approach in fuzzy logic and a number of bins that appeared to work well on our data. However, we have not devised a method to systematically obtain an optimal bin number or type of linear or non-linear fuzzy logic function, which needs to be investigated in studies with large sample sizes. For both shape and texture analyses, we have selected the feature dimensions that appeared reasonable to the dataset of this study. However, selecting appropriate feature dimensions and cluster numbers is still a challenging problem in the field of pattern recognition (Steinbach et al., 2004). Common approach is data-driven trial and error. For a large dataset, a supervised machine learning via artificial neural network might lead to identification of optimized feature dimensions as well as the number of group clusters (Raschka, 2015).

PGI was developed to explore the possibility of predicting WMH progression by quantification of image characteristics of WMH penumbras (Maillard et al., 2014). To do this, multiple layers surrounding a lesion mask was used to calculate PGI with a linear weighted function based on the layer locations of the "growth voxels." The choice of a linear weighted function is consistent with the probable locations of WMH lesion development found in recent studies (Maillard et al., 2014; Promjunyakul et al., 2016). In our study, we used three layers sounding the WMH lesions to demonstrate the potential growth. A large dataset with repeated measures in longitudinal studies is needed to identify a more appropriate number of layers and devise an optimal weighting function.

We are fully aware that WMH lesion growth is likely affected by multiple factors besides the shape, texture and PGI. In this regard, the potential effects of anatomical locations of WMH on its progression rate have been investigated in prior works (DeCarli et al., 2005; Wardlaw et al., 2013). Identification of other key contributors to WMH growth and the underlying biological mechanisms are warranted for future studies.

The objective of this paper is to formulate concepts and to demonstrate the feasibility of the methods used to analyze the WMH shape, texture, and potential growth. To accomplish this object, we selected high-quality T_2 FLAIR images which contain a large number of lesions with various sizes from six subjects as sample cases to develop our theoretical framework. While only small number of subjects was used in this study, a relatively large number of lesion (a total of 993) was used in our development and analyses. Nevertheless, the algorithms and parameters used for texture feature extraction and potential growth index estimation in this work were empirical based on trial and error, or were optimized based on the relatively small dataset. The algorithms and parameters used in this work need to be optimized based on larger datasets covering various type of lesions in future studies. Currently, we are working on the application of our methods to over 500 subjects with more than 2 years of brain imaging data from the ADNI (Alzheimer's Disease Neuroimaging Initiative) database.

Lastly, due to widely available 2D T_2 FLAIR images in clinical practice and research, we decided to develop our concept in 2D T_2 FLAIR first. On the other hand, we have also begun to expand our work to 3D imaging to capture the lesion shape, texture and potential growth in all spatial directions, which benefits from the recent development in 3D high-resolution T_2 FLAIR acquisition technique (Wiggermann et al., 2016).

In summary, our work demonstrated the concept and the feasibility that shape and texture features of WMH lesions observed on T_2 FLAIR images can be quantitatively characterized which are related to the potential growth index of white matter lesions. Future studies of large datasets and longitudinal studies based on the systematic framework proposed in this study are warranted to further optimize the algorithms and parameters used for white matter lesion shape and texture feature extraction and classification as well as PGI estimation. Furthermore, our approaches for image feature extraction and classification can potentially be generalized to other types of brain lesions and imaging modalities.

AUTHOR CONTRIBUTIONS

C-YG conducted experiments, wrote code to analyze the data, interpreted the data, and wrote the manuscript. DZ prepared brain images and lesion segmentation. DZ and RZ interpreted the data, participated in the scientific discussions, and provided critical insights. All authors reviewed the manuscript and approved it for publication.

REFERENCES

Ball, G. H., and Hall, D. J. (1965). *Isodata: A Novel Method of Data Analysis and Pattern Classification*. Menlo Park, CA: Stanford Research Institute.

Bauckhage, C., and Tsotsos, J. K. (2005). "Bounding box splitting for robust shape classification, II-478," in *IEEE International Conference on Image Processing 2005: IEEE.*

Bombois, S., Debette, S., Delbeuck, X., Bruandet, A., Lepoittevin, S., Delmaire, C., et al. (2007). Prevalence of subcortical vascular lesions and association with executive function in mild cognitive impairment subtypes. *Stroke* 38, 2595–2597. doi: 10.1161/STROKEAHA.107.486407

Calinski, T., and Harabasz, J. (1974). A dendrite method for cluster analysis. *Commun. Stat. Theory Methods* 3, 1–27.

Carmichael, O., and Hebert, M. (2004). Shape-based recognition of wiry objects. *IEEE Transac. Pattern. Anal. Mach. Intell.* 26, 1537–1552. doi: 10.1109/TPAMI.2004.128

Castellano, G., Bonilha, L., Li, L. M., and Cendes, F. (2004). Texture analysis of medical images. *Clin. Radiol.* 59, 1061–1069. doi: 10.1016/j.crad.2004.07.008

Celebi, M. E., and Aslandogan, Y. A. (2005). "A comparative study of three moment-based shape descriptors," in *International Conference on Information Technology: Coding and Computing (ITCC'05)-Volume II: IEE* (Washington, DC), 788–793.

Charman, W. N. (2005). Wavefront technology: past, present, and future. *Contact Lens Anterior Eye* 28, 75–92. doi: 10.1016/j.clae.2005.02.003

Chen, C.-C., Daponte, J. S., and Fox, M. D. (1989). Fractal feature analysis and classification in medical imaging. *IEEE Transac. Med. Imaging* 8, 133–142. doi: 10.1109/42.24861

Chen, G., and Bui, T. D. (1999). Invariant fourier-wavelet descriptor for pattern recognition. *Pattern Recogn.* 32, 1083–1088.

Chow, T. W. S., and Rahman, M. K. M. (2007). A new image classification technique using tree-structured regional features. *Neurocomputing*, 70, 1040–1050. doi: 10.1016/j.neucom2006.01.033

De Leeuw, F., de Groot, J. C., Achten, E., Oudkerk, M., Ramos, L., Heijboer, A., et al. (2001). Prevalence of cerebral white matter lesions in elderly people: a population based magnetic resonance imaging study. The rotterdam scan study. *J. Neurol. Neurosurg. Psychiatry* 70, 9–14. doi: 10.1136/jnnp.70.1.9

DeCarli, C., Fletcher, E., Ramey, V., Harvey, D., and Jagust, W. J. (2005). Anatomical mapping of white matter hyperintensities (WMH). *Stroke* 36, 50–55. doi: 10.1161/01.STR.0000150668.58689.f2

Desgraupes, B. (2013). *Clustering Indices*. Nanterre: University of Paris Ouest-Lab Modal'X, 1–34.

Godin, O., Tzourio, C., Maillard, P., Mazoyer, B., and Dufouil, C. (2011). Antihypertensive treatment and change in blood pressure are associated with the progression of white matter lesion volumes. *Circulation* 123:266–73. doi: 10.1161/CIRCULATIONAHA.110.961052

Greenberg, S. M. (2006). Small vessels, big problems. *N. Engl. J. Med.* 354, 1451–1453. doi: 10.1056/NEJMp068043

Guru, D., and Nagendraswamy, H. (2007). Symbolic representation of two-dimensional shapes. *Pattern Recogn. Lett.* 28, 144–155. doi: 10.1016/j.patrec.2006.06.017

Gwo, C., and Wei, C.-H. (2013). Plant identification through images: Using feature extraction of key points on leaf contours. *Appl. Plant Sci.* 1:apps.1200005. doi: 10.3732/apps.1200005

Gwo, C., and Wei, C.-H. (2016). Shoeprint retrieval: core point alignment for pattern comparison. *Sci. Justice* 56, 341–350. doi: 10.1016/j.scijus.2016.06.004

Haralick, R., Shanmugan, K., and Dinstein, I. (1973). Textural features for image classification. *IEEE Transac. Syst. Man Cyber.* 3, 610–621. doi: 10.1109/TSMC.1973.4309314

Hartigan, J. A., and Wong, M. A. (1979). Algorithm AS 136: a k-means clustering algorithm. *J. R. Stat. Soc.* 28, 100–108.

Hughes, G. (1968). On the mean accuracy of statistical pattern recognizers. *IEEE Transac. Inf. Theory* 14, 55–63. doi: 10.1109/TIT.1968.1054102

Hung, M.-C., Wu, J., Chang, J.-H., and, Yang, D.-L. (2005). An efficient k-means clustering algorithm using simple partitioning. *J. Inf. Sci. Eng.* 21, 1157–1177.

Iivarinen, J., Rauhamaa, J., and Visa, A. (1996). "Unsupervised segmentation of surface defects," in *International Conference on Pattern Recognition* (Vienna), 356–360.

Kauppinen, H., Seppanen, T., and Pietikainen, M. (1995). An experimental comparison of autoregressive and Fourier-based descriptors in 2D shape classification. *IEEE Transac. Pattern Anal. Mach. Intell.* 17, 201–207.

Khotanzad, A., and Hong, Y. H. (1990). Invariant image recognition by Zernike moments. *IEEE Transac. Pattern. Anal. Mach. Intell.* 12, 489–497. doi: 10.1109/34.55109

Kloppenborg, R. P., Nederkoorn, P. J., Geerlings, M. I., and van den Berg, E. (2014). Presence and progression of white matter hyperintensities and cognition A meta-analysis. *Neurology* 82, 2127–2138. doi: 10.1212/WNL.0000000000000505

Kpalma, K., and Ronsin, J. (2006). Multiscale contour description for pattern recognition. *Pattern Recogn. Lett.* 27, 1545–1559. doi: 10.1016/j.patrec.2006.03.003

Lee, S., Viqar, F., Zimmerman, M., E., Narkhede, A., Tosto, G., Benzinger, D. S., et al. (2016). White matter hyperintensities are a core feature of Alzheimer's disease: evidence from the dominantly inherited Alzheimer network. *Ann. Neurol.* 79, 929–939. doi: 10.1002/ana.24647

Loizou, C., Petroudi, S., Seimenis, I., Pantziaris, M., and Pattichis, C. (2015). Quantitative texture analysis of brain white matter lesions derived from T2-weighted MR images in MS patients with clinically isolated syndrome. *J. Neuroradiol.* 42, 99–114. doi: 10.1016/j.neurad.2014.05.006

Maillard, P., Fletcher, E., Lockhart, S. N., Roach, A. E., Reed, B., Mungas, D., et al. (2014). White matter hyperintensities and their penumbra lie along a continuum of injury in the aging brain. *Stroke* 45, 1721–1726. doi: 10.1161/STROKEAHA.113.004084

Maldjian, J. A., Whitlow, C. T., Saha, B. N., Kota, G., Vandergriff, C., Davenport, E. M., et al. (2013). Automated white matter total lesion volume segmentation in diabetes. *AJNR Am. J. Neuroradiol.* 34, 2265–70. doi: 10.3174/ajnr.A3590

Mikolajczyk, K., Zisserman, A., and Schmid, C. (2003). "Shape recognition with edge-based features," in *British Machine Vision Conference (BMVC'03)* (Norwich), 779–788.

Mukundan, R. (2004). "A new class of rotational invariants using discrete orthogonal moments," in *6th IASTED International Conference on Signal and Image Processing*, 80–84.

Newton, B. D., Wright, K., Winkler, M. D., Bovis, F., Takahashi, M., Dimitrov, I. E., et al. (2017). Three-dimensional shape and surface features distinguish multiple sclerosis lesions from nonspecific white matter disease. *J. Neuroimaging.* 27, 613–619. doi: 10.1111/jon.12449

Papakostas, G. A., Boutalis, Y. S., Karras, D. A., and Mertzios, B. G. (2007). A new class of Zernike moments for computer vision applications. *Inf. Sci.* 177, 2802–2819. doi: 10.1016/j.ins.2007.01.010

Poels, M. M., Zaccai, K., Verwoert, G. C., Vernooij, M. W., Hofman, A., van der Lugt, A., et al. (2012). Arterial stiffness and cerebral small vessel disease. *Stroke* 43:2637–42. doi: 10.1161/STROKEAHA.111.642264

Promjunyakul, N.-O., Lahna, D. L., Kaye, J. A., Dodge, H. H., Erten-Lyons, D., Rooney, W. D., et al. (2016). Comparison of cerebral blood flow and structural penumbras in relation to white matter hyperintensities: a multi-modal magnetic resonance imaging study. *J. Cereb. Blood Flow Metab.* 36, 1528–1536. doi: 10.1177/0271678X16651268

Raschka, S. (2015). *Python Machine Learning.* Birmingham: Packt Publishing.

Sachdev, P., Wen, W., Chen, X., and Brodaty, H. (2007). Progression of white matter hyperintensities in elderly individuals over 3 years. *Neurology* 68, 214–222. doi: 10.1212/01.wnl.0000251302.55202.73

Schmidt, R., Schmidt, H., Haybaeck, J., Loitfelder, M., Weis, S., Cavalieri, M., et al. (2011). Heterogeneity in age-related white matter changes. *Acta Neuropathol.* 122, 171–185. doi: 10.1007/s00401-011-0851-x

Sebastian, T. B., Klein, P. N., and Kimia, B. B. (2004). Recognition of shapes by editing their shock graphs. *IEEE Transac. Pattern Anal. Mach. Intell.* 26, 550–571. doi: 10.1109/TPAMI.2004.1273924

Shapiro, L., and Stockman, G. C. (2001). *Computer Vision. 2000.* New Jersey, NJ: Prentice Hall, 239–240.

ShuiHua, H., and ShuangYuan, Y. (2005). "An invariant feature representation for shape retrieval," in *Sixth International Conference on Parallel and Distributed Computing Applications and Technologies (PDCAT'05): IEEE*, 1052–1054.

Steinbach, M., Ertöz, L., and Kumar, V. (2004). "The challenges of clustering high dimensional data," In *New Directions in Statistical Physics: Econophysics, Bioinformatics, and Pattern Recognition*, ed L. T. Wille (Berlin, Heidelberg: Springer Berlin Heidelberg), 273–309.

Tahmasbi, A., Saki, F., and Shokouhi, S. B. (2011). Classification of benign and malignant masses based on zernike moments. *Comput. Biol. Med.* 41, 726–735. doi: 10.1016/j.compbiomed.2011.06.009

Tarumi, T., Khan, M. A., Liu, J., Tseng, B., M., Parker, R., Riley, J., et al. (2014). Cerebral hemodynamics in normal aging: central artery stiffness, wave reflection, and pressure pulsatility. *J. Cereb. Blood Flow Metab.* 34, 971–978. doi: 10.1038/jcbfm.2014.44

Taubin, G., and Cooper, D. B. (1991). "Recognition and positioning of rigid objects using algebraic moment invariants," in *Geometric Methods in Computer Vision: International Society for Optics and Photonics*, 175–187.

Teague, M. R. (1980). Image analysis via the general theory of moments. *J. Optic. Soc. Am.* 70, 920–930. doi: 10.1364/JOSA.70.000920

Teh, C.-H., and Chin, R. T. (1988). On image analysis by the methods of moments. *IEEE Transac. Pattern Anal. Mach. Intell.* 10, 496–513. doi: 10.1109/34.3913

Tibshirani, R., Walther, G., and Hastie, T. (2001). Estimating the number of clusters in a data set via the gap statistic. *J. R. Stat. Soc. Ser. B* 63, 411–423. doi: 10.1111/1467-9868.00293

Tsai, D.-M., and Hsiao, B. (2001). Automatic surface inspection using wavelet reconstruction. *Pattern Recogn.* 34, 1285–1305. doi: 10.1016/S0031-3203(00)00071-6

Tseng, B. Y., Gundapuneedi, T., Khan, M., Diaz-Arrastia, R., Levine, B., Lu, H., et al. (2013). White matter integrity in physically fit older adults. *Neuroimage* 82, 510–516. doi: 10.1016/j.neuroimage.2013.06.011

Wardlaw, J., Smith, E., Biessels, G., Cordonnier, C., Fazekas, F., Frayne, R., et al. (2013). Standards for reporting vascular changes on neuroimaging (STRIVE v1). Neuroimaging standards for research into small vessel disease and its contribution to ageing and neurodegeneration. *Lancet Neurol.* 12, 822–838. doi: 10.1016/S1474-4422(13)70124-8

Wee, C.-Y., and Paramesran, R. (2007). On the computational aspects of Zernike moments. *Image Vis. Comput.* 25, 967–980. doi: 10.1016/j.imavis.2006.07.010

Wen, W., and Sachdev, P. (2004). The topography of white matter hyperintensities on brain MRI in healthy 60-to 64-year-old individuals. *Neuroimage.* 22, 144–154. doi: 10.1016/j.neuroimage.2003.12.027

Wiggermann, V., Hernandez-Torres, E., Traboulsee, A., Li, D. K., and Rauscher, A. (2016). FLAIR2: a combination of FLAIR and T2 for improved MS lesion detection. *AJNR Am. J. Neuroradiol.* 37, 259–65. doi: 10.3174/ajnr.A4514

Xu, L. (1997). Bayesian Ying-Yang machine, clustering and number of clusters. *Pattern Recogn. Lett.* 18, 1167–1178. doi: 10.1016/S0167-8655(97)00121-9

Yadav, R. B., Nishchal, N. K., Gupta, A. K., and Rastogi, V. K. (2007). Retrieval and classification of shape-based objects using fourier, generic fourier, and wavelet-fourier descriptors technique: a comparative study. *Optics Lasers Eng.* 45, 695–708. doi: 10.1016/j.optlaseng.2006.11.001

Zernike, V. F. (1934). Beugungstheorie des Schneidenverfahrens und seiner verbesserten Form, der Phasenkontrastmethode. *Physica* 1, 689–704.

Zhang, D., and Lu, G. (2002). "A comparative study of fourier descriptors for shape representation and retrieval," in *Proceedings of 5th Asian Conference on Computer Vision* (Citeseer).

Zhang, D., and Lu, G. (2002). "Enhanced generic fourier descriptors for object-based image retrieval," in: *2002 IEEE International Conference on Acoustics, Speech, and Signal Processing: IEEE* (Orlando, FL).

Zhang, D., and Lu, G. (2003). A comparative study of curvature scale space and Fourier descriptors for shape-based image retrieval. *J. Vis. Commun. Image Represent.* 14, 39–57. doi: 10.1016/S1047-3203(03)00003-8

Zhao, Q. (2012). *Cluster Validity in Clustering Methods.* Joensuu: Publications of the University of Eastern Finland.

13

Topological Properties of Resting-State fMRI Functional Networks Improve Machine Learning-Based Autism Classification

Amirali Kazeminejad [1,2]* *and Roberto C. Sotero* [1,2,3]

[1] *Hotchkiss Brain Institute, University of Calgary, Calgary, AB, Canada,* [2] *Biomedical Engineering Graduate Program, University of Calgary, Calgary, AB, Canada,* [3] *Department of Radiology, University of Calgary, Calgary, AB, Canada*

Correspondence:
Amirali Kazeminejad
amirali.kazeminejad@ucalgary.ca;
roberto.soterodiaz@ucalgary.ca

Automatic algorithms for disease diagnosis are being thoroughly researched for use in clinical settings. They usually rely on pre-identified biomarkers to highlight the existence of certain problems. However, finding such biomarkers for neurodevelopmental disorders such as Autism Spectrum Disorder (ASD) has challenged researchers for many years. With enough data and computational power, machine learning (ML) algorithms can be used to interpret the data and extract the best biomarkers from thousands of candidates. In this study, we used the fMRI data of 816 individuals enrolled in the Autism Brain Imaging Data Exchange (ABIDE) to introduce a new biomarker extraction pipeline for ASD that relies on the use of graph theoretical metrics of fMRI-based functional connectivity to inform a support vector machine (SVM). Furthermore, we split the dataset into 5 age groups to account for the effect of aging on functional connectivity. Our methodology achieved better results than most state-of-the-art investigations on this dataset with the best model for the >30 years age group achieving an accuracy, sensitivity, and specificity of 95, 97, and 95%, respectively. Our results suggest that measures of centrality provide the highest contribution to the classification power of the models.

Keywords: graph theoiy, SVM–support vector machine, machine learing, fMRI, ABIDE, brain connectitvity

INTRODUCTION

Autism Spectrum Disorder (ASD) is a neurodevelopmental disease which manifests in early childhood and persists into adulthood. Recent studies show that 1 in 45 children is diagnosed with autism (Zablotsky et al., 2015). While there is no cure for ASD (Brentani et al., 2013), early diagnosis of autistic individuals is proven to improve quality of life (Fernell et al., 2013). To better detect ASD, biomarkers characterizing the disorder need to be identified. It has been shown that by using topological biomarkers extracted from the brain functional network, machine learning (ML) algorithms can be trained to aid in ASD diagnosis (Plitt et al., 2015). However, there are many variables, such as different methods to construct the functional network and carry out the topological measurements that can affect the extraction of these biomarkers. One goal of this study was to find the best combination of these variables to tackle the task of ASD classification. For this goal, we used 5 different network extraction pipelines with 12 graph theoretical topological measurements and preformed a statistical analysis to compare the classification results between the pipeline. The second goal was to identify the top topological measures in each pipeline and investigate their relation to ASD in order to attempt and further understand the disorder.

Our brains can be viewed as a network of functionally interconnected regions. To measure the strength of these connections, the temporal dynamics of brain activity is needed. Modalities such as Electroencephalography (EEG) and magnetoencephalography (MEG) provide this information, however, they suffer from poor spatial resolution when compared to Functional Magnetic Resonance Imaging (fMRI). In fMRI, brain activity is usually monitored by the changes in blood oxygenation which changes the magnetic properties of blood. The resulting signal is called the Blood-oxygen-level dependent (BOLD) signal. At the turn of the century, researchers provided evidence that fMRI can be used to identify functional connections of the brain while the subject was in a "resting-state" and not doing any specific task (Lowe et al., 2000). Later studies found many different functional networks can be identified using the resting-state connectivity derived from fMRI (van den Heuvel and Hulshoff Pol, 2010). Information from these networks can be extracted and used as an input to ML algorithms to automatically identify the best biomarkers distinguishing between healthy and diseased networks (Nielsen et al., 2013; Plitt et al., 2015; Hazlett et al., 2017; Heinsfeld et al., 2018).

ML has proven to be a powerful tool for automatic disease diagnosis in neurodegenerative disorders such as Alzheimer's Disease (AD) (Chen et al., 2011) and Parkinson's Disease (Kazeminejad et al., 2017; Talai et al., 2017). In recent years, researchers began investigating how the same principles can be used for automatic ASD diagnosis. Promising results with accuracies over 90% were observed using invasive methods and blood analysis (Howsmon et al., 2017). However, the classification studies conducted using non-invasive data acquisition such as brain imaging, while above chance levels, generally report lower accuracies. By using fMRI data acquired in the Autism Brain Imaging Data Exchange (ABIDE) (Nielsen et al., 2013) extracted the pairwise functional connectivity of 7,266 Regions of interest (ROI) using Pearson correlation and used a leave-one-out general linear model classifier to achieve a ASD vs. Healthy Controls (HC) classification accuracy of 60%. More recently, by applying and comparing different ML algorithms to the same dataset, the accuracy has reached 70%. Heinsfeld et al. used the Pearson correlation of fMRI activity of region pairs in CC200 atlas (Craddock et al., 2012) as the inputs to a multi-layer perceptron to achieve this result (Heinsfeld et al., 2018). Other research groups using their own datasets have reported higher accuracies. One study using cortical thickness, total brain volume, and surface area of different brain regions was able to achieve an accuracy of 81% using a neural network as their classifier (Hazlett et al., 2017).

Another emerging methodology in understanding different neurological disorders is graph theory, a mathematical tool used to explain network characteristics that can also be applied to the human brain network (Iturria-Medina et al., 2008; Bullmore and Sporns, 2009; Rubinov and Sporns, 2010; Sotero, 2016; Sanchez-Rodriguez et al., 2018). Graph theory can be used to measure the brain network segregation (clustering coefficient and transitivity), integration (characteristic path length and efficiency), and centrality (betweenness centrality, eigenvector centrality, participation coefficient and within module z-score). Recent brain imaging studies have found topological differences between ASD and normal brains which can be quantified using graph theory, such as global alterations of characteristic path length and efficiency in ASD (Rudie et al., 2013; Itahashi et al., 2014; Zeng et al., 2017; Qin et al., 2018) as well as alterations to segregation measures (Barttfeld et al., 2011; Rudie et al., 2013; Leung et al., 2014; Keown et al., 2017; Zeng et al., 2017) and centrality measures(Di Martino et al., 2013; Leung et al., 2014; Balardin et al., 2015).

Previous studies in AD patients have used topological properties of brain networks as features for a ML algorithm, achieving classification accuracies of 85% (Dyrba et al., 2015). However, this methodology hasn't been tested in ASD. With the emergence of the ABIDE dataset, large amounts of imaging and clinical data has become available to researchers (Di Martino et al., 2014). More than 1,000 datasets are available for individuals with ASD and HC each. This data is collected from multiple sites with slightly varying machinery and imaging parameters. Therefore, a well-developed preprocessing pipeline is essential to minimize the effects of site and imaging parameter changes, but further data manipulations may be needed to standardize the data from different sites.

One explanation for the lower accuracies of studies using the ABIDE dataset is that it covers a large age range (5–65). Age has been proposed as a factor attributing to the different results reported on resting-state fMRI analysis of ASD (Hull et al., 2016). Another study focusing on using multi-scale image textures to study neuroanatomical texture features in autism has found correlations between age and texture features (Chaddad et al., 2017). Therefore, any study that uses all this data will have to take aging effects into consideration. If these issues are correctly addressed, the ABIDE initiative will provide a suitable database for ML centered research on ASD. Another limitation that can be associated with the previously mentioned studies is that they use a simple connectivity matrix such as one computed by Pearson correlation as their features for the classification algorithms. The connectivity matrix is interpreted as the strengths of the connection between ROIs and the changes in these connection strengths are used to classify between ASD and HCs. We hypothesize that by applying graph theoretical measurement of network segregation (clustering coefficient and transitivity), integration (characteristic path length and efficiency), and centrality (betweenness centrality, eigenvector centrality, participation coefficient and within module z-score) for extracting features from the connectivity matrix, the performance of ML algorithm on this dataset will be improved.

In this study, we use fMRI BOLD signals to estimate functional connectivity matrices using different network extraction methods. Using these matrices, we construct a brain network modeling the functional connectivity of a subject's brain. Topological properties such as integration, segregation, and centrality of the obtained networks are then used as features (for a total of 817 features for each network extraction method) fed to a gaussian kernel Support Vector Machine (SVM) to classify whether a subject is suffering from ASD or not. We then use a sequential feature selection technique to choose the top 10 features that contribute to this classification. To control for the effects of aging, we separated our data into 5 age groups. Our best model, for the >30 age range achieved a classification accuracy, sensitivity, and specificity of ~95, 97, and 95%, respectively. Most regions that the features were extracted from had been previously shown to undergo structural and/or functional changes in ASD.

MATERIALS AND METHODS

Dataset and Preprocessing

In order to ensure replicability, we used the preprocessed version of ABIDE I (Di Martino et al., 2014) data publicly available via the Preprocessed Connectome Project (Cameron et al., 2013b). The preprocessing pipeline we used for this study is the Configurable Pipeline for the Analysis of Connectomes (CPAC) (Cameron et al., 2013a). Regions of interests (ROIs) were defined as the 116 regions in the automatic anatomical labeling (AAL) atlas (Tzourio-Mazoyer et al., 2002).

The preprocessing included the following steps. AFNI was used for removing the skull from the images. The brain was segmented into three tissues using FSL. The images were then normalized to the MNI 152 stereotactic space using ANTs. Functional preprocessing included motion and slice-timing correction as well as the normalization of voxel intensity. Nuisance signal regression included 24 parameters for head motion, CompCor with 5 principal components for tissue signal in CSF, and white matter, linear and quadratic trends for Low-frequency drifts and a global bandpass filter (0.01–0.1 Hz). These images where then co-registered to their anatomical counterpart by FSL. They were then normalized to the MNI 152 space using ANTs. The average voxel activity in each ROI was then extracted as the time-series for that region. Any subject that had a consistently 0 time-series was omitted from the dataset. To minimize the effects of age on the results, the dataset was split into 5 age ranges with 5-year increments for the first three step and a 10 year and unlimited increment for the final two. This was done in order to ensure that no age range will have a very small number of subjects. The distribution of the subjects in each age range can be seen in **Table 1**. Further breakdown of the subject's demographics is shown in **Supplementary Table A**.

TABLE 1 | Distribution of the data.

Site (# Samples in fMRI time series)	5–10 years	10–15 years	15–20 years	20–30 years	30–65 years	All
CALTECH (146)	0	0	3	13	5	20
CMUA (236)	0	0	0	1	0	1
KKI (152)	20	18	0	0	0	38
LEUVEN1 (246)	0	0	8	21	1	29
LEUVEN2 (246)	0	24	7	0	0	31
MAXMUNA (116)	0	0	1	3	7	11
MAXMUNB (116)	0	0	0	2	5	6
MAXMUNC (116)	0	0	0	13	3	14
MAXMUND (196)	2	5	1	0	2	9
NYU (176)	35	66	26	34	5	166
OHSU (78)	7	15	1	0	0	23
OLIN (206)	0	9	14	7	0	25
PITT (196)	0	16	4	7	5	32
SBL (196)	0	0	0	3	6	8
SDSU (176)	1	17	9	0	0	27
STANFORD (176–236)	21	15	0	0	0	36
TRINITY (146)	0	14	20	9	0	43
UCLA1 (116)	3	38	14	0	0	55
UCLA2 (116)	1	18	1	0	0	20
UM1 (296)	9	42	32	0	0	82
UM2 (296)	0	13	16	2	0	31
USM (236)	0	6	21	22	12	61
YALE (196)	10	26	12	0	0	48
All Sites	109	342	190	137	51	816

Number of participants from each site for each age group as well as the overall number of participants in a site that were used for this study. Last row shows the total number of subjects in each age-range. The number of MRI samples per fMRI time-series is annotated in brackets in the first column. The Stanford time-series did not have a consistent number of samples thus the number is presented as a range.

Creating the Functional Connectivity Network

To extract the whole-brain functional connectivity network of each subject, each ROI is seen as a network node and a measure of connectivity is used to connect these nodes (Bullmore and Sporns, 2009). This connectivity measure (w_{ij}) must be able to quantify the relationship between the time-series of ROI i and j. Correlation and mutual information metrics have been extensively used for this purpose (Rubinov and Sporns, 2010). We have used spearman's rank correlation coefficient, the percentage-bend correlation (Wilcox, 1994; Pernet et al., 2012) and partial correlation (Marrelec et al., 2006) as our correlation based measures of connectivity. We also used Sparse Inverse Covariance Estimation (SICE) (Huang et al., 2010) and mutual information as alternative measures of connectivity. More details on each method can be found in the **Supplementary Material**. The implementations used in the open source GraphVar Matlab toolbox (Kruschwitz et al., 2015) was used to compute these connectivity measures.

Graph Extraction

Once the whole-brain network is available, numerous methods can be used to express it in terms of a graph. The easiest way is to treat each ROI as a node and the connectivity matrix as connection weights. Another approach is to define a threshold T and disregard any edges with values $w_{ij} < T$ by changing them to 0. One can then either keep the edge weights for $w_{ij} > T$ or change them to 1 to construct a binary graph. It has been shown that binary graphs are easier to characterize using graph theoretical metrics and usually have better defined null models for statistical analysis (Rubinov and Sporns, 2010). As there is no proved way to calculate the value of T for a specific application, a proportional approach is usually used in its place. In this paper, the highest 20% of the weights were changed to 1 and the rest were disregarded as 0.

Graph Metrics

Graph theoretical analysis was performed on the extracted brain graph for each subject. The calculated graph properties consisted of measures of segregation (Clustering Coefficient, Transitivity), integration (Characteristic Path Length, Efficiency), and centrality (Betweenness centrality, within module degree Z-score, Participation coefficient) of the brain network. Formulas for each metric are presented in **Table A1** (Rubinov and Sporns, 2010). This resulted in a feature space of 817 variables for each subject. More information on this step is available in the **Supplementary Material.**

All steps from Graph extraction to this point were done using the openly available MATLAB toolbox GraphVar (Kruschwitz et al., 2015).

Classification, Validation, and Comparison

In this study, we used the python Scikit-learn implementation of the gaussian SVM as our classifier. Features were selected using a sequential forward floating algorithm (Pudil et al., 1994). This was done over 10 successive iterations. In the first iteration, all features in the feature space were individually used for classification and the best performing feature was added to a feature subset while being removed from the feature space. In each consecutive iteration, individual components of the feature space are added to feature subset and the best performing feature in combination with previous results is kept for future use. This resulted in 10 features being chosen as the best graph characteristics that distinguish between ASD and HC.

All classification metrics were acquired using a 10-fold stratified cross validation test with the data folds being the same for all algorithms. To further validate our results, the confusion matrix of each model was evaluated to determine model sensitivity and specificity.

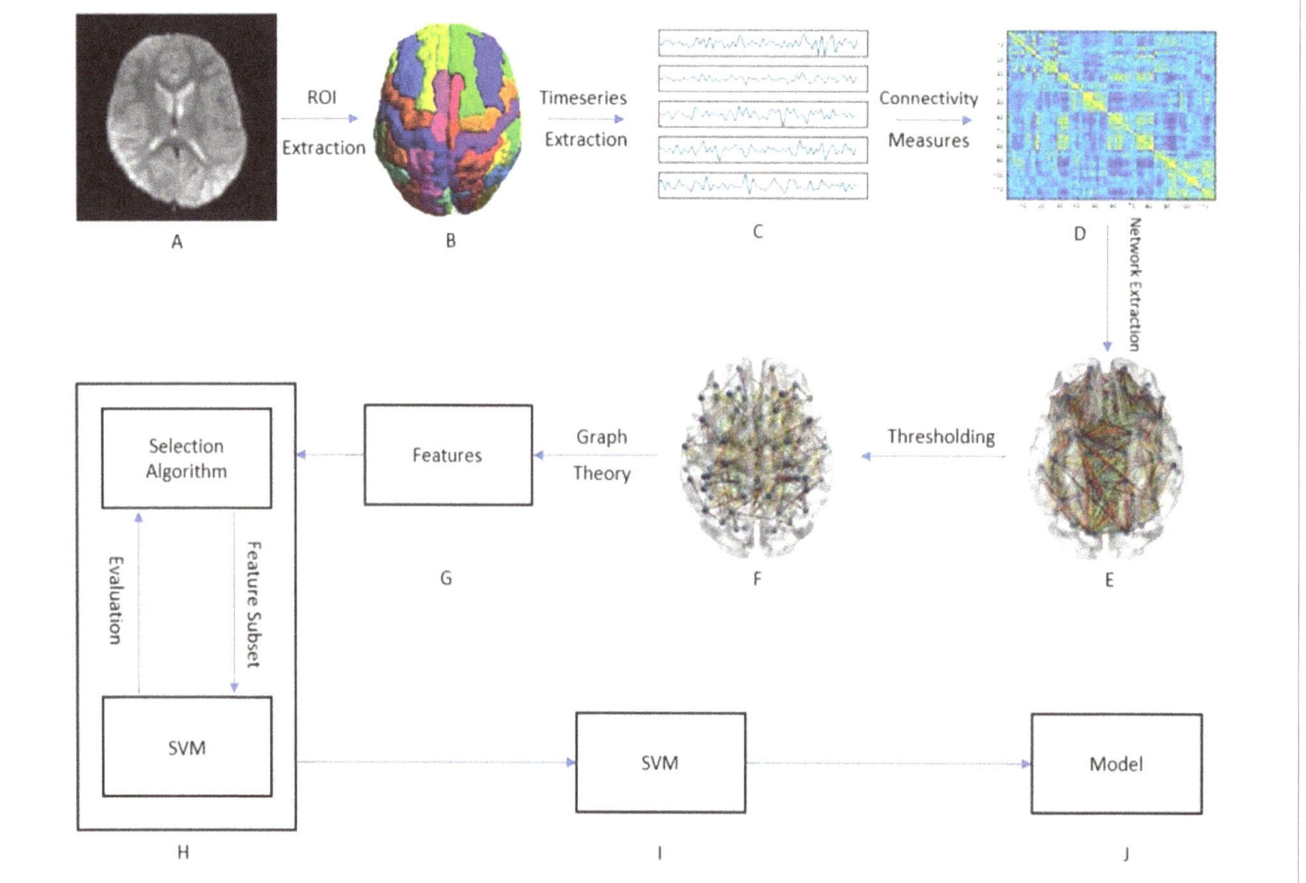

FIGURE 1 | Graphical framework of the experiment. **(A)** Raw fMRI images of subjects; **(B)** After preprocessing the brain is divided into 116 regions of interest (ROI); **(C)** By averaging the BOLD activity in each ROI, a time-series is extracted representing brain activity in that region; **(D)** Using different measures of connectivity, a connectivity matrix is generated from the ROI time-series quantifying the connectivity level between individual ROIs; **(E)** By treating the ROIs as graph nodes and the connectivity matrix as graph weights the brain network is expressed in graph form; **(F)** A threshold is applied to keep only the strongest connections; **(G)** Graph theoretical analysis is applied to the resulting graph from part F to obtain a feature vector for each subject; **(H)** A wrapper method called sequential feature selection is applied to choose a handful of features that contribute to the highest classification accuracy; **(I,J)** The resulting feature subset is passed to a linear SVM which trains a model to distinguish between ASD and HC.

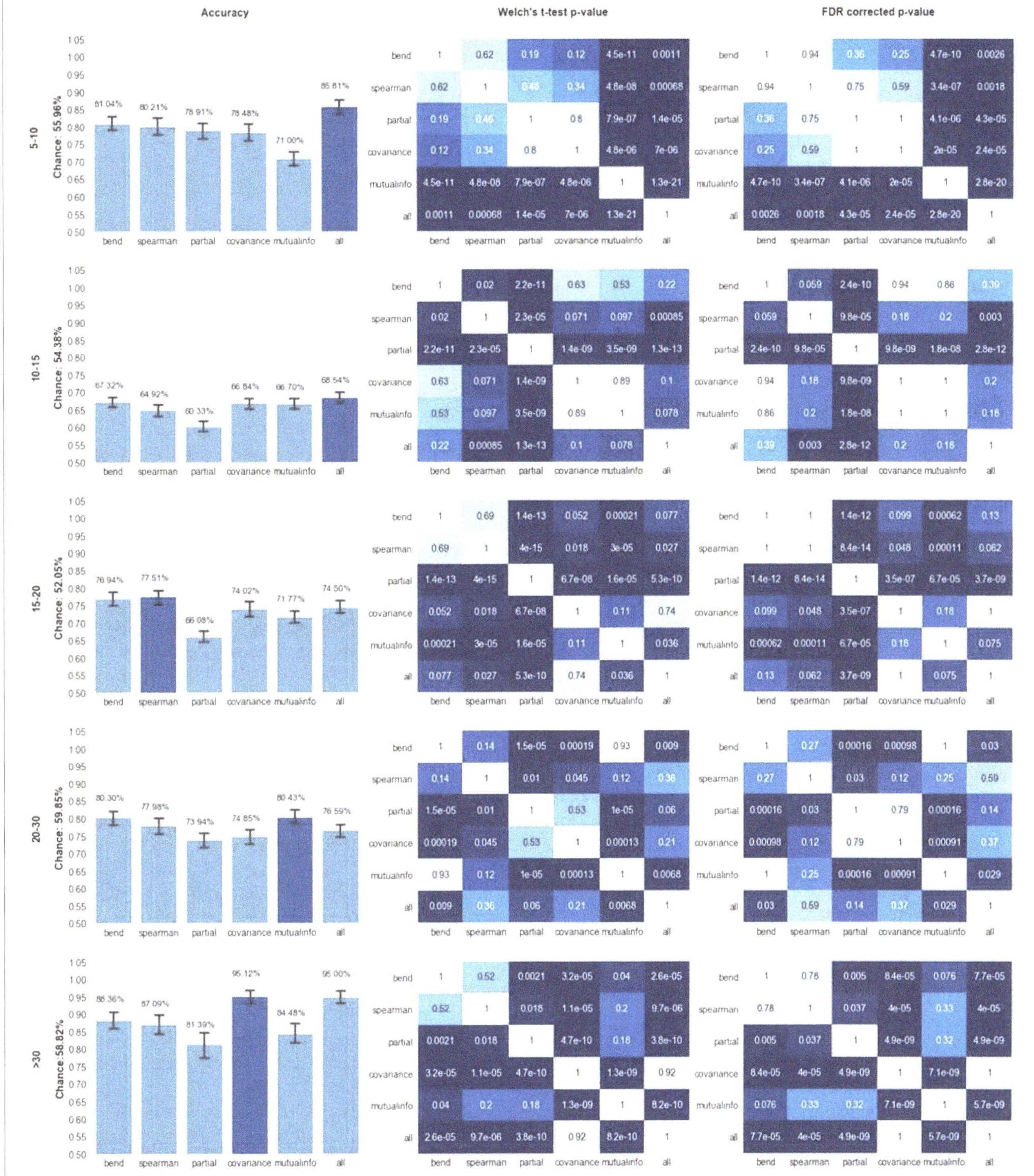

FIGURE 2 | Comparison of Model Performance; Left Column: Accuracy of the models trained using features extracted from the pipeline specified on the X axis for the age range specified on the far left (in years). Y axis labels specify the chance level for the classification task. Top preforming model is highlighted in dark blue; Middle Column: *p*-values of the Welch's *t*-test preformed on the models trained on different pipelines. Statistical significance ($p < 0.05$) is highlighted in dark blue; Right Panel: FDR corrected *p*-values based on the Benjamini, Hochberg method (Benjamini and Hochberg, 1995). The corrected *p*-values were capped at 1 therefore any value over that threshold was set to 1.

We minimized the risk of overfitting by using three limiting approaches. First, the simplest kernel (linear) was used for the SVM. Second, only 10 features were used to learn to classify between 104 subjects. Finally, using 10-fold cross validation ensured the model is only evaluated on data points that it has not experienced before.

As cross validation is inevitably dependent on how the data was randomly separated, we used a 10×10 Welch's t-tests to compare our models. The null hypothesis for these tests was that the two models have equal accuracies. To address the issue of multiple comparisons, we also reported the false discovery rate (FDR) corrected p-values for these tests.

Figure 1 presents a graphical depiction of the methodology proposed here.

RESULTS

Performance of the Classifiers

Our models were able to consistently perform better than the chance level calculated for their respective age ranges. Chance level was evaluated by assuming the model always chooses the most populous group. The left panel of **Figure 2** compares the performance of the different pipelines in each age range. The best preforming model for each age-range is highlighted.

The top preforming pipeline model was generally shown to have a statistically higher ($p < 0.05$) mean than most of the other pipelines. The only exception occurs in the case of the 10–15 age range in which the concatenation pipeline's accuracy fails to achieve a statistically significance difference with three other pipelines: mutual information, covariance, and bend correlation. The details of this statistical analysis are illustrated on the middle and right panels of **Figure 2**.

To further analyze the performance of the best models, we calculated their respective sensitivity and specificity (**Table 2**). All models exhibited a specificity of $> = 80\%$. The 10–15 age range showed relatively low sensitivity. Specificity shows the percentage of times that a Negative prediction (in this case HC is correct while sensitivity shows the percentage of times that a Positive prediction (ASD) is correct.

Analysis of Selected Features

To further understand the results, we plotted the regions from which the selected features were derived (**Figure 3**). The results for the top-preforming pipeline for each age range will be presented in the main body of this article. More details about the performance of all other pipelines for a given age range is given in the **Supplementary Material**. The size of the nodes in **Figure 3** correspond to the rank at which that feature was selected. The abbreviations of the node labels can be found in the **Supplementary Table B**. **Supplementary Table B** also tabulates the exact features for each age range as well as the p-value corresponding to the between group difference of that feature. The top group of measures as well as the top measure based on repetition is as follows: Measures of segregation, specifically clustering coefficient for the 5–10 years range. Measures of centrality for all other age ranges, with the most repeated measure being betweenness centrality for the 10–15 years range, eigenvector centrality for the 15–20 years range, within module degree z-score for the 20–30 years range and betweenness centrality for the >30 years range.

TABLE 2 | Classification performance of the best models.

Age range (years)	Best pipeline	Accuracy%	Specificity%	Sensitivity%
5–10	Concatenation	86	91	79
10–15	Concatenation	69	80	55
15–20	Spearman	78	80	76
20–30	Mutual information	80	87	69
>30	Covariance	95	91	97

DISCUSSION

Comparison With Previous Literature

In this study, we examined several different pipelines for ASD classification. These included 6 different network extraction techniques over 5 age ranges. Furthermore, we used 10-fold cross validation to examine the accuracy of the algorithm for each pipeline which is shown to be better than the leave-one-out cross validation used in previous studies (Kohavi, 1995). In addition, 10-fold cross validation may be used as a substitute for having a separate testing set because the model is evaluated on datapoints it has not seen before. Because of not having the exact models trained in previous studies, we compare our findings with them only by using the reported accuracy, specificity, and sensitivity. All models trained in this study were statistically compared with each other using a 10 by 10 cross validation t-test.

Previous studies were not able to report high prediction accuracies for the ABIDE dataset relative to similar studies on other neurological diseases such as AD. This can be related to the fact that this dataset consists of recordings conducted over multiple sites, some with slightly different image acquisition parameters. Moreover, the whole dataset covers a wide age range (5–64 years). To minimize the effects of age, we separated the dataset into 5 age ranges and trained separate models on each range. To allow for easier reproducibility and thus more meaningful comparisons, we chose to use a publicly available preprocessed version of the data through the Preprocessed Connectomes Project (http://preprocessed-connectomes-project.org/).

Table 3 shows a detailed comparison with previously reported ASD classification models. It is necessary to state all of the mentioned papers other than Chen et al. (2015) used the complete dataset to train their model while in this study separate models where trained for different age ranges. The cross-validation results in this study provide an estimate of how the models would perform if data from their respective age ranges were fed to them. Therefore, it can be hypothesized that the performance over the entire dataset would not be worse than the worst preforming age-range if, based on the subject's age, the correct model is used for a previously unseen dataset. Additional

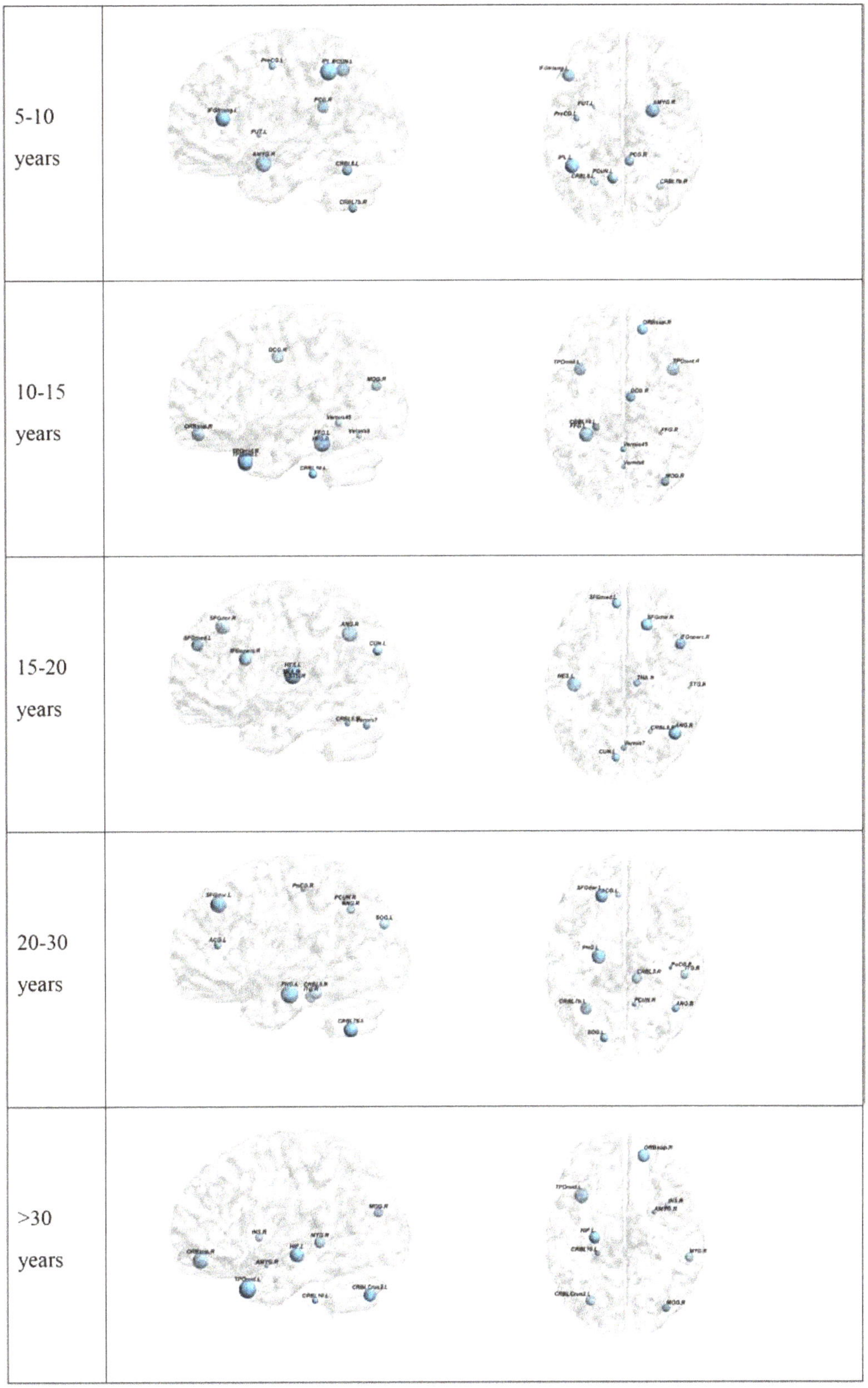

FIGURE 3 | Visualization of the top 10 selected features for each Age range. Two age-ranges show only 9 features. This is because in the 5–10 range PreCG.L was selected two times. In the >30 group the last selected feature was the global Characteristic path length. The full region names along with the abbreviations can be found in **Supplementary Table B**.

TABLE 3 | Previous model performance on the ABIDE dataset.

Accuracy %	Sensitivity %	Specificity %	Algorithm	References
69	72	67	Linear SVM	Plitt et al., 2015
66	60	72	Gaussian SVM	Chen et al., 2015
90.8	89	93	Random forest	Chen et al., 2015
67	NA	NA	SVC	Abraham et al., 2017
70	74	63	Deep neural network	Heinsfeld et al., 2018

data is needed to confirm this hypothesis. Our worst preforming model, the model for the 10–15 age range, outperformed almost all the previous models in specificity while having an accuracy comparable to that of the other SVM models. All other age ranges showed higher accuracy than all previous models except the Chen et al. random forest. This could be attributed to the fact that the performance metrics for the random forest model were assessed using a different scheme called out of bag prediction errors as opposed to the cross validation used in our models and all other previously reported studies mentioned here.

Comparison Between Pipelines

While in all age ranges except the 10–15 range, the top model showed a statistical significance in performance than most of the other models, our results do not reach a consensus about what network creation pipeline preforms best in all cases. However, the bend correlation pipeline's model was the second best model over all age range but the >30 range. Furthermore, it did not show any statistically significant difference in model performance from the top preforming model for the 10–15, 15–20, and 20–30 age ranges. Based on this, we would suggest bend correlation to be the first network construction pipeline for graph theoretical analysis of the ABIDE dataset if computational time is limited.

A possible explanation for the relatively lower performance of the 10–15 range compared to other age ranges is that the larger number of subjects in this group translated into higher between site variability in the data. Therefore, even though our model achieved higher specificity than most previous studies, further steps are needed to address the inherent heterogeneity of the ABIDE dataset.

Analysis of the Selected Features

Centrality measures were shown to be most operative in providing features for the classification tasks in the top 10 selected features. This also held true when selecting the top 5 features. Centrality measures have been shown to undergo changes in ASD. A previous study on the structural network of the brain found that autism is accompanied by centrality alterations in regions relevant for social and sensorimotor processing (Balardin et al., 2015). Another study found changes in hubness of ASD brain networks using resting-state fMRI (Itahashi et al., 2014). Our results suggest that the changes in centrality measures play a key role in being able to differentiate between ASD and HC. The only exception was observed for the 5–10 years age range where clustering coefficient, a measure of segregation, was chosen more times than the rest. This also held true when only looking at the top 5 features. This suggests that at a young age, there may not be many changes to the hubs of the brain network but the organization of the network into sub-networks is altered.

LIMITATIONS

There are several limitations in the current study. First, ABIDE I data was used in different age ranges to investigate the prediction accuracy of our pipelines while minimizing the effects of aging on the resting-state networks. Furthermore, although to the best of our knowledge ABIDE is the most comprehensive database for ASD functional imaging, further analyses are needed to confirm its representability of the whole ASD population. Second, we relied on a single preprocessing pipeline for the sake of easier comparison between our work and previous studies. It is entirely possible that another preprocessing pipeline is better suited to this graph theoretical approach. Future studies will need to investigate this limitation. Additionally, the comparison between our models and previous studies only used three metrics (accuracy, sensitivity, and specificity). A statistical test may be needed to further analyze the significance of our findings. However, this is not possible without access to the exact cross validation folds or out of bag sample errors of those studies. Nevertheless, due to the observed improvement, we suspect that our algorithm has reached a statistically significant improvement over previous results.

Another shortcoming that is not limited to this study is related to how the classification task is formulated. To the best of our knowledge, all research in this field including the present study have focused on distinguishing HCs from ASDs. However, as the name suggests, ASD is a spectrum and individual cases can vary greatly in how the disorder affects them. To address this issue, databases such as ABIDE will play a vital role. Extensive detailed clinical analysis data will be needed to correctly approximate the position of an individual on the spectrum.

Finally, variability present in the ABIDE dataset, such as different imaging parameters and devices, due to it being a multi-site initiative may lead to uncontrolled variations in the data or model being biased toward better represented sites. While the normalization steps in the preprocessing help reduce the variations, further investigations will be needed to confirm if they have been eliminated to a sufficient degree. Our results show better overall performance over previous investigations which suggests these limitations may have been addressed in a satisfactory manner.

CONCLUSION

In this study we utilized graph theory and ML to propose a novel pipeline for automatic diagnosis of ASD which significantly improved performance over previously proposed models. The relative strength of our method suggests graph theoretical analysis paired with the right preprocessing pipeline can nullify the effects of multi-site and multi-device image acquisition to a good degree and is more robust than previous methods. Our pipeline automatically selected 10 biomarkers for each age range being investigated. Measures of centrality were shown to be most operative in distinguishing between ASD and HC.

ETHICS STATEMENT

We used the data collected as part of the ABIDE database and complied with everything that they have asked to be included in any manuscript using that data. The original ethics statement form the (Di Martino et al., 2014) paper is as follows: All contributions were based on studies approved by local IRBs, and data were fully anonymized (removing all 18 HIPAA protected health information identifiers, and face information from structural images). All data distributed were visually inspected prior to release.

AUTHOR CONTRIBUTIONS

The work presented here was carried out in collaboration between all authors. The research was designed by both authors. AK acquired and analyzed the data and carried out the experiment with RS providing supervision and guidance. The manuscript was written by AK and revised by RS. All authors have read and approved the submission of the manuscript.

ACKNOWLEDGMENTS

This work was partially supported by the Biomedical engineering research scholarship of the University of Calgary. The database used in this study was part of the openly available ABIDE I. The funding source for that project is as follows. Primary support for the work by Adriana Di Martino was provided by the NIMH (K23MH087770) and the Leon Levy Foundation. Primary support for the work by Michael P. Milham and the INDI team was provided by gifts from Joseph P. Healy and the Stavros Niarchos Foundation to the Child Mind Institute, as well as by a NIMH award to MPM (R03MH096321).

REFERENCES

Abraham, A., Milham, M. P., Di Martino, A., Craddock, R. C., Samaras, D., Thirion, B., et al. (2017). Deriving reproducible biomarkers from multi-site resting-state data: an autism-based example. *NeuroImage* 147, 736–745. doi: 10.1016/j.neuroimage.2016.10.045

Balardin, J. B., Comfort, W. E., Daly, E., Murphy, C., Andrews, D., Murphy, D. G., et al. (2015). Decreased centrality of cortical volume covariance networks in autism spectrum disorders. *J. Psychiatr. Res.* 69, 142–149. doi: 10.1016/j.jpsychires.2015.08.003

Barttfeld, P., Wicker, B., Cukier, S., Navarta, S., Lew, S., and Sigman, M. (2011). A big-world network in ASD: dynamical connectivity analysis reflects a deficit in long-range connections and an excess of short-range connections. *Neuropsychologia* 49, 254–63. doi: 10.1016/j.neuropsychologia.2010.11.024

Benjamini, Y., and Hochberg, H. (1995). Controlling the false discovery rate: a practical and powerful approach to multiple testing. *J. R. Stat. Soc. Seri B* 57, 289–300. doi: 10.1111/j.2517-6161.1995.tb02031.x

Brentani, H., Paula, C. S., Bordini, D., Rolim, D., Sato, F., Portolese, J., et al. (2013). Autism spectrum disorders: an overview on diagnosis and treatment. *Revista Brasileira de Psiquiatria* 35 (Suppl. 1), S62–72. doi: 10.1590/1516-4446-2013-S104

Bullmore, E., and Sporns, O. (2009). Erratum: complex brain networks: graph theoretical analysis of structural and functional systems. *Nat. Rev. Neurosci.* 10, 312–312. doi: 10.1038/nrn2618

Cameron, C., Sharad, S., Brian, C., Ranjeet, K., Satrajit, G., Chaogan, Y., et al. (2013a). Towards automated analysis of connectomes: the configurable pipeline for the analysis of connectomes (C-PAC). *Front. Neuroinform.* 7:4. doi: 10.3389/conf.fninf.2013.09.00042

Cameron, C., Yassine, B., Carlton, C., Francois, C., Alan, E., András, J., et al. (2013b). The neuro bureau preprocessing initiative: open sharing of preprocessed neuroimaging data and derivatives. *Front. Neuroinform.* 7:41. doi: 10.3389/conf.fninf.2013.09.00041

Chaddad, A., Desrosiers, C., and Toews, M. (2017). Multi-scale radiomic analysis of sub-cortical regions in mri related to autism, gender and age. *Sci. Rep.* 7:45639. doi: 10.1038/srep45639

Chen, C. P., Keown, C. L., Jahedi, A., Nair, A., Pflieger, M. E., Bailey, B. A., et al. (2015). Diagnostic classification of intrinsic functional connectivity highlights somatosensory, default mode, and visual regions in autism. *NeuroImage* 8, 238–45. doi: 10.1016/j.nicl.2015.04.002

Chen, G., Ward, B. D., Xie, C., Li, W., Wu, Z., Jones, J. L., et al. (2011). Classification of alzheimer disease, mild cognitive impairment, and normal cognitive status with large-scale network analysis based on resting-state functional MR imaging. *Radiology* 259, 213–221. doi: 10.1148/radiol.101 00734

Craddock, R. C., James, G. A., Holtzheimer, P. E., Hu, X. P., and Mayberg, H. S. (2012). A whole brain fMRI atlas generated via spatially constrained spectral clustering. *Hum. Brain Mapp.* 33, 1914–28. doi: 10.1002/hbm.21333

Di Martino, A., Yan, C. G., Li, Q., Denio, E., Castellanos, F. X., Alaerts, K., et al. (2014). The autism brain imaging data exchange: towards a large-scale evaluation of the intrinsic brain architecture in autism. *Molecul. Psychiatr.* 19, 659–667. doi: 10.1038/mp.2013.78

Di Martino, A., Zuo, X. N., Kelly, C., Grzadzinski, R., Mennes, M., Schvarcz, A., et al. (2013). Shared and distinct intrinsic functional network centrality in autism and attention-deficit/hyperactivity disorder. *Biol. Psychiatr.* 74, 623–32. doi: 10.1016/j.biopsych.2013.02.011

Dyrba, M., Grothe, M., Kirste, T., and Teipel, S. J. (2015). Multimodal analysis of functional and structural disconnection in alzheimer's disease using multiple kernel SVM. *Hum. Brain Mapp.* 36, 2118–2131. doi: 10.1002/hbm.22759

Fernell, E., Eriksson, M. A., and Gillberg, C. (2013). Early diagnosis of autism and impact on prognosis: a narrative review. *Clin. Epidemiol.* 5, 33–43. doi: 10.2147/CLEP.S41714

Hazlett, H. C., Gu, H., Munsell, B. C., Kim, S. H., Styner, M., Wolff, J. J., et al. (2017). Early brain development in infants at high risk for autism spectrum disorder. *Nature* 542, 348–351. doi: 10.1038/nature21369

Heinsfeld, A. S., Franco, A. R., Craddock, R. C., Buchweitz, A., and Meneguzzi, F. (2018). Identification of autism spectrum disorder using deep learning and the ABIDE dataset. *NeuroImage* 17, 16–23. doi: 10.1016/j.nicl.2017.08.017

Howsmon, D. P., Kruger, U., Melnyk, S., James, S. J., and Hahn, J. (2017). Classification and adaptive behavior prediction of children with autism spectrum disorder based upon multivariate data analysis of markers of oxidative stress and DNA methylation. *PLOS Comput. Biol.* 13:e1005385. doi: 10.1371/journal.pcbi.1005385

Huang, S., Li, J., Sun, L., Ye, J., Fleisher, A., Wu, T., et al. (2010). Learning brain connectivity of alzheimer's disease by sparse inverse covariance estimation. *NeuroImage* 50, 935–949. doi: 10.1016/j.neuroimage.2009.12.120

Hull, J. V., Dokovna, L. B., Jacokes, Z. J., Torgerson, C. M., Irimia, A., and Darrell Van Horn, J. (2016). Resting-state functional connectivity in autism spectrum disorders: a review. *Front. Psychiatry* 7:205.

Itahashi, T., Yamada, T., Watanabe, H., Nakamura, M., Jimbo, D., Shioda, S., et al. (2014). Altered network topologies and hub organization in adults with autism: a resting-state fMRI study. *PLoS ONE* 9:e94115. doi: 10.1371/journal.pone.0094115

Iturria-Medina, Y., Sotero, R. C., Canales-Rodríguez, E. J., Alemán-Gómez, Y., and Melie-García, L. (2008). Studying the human brain anatomical network via diffusion-weighted MRI and graph theory. *NeuroImage* 40, 1064–1076. doi: 10.1016/j.neuroimage.2007.10.060

Kazeminejad, A., Golbabaei, S., and Soltanian-Zadeh, H. (2017). "Graph theoretical metrics and machine learning for diagnosis of Parkinson's disease using Rs-fMRI," in *2017 Artificial Intelligence and Signal Processing Conference (AISP)* (Shiraz: IEEE), 134–139. doi: 10.1109/AISP.2017.8324124

Keown, C. L., Datko, M. C., Chen, C. P., Maximo, J. O., Jahedi, A., and Müller, R. A. (2017). Network organization is globally atypical in autism: a graph theory study of intrinsic functional connectivity. *Biol. Psychiatr.* 2, 66–75. doi: 10.1016/j.bpsc.2016.07.008

Kohavi, R. (1995). *A Study of Cross-Validation and Bootstrap for Accuracy Estimation and Model Selection.* Available online at: http://ai.stanford.edu/~ronnyk/accEst.pdf

Kruschwitz, J. D., List, D., Waller, L., Rubinov, M., and Walter, H. (2015). GraphVar: a user-friendly toolbox for comprehensive graph analyses of functional brain connectivity. *J. Neurosci. Methods* 245, 107–115. doi: 10.1016/j.jneumeth.2015.02.021

Leung, R. C., Ye, A. X., Wong, S. M., Taylor, M. J., and Doesburg, S. M. (2014). Reduced beta connectivity during emotional face processing in adolescents with autism. *Molecul. Autism* 5:51. doi: 10.1186/2040-2392-5-51

Lowe, M. J., Dzemidzic, M., Lurito, J. T., Mathews, V. P., and Phillips, M. D. (2000). Correlations in low-frequency BOLD fluctuations reflect cortico-cortical connections. *NeuroImage* 12, 582–87. doi: 10.1006/nimg.2000.0654

Marrelec, G., Krainik, A., Duffau, H., Pélégrini-Issac, M., Lehéricy, S., Doyon, J., et al. (2006). Partial correlation for functional brain interactivity investigation in functional MRI. *Neuroimage* 32, 228–237. doi: 10.1016/j.neuroimage.2005.12.057

Nielsen, J. A., Zielinski, B. A., Fletcher, P. T., Alexander, A. L., Lange, N., Bigler, E. D., et al. (2013). Multisite functional connectivity MRI classification of autism: ABIDE results. *Front. Hum. Neurosci.* 7:599. doi: 10.3389/fnhum.2013.00599

Pernet, C. R., Wilcox, R., and Rousselet, G. A. (2012). Robust correlation analyses: false positive and power validation using a new open source matlab toolbox. *Front. Psychol.* 3:606. doi: 10.3389/fpsyg.2012.00606

Plitt, M., Barnes, K. A., and Martin, A. (2015). Functional connectivity classification of autism identifies highly predictive brain features but falls short of biomarker standards. *YNICL* 7, 359–366. doi: 10.1016/j.nicl.2014.12.013

Pudil, P., Novovičová, J., and Kittler, J. (1994). Floating search methods in feature selection. *Pattern Recogn. Lett.* 15, 1119–1125. doi: 10.1016/0167-8655(94)90127-9

Qin, B., Wang, L., Zhang, Y., Cai, J., Chen, J., and Li, T. (2018). Enhanced topological network efficiency in preschool autism spectrum disorder: a diffusion tensor imaging study. *Front. Psychiatr.* 9:278.

Rubinov, M., and Sporns, O. (2010). Complex network measures of brain connectivity: uses and interpretations. *NeuroImage* 52, 1059–1069. doi: 10.1016/j.neuroimage.2009.10.003

Rudie, J. D., Brown, J. A., Beck-Pancer, D., Hernandez, L. M., Dennis, E. L., Thompson, P. M., et al. (2013). Altered functional and structural brain network organization in autism. *NeuroImage* 2, 79–94. doi: 10.1016/j.nicl.2012.11.006

Sanchez-Rodriguez, L. M., Iturria-Medina, Y., Baines, E. A., Mallo, S. C., Dousty, M., Sotero, R. C., et al. (2018). Design of optimal nonlinear network controllers for alzheimer's disease. *PLoS Comput. Biol.* 14:e1006136. doi: 10.1371/journal.pcbi.1006136

Sotero, R. C. (2016). Topology, cross-frequency, and same-frequency band interactions shape the generation of phase-amplitude coupling in a neural mass model of a cortical column. *PLOS Comput. Biol.* 12:e1005180. doi: 10.1371/journal.pcbi.1005180

Talai, S., Boelmans, K., Sedlacik, J., and Forkert, N. D. (2017). "Automatic classification of patients with idiopathic Parkinson's disease and progressive supranuclear palsy using diffusion MRI datasets," in *International Society for Optics and Photonics*, eds G. Samuel, Armato, Nicholas, and A. Petrick, 10134:101342H.

Tzourio-Mazoyer, N., Landeau, B., Papathanassiou, D., Crivello, F., Etard, O., Delcroix, N., et al. (2002). Automated anatomical labeling of activations in SPM using a macroscopic anatomical parcellation of the MNI MRI single-subject brain. *NeuroImage* 15, 273–289. doi: 10.1006/nimg.2001.0978

van den Heuvel, M. P., and Hulshoff Pol, H. E. (2010). Exploring the brain network: a review on resting-state fMRI functional connectivity. *Eur. Neuropsychopharmacol.* 20, 519–34. doi: 10.1016/j.euroneuro.2010.03.008

Wilcox, R. R. (1994). The percentage bend correlation coefficient. *Psychometrika* 59, 601–16. doi: 10.1007/BF02294395

Zablotsky, B., Black, L. I., Maenner, M. J., Schieve, L. A., and Blumberg, S. J. (2015). Estimated prevalence of autism and other developmental disabilities following questionnaire changes in the 2014 national health interview survey. *Natl. Health Stat. Rep.* 87, 1–20.

Zeng, K., Kang, J., Ouyang, G., Li, J., Han, J., Wang, Y., et al. (2017). Disrupted brain network in children with autism spectrum disorder. *Sci. Rep.* 7:16253. doi: 10.1038/s41598-017-16440-z

14

Improved Wavelet Threshold for Image De-Noising

Yang Zhang [1*], *Weifeng Ding* [2], *Zhifang Pan* [3] *and Jing Qin* [4]

[1] School of Information and Engineering, The First Affiliated Hospital of WenZhou Medical University, WenZhou Medical University, WenZhou, China, [2] The Chinese People's Liberation Army 118 Hospital, WenZhou, China, [3] School of Information and Engineering and Information Technology Centre, WenZhou Medical University, WenZhou, China, [4] School of Nursing, Hong Kong Polytechnic University, Kowloon, Hong Kong

***Correspondence:**
Yang Zhang
zhangyang0408@wmu.edu.cn

With the development of communication technology and network technology, as well as the rising popularity of digital electronic products, an image has become an important carrier of access to outside information. However, images are vulnerable to noise interference during collection, transmission and storage, thereby decreasing image quality. Therefore, image noise reduction processing is necessary to obtain higher-quality images. For the characteristics of its multi-analysis, relativity removal, low entropy, and flexible bases, the wavelet transform has become a powerful tool in the field of image de-noising. The wavelet transform in application mathematics has a rapid development. De-noising methods based on wavelet transform is proposed and achieved with good results, but shortcomings still remain. Traditional threshold functions have some deficiencies in image de-noising. A hard threshold function is discontinuous, whereas a soft threshold function causes constant deviation. To address these shortcomings, a method for removing image noise is proposed in this paper. First, the method decomposes the noise image to determine the wavelet coefficients. Second, the wavelet coefficient is applied on the high-frequency part of the threshold processing by using the improved threshold function. Finally, the de-noised images are obtained to rebuild the images in accordance with the estimation in the wavelet-based conditions. Experiment results show that this method, discussed in this paper, is better than traditional hard threshold de-noising and soft threshold de-noising methods, in terms of objective effects and subjective visual effects.

Keywords: wavelet threshold, wavelet transform, image de-noising, MSE, PSNR

INTRODUCTION

The transmission, detection and collection of signals are subject to pollution of varying degrees of random noise, influenced by the environment and due to the nature of the work. Thus, the implementation of signal de-noising is necessary. How to filter out the noise in the real signal to obtain effective information, is a current research hotspot. Wavelet transform has a time-frequency local analysis function, and its de-noising results are relatively good. Thus, its application is also very extensive.

In recent years, with the deepening of the intersection and research, along with the application of mathematics and other disciplines, the application of fuzzy mathematics, mathematical morphology, intelligent optimization, neural network, and wavelet theory and technology in image processing, as well as some new methods of noise resistance have emerged. In the early stage, the traditional de-noising method has a low pass filter method, which mainly includes median filtering, linear filtering and adaptive filtering.

During image collection, coding and transmission, all images are visible or invisible to varying degrees of noise. The image noise is divided into three main categories. The first is Gauss noise, which belongs to the category of electronic noise that is produced by a sensitive element caused by the random thermal motion of the electronic components. The second is Poisson noise, which is produced during the process of photoelectric conversion; it has an apparent effect under a weakened light. The third is particle noise, which is produced during the process of photography and can be found under a microscope. The smooth images that can be seen in the photo will display random particle images under the microscope (Auber and Kornprobst, 2006). The purpose of image processing is to perform some operations or processing on the digitized image information, in order to improve the image quality or to achieve a desired effect. For example, the non-uniformity of the sensitivity of sensitive components in photoelectric conversion, transmission error and human factors during the digitization diminishes the quality of an image, which contains various random noises. Sometimes, this random noise will greatly affect the image quality. The noise image affects not only the visual effect of the viewed image, but also affects image processing. Image de-noising aims to retain useful information and reduce or eliminate the interference of noise in the image. De-noising is a key link in image processing. In practical applications, this process is often used as a pretreatment of image processing and recognition, which is the basis of subsequent high-level image processing. Thus far, all studies on image de-noising have focused on this effect and has achieved great progress. However, with the emergence of new problems, people have higher standards of image quality. The traditional image noise removal algorithm is based on the spectrum distribution. In frequency, wavelet de-noising is the commonly used method to separate useful information and noise from images (Johnstone and Silverman, 2005, Othman and Qian, 2006). Other methods include the Markov field model, partial differential equation and LP regularization method (Baske, 2011). This method is also a drawback on regularizing noise. The convergence rate is slow in regions with minimal changes. Sinha and Dougherty (Thomas Asaki and Kevin Vixie, 2010) combined fuzzy mathematics with mathematical morphology and applied it to image processing. In recent years, the feed forward BP neural network was proposed as a filter to de-noise (Noh et al., 2011; Swami et al., 2017). Wavelet transform has also greatly contributed to image de-noising (Michal et al., 2006; Apotsos et al., 2008; Patil, 2015). The correlation coefficient method is based on the correlation between the wavelet coefficients at the corresponding positions for each scale, whereas the noise is neither correlated nor has a weak correlation on each scale to remove the noise. Noise is mainly concentrated in high frequencies, provided that high-frequency processing can achieve the effect of noise reduction. In 2006, Elad and Aharon (2006) proposed a de-noising method on the basis of sparse representation and KSVD dictionary learning. The dictionary learned by the KSVD algorithm (Oey et al., 2013) was used for image de-noising. However, the KSVD algorithm ignores the similarity of the image, and the KSVD algorithm cannot use the detailed information of the image when learning the dictionary on a single scale. At present, the popular multi-scale directional transformation mainly includes: curved wave transformation (Palakkal and Prabhu, 2012), contour wave trans-formation and non-sub sampling contour wave transformation (Amisha et al., 2013). The multi-scale transformation methods can use the inherent geometric features of the natural image data, and all relative wavelet transforms have remarkably improved in direction selection. The 3D block matching algorithm (BM3D) (Lebrun, 2012) is an effective de-noising method for Gauss noise. This algorithm can preserve information such as edge and texture. BM3D comprehensively utilizes non-locality, linear transformation threshold, Wiener filtering, and sparse representation. BM3D also reveals details of different sub-block classes and retains the basic characteristics of each sub-block. This method can improve the resolution in noisy images, however the computation is very large, as each similar block needs to be computed. Pizarro et al. (2010) selected non-local constraints as fidelity items. In similarity measure, the error of noise image and real images was minimal. Moreover, the high-order smoothing of the de-noised image was used as a regularization term, and a non-local data smoothing model was proposed. The model was applied to the similarity between images to obtain a further general model. A selected unsuitable threshold can easily present a Gibbs phenomenon (Huang et al., 2005, Chen et al., 2005). Mallat presented alternating projection (AP) for de-noising. The AP (Mallat and Hwang, 1992; Zhu et al., 2017) method obtains the modulus maxima at each scale after the signal is differentiated on each scale. Then, the non-propagating modulus maxima should restore the signal. The disadvantage of the alternating projection method is that the computation is very large and, the iteration is prone to instability. Li proposed a novel hybrid model based on an extreme learning machine, k-nearest neighbor regression and wavelet de-noising (Li et al., 2017).Using the linear mode to reduce noise will lead to the loss of detail in textured images. The static wavelet transforms (SWT) use time invariance to achieve image de-noising (Wang et al., 2003). Some researchers (Zou et al., 2015; Liu et al., 2017) proposed an approach that searches for candidate matching blocks along the edges that are well-adapted to image details. All similar blocks form a 3D group. De-noising is performed by shrinking the coefficients of the 3D transform applied on these groups. The non-linear diffusion filtering method based on PDE, is a non-linear anisotropic de-noising method (Lee et al., 2005). A non-linear model for de-noising can be excessive in the smoothing of images. Scholars have also studied how to improve the speed of de-noising. The Non-linear Diffusion techniques and PDE-based variational models are very popular in image restoring and processing. The researchers proposed (Fazli et al., 2010; Zeng et al., 2012, 2018) that a heuristic method such as Particle Swarm Optimization (PSO), be used for Complex PDE parameter tuning by minimizing the Structural SIMilarity (SSIM) measure. Tasdizen (2009) enhanced the algorithm efficiency by clustering the blocks with PCA, selecting the similarity between block features as the measurement of block similarity, and optimally estimating the parameters. Mahmoudi and Sapiro (2005) proposed to accelerate the algorithm by eliminating irrelevant neighborhoods in the weighted averaging process. Currently, many researchers have proposed a combination of ways for de-noising. For example, machine learning and random walks are combined with traditional noise removal methods (Huang et al., 2006; Jieru et al., 2016; Liu et al., 2018). Zeng et al. (2017), proposed de-noising and de-blurring gold immune chromatographic strip images via gradient projection algorithms.

Presently, details of images and how to remove noise from them has received increased attention. In this paper, we present an improved threshold to de-noising of MRI images. Experimental results show that the de-noising effect is better than the hard and soft threshold.

PRINCIPLE OF WAVELET DE-NOISING MEDTHOD

In current research, there are numerous ways to eliminate noise from images. The application of wavelet de-noising is very extensive. The wavelet method for removing noise has numerous advantages. Not only is the algorithm simple to implement, but it also has a particularly superb effect of de-noising. This method has therefore achieved great results in practical applications. The main principle of wavelet threshold de-noising is based on the strong correlation of the wavelet. The energy concentration of the signal after wavelet transform is often concentrated on the large wavelet coefficient. The noise energy after wavelet transform does not have concentrated characteristics, because the noise does not have the correlation of wavelets. Wavelet coefficients with large amplitude values are mostly signals, whereas the coefficients with small amplitude values are largely noise. The threshold is set on the basis of this property. The hard and soft threshold function method was proposed by Donoho (Donoho, 1995) et al.

The hard threshold is expressed as follows:

$$\hat{w}_{j,k} = \begin{cases} w_{j,k}, |w_{j,k}| >= \lambda \\ 0, |w_{j,k}| < \lambda \end{cases} \tag{1}$$

The soft threshold is calculated as follows:

$$\hat{w}_{j,k} = \begin{cases} \mathrm{sgn}\,(w_{j,k})(|w_{j,k}| - \lambda), |w_{j,k}| >= \lambda \\ 0, |w_{j,k}| < \lambda \end{cases} \tag{2}$$

The Semi-threshold function is expressed as follows:

$$\hat{w}_{j,k} = \begin{cases} 0, |w_{j,k}| <= \lambda \\ \mathrm{sgn}\,(w_{j,k})\frac{\lambda_2(|w_{j,k}|-\lambda_1)}{\lambda_2-\lambda_1}, \lambda_1 < |w_{j,k}| < \lambda_2 \\ w_{j,k}, |w_{j,k}| > \lambda \end{cases} \tag{3}$$

Although the soft, hard thresholds and semi- thresholds have achieved some results, they all still have drawbacks. The hard threshold function can better preserve boundary information however, the hard threshold function is discontinuous at closed values, thus removing the noise cancellation effect remains rough. Furthermore, its application has some limitations; this function only processes wavelet coefficients smaller than the threshold and does not manage wavelet coefficients larger than the threshold. Therefore, the de-noising result is relatively different. The resulting estimated signal produces additional oscillations. Furthermore, the interference of the noise signal is often mixed in with the wavelet coefficients greater than the closed value function. The soft threshold function has improved overall continuity, and the de-noising result is relatively smooth. However, after noise cancellation, the signal is easily overwhelmed by noise, thereby resulting in difficulties at higher-order derivatives, causing de-noising distortion. Moreover, the soft threshold function performs constant value compression on the wavelet coefficients rather than the threshold. This function directly affects the degree of approximation of the reconstructed signals. The semi-threshold function not only retains a large coefficient, but also has continuity.

The calculation of complexity through this function is higher. In the semi-threshold function, determining the threshold is a difficult point. Therefore, the traditional threshold function has its own defects and has certain limitations in its application, which affects the effect of de-noising.

In this article, we proposed a new threshold function. We improved the threshold to compensate for the deficiency of soft and hard thresholds. In our experiment, we analyzed the experimental results of subjective and objective experiments and concluded that the improved threshold function de-noising effect is better than the hard and soft threshold de-noising.

IMPROVED WAVELET THRESHOLD DE-NOISING METHOD

For the method of threshold de-noising, using hard and soft closed-valued functions, the basic idea is to remove relatively small wavelet coefficients as much as possible. When a hard threshold function is used to de-noise, although it can save the effective part of the original signal relatively well, the reconstructed signal after the noise processing will be very rough. When de-noising with a soft threshold function, the reconstructed signal will easily lose useful signals.

The key to threshold shrinkage is the determination of threshold and threshold functions. If the threshold is selected as large, details will be lost. If the threshold is selected small, then the noise still exists. Although a hard threshold de-noising is simple and easy to implement, it will generate a pseudo-Gibbs phenomenon at the image boundary. In comparison with hard thresholds, soft thresholds are continuous, and the structure of wavelet coefficients is maintained, thereby effectively reducing the pseudo Gibbs phenomenon. However, when wavelet coefficients with an absolute value greater than the threshold value are processed, the image edges will become blurred. To achieve improved results for de-noising, we have enhanced the threshold functions.

Improved Threshold Functions

The improved threshold function is as follows:

$$\hat{w}_{j,k} = \begin{cases} w_{j,k} - \frac{w_{j,k}}{2} \cdot \frac{1}{100^{|w_{j,k}|\lambda} - 99}, |w_{j,k}| > \lambda \\ \frac{w_{j,k}}{2} \cdot \frac{1}{1 - \log_{100}^{|w_{j,k}|/\lambda}}, |w_{j,k}| <= \lambda \end{cases} \quad (4)$$

The threshold function after adding an adjustment factor is as follows:

$$\hat{w}_{j,k} = \begin{cases} w_{j,k} - \frac{w_{j,k}.m}{2} \cdot \frac{1}{100^{|w_{j,k}|\lambda} - 99}, |w_{j,k}| > \lambda \\ \frac{w_{j,k}.m}{2} \cdot \frac{1}{1 - \log_{100}^{|w_{j,k}|/\lambda}}, |w_{j,k}| <= \lambda \end{cases} \quad (5)$$

Where$m \in Z$.

When$|w_{j,k}| \rightarrow \lambda^+$, the first inequality of Equation (4) can be written as:

$$\lim_{|w_{j,k}| \rightarrow \lambda^+} \left(\frac{w_{j,k}m}{2} \cdot \frac{1}{100^{|w_{j,k}|\lambda} - 99}\right) = \frac{\lambda}{2} \quad (6)$$

When$|w_{j,k}| \rightarrow \lambda^-$, the second inequality of formula (4) can be written:

$$\lim_{|w_{j,k}| \rightarrow \lambda^-} \left(\frac{w_{j,k}.m}{2} \cdot \frac{1}{1 - \log_{100}^{|w_{j,k}|/\lambda}}\right) = \frac{\lambda}{2} \quad (7)$$

The threshold is continuous at the $\pm\lambda$ point and has high-order derivatives. The threshold function is continuous, and the high order is steerable. The second inequality slowly approaches zero. Here *in* adjusts the shape of the threshold function; m adjusts the variation of wavelet coefficient; k determines the asymptote of the threshold function. When $k = 1$,we proposed that the threshold function approaches the hard threshold function. When $k = 0$, the threshold function approaches the soft threshold function. Thus, the parameter k was adjusted; we proposed that the threshold function can vary between the interval values of soft threshold function and hard threshold function.

The new threshold function proposed in this paper combines the advantages of soft and hard threshold functions. This approach enables the smooth transition of the wavelet threshold curve. The same continuity is achieved in the wavelet domain as the traditional soft threshold function, which improves the shortcomings of hard threshold function discontinuity. Moreover, pseudo-Gibbs phenomenon can be avoided. The new threshold function is a high-order steerable between the intervals of $|w_{j,k}| > \lambda$ and $|w_{j,k}| <= \lambda$. This type of conductivity enables the elimination of the generated oscillation phenomenon in threshold de-noising and the improves the suppression of overkill of the detail coefficient. Thus, the signal after reconstruction can be made smoother.

Improved Threshold Selection

The threshold is vital in image threshold de-noising, and Donoho (1995) proposed a unified threshold method.

$$\lambda = \delta\sqrt{2\log(M * N)} \quad (8)$$

However, this method is not ideal in practical applications and causes over-segmentation (Grace et al., 2000). Through analysis, it was found that the decomposition of the image by wavelet increases with the number of decomposition layers. The energy of noise will become smaller and smaller, and the energy of image information will become increasingly larger. Wavelet decomposition is performed in accordance with the high and low frequency characteristics of a wavelet. This method proposes the following hierarchical threshold estimation.

$$\lambda = \delta\sqrt{2\log M * N} * (1 - \alpha^* j) \quad (9)$$

Where j is the resolution scale. $M \times N$ represents image size. $0 < \alpha < 1$, and α denotes the adjustment parameter. When we calculate the high-frequency threshold, α is a smaller value, resulting in a slightly larger threshold. When we calculate the low-frequency, α is a larger value, resulting in a slightly smaller threshold. By adjusting α to the threshold parameter α, the accuracy of the threshold estimation is microscopically improved.

EXPERIMENT ANALYSIS

In this paper, the experimental analysis consists mainly of two parts. The objective and subjective evaluation.

Objective Evaluation

To illustrate the effectiveness of the wavelet threshold algorithm in medical image de-noising, the traditional threshold method and the proposed method was compared. Objective evaluation index is described by peak signal-to-noise ratio (PSNR) and mean square error (MSE).

The PSNR is expressed as follows:

$$PSNR = 10 * \lg\left(\frac{255^2}{MSE}\right) \quad (10)$$

The MSE is calculated as follows:

$$MSE = \frac{1}{M * N}\left[\sum_{i=1}^{M}\sum_{j=1}^{M}((g(i,j) - \hat{g}(i,j)))^2\right] \quad (11)$$

Where $M * N$ is the size of image; $g(i,j)$denotes original image, and $\hat{g}(i,j)$represents the restoration image. Our data were obtained from the Chinese People's Liberation Army 118 Hospital. The results shown in **Table 1** compare the hard threshold method, the soft threshold method and the proposed method.

Through simulation experiments, the data in **Tables 1–3** show that the proposed method obtains a large peak signal-to-noise ratio and a smaller mean square error. Thus, our improved wavelet de-noising effect is better.

Subjective Evaluation

The experiment was programmed in MATLAB2014 (b). MRI brain images were used to prove the effectiveness of the improved threshold function in medical image de-noising. After

TABLE 1 | De-noising results in different ways of MRI 1.

MSE	0.01	0.03	0.05	0.1	PSNR	0.01	0.03	0.05	0.1
Hard threshold	310	603	643	1,495		23.21	20.33	20.05	16.49
Soft threshold	386	765	771	1,627		22.64	19.29	19.26	16.01
Proposed	147	311	341	625		26.46	23.20	23.20	20.17

TABLE 2 | De-noising results in different ways of MRI 2.

MSE	0.01	0.03	0.05	0.1	PSNR	0.01	0.03	0.05	0.1
Hard threshold	624	780	910	1,136		20.18	19.21	18.54	16.49
Soft threshold	740	952	1080	1,530		22.64	19.29	19.26	16.01
Proposed	206	338	483	668		24.99	22.84	21.29	19.83

TABLE 3 | De-noising results in different ways of MRI 3.

MSE	0.01	0.03	0.05	0.1	PSNR	0.01	0.03	0.05	0.1
Hard threshold	387	350	549	1,022		22.53	22.67	20.74	17.77
Soft threshold	465	422	647	1,308		21.46	21.88	20.02	16.96
Proposed	180	133	287	631		25.58	26.89	23.55	20.13

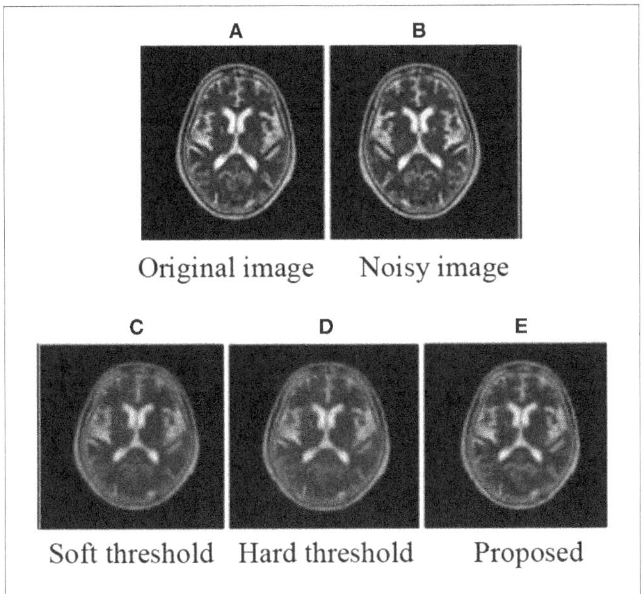

FIGURE 1 | MRI 1 of subjective results.

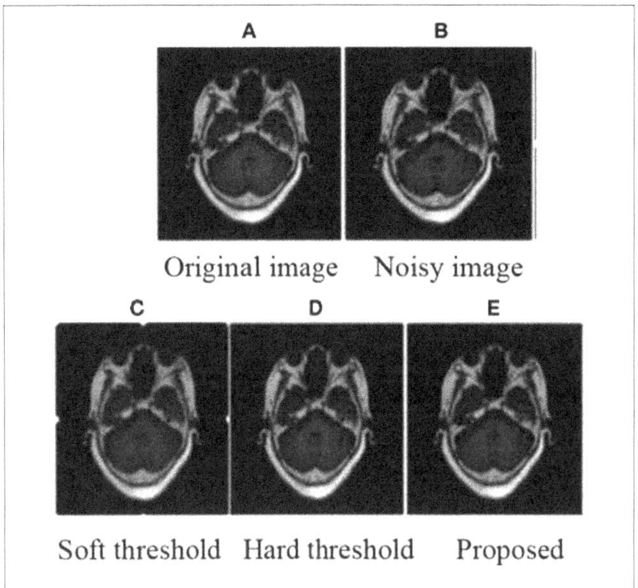

FIGURE 2 | MRI 2 of subjective results.

decomposition, the threshold was calculated using Equation (9) and processed by the corresponding threshold. Finally, the image was reconstructed to obtain the image after de-noising. The subjective experimental results show that the method proposed in this paper can achieve improved de-noising effects. De-noising effects are achieved when the mean value is 0 and the variance is as follows: 0.01, 0.03, 0.05, and 0.1. The experimental results are shown in **Figures 1–3**

After adding noise, the original image was almost drowned by noise. Using soft and hard thresholds to remove noise, considerable noises remained in the image. Given the increase in noise, the image appears smoother by using soft and hard thresholds to remove noise. The method in this paper, removed all the noise in the image, and the image was relatively clear. By contrasting the experiments, we suggest that the proposed method has a better effect than hard and soft threshold methods.

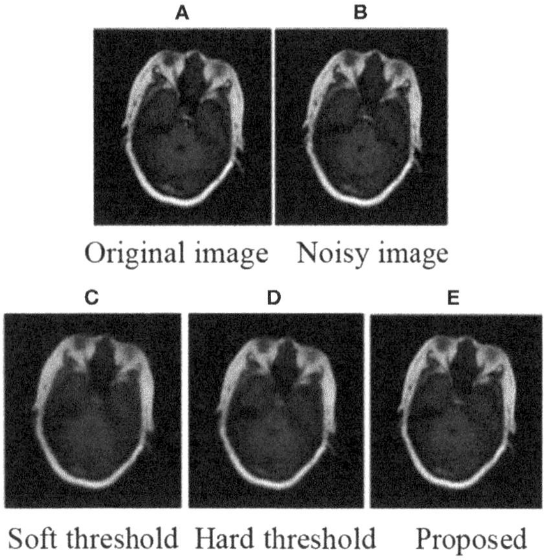

FIGURE 3 | MRI 3 of subjective results.

CONCLUSION

In this study, we analyzed the shortcomings of traditional hard and soft threshold functions for medical image de-noising. We proposed an improved threshold function for de-noising. The mediation factor was increased to find the best estimate of the wavelet coefficient function. The wavelet coefficients were smoothed by the soft threshold function. Thus, the image looks smooth when noise is removed via soft threshold. Through subjective and objective evaluations, the results show that the effect of the hard threshold function is better than that of the soft threshold. However, the signal will produce jumping points when generating additional shocks and the original signal will not be the smooth. The hard threshold method will predict the ringing effect. Improved threshold selection based on the multi-layer wavelet transform, overcomes the disadvantages of soft and hard thresholds. Experimental results showed that the proposed method in this paper can effectively improve the de-noising performance of both soft and hard threshold functions.

AUTHOR CONTRIBUTIONS

YZ conceived the study, designed model, and wrote the draft. WD provided data, acquired the pre-processed the data and analyzed the data. ZP and JQ gave critical revision. All authors consent for this submission.

FUNDING

This work was supported by Scientific Research Task in Department Education of ZheJiang (Y201328002 & kg2015243). Talents stating Task of WenZhou Medical University (QTJ11008). Wenzhou Science and technology bureau (Y20150086 & 2018ZG016), Zhejiang Provincial Natural Science foundation of China (LY16F030010).

REFERENCES

Amisha, J. S., Makwana, R., and Gupta, S. B. (2013). Single image super-resolution via non sub-sample contourlet transform based learning and a gabor prior. *Int. J. Comput. Appl.* 18, 32–38. doi: 10.5120/10735-5580

Apotsos, A., Raubenheimer, B., Elgar, S, and Guza, R. T. (2008).Testing and calibrating parametric wave transformation models on natural beaches. *Coastal Eng.* 3, 224–233. doi: 10.1016/j.coastaleng.2007.10.002

Auber, G., and Kornprobst, P. (2006). *Mathematical Problems in Images Processing. Partial Differential Equations and the Calculus of Variations*. New York, NY: Springer Press.

Baske, A. (2011). *Markov Random Fields for Vision and Image Processing*. Massachusetts; London: MIT Press, 31–59.

Chen, G. Y., Bui, T. D., and Krzyak, A. (2005). Image denoising with neighbor dependency and customized wavelet and threshold. *Pattern Recogn.* 1, 115–124. doi: 10.1016/j.patcog.2004.05.009

Donoho, D. L. (1995). De-noising by Soft-thresholding. *Trans. Inform. Theory* 3, 613–627. doi: 10.1109/18.382009

Elad, M., and Aharon, M. (2006). "Image De-noising via Learned Dictionaries and Sparse representation," in *Computer society Conference on Computer Vision and Pattern Recognition* (New York, NY), 1–6. doi: 10.1109/CVPR.2006.142

Fazli, S., Bouzari, H., and Moradi pour, H. (2010). "Complex PDE image denoising based on Particle Swarm Optimization," in *2nd International Congress on Ultra Modern Telecommunications and Control Systems* (Moscow), 364–370. doi: 10.1109/ICUMT.2010.5676612

Grace, S. C., Bin, Y., and Vetterli, M. (2000). Adaptive wavelet threshold for image de-noising and compression. *Trans. Image Process.* 9, 1532–1154. doi: 10.1109/83.862633

Huang, G. B., Zhu, Q. Y., and Siew, C. K. (2006). Extreme learning machine: theory and applications. *Neuro Comput.* 1, 489–501. doi: 10.1016/j.neucom.2005.12.126

Huang, K. Q., Wu, Z. Y., Fung George, S. K., and Chan Francis, H. Y. (2005). Color image denoising with wavelet thresholding based on human visual system model. *Image Commun.* 2, 115–127. doi: 10.1016/j.image.2004.08.002

Jieru, Z., Ju, Y., Lu, H., Xuan, P., and Zou, Q. (2016). Accurate identification of cancer lections through hybrid machine learning technology. *Int. J. Genomics* 2016, 1–11. doi: 10.1155/2016/7604641

Johnstone, I., and Silverman, B. (2005). Empirical byes selection of wavelet thresholds. *Annals Statist.* 4, 1700–1752. doi: 10.1214/009053605000000345

Lebrun, M. (2012). An Analysis and Implementation of the BM3D Image De-noising Method. *Image Process.* 2, 175–213. doi: 10.5201/ipol.2012.1-bm3d

Lee, B. I., Lee, S. H., Kim, T. S., Kwon, O., Woo, E. J., and Seo, J. K. (2005). Harmonic decomposition in PDE based de-noising technique for magnetic resonance electrical impedance tomography. *Biomed. Eng.* 52, 1912–1920. doi: 10.1109/TBME.2005.856258

Li, W., Kong, D., and Wu, J. (2017). A novel hybrid model based on extreme learning machine, k-nearest neighbor regression and wavelet de-noising applied to short-term electric load forecasting. *Energies* 10, 1–16. doi: 10.3390/en10050694

Liu, D., Wen, B., Liu, X., Wang, Z., and Huang, T. (2018). "When image denoising meets high-level vision tasks: a deep learning approach," in *Proceedings of the Twenty-Seventh International Joint Conference on Artificial Intelligence*, 842–848. doi: 10.24963/ijcai.2018/117

Liu, J., Liu, R., Wang, Y., Chen, J., Yang, Y., and Ma, D. (2017). Image denoising searching similar blocks along edge directions. *Image Commun.* 57, 33–45. doi: 10.1016/j.image.2017.05.001

Mahmoudi, M., and Sapiro, G. (2005). Fast image and video denoising via non local means of similar. *Signal Process. Lett.* 2, 839–842. doi: 10.1109/LSP.2005.859509

Mallat, B. S., and Hwang, W. L. (1992). Singularity detection and processing with wavelets. *Inform. Theory* 2, 617–643. doi: 10.1109/18.119727

Michal., A., Elad, M., and Bruckstein, A. (2006). An algorithm for designing over completes dictionaries for sparse representation. *Trans. Signal Process.* 11, 4311–4322. doi: 10.1109/TSP.2006.881199

Noh, H., You, T., Mun, J., and Han, B. (2011). Deep neural networks by noise: its interpretation and optimization. *Machine Learn.* 11, 1–10. doi: 10.arxiv.org/abs/1710.05179

Oey, E., Junius, E., Alfiansyah, R., and Hedwing, R. (2013). Image de-noising by enhancing K-SVD algorithm. *Internetwork. Ind. J.* 2, 9–13. Available online at: http://www.internetworkingindonesia.org/Issues/Vol5-No2-B-2013/iij_vol5_no2_b_2013_oey.pdf

Othman, H., and Qian, S. E. (2006). Noise reduction of hyper spectral imagery using hybrid spatial spectral derivative domain wavelet shrinkage. *Geosci. Remote Sensin.* 4, 397–408. doi: 10.1109/TGRS.2005.860982

Palakkal, S., and Prabhu, K. M. M. (2012). Poisson image denoising using fast discrete curvelet transform and wave atom. *Signal Process.* 9, 2002–2017. doi: 10.1016/j.sigpro.2012.01.008

Patil, R. (2015). Noise reduction using wavelet transform and singular vector decomposition. *Proc. Comput. Sci.* 54, 849–853. doi: 10.1016/j.procs.2015.06.099

Pizarro, L., Mrazek, P., and Didas, S. (2010). Generalized nonlocal image smoothing. *Int. J. Comput. Vision* 90, 62–87. doi: 10.1007/s11263-010-0337-7

Swami, S., Jain, A., Chellappa, R., and Lim, S. N. (2017). Regularizing deep networks using efficient layerwise adversarial training. *arxiv:1705.07819.*

Tasdizen, T. (2009). Principal neighborhood dictionaries for nonlocal means image de-noising. *Image Process.* 18, 2649–2660. doi: 10.1109/TIP.2009.2028259

Thomas Asaki, J., and Kevin Vixie, R. (2010). Image De-noising by regularization on characteristic graphs. *Appl. Math. Sci.*4, 2541–2560. https://www.researchgate.net/publication/265273866

Wang, X. H., Istepanian, R. S. H., and Song, Y. H. (2003). Microarray image enhancement by de-noising using stationary wavelet transform. *Nanobioscience* 2, 184–189. doi: 10.1109/TNB.2003.816225

Zeng, N., Qiu, H., Wang, Z., Liu, W., Zhang, H., and Li, Y. (2018). A new switching-delayed-PSO-based optimized SVM algorithm for diagnosis of Alzheimer's disease. *Neurocomputing* 320, 195–220. doi: 10.1016/j.neucom.2018.09.001

Zeng, N., Wang, Z., Li, Y., Du, M., and Liu, X. (2012). A hybrid EKF and switching PSO algorithm for joint state and parameter estimation of lateral flow immunoassay models. *Comput. Biol. Bioinform.* 9, 321–329. doi: 10.1109/TCBB.2011.140

Zeng, N., Zhang, H., Li, Y., Liang, J., and Dobaie, A. M. (2017). Denoising and deblurring gold immunochromatographic strip images via gradient projection algorithms. *Neurocomputing* 247, 165–172. doi: 10.1016/j.neucom.2017.03.056

Zhu, L., Su, F., Xu, Y., and Zou, Q. (2017). Network-based method for mining novel HPV infection related genes using random walk with restart algorithm. *Mol. Basis Dis.* 6, 2376–2383. doi: 10.1016/j.bbadis.2017.11.021

Zou, Q., Li, J., Song, L., Zeng, X., and Wang, G. (2015). Similarity computation strategies in the microRNA-disease network: a survey. *Brief. Funct. Genomics* 15, 55–64. doi: 10.1093/bfgp/elv024

15

Nested Dilation Networks for Brain Tumor Segmentation Based on Magnetic Resonance Imaging

Liansheng Wang[1,2]*, Shuxin Wang*[2]*, Rongzhen Chen*[2]*, Xiaobo Qu*[3]*, Yiping Chen*[1,2]*, Shaohui Huang*[2*] *and Changhua Liu*[4*]

[1] Fujian Key Laboratory of Sensing and Computing for Smart City, School of Information Science and Engineering, Xiamen University, Xiamen, China, [2] Department of Computer Science, School of Information Science and Engineering, Xiamen University, Xiamen, China, [3] Department of Electronic Science, Fujian Provincial Key Laboratory of Plasma and Magnetic Resonance, School of Electronic Science and Engineering (National Model Microelectronics College), Xiamen University, Xiamen, China, [4] Department of Medical Imaging, Chenggong Hospital Affiliated to Xiamen University, Xiamen, China

Correspondence:
Shaohui Huang
hsh@xmu.edu.cn
Changhua Liu
liuxingc@126.com

Aim: Brain tumors are among the most fatal cancers worldwide. Diagnosing and manually segmenting tumors are time-consuming clinical tasks, and success strongly depends on the doctor's experience. Automatic quantitative analysis and accurate segmentation of brain tumors are greatly needed for cancer diagnosis.

Methods: This paper presents an advanced three-dimensional multimodal segmentation algorithm called nested dilation networks (NDNs). It is inspired by the U-Net architecture, a convolutional neural network (CNN) developed for biomedical image segmentation and is modified to achieve better performance for brain tumor segmentation. Thus, we propose residual blocks nested with dilations (RnD) in the encoding part to enrich the low-level features and use squeeze-and-excitation (SE) blocks in both the encoding and decoding parts to boost significant features. To prove the reliability of the network structure, we compare our results with those of the standard U-Net and its transmutation networks. Different loss functions are considered to cope with class imbalance problems to maximize the brain tumor segmentation results. A cascade training strategy is employed to run NDNs for coarse-to-fine tumor segmentation. This strategy decomposes the multiclass segmentation problem into three binary segmentation problems and trains each task sequentially. Various augmentation techniques are utilized to increase the diversity of the data to avoid overfitting.

Results: This approach achieves Dice similarity scores of 0.6652, 0.5880, and 0.6682 for edema, non-enhancing tumors, and enhancing tumors, respectively, in which the Dice loss is used for single-pass training. After cascade training, the Dice similarity scores rise to 0.7043, 0.5889, and 0.7206, respectively.

Conclusion: Experiments show that the proposed deep learning algorithm outperforms other U-Net transmutation networks for brain tumor segmentation. Moreover, applying cascade training to NDNs facilitates better performance than other methods. The findings of this study provide considerable insight into the automatic and accurate segmentation of brain tumors.

Keywords: brain tumor segmentation, nested dilation networks, residual blocks nested with dilations, squeeze-and-excitation blocks, coarse-to-fine

1. INTRODUCTION

Brain tumors are one of the deadliest cancers worldwide. Gliomas are the most common primary craniocerebral tumor and are caused by the carcinogenesis of glial cells in the brain and spinal cord (Bauer et al., 2013). In pathology, gliomas can be classified as low-grade or high-grade according to the malignant degree of the tumor cells (Cho and Park, 2017; Wang et al., 2018b). Low-grade gliomas are mainly represented by low-speed cell division and proliferation, whereas high-level gliomas are characterized by rapid cell division and proliferation accompanied by angiogenesis, hypoxia, and necrosis (Gerlee and Nelander, 2012; Bogdańska et al., 2017). Although significant advances have been made in healthcare so far, the vast majority of gliomas are incurable, except for a small number of low-grade gliomas, which can be completely resected surgically. Gliomas can be further divided into different tumor sub-regions according to the severity of the tumor cells, such as edemas, non-enhancing tumors, and enhancing tumors. Magnetic resonance imaging (MRI) is the most frequently used and most effective noninvasive auxiliary diagnostic tool (Wen et al., 2010; Yang et al., 2018), providing a reference for the formulation of treatment programs (Mazzara et al., 2004). Brain tumors are usually imaged with different MRI modalities, and these images are interpreted by image analysis methods (Bauer et al., 2013). The MRI sequence usually includes four different modalities: T1-weighted, T2-weighted, post-contrast T1-weighted, and fluid-attenuated inversion-recovery (FLAIR). Different MRI modalities are employed for different diagnosis tasks in clinical diagnosis and treatment. However, it is still a daunting task for clinicians to diagnose diseases with MRI, because there is a wide variation in the size, shape, regularity, location, and heterogeneous appearance of brain tumors (Dong et al., 2017). Therefore, automatic quantitative analysis and accurate segmentation of brain tumors are greatly needed clinically to help doctors make accurate diagnoses.

CNNs have become a prominent deep learning method and have been used to make a series of breakthroughs in different tasks, including computer vision (Krizhevsky et al., 2012; Long et al., 2015; Ren et al., 2015). The success of CNNs is credited to their ability to independently learn deep features instead of relying on manual features. With historical opportunities provided by a strong calculation capability and large numbers of annotations, the development of CNNs has been explosive. The original LeNet5 (LeCun et al., 1998) was proposed in 1998 with five layers, establishing the modern structure of CNNs. Krizhevsky et al. (2012) presented a classical CNN structure called "AlexNet, and made a historic breakthrough. The great success of AlexNet stimulated new research on CNNs. ZFNet (Zeiler and Fergus, 2014), VGGNet (Simonyan and Zisserman, 2014), GoogLeNet (Szegedy et al., 2015), and ResNet (He et al., 2016) were successively presented with more layers and better performances. Huang et al. (2017) used a more radical dense connection mechanism to maximize the flow of information. Hu et al. (2017) proposed an SE network that modeled the interdependencies between feature channels, adaptively learning important information. All of these CNN studies made it possible to apply neural networks to medical image processing.

Recent reports have shown that CNNs outperform state-of-the-art medical image analyses (Li et al., 2017; Lin et al., 2018). MRI-based brain tumor segmentation is a task that still requires extensive attention. Extant methods for automatic brain tumor segmentation are diverse. DeepMedic (Kamnitsas et al., 2016b) was designed as a dual-pathway three-dimensional (3D) network with 11 layers, to simultaneously process images at different scales and combine the results with fully connected layers. Kamnitsas et al. (2016a) and Castillo et al. (2017) further improved the architecture of DeepMedic by adding residual connections and parallel pathways. U-Net (Ronneberger et al., 2015) was proposed to train an end-to-end network with few images for the accurate segmentation of biomedical images. Many architectures similar to U-Net have been widely adopted for brain tumor segmentation. Kayalibay et al. (2017) and Isensee et al. (2017) employed deep supervision by combining segmentation layers from different levels in the localization pathway. Iqbal et al. (2018) increased the number of U-Net layers and trained the network with the Dice loss. Le and Pham (2018) used the U-Net architecture to extract features and put them into an ExtraTrees classifier. Zhao et al. (2018) integrated fully convolutional neural network (FCNN) and conditional random field (CRF) and trained three models using two-dimensional (2D) image patches obtained from axial, coronal, and sagittal views. A voting-based fusion strategy was used to obtain segmentation results. To deal with the class imbalance problem, Wang et al. (2017) proposed a triple-cascaded framework for brain tumor segmentation. Three similar networks were used to segment the entire tumor (all lesions, including edema, non-enhancing tumors, and enhancing tumors), and the tumor core (all lesions except edema). They then sequentially enhanced tumor core. Zhou et al. (2018) drew upon lesions with coarse-to-fine medical image segmentation methods and proposed a single multitask CNN that could learn correlations between different categories. Partial model parameters can be shared when different tasks are being trained according to different sets of training data to utilize the underlying correlation among classes.

We propose a CNN-based 3D segmentation algorithm, the NDN, which can handle multimodal images. Instead of simple convolution layers, residual blocks are stacked in the U-Net architecture to simplify optimization. The SE blocks used in NDNs fuse the global information and adaptively learn important information from each channel. A new block i.e., residual blocks nested with dilations (RnD) enlarges the receptive fields and avoids the gridding effect. RnD blocks can enrich information in shallow layers by using dilation convolutions while retaining detailed information during the rapid expansion of receptive fields by using residual connections. The cascade training strategy is adopted to train three tasks individually to deal with the class imbalance problem.

2. MATERIALS AND METHODS

This section describes the proposed NDNs algorithm for detailed brain tumor segmentation, including the data preprocessing, network architecture, training strategy, and post-processing methods. We also concisely describe the experimental design.

2.1. Data Acquisition and Preprocessing

2.1.1. Data Acquisition

Most of the data used in this work are downloaded from the Medical Segmentation Decathlon (MSD) organized by the 21st Annual Conference on Medical Image Computing and Computer-Assisted Intervention (MICCAI) 2018. A small number of low-grade glioma data are abstained from MICCAIs Multimodal Brain Tumor Segmentation (BraTS) Challenge of the same year. These are used to test the stability of the proposed algorithm. The images for each patient comprise four scanning sequences: T1-weighted, T2-weighted, post-contrast T1-weighted, and FLAIR. Every scan is aligned to the same anatomical template space and interpolated into $1 \times 1 \times 1mm^3$ with an image size of $240 \times 240 \times 155$ voxels. The purpose of the study is to segment brain tumors (i.e., gliomas) into three different classes: edemas, non-enhancing tumors, and enhancing tumors. All data are labeled and verified by an expert human rater. Efforts were made to mimic the accuracy required for clinical use.

2.1.2. Data Preprocessing and Augmentation

Training an effective neural network requires thousands or even tens of thousands of data. However, the quantity of available medical images is usually well short of that. To avoid overfitting, more training data need to be generated from the limited images and annotations. Our method applies the following data augmentation techniques to make reasonable changes to the image shapes: flip the x-, y-, or z-axis with a probability of 50%; rotate the images with a rotation angle of $-15°$ to $15°$; apply gamma correction with the gamma value varied randomly from 0.4 to 1.6; and apply elastic distortion. **Figure 1** shows the data augmentation.

Images from multiple modalities may have varying intensity ranges. When the intensity values are not standardized, it is detrimental to the training of the neural network. Normalization is critical to allow images from different modalities to be trained with one algorithm. In our study, each modality is normalized individually by subtracting the mean from the value for each patient and dividing it by the standard deviation. The useless black borders in the images along the x- and y-axes are also removed. On the z-axis, we note that the head and tail of the image slices are uninformative. Therefore, 70% of the slices used for the network input are captured from the middle.

2.2. Residual Blocks

He et al. (2016) reformulated the layers as residual blocks and yielded unusually brilliant results in the 2015 ImageNet competition. Instead of simply stacking convolution layers to fit a desired underlying mapping, they added identity mapping, which was easier to optimize. The residual blocks depicted in **Figure 2A** are achieved by a shortcut connection and element-wise addition operation, performed on the input and output feature maps of the blocks, channel-by-channel. The operating principle of the residual blocks can be defined as

$$y = F(x, W_i) + x, \tag{1}$$

where x and y are the input and output vectors of the relevant layers; and $F(x, W_i)$ is the mapping function for the residual path. The results of $F(x, W_i)$ should have the same dimensions as x. Otherwise, we can perform linear mapping on the shortcut connection (**Figure 2B**). This simple algorithm does not add additional parameters or computations to the network, but it greatly increases the training speed of the model and improves the training effect.

The standard convolutional layers of a U-Net are replaced by the residual structure shown in **Figure 2A**. The residual path comprises two convolution layers with a kernel size of 3, followed by a batch normalization (BN) operation (Ioffe and Szegedy, 2015) and a rectified linear unit (ReLU). The input and output of the residual path are added element by element. The results of the residual blocks are fed directly into subsequent network layers.

2.3. SE Blocks

A lot of research has recently been accomplished to strengthen the learning power of CNNs and to improve their performance. Hu et al. (2017) introduced the SE blocks to enhance the representations of features produced by a convolutional network. SE blocks embed the global spatial information into the channel vector by encoding each channel dependency with a fully connected operation. It allows the network to pay different amounts of attention to each channel according to the importance of the feature maps. **Figure 3A** illustrates the structure of SE blocks. The features are first passed through a squeeze operation achieved by a global average pooling layer to aggregate global information per channel for the whole image. Then, the outputs are fed into an excitation operation to get the final weights for each channel. The excitation operation is achieved by using two fully connected layers: one with ReLU activation and another with a sigmoid. Finally, the weight vectors are reshaped to $(1, 1, 1, C)$, where C is the number of the feature maps and are applied to each feature map by the multiply operation. The SE blocks emphasize useful features and suppress useless features through weights like an attention mechanism.

SE blocks have a simple structure and can be used directly in existing state-of-the-art architectures. We draw on experience with the attention mechanism and nested SE blocks in the architecture to help the network focus on important feature maps. As shown in **Figure 3B**, feature maps with size (X, Y, Z, C) are put into SE blocks. Then, the blocks generate a significant coefficient for each channel, finally gaining outputs with different weights and the same size as the inputs.

2.4. RnD Blocks

The traditional up-sampling and down-sampling structures lead to a loss of internal structure, and the information of small objects cannot be reconstructed. To solve this problem, Yu and Koltun (2015) presented a model with dilated convolutions that can increase the receptive fields without reducing the resolution or increasing the parameters. Chen et al. (2014,

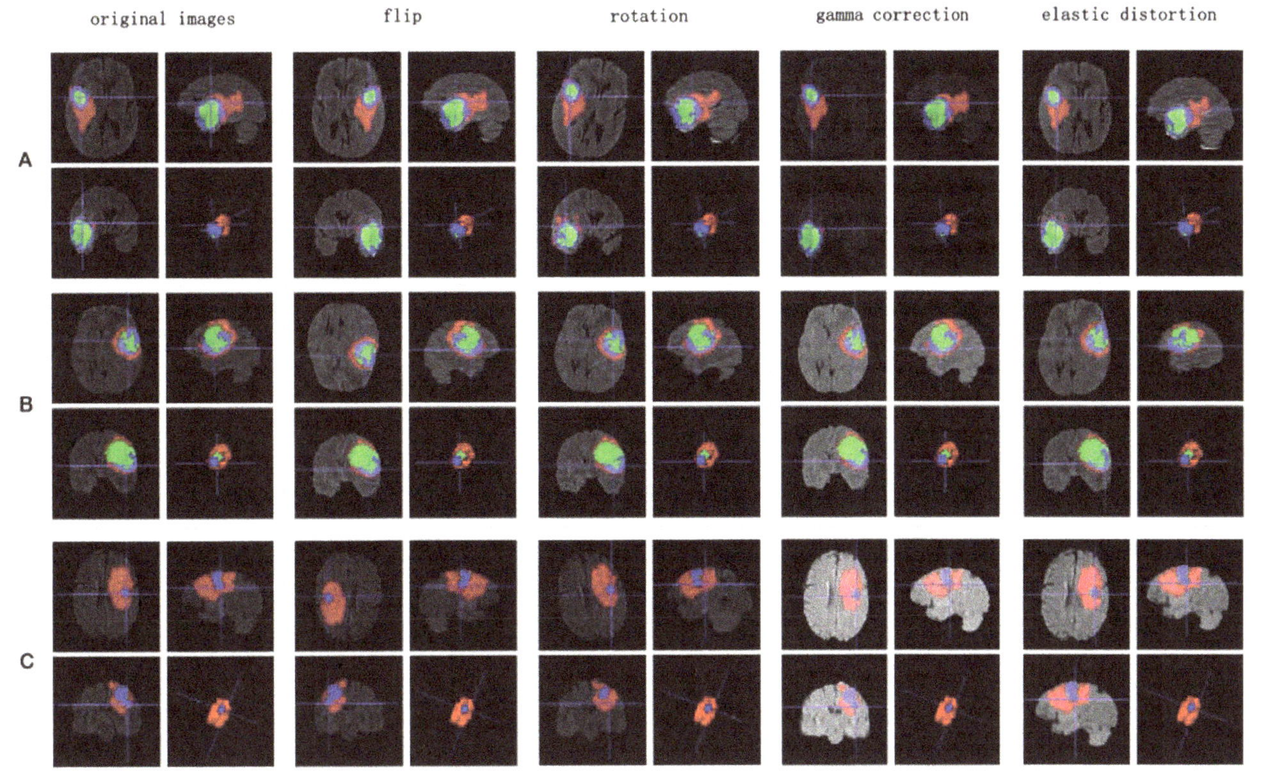

FIGURE 1 | Data augmentation results. Rows list three samples for different patients. Columns represent different data augmentation operations. **(A-C)** list three samples for different patients.

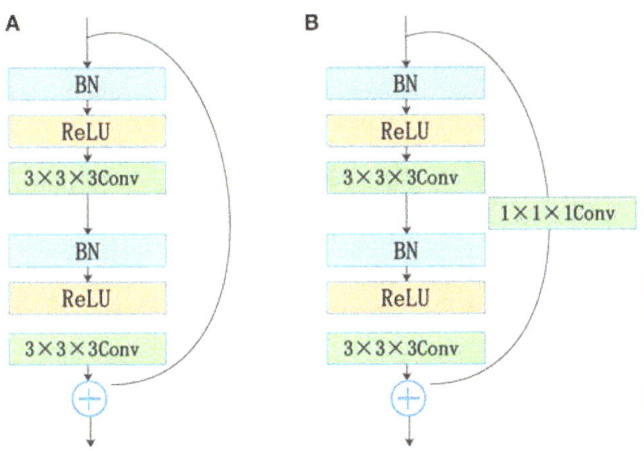

FIGURE 2 | Residual blocks: **(A)** shortcut connection and **(B)** shortcut connection with the convolution layer.

2017, 2018) used dilated convolutions in their networks and achieved good performance for dense prediction tasks. However, standard dilated convolution causes a gridding issue that will harm small objects. Wang et al. (2018a) proposed a hybrid dilated convolution (HDC) framework, which can not only expand receptive fields but also mitigate the gridding issue. Implementing the HDC framework requires two conditions to be met. First, the dilation rates of a groups dilated convolutions should not have a common divisor > 1. The maximum distance between two nonzero values is defined as follows:

$$M_i = max[M_{i+1} - 2r_i, M_{i+1} - 2(M_{i+1} - r_i), r_i], \quad (2)$$

where r_i is the dilation rate in layer i, and M_i is the maximum dilation rate from layer 0 to layer i. The second condition requires satisfying $M_i < K$, where K is the kernel size.

The standard U-Net architecture does not get enough semantic information in the shallow layers because of the limited receptive fields. This is harmful to feature fusion in the first few cross-layer connections. To resolve this issue and avoid the gridding effect, we draw on an idea from the HDC framework. RnD blocks (**Figure 4**) are built to enlarge receptive fields in the first two layers of the network. This new type of block can obtain more extensive local information via 3 convolution layers with different dilation rates (e.g., 1, 2, 5). The kernel size is 3 for all dilated convolutions, which are followed by a ReLU activation. The residual connection in RnD blocks helps retain information and fill details during the rapid expansion of receptive fields.

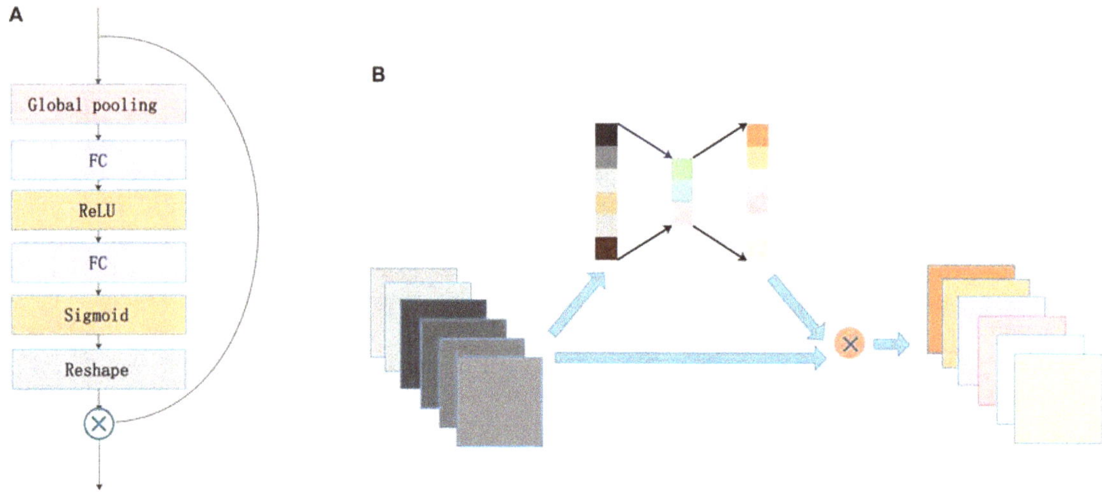

FIGURE 3 | SE blocks: **(A)** architecture and **(B)** concept map.

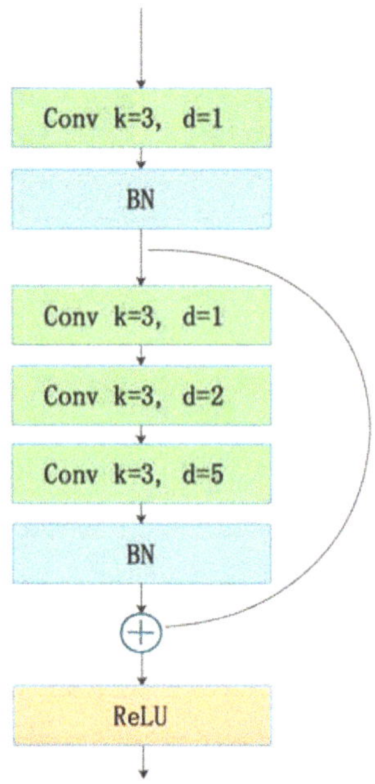

FIGURE 4 | Architecture of RnD blocks with different dilation rates.

2.5. NDNs

The structure of our proposed NDNs is shown in **Figure 5**. The architecture is inspired by U-Net, which is a stable encoder–decoder network designed for limited data training, especially for medical images. Here, we carefully modify the standard U-Net to make it perform better for the brain tumor segmentation task. First, we use 3D convolution layers rather than 2D to adapt images from multiple modalities. The classic encoder–decoder structure that fuses the lower features in the shallow layers and higher features in the deep layers is retained to ensure the stability of the proposed network. The architecture comprises three max-pooling layers to capture context and three up-sampling layers to enable precise localization. To obtain enough receptive fields, the first two encoder modules adopt RnD blocks to enrich the low-level features. This is followed by an SE block and a max-pooling layer. In the decoder part, each module comprises a stack of residual blocks, an SE block, and an up-sampling layer. The BN is employed immediately after each convolution and before activation. As shown in **Figure 5**, the network can obtain rich information to boost essential features and achieve a stable effect.

2.6. Cascade Training

The cascade strategy trains different models for each category sequentially, showing ideal results. Coarse-to-fine medical image segmentation is becoming increasingly popular because of the class imbalance problem. Cascaded models decompose complex problems into simple ones and capitalize on the hierarchical structure of tumor sub-regions. A single model is trained repeatedly to segment substructures of brain tumors hierarchically and sequentially. Each sequence is handled as a binary segmentation problem. The first task is to segment the entire tumor including edemas, enhancing tumors, and non-enhancing tumors. These three classes are regarded as a binary segmentation problem. Then, NDNs are trained to crop the target. After the first stage of training, the entire tumor region is segmented in the 3D volumes of a patient. A cuboid sub-region, based on the entire tumor, is used as inputs to the network to segment the enhancing and non-enhancing tumors together. Similarly, the third training differentiates enhancing tumors from non-enhancing ones by using the cuboid sub-region produced by the second stage as input.

In the training, the input of the network is generated based on the ground truth, as shown in **Figure 6A**. In the testing, the results of the previous stage are extended by 32 pixels on the x- and y-axes, and 8 slices on the z-axis as the input for the

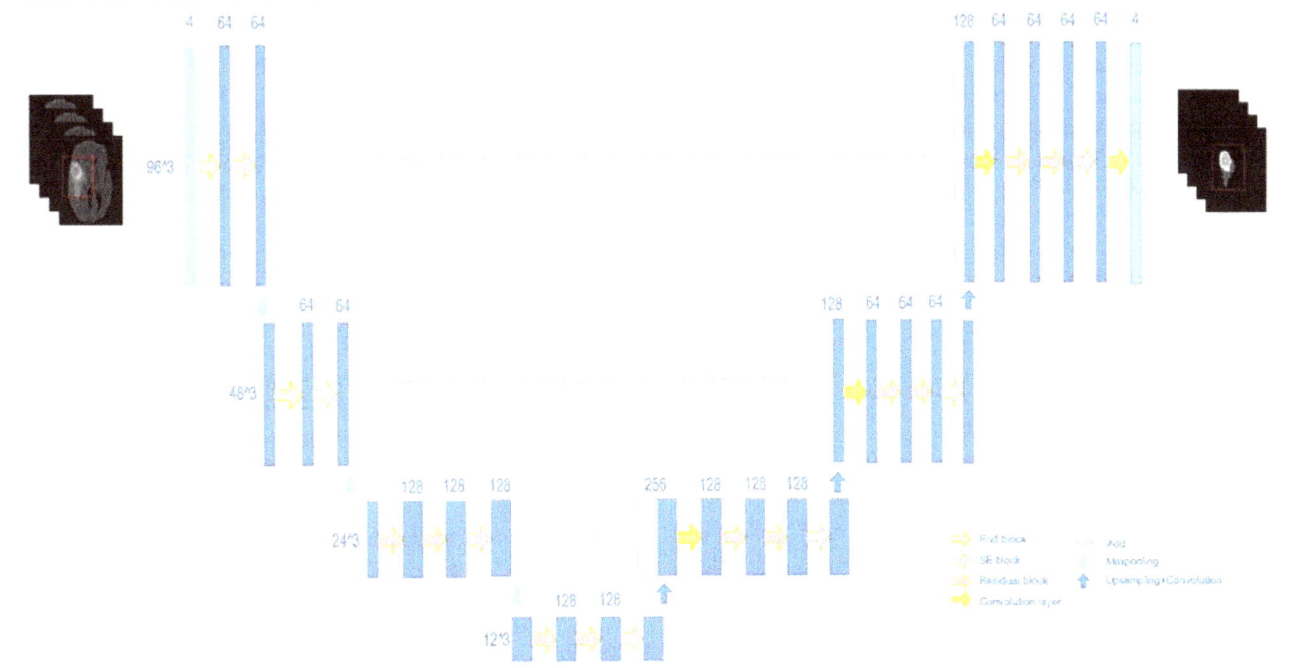

FIGURE 5 | Architecture of the proposed NDNs with SE blocks and RnD blocks.

next stage. The process is described in **Figure 6B**. Finally, we integrate the three binary segmentation tasks to obtain the final segmentation results of multiple classes. Cascade training offers a way to adaptively alleviate the class imbalance problem of brain tumor segmentation.

2.7. Post-processing

Post-processing is further used to improve the segmentation results of NDNs. During data processing, we noticed that the brain tumors for all patients in the 3D volumes were of a single connected domain. Thus, isolated small clusters should be removed from the results. More specifically, connected domain analysis should be performed to retain the maximal region and remove other smaller clusters to better fit the ground truth. Moreover, some patients are observed to have benign tumors, which means that the gliomas only comprise edemas and non-enhancing tumors. Some small clusters are erroneously classified as enhancing tumors in our task instead of benign tumors, which harms the segmentation results. To deal with this issue, we impose volumetric constraints by removing enhancing tumor clusters in the segmentation that are smaller than a predefined threshold.

2.8. Dice Similarity Score

In our work, the Dice similarity score is calculated for quantitative evaluation. This performance metric measures the similarity between the ground truth and predicted results. The Dice similarity score is defined as follows:

$$DSC = \frac{2TP}{(FP + 2TP + FN)}, \tag{3}$$

where TP, FP, and FN are the numbers of true positives, false positives, and false negatives, respectively.

MSD and BraTS 2018 provide three different tumor regions that can be described as edemas, enhancing tumors, and non-enhancing tumors. The Dice similarity scores are calculated for each tumor region to evaluate the segmentation results, and the scores are compared with those of other methods.

2.9. Experimental Design

We conduct three groups of experiments according to different requirements, which we describe in this section.

Experiment 1: We explored the effects of different network structures on brain tumor segmentation. Ronneberger et al. (2015) developed a U-Net architecture based on the fully convolutional network (FCN) (Long et al., 2015), which can work with very few training images and yield more precise segmentation. Some new architectures derived from U-Net have appeared and have been applied to the field of medical image processing. In Experiment 1, the standard Conv + BN + ReLU module in U-Net was replaced by frequently used blocks, such as residual blocks and dense blocks separately for comparison with the proposed NDNs.

Experiment 2: Different loss functions were attempted with NDNs to improve segmentation results. The loss function quantifies the amount by which the predicted value deviates from the actual value. Choosing a suitable loss function benefits both the training process and the results of brain tumor segmentation. In Experiment 2, different loss functions were applied to the brain tumor segmentation task: the categorical cross-entropy loss, Dice loss, and focal loss. The Dice similarity scores are calculated for each task.

Experiment 3: The proposed method was compared with other state-of-the-art methods. We implemented several previously published algorithms and trained the networks with the same datasets. The brain tumors comprise of edemas, enhancing tumors, and non-enhancing tumors with very different volumes, resulting in an imbalanced number of samples in each class. This category imbalance problem impairs the performance of a deep network. In Experiment 3, a cascade strategy was used to train NDNs, which decomposed a multiple classification problem into multiple binary classification problems. The segmentation results of the cascaded NDNs were compared with several state-of-the-art methods according to the Dice similarity score.

2.10. Implementation Details

All networks were implemented in Keras (Chollet et al., 2015) 2.1.2 using the Tensorflow (Abadi et al., 2016) 1.4.0 backend. Adaptive moment estimation (Kingma and Ba, 2014) was used as an optimizer with an initial learning rate of 0.0001, a momentum of 0.9, and a weight decay of 0.00001. Training was implemented on an NVIDIA 1080 Ti GPU with a version of CUDA 8.0 for 300 epochs. We did not use a dropout (Hinton et al., 2012) but rather L2 regularization and BN for the whole network structure. We cropped $96 \times 96 \times 48$ patches as inputs close to the ground truth from images and annotations. All networks were trained from scratch with a batch size of 4.

3. EXPERIMENTS AND RESULTS

In this section, we explain the advantages of the proposed algorithm with regard to brain tumor segmentation. The Dice similarity score is adopted as the evaluation criterion for each model. Edemas, non-enhancing tumors, and enhancing tumors were trained together with single NDNs in Experiments 1 and 2 for the sake of fairness. In Experiment 3, however, the cascade training strategy was used to train NDNs for each class, which was then compared with the state-of-the-art methods.

3.1. Experiment 1

To prove the effectiveness of the NDNs structure, different U-Net-like networks were trained with the same brain tumor dataset for comparison. A traditional 3D U-Net with three down-sampling layers and three symmetric up-sampling layers was trained first. It consisted of two convolution layers used repeatedly with a kernel size of 3, similar to the standard 2D U-Net structure presented by Ronneberger et al. (2015). The

TABLE 1 | Comparison of different U-Net-like architectures: (A) standard 3D U-Net; (B) U-Net with residual blocks; (C) U-Net with dense blocks; (D) NDNs without SE blocks; (E) NDNs without RnD blocks; and (F) NDNs network.

Methods \ Dice		Edema	Non-enhancing tumor	Enhancing tumor
A		0.6686	0.4734	0.6169
B	ResNet18	0.6645	0.5022	0.6455
	ResNet50	**0.6792**	0.5314	0.6289
	ResNet101	0.6752	0.5617	0.6342
C		0.6734	0.5527	0.6287
D		0.6590	0.5612	0.6305
E		0.6725	0.536	0.638
F		0.6652	**0.5880**	**0.6682**

The bold values mean the best result (the highest dice value) for each class.

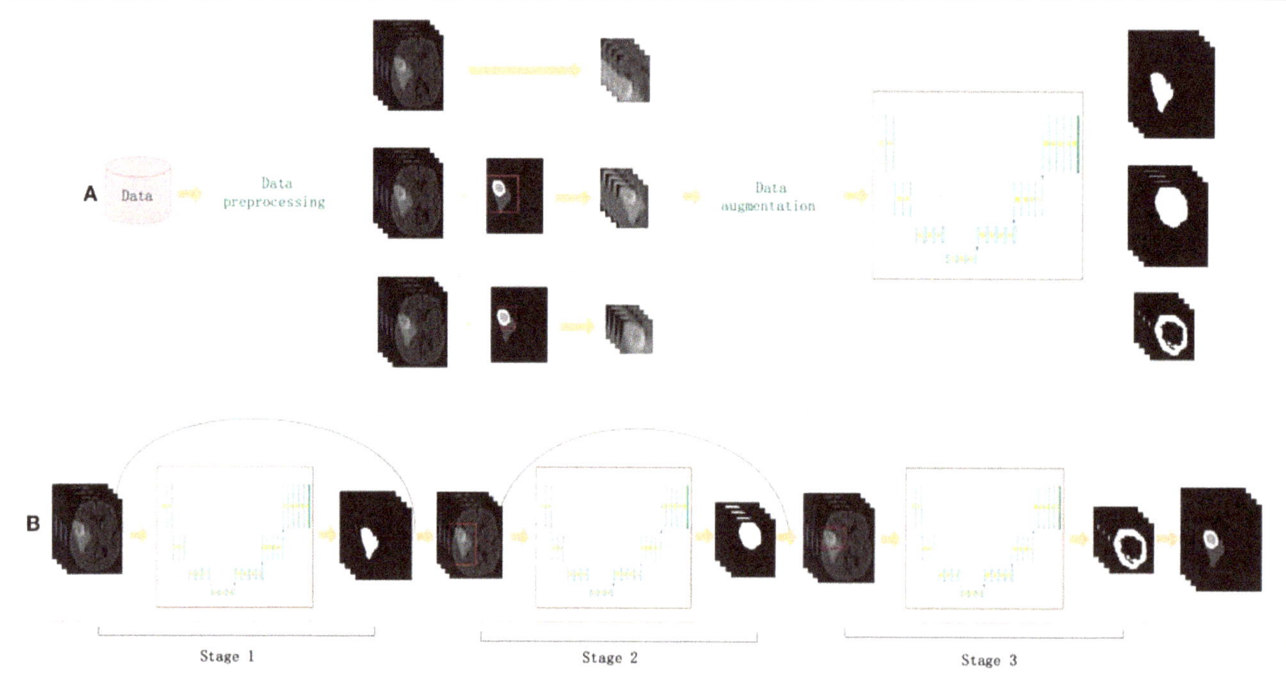

FIGURE 6 | Cascade strategy applied to NDNs: **(A)** training and **(B)** testing.

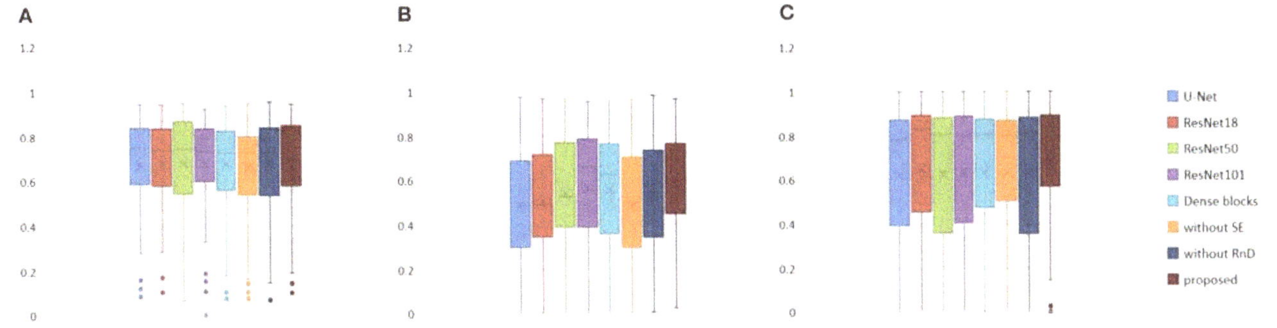

FIGURE 7 | Boxplots for each method in **Table 1**. Dice similarity scores for **(A)** edema, **(B)** non-enhancing tumors, and **(C)** enhancing tumors. The symbol "×" marks the mean.

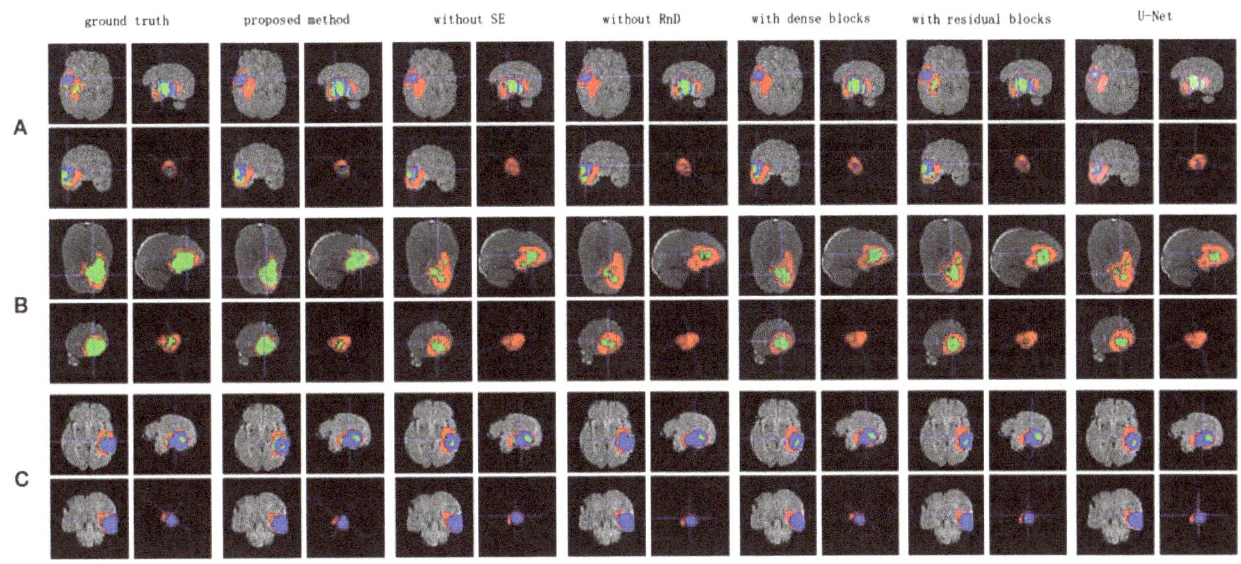

FIGURE 8 | Brain tumor segmentation results predicted by different U-Net-like networks. The rows represent three samples from different patients, and the columns represent results predicted by each U-Net-like network. The organizers provided the ground truth images. **(A-C)** list three samples for different patients.

filter number was doubled at the end of each down-sampling layer and halved after each up-sampling layer. Then, the repeated convolution layers were replaced by residual blocks and dense blocks to be trained. ResNet18, ResNet50, and ResNet101 were each employed as an encoder path, and the decoder path was consistent with the expanding path in 3D U-Net. For the dense U-Net, dense blocks were used as substitutes for the two repeated convolution layers, and each dense block had four dense connected convolution layers. Finally, we studied the effect of the NDNs architecture with SE blocks or RnD blocks only. **Table 1** lists the Dice similarity scores calculated for brain tumor segmentation with these networks, and **Figure 7** presents the boxplots for each class. Note that all networks were trained with the Dice loss in Experiment 1.

We achieved better results for non-enhancing tumor segmentation and enhancing tumor segmentation with NDNs than with the other U-Net-like architectures. According to **Table 1**, the non-enhancing tumor results segmented by NDNs are about 2.6% better than U-Net with ResNet101, and the enhancing tumor segmentation results are at least 2.0% better than the other methods. However, the proposed algorithm lacked the ability to segment the edema part with a result of 0.6652, which is worse than the other U-Net-like algorithms. **Figure 8**

TABLE 2 | Comparison with different losses: (A) categorical cross-entropy; (B) weighted categorical cross-entropy loss; (C) focal loss; and (D) Dice loss.

Methods \ Dice	Edema	Non-enhancing tumor	Enhancing tumor
A	**0.6708**	0.5321	0.6579
B	0.6634	0.5774	0.6604
C	0.5905	0.5721	0.6445
D	0.6652	**0.5880**	**0.6682**

The bold values mean the best result (the highest dice value) for each class.

presents the ground truth and prediction results for different U-Net-like architectures from different perspectives.

3.2. Experiment 2

Class imbalance is a severe issue in medical image segmentation and needs to be carefully tackled. The data provided by MSD and BraTS 2018 are heavily imbalanced, especially the classes of the non-enhancing tumors and enhancing tumors. To alleviate the class imbalance, we use a Dice loss function. We also explore the effects of other loss functions on NDNs for comparison. The categorical cross-entropy is used as a base loss function:

$$Crossentropy(p,q) = -\frac{1}{N}\sum_{x,y,z}\sum_{k} p^k_{x,y,z}\log q^k_{x,y,z}, \quad (4)$$

where $p^k_{x,y,z}$ and $q^k_{x,y,z}$ correspond to the ground truth and predicted results for class k, and N is the total number of samples. Based on previous experience, the class imbalance can be addressed by associating different weights with individual classes. Therefore, the weighted categorical cross-entropy is also used:

$$W\_Crossentropy(p,q) = -\frac{1}{N}\sum_{x,y,z}\sum_{k} w^k p^k_{x,y,z}\log q^k_{x,y,z}, \quad (5)$$

where w^k is the weight for class k. Here the weights for the background, edema, non-enhancing tumors, and enhancing tumors are defined as $(1, 1, 2, 1)$ respectively. The focal loss function described by Lin et al. (2017) for dense object detection is a modified version of binary cross-entropy and is aimed toward low-confidence labels. We adopt a multiclass focal loss for the segmentation task:

$$Focal(p,q) = -\frac{\sum_{x,y,z}\sum_k p^k_{x,y,z}(1-q^k_{x,y,z})^{\gamma}\log q^k_{x,y,z}}{\sum_{x,y,z}\sum_k p^k_{x,y,z}}, \quad (6)$$

where $(1-q^k_{x,y,z})^{\gamma}$ is a modulating factor and the value of γ is set to 2.0 in our algorithm. Finally, our proposed model is trained with the following Dice loss to segment different parts of the brain tumors:

$$Dice(p,q) = 1 - \frac{1}{N}\frac{2\sum_{x,y,z}\sum_k p^k_{x,y,z} * q^k_{x,y,z}}{\sum_{x,y,z}\sum_k p^k_{x,y,z} + \sum_{x,y,z}\sum_k q^k_{x,y,z}}. \quad (7)$$

The Dice similarity scores for the different loss functions used in NDNs are presented in **Table 2** and **Figure 9**. We obtain final scores of 0.6652, 0.5880, and 0.6682 for edemas, non-enhancing tumors, and enhancing tumors, respectively, using the Dice loss. Normal loss functions like the categorical cross-entropy may achieve good results for balanced datasets, but datasets with a massive imbalance among classes require special attention. We avoid weighted categorical cross-entropy as much as possible, because it needs additional hyperparameters that may introduce another difficult problem for network optimization. The results show that the focal loss may be good for binary classification problems to solve intra-class imbalance. However, it is less helpful for inter-class imbalance. The Dice loss is calculated based on the Dice coefficient and can deal with situations with large amounts of class imbalance. **Figure 10** shows the ground truth and prediction results for the different loss functions used in NDNs.

TABLE 3 | Comparison of methods for the same dataset: (A) Isensee et al. (2017); (B) Iqbal et al. (2018); (C) Wang et al. (2017); (D) Zhou et al. (2018); and (E) our proposed method training with the cascade strategy.

Methods \ Dice	Edema	Non-enhancing tumor	Enhancing tumor
A	0.6574	0.5418	0.6943
B	0.6808	0.5727	0.6661
C	0.6919	0.5504	0.6793
D	0.6894	0.5376	0.6861
E	**0.7043**	**0.5889**	**0.7206**

The bold values mean the best result (the highest dice value) for each class.

3.3. Experiment 3

We reproduced several state-of-the-art methods for brain tumor segmentation for comparison with our algorithm. Isensee et al. (2017) achieved a high Dice score in the BraTS 2017 Challenge by using a U-Net-like architecture. They employed deep supervision in the localization pathway to integrate segmentation layers at different levels of the network and combined them via element-wise summation to form the final network output. Iqbal et al. (2018) adopted SE blocks at the end of the decoder part and fused its output with the output of encoder blocks. These two methods were chosen for comparison, because they have similarities with our network structure. Wang et al. (2017) proposed a triple-cascaded framework to segment the entire tumor, tumor core, and enhancing tumor core sequentially. They used dilated convolutions after the down-sampling layers and set the dilation parameter from 1 to 3. Zhou et al. (2018) presented a one-single multitask CNN that can learn the correlations between different categories. These two methods used a cascade or cascade-like training strategy like our training process, and they both obtained high Dice scores in the brain tumor segmentation task. In this experiment, a multiclass segmentation problem was decomposed into three binary segmentation problems by repeated training of NDNs with the coarse-to-fine method just like (Wang et al., 2017). **Table 3** and **Figure 11** present the quantitative evaluation according to the Dice similarity scores for the same datasets.

Table 3 indicates that the Dice similarity scores of our proposed method are 0.7043, 0.5889, and 0.7206 for edemas, non-enhancing tumors, and enhancing tumors, respectively, which are higher than those of all comparison methods for every class. Moreover, the results are 3.9 and 5.2% higher for edemas and enhancing tumors than when the three classes are trained together, and the results for the non-enhancing tumors do not worsen. These results prove that the cascade training strategy can improve the accuracy for brain tumor segmentation. **Figure 12** shows the ground truth and prediction results for different state-of-the-art methods.

4. DISCUSSION

4.1. Competitive Segmentation Results

U-Net increases the number of up-sampling and skip connections compared with FCN, which can supplement more location information for semantic information. The U-Net architecture has received increasing attention recently and has been shown that it is a stable algorithm for many segmentation tasks. Despite its great success, however, U-Net still has limitations for some specialized tasks.

We found that stacking residual blocks instead of simple convolution layers can improve the brain tumor segmentation performance. This is because residual blocks can fuse receptive fields of different sizes and ease the training of the networks. Attention mechanisms have shown their utility for many computer vision tasks. SE blocks work as an attention mechanism that can explore the relationship between channels to suppress useless information and enhance useful information by fusing global information. They can help a network notice essential features and make correct decisions. Nesting the SE blocks into our base structure causes the corresponding Dice similarity

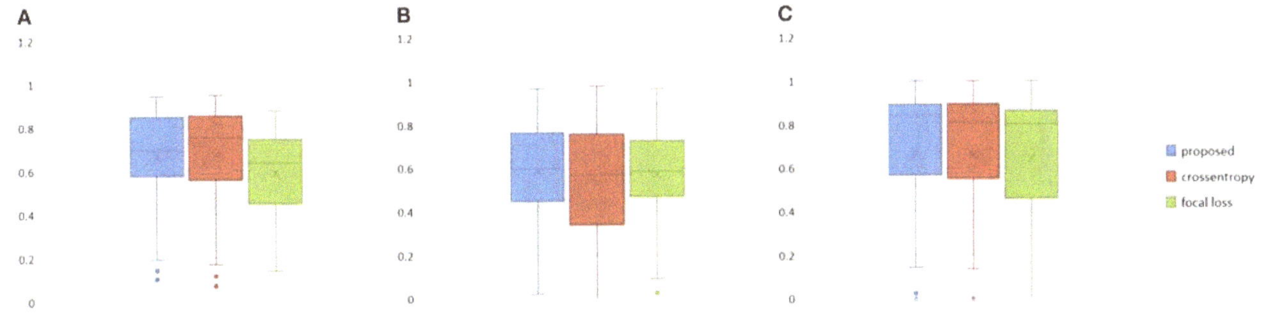

FIGURE 9 | Boxplots for each method in **Table 2**. Dice similarity scores for **(A)** edemas, **(B)** non-enhancing tumors, and **(C)** enhancing tumors. The symbol "×" marks the mean.

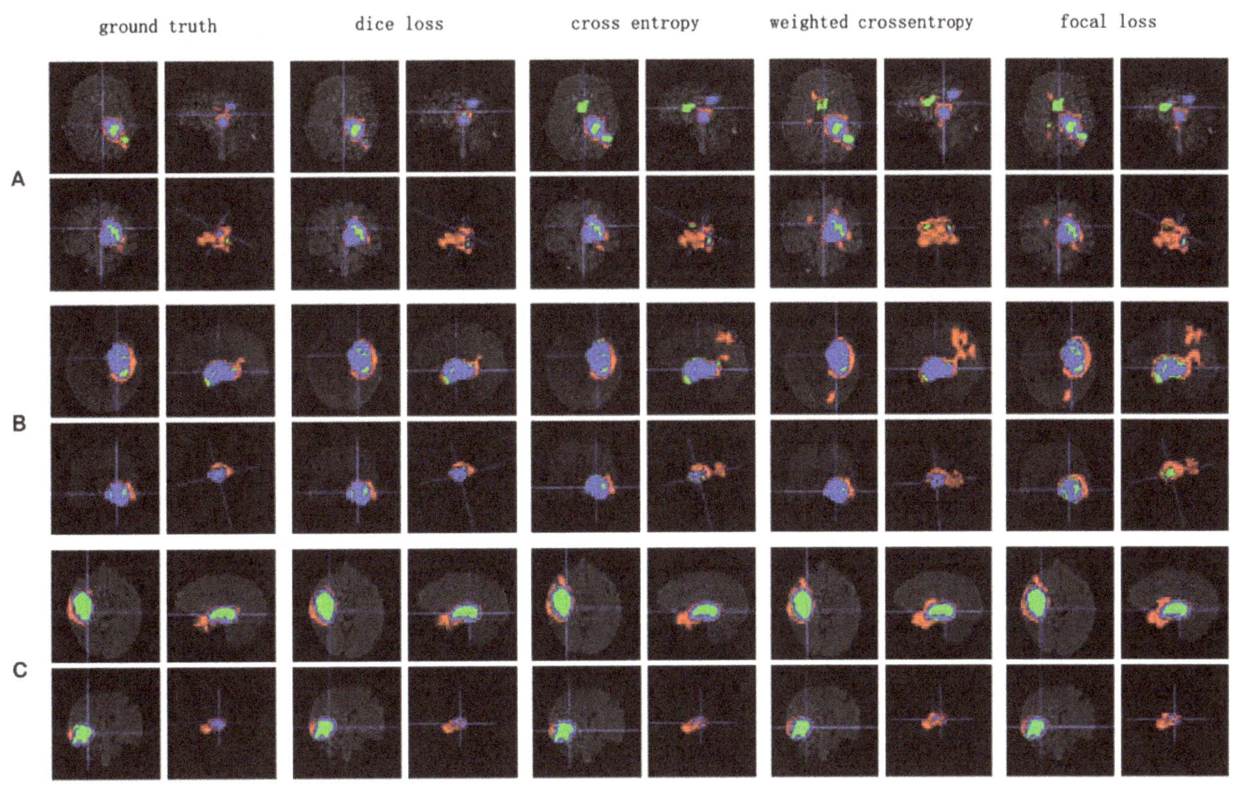

FIGURE 10 | Brain tumor segmentation results predicted by NDNs with different loss functions. The rows represent three samples from different patients, and the columns represent results predicted by NDNs with different losses. Organizers provided ground truth images. **(A-C)** list three samples for different patients.

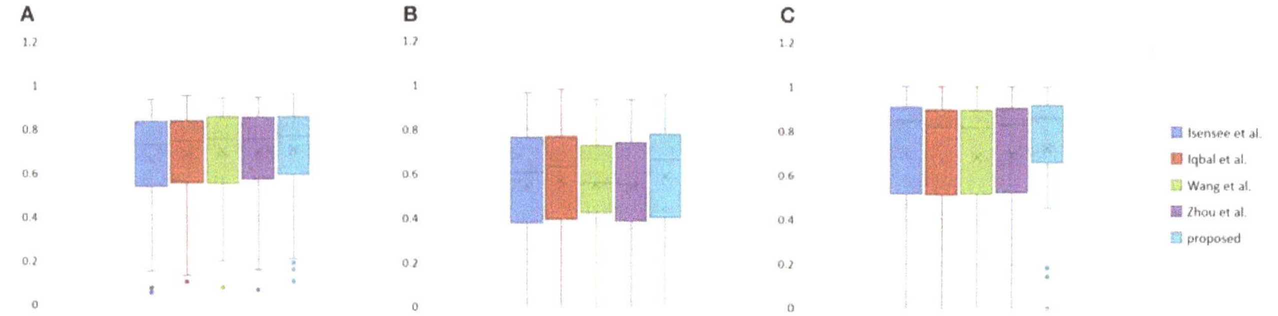

FIGURE 11 | Boxplots for each method in **Table 3**. Dice similarity scores for **(A)** edemas, **(B)** non-enhancing tumors, and **(C)** enhancing tumors. The symbol "×" marks the mean.

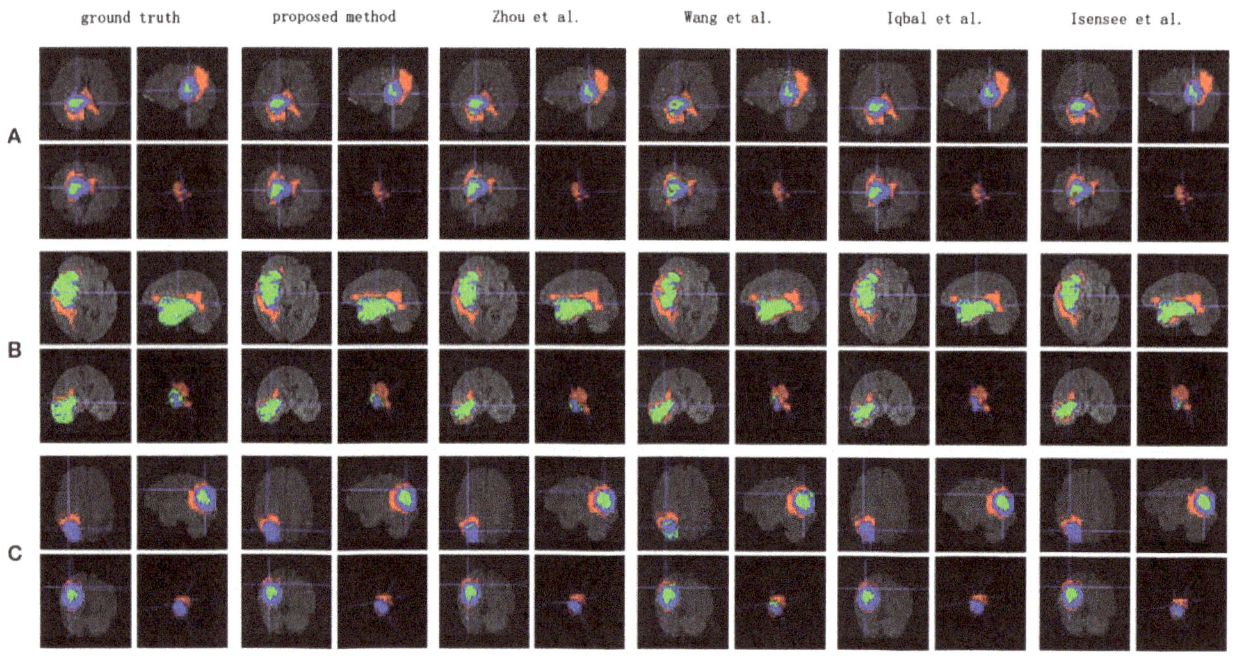

FIGURE 12 | Brain tumor segmentation results predicted by the different algorithms. The rows represent three samples from different patients, and the columns represent algorithms from published papers. Organizers provided the ground truth images. **(A-C)** list three samples for different patients.

scores of the edemas, non-enhancing tumors, and enhancing tumors to reach 0.6725, 0.536, and 0.638, respectively. To solve the problem of insufficient receptive fields and to simultaneously avoid the gridding issue, we add RnD blocks to the network. By learning from the HDC framework, RnD blocks can enlarge receptive fields by using dilated convolutions with different dilation rates. Based on this, our method obtains results of 0.6652, 0.5880, and 0.6682, respectively.

An extreme imbalance between categories affects the segmentation results, especially for edemas, and needs to be addressed. Non-enhancing tumors usually have smaller regions than the other two classes, as shown in **Figure 14**, which will have a negative effect on the segmentation results. In order to alleviate the class imbalance, two measures are taken. First, different losses are employed by NDNs to determine the best performance, and a Dice loss function is eventually selected. Moreover, we borrowed the cascade training strategy adopted by many state-of-the-art methods for brain tumor segmentation. Cascade training can balance the quantitative differences among different classes to some extent. The final results obtained by our proposed method were 0.7043 for edema, 0.5889 for non-enhancing tumors, and 0.7206 for enhancing tumors. The experimental results are shown in **Figure 13**. These reasonable results are attributed to both the network structure and training strategies.

4.2. Limitations

This study is limited by the class imbalance problem, even though some measures have been taken to alleviate it. Some small

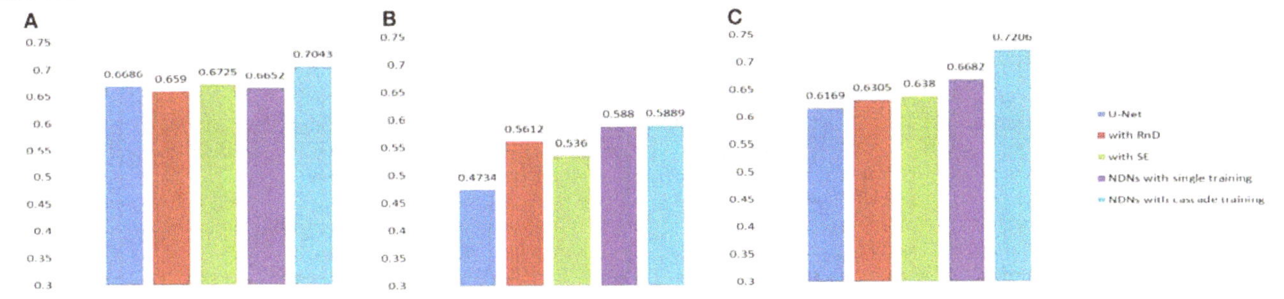

FIGURE 13 | Histogram for each method. Dice similarity scores for **(A)** edemas, **(B)** non-enhancing tumors, and **(C)** enhancing tumors.

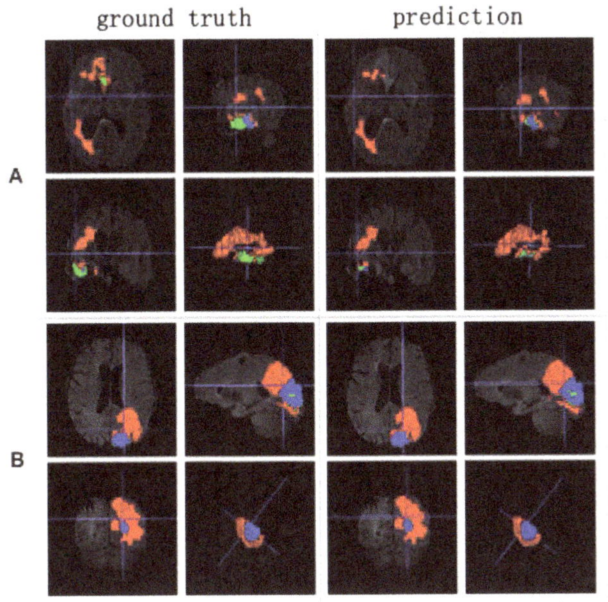

FIGURE 14 | Limitations caused by the class imbalance problem. **(A,B)** present two different samples.

regions in brain tumors like non-enhancing tumors could not be predicted very well. For example, in the two samples in **Figure 14**, only 8.5% of the entire tumor is non-enhancing in sample A and 2.25% in sample B. This huge category imbalance lead to inaccurate segmentation results of 0.279 and 0.402 for non-enhancing tumors in samples A and B, respectively. The class imbalance problem remains a challenge that should be addressed in the future.

5. CONCLUSION

Clinical applications of computer-aided systems have gained a great deal of research attention. Supremely accurate brain tumor segmentation is a tedious but vital task for clinicians because of various sizes and shapes of tumors. Quantitative analysis of brain tumors is critical to relieve pressure on doctors and obtain more accurate segmentation results. We developed a new deep learning framework based on U-Net, NDNs, for segmenting brain tumors. Our results showed that NDNs can extract discriminative features of edemas, non-enhancing tumors, and enhancing tumors by obtaining large receptive fields and integrating channel information. Compared with other state-of-the-art methods, NDNs obtained higher Dice similarity scores. The proposed method makes it possible to generate accurate segmentation result for brain tumors without manual interference and provides considerable insight on the application of computer-aided systems to clinical tasks.

AUTHOR'S NOTE

All data are made available online with a permissive copyright-license (CC-BY-SA 4.0), allowing for data to be shared, distributed and improved upon.

AUTHOR CONTRIBUTIONS

LW, SW, and RC conceptualized the algorithm design. LW, SW, and SH designed the study. LW, SW, RC, SH, and CL collected the data. LW, SW, SH, and CL analyzed the data. LW, SW, and CL interpreted the data. LW, SW, and SH sourced the literature. LW, SW, RC, and SH wrote the draft. LW, SH, XQ, YC, and CL edited the manuscript. LW and CL acquired the funding and supervised the whole study.

FUNDING

This work was partially supported by the National Natural Science Foundation of China (Grant No. 61671399, 61601392, 61571380), National Key R&D Program of China (Grant No. 2017YFC0108703), and Fundamental Research Funds for the Central Universities (Grant No. 20720180056).

REFERENCES

Abadi, M., Barham, P., Chen, J., Chen, Z., Davis, A., Dean, J., et al. (2016). "Tensorflow: a system for large-scale machine learning," in *OSDI'16 Proceedings of the 12th USENIX Conference on Operating Systems Design and Implementation*, Vol. 16 (Savannah, GA), 265–283.

Bauer, S., Wiest, R., Nolte, L.-P., and Reyes, M. (2013). A survey of mri-based medical image analysis for brain tumor studies. *Phys. Med. Biol.* 58:R97. doi: 10.1088/0031-9155/58/13/R97

Bogdańska, M. U., Bodnar, M., Piotrowska, M. J., Murek, M., Schucht, P., Beck, J., et al. (2017). A mathematical model describes the malignant transformation of low grade gliomas: prognostic implications. *PLoS ONE* 12:e0179999. doi: 10.1371/journal.pone.0179999

Castillo, L. S., Daza, L. A., Rivera, L. C., and Arbeláez, P. (2017). "Volumetric multimodality neural network for brain tumor segmentation," in *13th International Conference on Medical Information Processing and Analysis*, Vol. 10572 (International Society for Optics and Photonics), 105720E.

Chen, L.-C., Papandreou, G., Kokkinos, I., Murphy, K., and Yuille, A. L. (2014). Semantic image segmentation with deep convolutional nets and fully connected crfs. *arXiv preprint arXiv:1412.7062.*

Chen, L.-C., Papandreou, G., Kokkinos, I., Murphy, K., and Yuille, A. L. (2018). Deeplab: semantic image segmentation with deep convolutional nets, atrous convolution, and fully connected crfs. *IEEE Trans. Pattern Anal. Mach. Intel.* 40, 834–848. doi: 10.1109/TPAMI.2017.2699184

Chen, L.-C., Papandreou, G., Schroff, F., and Adam, H. (2017). Rethinking atrous convolution for semantic image segmentation. *arXiv preprint arXiv:1706.05587.*

Cho, H.-H., and Park, H. (2017). "Classification of low-grade and high-grade glioma using multi-modal image radiomics features," in *Engineering in Medicine and Biology Society (EMBC), 2017 39th Annual International Conference of the IEEE* (Jeju Island: IEEE), 3081–3084.

Chollet, F., Rahman, F., Lee, T., de Marmiesse, G., Zabluda, O., and Pumperla, M. (2015). *Keras.* https://github.com/fchollet/keras (accessed February 02, 2019).

Dong, H., Yang, G., Liu, F., Mo, Y., and Guo, Y. (2017). "Automatic brain tumor detection and segmentation using u-net based fully convolutional networks," in *Annual Conference on Medical Image Understanding and Analysis* (Edinburgh: Springer), 506–517.

Gerlee, P., and Nelander, S. (2012). The impact of phenotypic switching on glioblastoma growth and invasion. *PLoS Comp. Biol.* 8:e1002556. doi: 10.1371/journal.pcbi.1002556

He, K., Zhang, X., Ren, S., and Sun, J. (2016). "Deep residual learning for image recognition," in *Proceedings of the IEEE Conference on Computer Vision and Pattern Recognition* (Las Vegas, NV), 770–778.

Hinton, G. E., Srivastava, N., Krizhevsky, A., Sutskever, I., and Salakhutdinov, R. R. (2012). Improving neural networks by preventing co-adaptation of feature detectors. *arXiv preprint arXiv:1207.0580.*

Hu, J., Shen, L., and Sun, G. (2017). Squeeze-and-excitation networks. *arXiv preprint arXiv:1709.01507.*

Huang, G., Liu, Z., Van Der Maaten, L., and Weinberger, K. Q. (2017). "Densely connected convolutional networks," in *Computer Vision and Pattern Recognition*, Vol. 1 (Honolulu), 3.

Ioffe, S., and Szegedy, C. (2015). Batch normalization: accelerating deep network training by reducing internal covariate shift. *arXiv preprint arXiv:1502.03167.*

Iqbal, S., Ghani, M. U., Saba, T., and Rehman, A. (2018). Brain tumor segmentation in multi-spectral mri using convolutional neural networks (cnn). *Microsc. Res. Tech.* 81, 419–427. doi: 10.1002/jemt.22994

Isensee, F., Kickingereder, P., Wick, W., Bendszus, M., and Maier-Hein, K. H. (2017). "Brain tumor segmentation and radiomics survival prediction: Contribution to the brats 2017 challenge," in *International MICCAI Brainlesion Workshop*, (Quebec City, QC: Springer), 287–297.

Kamnitsas, K., Ferrante, E., Parisot, S., Ledig, C., Nori, A. V., Criminisi, A., et al. (2016a). "Deepmedic for brain tumor segmentation," in *International Workshop on Brainlesion: Glioma, Multiple Sclerosis, Stroke and Traumatic Brain Injuries* (Athens: Springer), 138–149.

Kamnitsas, K., Ledig, C., Newcombe, V. F., Simpson, J. P., Kane, A. D., Menon, D. K., et al. (2016b). Efficient multi-scale 3d cnn with fully connected crf for accurate brain lesion segmentation. *arXiv [Preprint]. arXiv:1603. 05959.*

Kayalibay, B., Jensen, G., and van der Smagt, P. (2017). Cnn-based segmentation of medical imaging data. *arXiv [Preprint]. arXiv:1701.03056.*

Kingma, D. P. and Ba, J. (2014). Adam: A method for stochastic optimization. *arXiv [Preprint]. arXiv:1412.6980.*

Krizhevsky, A., Sutskever, I., and Hinton, G. E. (2012). "Imagenet classification with deep convolutional neural networks," in *Advances in Neural Information Processing Systems*, (Lake Tahoe, NV), 1097–1105.

Le, H. T. and Pham, H. T.-T. (2018). Brain tumour segmentation using u-net based fully convolutional networks and extremely randomized trees. *Vietnam J. Sci. Tech. Eng.* 60, 19–25. doi: 10.31276/VJSTE.60(3).19

LeCun, Y., Bottou, L., Bengio, Y., and Haffner, P. (1998). Gradient-based learning applied to document recognition. *Proc. IEEE* 86, 2278–2324.

Li, X., Chen, H., Qi, X., Dou, Q., Fu, C.-W., and Heng, P. A. (2017). H-denseunet: Hybrid densely connected unet for liver and liver tumor segmentation from ct volumes. *arXiv [Preprint.] arXiv:1709.07330.* doi: 10.1109/TMI.2018.28 45918

Lin, T. Y., Goyal, P., Girshick, R., He, K., and Dollar, P. (2017). Focal loss for dense object detection. *IEEE Trans. Pattern Anal. Mach. Intel.* 99, 2999–3007. doi: 10.1109/TPAMI.2018.2858826

Lin, W., Tong, T., Gao, Q., Guo, D., Du, X., Yang, Y., et al. (2018). Convolutional neural networks-based mri image analysis for the alzheimers disease prediction from mild cognitive impairment. *Front. Neurosci.* 12:777. doi: 10.3389/fnins.2018.00777

Long, J., Shelhamer, E., and Darrell, T. (2015). "Fully convolutional networks for semantic segmentation," in *Proceedings of the IEEE Conference on Computer Vision and Pattern Recognition* (Boston, MA), 3431–3440.

Mazzara, G. P., Velthuizen, R. P., Pearlman, J. L., Greenberg, H., and Wagner, H. N. (2004). Brain tumor target volume determination for radiation treatment planning through automated mri segmentation. *Int. J. Radiat. Oncol. Biol. Phys.* 59, 300–312. doi: 10.1016/j.ijrobp.2004.1.026

Ren, S., He, K., Girshick, R., and Sun, J. (2015). "Faster r-cnn: towards real-time object detection with region proposal networks," in *Advances in Neural Information Processing Systems* (Montréal, QC), 91–99.

Ronneberger, O., Fischer, P., and Brox, T. (2015). "U-net: convolutional networks for biomedical image segmentation," in *International Conference on Medical Image Computing and Computer-Assisted Intervention*, (Springer), 234–241.

Simonyan, K., and Zisserman, A. (2014). Very deep convolutional networks for large-scale image recognition. *arXiv [Preprint]. arXiv:1409.1556.*

Szegedy, C., Liu, W., Jia, Y., Sermanet, P., Reed, S., Anguelov, D., et al. (2015). "Going deeper with convolutions," in *Proceedings of the IEEE Conference on Computer Vision and Pattern Recognition* (Boston, MA), 1–9.

Wang, G., Li, W., Ourselin, S., and Vercauteren, T. (2017). "Automatic brain tumor segmentation using cascaded anisotropic convolutional neural networks," in *International MICCAI Brainlesion Workshop* (Quebec City, QC), 178–190.

Wang, P., Chen, P., Yuan, Y., Liu, D., Huang, Z., Hou, X., et al. (2018a). "Understanding convolution for semantic segmentation," in *2018 IEEE Winter Conference on Applications of Computer Vision (WACV)* (Lake Tahoe, NV/CA: IEEE), 1451–1460.

Wang, X., Wang, D., Yao, Z., Xin, B., Wang, B., Lan, C., et al. (2018b). Machine learning models for multiparametric glioma grading with quantitative result interpretations. *Front. Neurosci.* 12:1046. doi: 10.3389/fnins.201 8.01046

Wen, P. Y., Macdonald, D. R., Reardon, D. A., Cloughesy, T. F., Sorensen, A. G., Galanis, E., et al. (2010). Updated response assessment criteria for high-grade gliomas: response assessment in neuro-oncology working group. *J. Clin. Oncol.* 28, 1963–1972. doi: 10.1200/JCO.2009.26.3541

Yang, Y., Yan, L.-F., Zhang, X., Han, Y., Nan, H.-Y., Hu, Y.-C., et al. (2018). Glioma grading on conventional mr images: a deep learning study with transfer learning. *Front. Neurosci.* 12:804. doi: 10.3389/fnins.2018.00804

Yu, F., and Koltun, V. (2015). Multi-scale context aggregation by dilated convolutions. *arXiv [Preprint]. arXiv:1511.07122.*

Zeiler, M. D., and Fergus, R. (2014). "Visualizing and understanding convolutional networks. in *European Conference on Computer Vision*, (Springer), 818–833.

Zhao, X., Wu, Y., Song, G., Li, Z., Zhang, Y., and Fan, Y. (2018). A deep learning model integrating FCNNs and CRFs for brain tumor segmentation. *Med. Image Anal.* 43, 98–111. doi: 10.1016/j.media.2017.10.002

Zhou, C., Ding, C., Lu, Z., Wang, X., and Tao, D. (2018). "One-pass multi-task convolutional neural networks for efficient brain tumor segmentation," in *International Conference on Medical Image Computing and Computer-Assisted Intervention*, (Springer), 637–645.

16

Convolutional Neural Networks-Based MRI Image Analysis for the Alzheimer's Disease Prediction From Mild Cognitive Impairment

*Weiming Lin[1,2,3], Tong Tong[3,4], Qinquan Gao[1,3,4], Di Guo[5], Xiaofeng Du[5], Yonggui Yang[6], Gang Guo[6], Min Xiao[2], Min Du[1,7]*and Xiaobo Qu[8]**

[1] College of Physics and Information Engineering, Fuzhou University, Fuzhou, China, [2] School of Opto-Electronic and Communication Engineering, Xiamen University of Technology, Xiamen, China, [3] Fujian Key Lab of Medical Instrumentation & Pharmaceutical Technology, Fuzhou, China, [4] Imperial Vision Technology, Fuzhou, China, [5] School of Computer & Information Engineering, Xiamen University of Technology, Xiamen, China, [6] Department of Radiology, Xiamen 2nd Hospital, Xiamen, China, [7] Fujian Provincial Key Laboratory of Eco-Industrial Green Technology, Nanping, China, [8] Department of Electronic Science, Xiamen University, Xiamen, China

***Correspondence:**
Min Du
dm_dj90@163.com
Xiaobo Qu
quxiaobo@xmu.edu.cn

[†] Data used in the preparation of this paper were obtained from the ADNI database (http://adni.loni.usc.edu/). As such, the investigators within the ADNI contributed to the design and implementation of ADNI and/or provided data but did not participate in analysis or writing of this report. A complete listing of ADNI investigators can be found at the website (http://adni.loni.usc.edu/wp-content/uploads/how_to_apply/ADNI_Acknowledgement_List.pdf).

Mild cognitive impairment (MCI) is the prodromal stage of Alzheimer's disease (AD). Identifying MCI subjects who are at high risk of converting to AD is crucial for effective treatments. In this study, a deep learning approach based on convolutional neural networks (CNN), is designed to accurately predict MCI-to-AD conversion with magnetic resonance imaging (MRI) data. First, MRI images are prepared with age-correction and other processing. Second, local patches, which are assembled into 2.5 dimensions, are extracted from these images. Then, the patches from AD and normal controls (NC) are used to train a CNN to identify deep learning features of MCI subjects. After that, structural brain image features are mined with FreeSurfer to assist CNN. Finally, both types of features are fed into an extreme learning machine classifier to predict the AD conversion. The proposed approach is validated on the standardized MRI datasets from the Alzheimer's Disease Neuroimaging Initiative (ADNI) project. This approach achieves an accuracy of 79.9% and an area under the receiver operating characteristic curve (AUC) of 86.1% in leave-one-out cross validations. Compared with other state-of-the-art methods, the proposed one outperforms others with higher accuracy and AUC, while keeping a good balance between the sensitivity and specificity. Results demonstrate great potentials of the proposed CNN-based approach for the prediction of MCI-to-AD conversion with solely MRI data. Age correction and assisted structural brain image features can boost the prediction performance of CNN.

Keywords: Alzheimer's disease, deep learning, convolutional neural networks, mild cognitive impairment, magnetic resonance imaging

INTRODUCTION

Alzheimer's disease (AD) is the cause of over 60% of dementia cases (Burns and Iliffe, 2009), in which patients usually have a progressive loss of memory, language disorders and disorientation. The disease would ultimate lead to the death of patients. Until now, the cause of AD is still unknown, and no effective drugs or treatments have been reported to stop or reverse AD progression. Early diagnosis of AD is essential for making treatment plans to slow down the progress to AD. Mild cognitive impairment (MCI) is known as the transitional stage between normal cognition and dementia (Markesbery, 2010), about 10–15% individuals with MCI progress to AD per year (Grundman et al., 2004). It was reported that MCI and AD were accompanied by losing gray matter in brain (Karas et al., 2004), thus neuropathology changes could be found several years before AD was diagnosed. Many previous studies used neuroimaging biomarkers to classify AD patients at different disease stages or to predict the MCI-to-AD conversion (Cuingnet et al., 2011; Zhang et al., 2011; Tong et al., 2013, 2017; Guerrero et al., 2014; Suk et al., 2014; Cheng et al., 2015; Eskildsen et al., 2015; Li et al., 2015; Liu et al., 2015; Moradi et al., 2015). In these studies, structural magnetic resonance imaging (MRI) is one of the most extensively utilized imaging modality due to non-invasion, high resolution and moderate cost.

To predict MCI-to-AD conversion, we separate MCI patients into two groups by the criteria that whether they convert to AD within 3 years or not (Moradi et al., 2015; Tong et al., 2017). These two groups are referred to as MCI converters and MCI non-converters. The converters generally have more severe deterioration of neuropathology than that of non-converters. The pathological changes between converters and non-converters are similar to those between AD and NC, but much milder. Therefore, it much more difficult to classify converters/non-converters than AD/NC. This prediction with MRI is challenging because the pathological changes related to AD progression between MCI non-converter and MCI converter are subtle and inter-subject variable. For example, ten MRI-based methods for predicting MCI-to-AD conversion and six of them perform no better than random classifier (Cuingnet et al., 2011). To reduce the interference of inter-subject variability, MRI images are usually spatially registered to a common space (Coupe et al., 2012; Young et al., 2013; Moradi et al., 2015; Tong et al., 2017). However, the registration might change the AD related pathology and loss some useful information. The accuracy of prediction is also influenced by the normal aging brain atrophy, with the removal of age-related effect, the performance of classification was improved (Dukart et al., 2011; Moradi et al., 2015; Tong et al., 2017).

Machine learning algorithms perform well in computer-aided predictions of MCI-to-AD conversion (Dukart et al., 2011; Coupe et al., 2012; Wee et al., 2013; Young et al., 2013; Moradi et al., 2015; Beheshti et al., 2017; Cao et al., 2017; Tong et al., 2017). In recent years, deep learning, as a promising machine learning methodology, has made a big leap in identifying and classifying patterns of images (Li et al., 2015; Zeng et al., 2016, 2018). As the most widely used architecture of deep learning, convolutional neural networks (CNN) has attracted a lot of attention due to its great success in image classification and analysis (Gulshan et al., 2016; Nie et al., 2016; Shin et al., 2016; Rajkomar et al., 2017; Du et al., 2018). The strong ability of CNN motivates us to develop a CNN-based prediction method of AD conversion.

In this work, we propose a CNN-based prediction approach of AD conversion using MRI images. A CNN-based architecture is built to extract high level features of registered and age-corrected hippocampus images for classification. To further improve the prediction, more morphological information is added by including FreeSurfer-based features (FreeSurfer, RRID:SCR_001847) (Fischl and Dale, 2000; Fischl et al., 2004; Desikan et al., 2006; Han et al., 2006). Both CNN and FreeSurfer features are fed into an extreme learning machine as classifier, which finally makes the decision of MCI-to-AD. Our main contributions to boost the prediction performance include: (1) Multiple 2.5D patches are extracted for data augmentation in CNN; (2) both AD and NC are used to train the CNN, digging out important MCI features; (3) CNN-based features and FreeSurfer-based features are combined to provide complementary information to improve prediction. The performance of the proposed approach was validated on the standardized MRI datasets from the Alzheimer's Disease Neuroimaging Initiative (ADNI – Alzheimer's Disease Neuroimaging Initiative, RRID:SCR_003007) (Wyman et al., 2013) and compared with other state-of-the-art methods (Moradi et al., 2015; Tong et al., 2017) on the same datasets.

MATERIALS AND METHODS

The proposed framework is illustrated in **Figure 1**. The MRI data were processed through two paths, which extract the CNN-based and FreeSurfer-based image features, respectively. In the left path, CNN is trained on the AD/NC image patches and then is employed to extract CNN-based features on MCI images. In the right path, FreeSurfer-based features which were calculated with FreeSurfer software. These features, which were further mined with dimension reduction and sparse feature selection via PCA and Lasso, respectively, were concatenated as a features vector and fed to extreme learning machine as classifier. Finally, to evaluate the performance of the proposed approach, the leave-one-out cross validation is then used.

ADNI Data

Data used in this work were downloaded from the ADNI database. The ADNI is an ongoing, longitudinal study designed to develop clinical, imaging, genetic, and biochemical biomarkers for the early detection and tracking of AD. The ADNI study began in 2004 and its first 6-year study is called ADNI1. Standard analysis sets of MRI data from ADNI1 were used in this work, including 188 AD, 229 NC, and 401 MCI subjects (Wyman et al., 2013). These MCI subjects were grouped as: (1) MCI converters who were diagnosed as MCI at first visit, but converted to AD during the longitudinal visits within 3 years (n = 169);

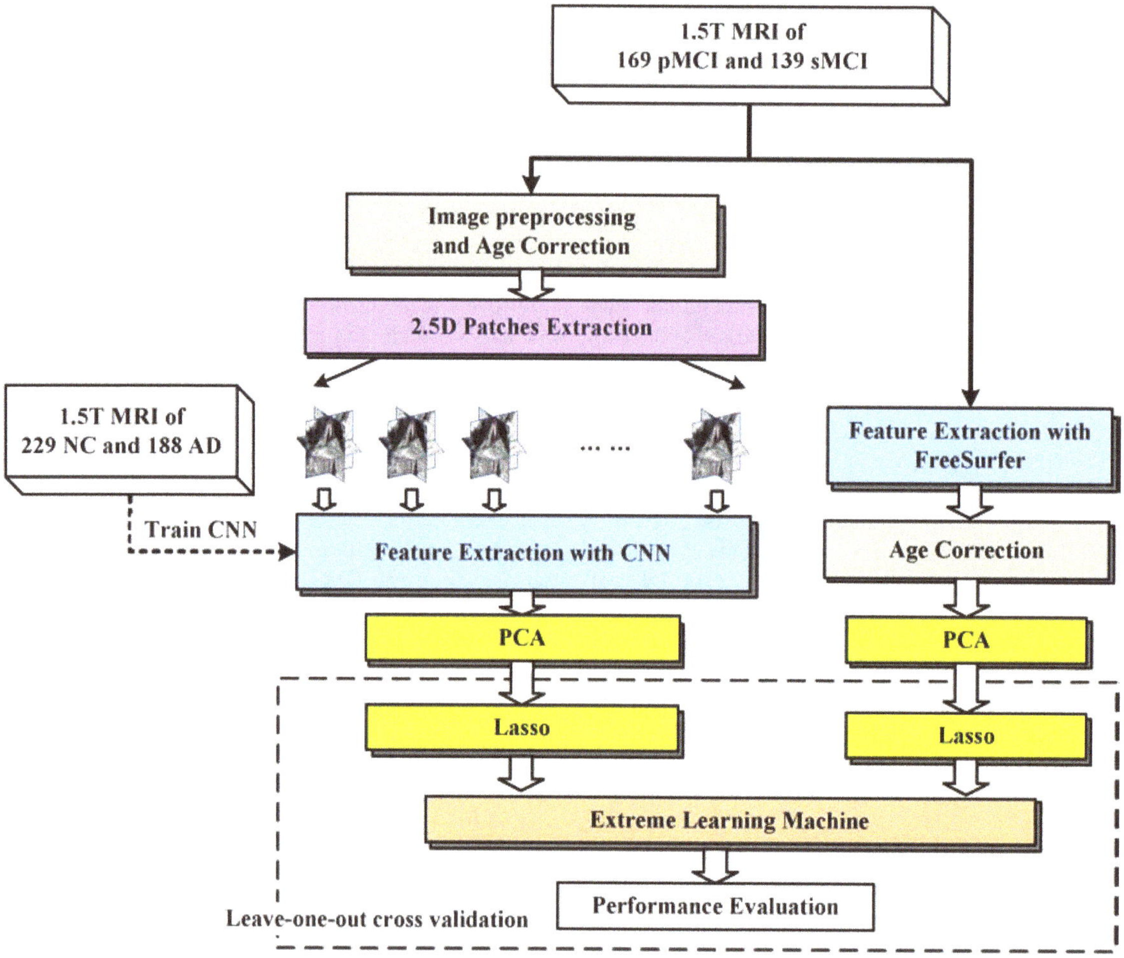

FIGURE 1 | Framework of proposed approach. The dashed arrow indicates the CNN was trained with 2.5D patches of NC and AD subjects. The dashed box indicates Leave-one-out cross validation was performed by repeat LASSO and extreme learning machine 308 times, in each time one different MCI subject was leaved for test, and the other subjects with their labels were used to train LASSO and extreme learning machine.

(2) MCI non-converters who did not convert to AD within 3 years (n = 139). The subjects who were diagnosed as MCI at least twice, but reverse to NC at last, are also considered as MCI non-converters; (3) Unknown MCI subjects who missed some diagnosis which made the last state of these subjects was unknown (n = 93). The demographic information of the dataset are presented in **Table 1**. The age ranges of different groups are similar. The proportions of male and female are close in AD/NC groups while proportions of male are higher than female in MCI groups.

Image Preprocessing

MRI images were preprocessed following steps in Tong et al. (2017). All images were first skull-stripped according to Leung et al. (2011), and then aligned to the MNI151 template using a B-spline free-form deformation registration (Rueckert et al., 1999). In the implementation, we follow the Tong's way to register images (Tong et al., 2017), showing that the effect of deformable registration with a control point spacing between 10 and 5 mm have the best performance in classifying AD/NC and converters/non-converters. After that, image intensities of

TABLE 1 | The demographic information of the dataset used in this work.

	AD	NC	MCIc	MCInc	MCIun
Subjects' number	188	229	169	139	93
Age range	55–91	60–90	55–88	55–88	55–89
Males/Females	99/89	119/110	102/67	96/43	60/33

MCIc means MCI converters. MCInc means MCI non-converters, MCIun means MCI unknown.

the subjects were normalized by deform the histogram of each subject's image to match the histogram of the MNI151 template (Nyul and Udupa, 1999). Finally, all MRI images were in the same template space and had the same intensity range.

Age Correction

Normal aging has atrophy effects similar with AD (Giorgio et al., 2010). To reduce the confounding effect of age-related atrophy, age correction is necessary to remove age-related effects, which is estimated by fitting a pixel regression model (Dukart et al., 2011) to the subjects' ages. We assume there are N healthy subjects and M voxels in each preprocessed MRI image, and denote $\mathbf{y}_m \in \mathbf{R}^{1 \times N}$ as the vector of the intensity values of N healthy subjects at mth voxel, and $\alpha \in \mathbf{R}^{1 \times N}$ as the vector of the ages of N healthy subjects. The age-related effect is estimated by fitting linear regression model $y_m = \omega_m \alpha + b_m$ at mth voxel. For nth subject, the new intensity of mth voxel can be calculated as $y'_{mn} = \omega_m(C - \alpha_n) + y_{mn}$, where y_{mn} is original intensity, α_n is age of nth subject. In this study, C is 75, which is the mean age of all subjects.

CNN-Based Features

A CNN was adopted to extract features from MRI Images of NC and AD subjects. Then, the trained CNN was used to extract image features of MCI subjects. To explore the multiple plane images in MRI, a 2.5D patch was formed by extracting three 32 × 32 patches from transverse, coronal, and sagittal plane centered at a same point (Shin et al., 2016). Then, three patches were combined into a 2D RBG patch. **Figure 2** shows an example of constructing 2.5D patch. For a given voxel point, three patches of MRI are extracted from three planes and then concatenated into a three channel cube, following the same way of composing a colorful patch with red/green/blue channels that are commonly used in computer vision. This process allows us to mine fruitful information form 3D views of MRI by feeding the 2.5D patch into the typical color image processing CNN network. Data augmentation (Shin et al., 2016) was used to increase training samples, by extracting multiple patches at different locations from MRI images. The choice of locations has three constraints, (1) The patches must be originated in either left or right hippocampus region which have high correlation with AD (van de Pol et al., 2006); (2) There must be at least two voxels distance between each location; (3) All locations were random chosen. With these constraints, 151 patches were extracted from each image and the sampling positions were fixed during experiments. The number of samples was expanded by a factor of 151, which could reduce over-fitting.

Typically extracted patches are presented in **Figure 3**. **Figure 3A** shows four 2.5D patches obtained from one subject. These patches are extracted from different positions and show different portions of hippocampus, which means these patches contain different information of morphology of hippocampus. When trained with these patches that spread in whole hippocampus, CNN learns the morphology of whole hippocampus. **Figure 3B** shows patches extracted in same position from four subjects of different groups, demonstrating that the AD subject has the most severe atrophy of hippocampus and expansion of ventricle. This implies that obvious differences are existed between AD and NC. However, the MCI subjects have the medium atrophy of hippocampus, and non-converter is more like NC rather than AD, and converter is more similar to AD. The difference between converter and non-converter is smaller than the difference between AD and NC.

The architecture of the CNN is summarized in **Figure 4**. The network has an input of 32 × 32 RGB patch. There are three convolutional layers and three pooling layers. The kernel size of convolutional layer is 5 × 5 with 2 pixels padding, and the kernel size and stride of pooling layers is 3 × 3 and 2. The input patch has a size of 32 × 32 and 3 RBG channels. The first convolutional layer generates 32 feature maps with a size of 32 × 32. After max pooling, these 32 feature maps were down-sampled into 16 × 16. The next two convolutional layers and average pooling layers finally generate 64 features maps with a size of 4 × 4. These features are concatenated as a feature vector, and then fed to full connection layer and softmax layer for classification. There are also rectified linear units layers and local response normalization layers in CNN, but are not shown for simplicity.

The CNN was trained with patches from NC and AD subjects, and there are 62967 (subject number 417 times 151) patches which are randomly split into 417 mini-batches. Mini-batch stochastic gradient descent was used to update the coefficients of CNN. In each step, a mini-batch was fed into CNN, and then error back propagation algorithm was carried out to computer gradient g_j of jth coefficient θ_j, and update the coefficient as $\theta'_j = \theta_j + \nabla\theta n\, j$, in which $\nabla\theta n\, j = m\nabla\theta n{-}1\, j - \eta(g_j + \lambda\theta_j)$ is the increment of θ_j at nth step. The momentum m, learning rate η and weight decay λ are set as 0.9, 0.001, and 0.0001, respectively, in this work. It is called one epoch with all mini-batches used to train CNN once. The CNN was trained with 30 epochs. Once the network was trained, CNN will be used to extract high level features of MCI subjects' images. The 1024 features output by the last pooling layer were taken as CNN-based features. Thus, CNN generates 154624 (1024 × 151) features for each image.

FreeSurfer-Based Features

The FreeSurfer (version 4.3) (Fischl and Dale, 2000; Fischl et al., 2004; Desikan et al., 2006; Han et al., 2006) was used to mine more morphological information of MRI images, such as cortical volume, surface area, cortical thickness average, and standard deviation of thickness in each region of interest. These features can be downloaded directly from ADNI website, and 325 features are used to predict MCI-to-AD conversion after age correction. The age correction for FreeSurfer-based features is similar as described above, but on these 325 features instead of on intensity values of MRI images.

Features Selection

Redundant features maybe exist among CNN-based features, thus we introduced the principle component analysis (PCA) (Avci and Turkoglu, 2009; Babaoğlu et al., 2010; Wu et al., 2013) and least absolute shrinkage and selection operator (LASSO) (Kukreja et al., 2006; Usai et al., 2009; Yamada et al., 2014) to reduce the final number of features.

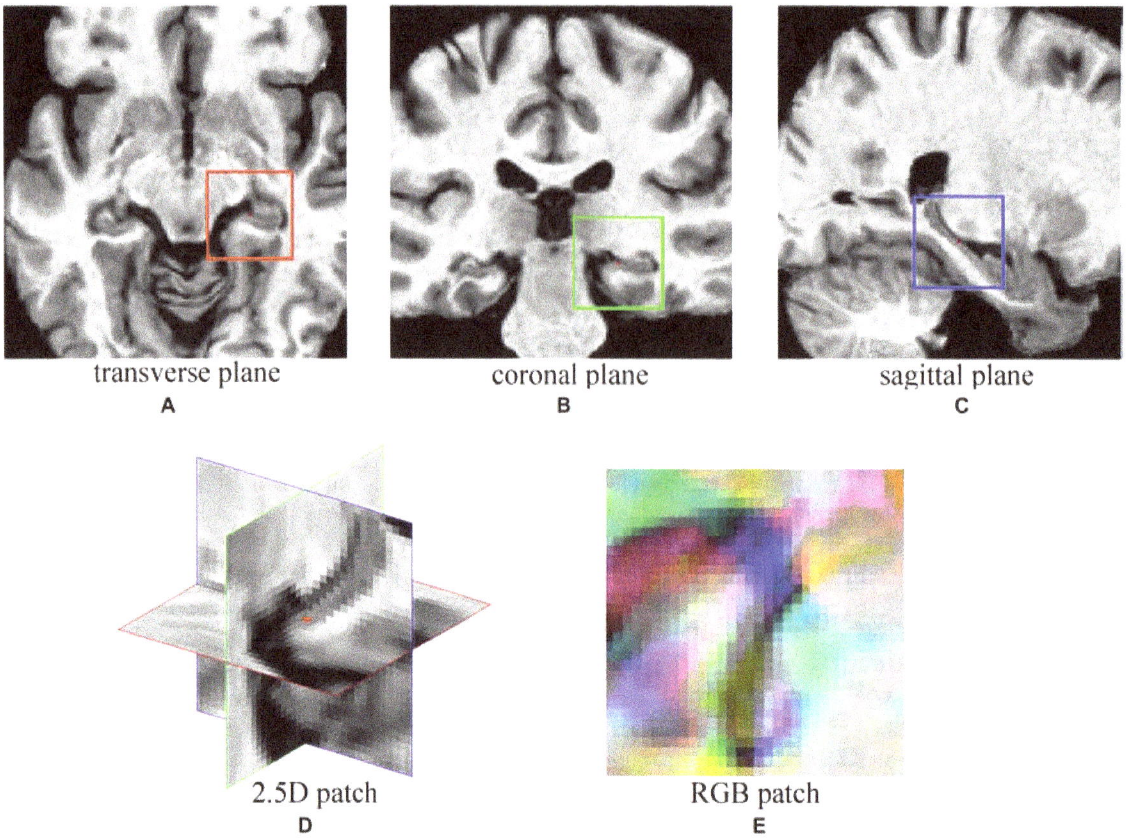

FIGURE 2 | The demonstration of 2.5D patch extraction from hippocampus region. **(A–C)** 2D patches extracted from transverse (red box), coronal (green box), and sagittal (blue box) plane; **(D)** The 2.5D patch with three patches at their spatial locations, red dot is the center of 2.5D patch; **(E)** Three patches are combined into RGB patch as red (red box patch), green (green box patch), and blue (blue box patch) channels.

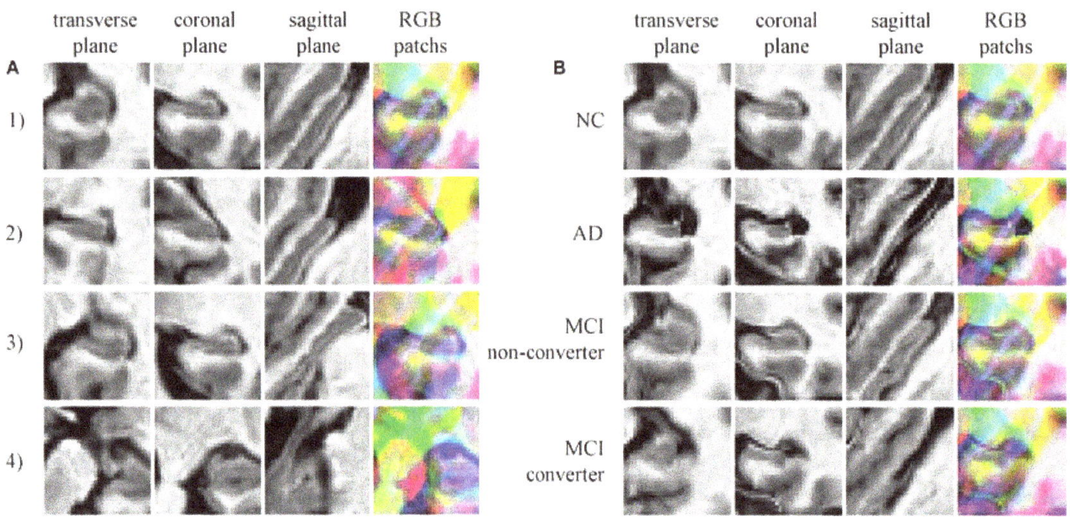

FIGURE 3 | **(A)** Four random chosen 2.5D patches of one subject (who is normal control, female and 76.3 years old), indicating that these patches contain different information of hippocampus; **(B)** The comparison of correspond 2.5D patches of four subjects from four groups, the different level of hippocampus atrophy can be found.

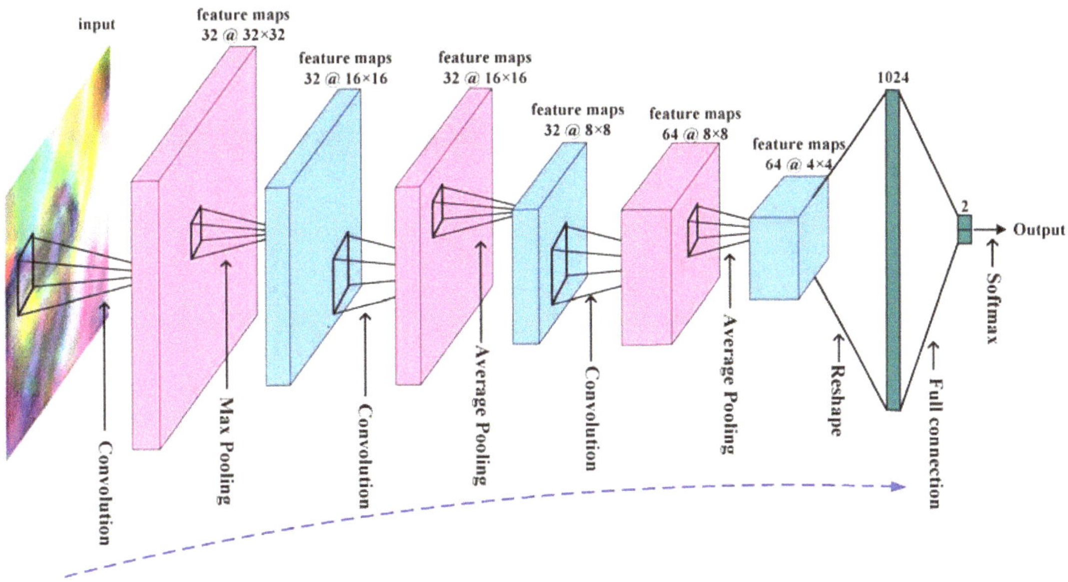

FIGURE 4 | The overall architecture of the CNN used in this work.

PCA is an unsupervised learning method that uses an orthogonal transformation to convert a set of samples consisting of possibly correlated features into samples consisting of linearly uncorrelated new features. It has been extensively used in data analysis (Avci and Turkoglu, 2009; Babaoğlu et al., 2010; Wu et al., 2013). In this work, PCA is adopted to reduce the dimensions of features. Parameters of PCA are: (1) For CNN-based features, there are 1024 features for each patch. After PCA, P_C features were left for each patch, since there are 151 patches for one subject, there are still $P_C \times 151$ features for each subject; (2) For FreeSurfer-based features, P_F features were left for each MCI subject.

LASSO is a supervised learning method that uses L_1 norm in sparse regression (Kukreja et al., 2006; Usai et al., 2009; Yamada et al., 2014) as follows:

$$\min_{\alpha} 0.5||\boldsymbol{y} - \mathbf{D}\boldsymbol{\alpha}||_2^2 + \lambda||\boldsymbol{\alpha}||_1 \quad (1)$$

Where $\boldsymbol{y} \in \mathbf{R}^{1 \times N}$ is the vector consisting of N labels of training samples, $\mathbf{D} \in \mathbf{R}^{N \times M}$ is the feature matrix of N training samples consisting of M features, λ is the penalty coefficient that was set to 0.1, and $\boldsymbol{\alpha} \in \mathbf{R}^{1 \times M}$ is the target sparse coefficients and can be used for selecting features with large coefficients. The LASSO was solved with least angle regression (Efron et al., 2004), and L features are selected after L iterations. Parameters of LASSO are: (1) For CNN-based features, L_C features were selected from $P_C \times 151$ features for each MCI subject; (2) For FreeSurfer-based features, L_F features were selected from P_F features. After PCA and LASSO, there were $L_C + L_F$ features.

Figure 5 shows more details of CNN-based features. 151 patches are extracted from all MRI images, including AD, NC, and MCI. First, the CNN is trained with patches of all AD and NC subjects. After that, the trained CNN is used to output 1024 features from each MCI patch. The 1024 features of each patch are reduced to P_C features by PCA, and then features of all 151 patches from one subject are concatenated, and Lasso is used to select L_C most informative features from them.

Extreme Learning Machine

The extreme learning machine, a feed-forward neural network with a single layer of hidden nodes, learns much faster than common networks trained with back propagation algorithm (Huang et al., 2012; Zeng et al., 2017). A special extreme learning machine, that adopts kernel (Huang et al., 2012) to calculates the outputs as formula (2) and avoids the random generation of input weight matrix, is chosen to classify converters/non-converters with both CNN-based features and FreeSurfer-based features. In formula (2), the $\boldsymbol{\Omega}$ is a matrix with elements $\Omega_{i,j} = \mathbf{K}(\boldsymbol{x}_i, \boldsymbol{x}_j)$, where $\mathbf{K}(\boldsymbol{a}, \boldsymbol{b})$ is a radial basis function kernel in this study, $[\boldsymbol{x}_1, \ldots, \boldsymbol{x}_N]$ are N training samples, $\boldsymbol{y}$ is the label vector of training samples, and $\boldsymbol{x}$ is testing sample. C is a regularization coefficient and was set to 1 in this study.

$$f(\mathbf{x}) = \begin{bmatrix} K(\mathbf{x}, \mathbf{x}_1) \\ \vdots \\ K(\mathbf{x}, \mathbf{x}_N) \end{bmatrix}^T (\Omega + 1/C)^T y \quad (2)$$

Implementation

In our implementation, CNN was accomplished with Caffe[1], LASSO was carried out with SPAMS[2], and extreme learning machine was performed with shared online code[3]. The hippocampus segmentation was implemented with MALPEM

[1] http://caffe.berkeleyvision.org/
[2] http://spams-devel.gforge.inria.fr/
[3] http://www.ntu.edu.sg/home/egbhuang/

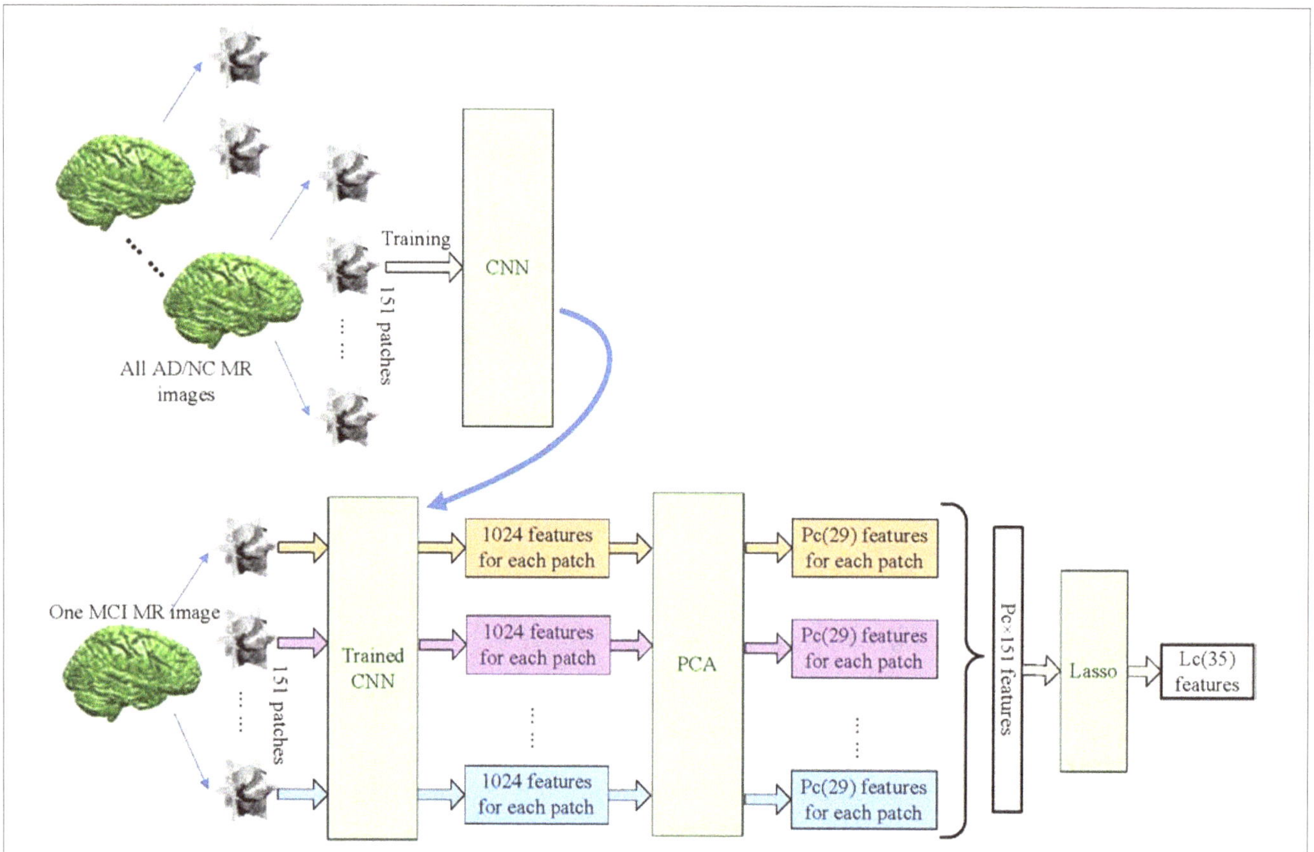

FIGURE 5 | The workflow of extracting CNN-based features. The CNN was trained with all AD/NC patches, and used to extract deep features from all 151 patches of MCI subject. The feature number of each patch is reduced to P_C (P_C = 29) from 1024 by PCA. Finally, Lasso selects L_C (L_C = 35) features from $P_C \times 151$ features for each MCI subject.

[4](Ledig et al., 2015) for all MRI images. Then all hippocampus masks were registered as corresponding MRI images, and then overlapped to create a mask containing hippocampus regions. All image features were normalized to have zero mean and unit variance before training or selection. To evaluate the performance, Leave-one-out cross validation was used as (Coupé et al., 2012; Ye et al., 2012; Zhang et al., 2012).

RESULTS

Validation of the Robustness of 2.5D CNN

To validate the robustness of the CNN, several experiments have been performed with the CNN. In experiments, the binary decisions of CNN for 151 patches were united to make final diagnosis of the testing subject. We compared the performance in four different conditions: (1) The CNN was trained with AD/NC patches and used to classify AD/NC subjects; (2) The CNN was trained with converters/non-converters patches and used to classify converters/non-converters; (3) The CNN was trained with AD/NC patches and used to classify converters/non-converters; (4) The condition is similar with (3), but with different sampling patches in each validation run.

The results are shown in **Table 2**. The CNN has a poor accuracy of 68.49% in classifying converters/non-converters when trained with converters/non-converters patches, but CNN has obtained a much higher accuracy of 73.04% when trained with AD/NC patches. This means that the CNN learned more useful information from AD/NC data than that from converters/non-converters data. And the prediction performance of CNN is close when different sampling patches are used.

Effect of Combining Two Types of Features

In this section, we present the performance of CNN-based features, FreeSurfer-based features, and their combinations. The P_C, P_F, L_C, and L_F parameters were set to 29, 150, 35, and 40, respectively, which were optimized in experiments. Finally, 75 features were selected and fed to the extreme learning machine.

Performance was evaluated by calculating accuracy (the number of correctly classified subjects divided by the total number of subjects), sensitivity (the number of correctly classified MCI converters divided by the total number of

[4]http://www.christianledig.com/

TABLE 2 | The performance of the 2.5D CNN.

	Classifying: AD/NC Trained with: AD/NC	Classifying: MCIc/MCInc Trained with: MCIc/MCInc	Classifying: MCIc/MCInc Trained with: AD/NC	Different patch Sampling
Accuracy	88.79%	68.68%	73.04%	72.75%
Standard deviation	0.61%	1.63%	1.31%	1.20%
Confidence interval	[0.8862, 0.8897]	[0.6821, 0.6914]	[0.7265, 0.7343]	[0.7252, 0.7299]

MCIc means MCI converters. MCInc means MCI non-converters. The results were obtained with 10-fold cross validations, and averaged over 50 runs.

TABLE 3 | The performance of different features used, and the performance without age correction.

Method	Accuracy	Sensitivity	Specificity	AUC
Proposed method (both features)	**79.9%**	**84%**	**74.8%**	**86.1%**
Only CNN-based features	76.9%	81.7%	71.2%	82.9%
Only FreeSurfer-based features	76.9%	82.2%	70.5%	82.8%
Without age correction	75.3%	79.9%	69.8%	82.6%

Bold values indicate the best performance in each column.

MCI converters), specificity (the number of correctly classified MCI non-converters divided by the total number of MCI non-converters), and AUC (area under the receiver operating characteristic curve). The performances of the proposed method and the approach with only one type of features are summarized in **Table 3**. These results indicates that the approaches with only CNN-based features or FreeSurfer-based features have similar performances, and the proposed method combining both features achieved best accuracy, sensitivity, specificity and AUC. Thus, it is meaningful to combine two features in the prediction of MCI-to-AD conversion. The AUC of the proposed method reached 86.1%, indicating the promising performance of this method. The receiver operating characteristic (ROC) curves of these approaches are shown in **Figure 6**.

Impact of Age Correction

We investigated the impact of age correction on the prediction of conversion here. The prediction accuracy in **Table 3** and the ROC curves in **Figure 6** implied that age correction can significantly improve the accuracy and AUC, Thus, age correction is an important step in the proposed method.

Comparisons to Other Methods

In this section, we first compared the extreme learning machine with support vector machine and random forest. The performances of three classifiers are shown in **Table 4**, indicating that extreme learning machine achieves the best accuracy and AUC among three classifiers.

Then we compared the proposed method with other state-of-the-art methods that use the same data (Moradi et al., 2015; Tong et al., 2017), which consists of 100 MCI non-converters and 164 MCI converters. In both methods, MRI images were first preprocessed and registered, but in different ways. After that, features selection was performed to select the most informative voxels among all MRI voxels. Moradi used regularized logistic regression algorithm to select a subset of MRI voxels, and Tong used elastic net algorithm instead. Both methods trained feature selection algorithms with AD/NC data to learn the most discriminative voxels and then used to selected voxels from MCI data. Finally, Moradi used low density separation to calculate MRI biomarkers and to predict MCI converters/non-converters. Tong used elastic net regression to calculate grading biomarkers from MCI features, and SVM was utilized to classify MCI converters/non-converters with grading biomarker.

For fair comparisons, both 10-fold cross validation and leave-one-out cross validation were performed on the proposed method and method of Tong et al. (2017) with only MRI data was used. Parameters of the compared approaches were optimized to achieve best performance. **Table 5** shows the performances of three methods in 10-fold cross validation and **Table 6** summarizes the performances in leave-one-out cross validations. These two tables demonstrate that the proposed method achieves the best accuracy and AUC among three methods, which means that the proposed method is more accurate in predicting MCI-to-AD conversion than other methods. The sensitivity of the proposed method is a little lower than the method of Moradi et al. (2015) but much higher than the method of Tong et al. (2017), and the specificity of the proposed method is between other two methods. Higher sensitivity means lower rate of missed diagnosis of converters, and higher specificity means lower rate of misdiagnosing non-converters as converters. Overall, the proposed method has a good balance between the sensitivity and specificity.

DISCUSSION

The CNN has a better performance when trained with AD/NC patches rather than MCI patches, we think the reason is that the pathological changes between MCI converters and non-converters are slighter than those between AD and CN. Thus, it is more difficult for CNN to learn useful information directly from MCI data about AD-related pathological changes than from AD/NC data. The pathological changes are also hampered by inter-subject variations for MCI data. Inspired by the work in Moradi et al. (2015) and Tong et al. (2017) which use information

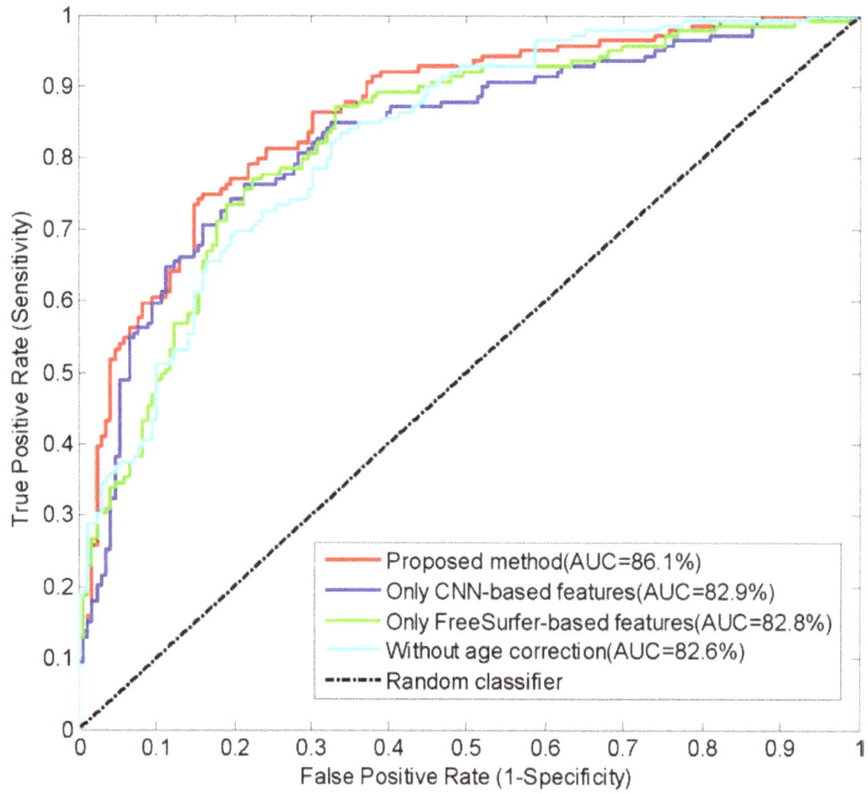

FIGURE 6 | The ROC curves of classifying converters/non-converters when different features used or without age correction.

TABLE 4 | Comparison of extreme learning machine with other two classifiers.

Method	Accuracy	Sensitivity	Specificity	AUC
SVM	**79.87%**	83.43%	**75.54%**	83.85%
Random forest	75.0%	82.84%	65.47%	81.99%
Extreme learning machine	**79.87%**	**84.02%**	74.82%	**86.14%**

Implementation of SVM was performed using third party library LIBSVM (https://www.csie.ntu.edu.tw/~cjlin/libsvm/), and the random forest was utilized with the third party library (http://code.google.com/p/randomforest-matlab). Both classifiers used the default settings.

TABLE 5 | Comparison with others methods on the same dataset in 10-fold cross validation.

Method	Accuracy	Sensitivity	Specificity	AUC
MRI biomarker in Moradi et al., 2015	74.7%	**88.9%**	51.6%	76.6%
Global grading biomarker in Tong et al., 2017	78.9%	76.0%	**82.9%**	81.3%
Proposed method	**79.5%**	86.1%	68.8%	**83.6%**

The performances of MRI biomarker and global grading biomarker are described in Moradi et al. (2015) and (Tong et al., 2017). The results are averages over 100 runs, and the standard deviation/confidence intervals of accuracy and AUC of the proposed method are 1.19%/[0.7922, 0.7968] and 0.83%/[0.8358, 0.8391]. Bold values indicate the best performance in each column.

TABLE 6 | Comparison with others methods on the same dataset in leave-one-out cross validation.

Method	Accuracy	Sensitivity	Specificity	AUC
MRI biomarker in Moradi et al., 2015	–	–	–	–
Global grading biomarker in Tong et al., 2017	78.8%	76.2%	**83%**	81.2%
Proposed method	**81.4%**	**89.6%**	68%	**87.8%**

The global grading biomarkers was download from the web described in Tong et al. (2017) and the experiment was performed with same method as in Tong et al. (2017). Bold values indicate the best performance in each column.

TABLE 7 | The 15 most informative FreeSurfer-based features for predicting MCI-to-AD conversion.

Number	FreeSurfer-based feature
1	Cortical Thickness Average of Left FrontalPole
2	Volume (Cortical Parcellation) of Left Precentral
3	Volume (Cortical Parcellation) of Right Postcentral
4	Volume (WM Parcellation) of Left AccumbensArea
5	Cortical Thickness Average of Right CaudalMiddleFrontal
6	Cortical Thickness Average of Right FrontalPole
7	Volume (Cortical Parcellation) of Left Bankssts
8	Volume (Cortical Parcellation) of Left PosteriorCingulate
9	Volume (Cortical Parcellation) of Left Insula
10	Cortical Thickness Average of Left SuperiorTemporal
11	Cortical Thickness Standard Deviation of Left PosteriorCingulate
12	Volume (Cortical Parcellation) of Left Precuneus
13	Volume (WM Parcellation) of CorpusCallosumMidPosterior
14	Volume (Cortical Parcellation) of Left Lingual
15	Cortical Thickness Standard Deviation of Right Postcentral

of AD and NC to help classifying MCI, we trained the CNN with the patches from AD and NC subjects and improved the performance.

After non-rigid registration, the differences between all subject's MRI brain image are mainly in hippocampus (Tong et al., 2017). So we extracted 2.5D patches only from hippocampus regions, that makes the information of other regions lost. For this reason, we included the whole brain features calculated by FreeSurfer as complementary information. The accuracy and AUC of classification are increased to 79.9 and 86.1% from 76.9 to 82.9% with the help of FreeSurfer-based features. To explore which FreeSurfer-based features contribute mostly when they are used to predict MCI-to-AD conversion, we used Lasso to select the most informative features, and the top 15 features are listed in **Table 7**, in which the features are almost volume and thickness average of regions related to AD. The thickness average of frontal pole is the most discriminative feature. The quantitative features of hippopotamus are not listed, indicating they contribute less than these listed features when predicting conversion. The CNN extract the deep features of hippopotamus morphology, rather than the quantitative features of hippopotamus, which are discriminative for AD diagnosis. Therefore, The CNN-based features and FreeSurfer-based features contain different useful information for classification of converters/non-converters, and they are complementary to improve the performance of classifier.

Different from the two methods used in Moradi et al. (2015) and Tong et al. (2017), which directly used voxels as features, the proposed method employs CNN to learn the deep features from the morphology of hippopotamus, and combined CNN-based features with the globe morphology features that were computed by FreeSurfer. We believe that the learnt CNN features might be more meaningful and more discriminative than voxels. When comparing with these two methods, only MRI data was used, but the performances of these two methods were improved when combined MRI data with age and cognitive measures, so investigating the combination of the propose approach with other modality data for performance improvement is also one of our future works.

We have also listed several deep learning-based studies in recent years for comparison in **Table 8**. Most of them have an accuracy of predicting conversion above 70%, especially the last three approaches (including the proposed one) have the accuracy above 80%. The best accuracy was achieved by Lu et al. (2018a), which uses both MRI and PET data. However, when only MRI data is used, Lu's method declined the accuracy to 75.44%. Although an accuracy of 82.51% was also obtained with PET data (Lu et al., 2018b), PET scanning usually suffers from contrast agents and more expensive cost than the routine MRI. In summary, our approach achieved the best performance when only MRI images were used and is expected to be improved by incorporating other modality data, e.g., PET, in the future.

In this work, the period of predicting conversion was set to 3 years, that separates MCI subjects into MCI non-converters and MCI converters groups by the criterion who covert to AD within 3 years. But not matter what the period for prediction is, there is a disadvantage that even the classifier precisely predict a MCI non-converters who would not convert to AD within a specific period, but the conversion might still happen half year or even 1 month later. Modeling the progression of AD and predicting the time of conversion with longitudinal data are more meaningful

TABLE 8 | Results of previous deep learning based approaches for predicting MCI-to-AD conversion.

Study	Number of MCIc/MCInc	Data	Conversion time	Accuracy	AUC
Li et al., 2015	99/56	MRI + PET	18 months	57.4%	–
Singh et al., 2017	158/178	PET	–	72.47%	–
Ortiz et al., 2016	39/64	MRI + PET	24 months	78%	82%
Suk et al., 2014	76/128	MRI + PET	–	75.92%	74.66%
Shi et al., 2018	99/56	MRI + PET	18 months	78.88%	80.1%
Lu et al., 2018a	217/409	MRI + PET	36 months	**82.93%**	–
Lu et al., 2018a	217/409	MRI	36 months	75.44%	–
Lu et al., 2018b	112/409	PET	–	82.51%	–
This study	164/100	MRI	36 months	81.4%	**87.8%**

MCIc means MCI converters. MCInc means MCI non-converters. Different subjects and modalities of data are used in these approaches. All the criteria are copied from the original literatures. Bold values indicate the best performance in each column.

(Guerrero et al., 2016; Xie et al., 2016). Our future work would investigate the usage of CNN in modeling the progression of AD.

CONCLUSION

In this study, we have developed a framework that only use MRI data to predict the MCI-to-AD conversion, by applying CNN and other machine learning algorithms. Results show that CNN can extract discriminative features of hippocampus for prediction by learning the morphology changes of hippocampus between AD and NC. And FreeSurfer provides extra structural brain image features to improve the prediction performance as complementary information. Compared with other state-of-the-art methods, the proposed one outperforms others in higher accuracy and AUC, while keeping a good balance between the sensitivity and specificity.

AUTHOR CONTRIBUTIONS

WL and XQ conceived the study, designed the experiments, analyzed the data, and wrote the whole manuscript. TT and QG provided the preprocessed data. WL, XQ, DG, XD, and MX carried out experiments. YY and GG helped to analyze the data and experiments result. MD and XQ revised the manuscript.

FUNDING

This work was partially supported by National Key R&D Program of China under Grants (No. 2017YFC0108703), National Natural Science Foundation of China under Grants (Nos. 61871341, 61571380, 61811530021, 61672335, 61773124, 61802065, and 61601276), Project of Chinese Ministry of Science and Technology under Grants (No. 2016YFE0122700), Natural Science Foundation of Fujian Province of China under Grants (Nos. 2018J06018, 2018J01565, 2016J05205, and 2016J05157), Science and Technology Program of Xiamen under Grants (No. 3502Z20183053), Fundamental Research Funds for the Central Universities under Grants (No. 20720180056), and the Foundation of Educational and Scientific Research Projects for Young and Middle-aged Teachers of Fujian Province under Grants (Nos. JAT160074 and JAT170406).

REFERENCES

Avci, E., and Turkoglu, I. (2009). An intelligent diagnosis system based on principle component analysis and ANFIS for the heart valve diseases. *Expert Syst. Appl.* 36, 2873–2878. doi: 10.1016/j.eswa.2008.01.030

Babaoğlu, I., Fındık, O., and Bayrak, M. (2010). Effects of principle component analysis on assessment of coronary artery diseases using support vector machine. *Expert Syst. Appl.* 37, 2182–2185. doi: 10.1016/j.eswa.2009.07.055

Beheshti, I., Demirel, H., Matsuda, H., and Alzheimer's Disease Neuroimaging Initiative (2017). Classification of Alzheimer's disease and prediction of mild cognitive impairment-to-Alzheimer's conversion from structural magnetic resource imaging using feature ranking and a genetic algorithm. *Comput. Biol. Med.* 83, 109–119. doi: 10.1016/j.compbiomed.2017.02.011

Burns, A., and Iliffe, S. (2009). Alzheimer's disease. *BMJ* 338:b158. doi: 10.1136/bmj.b158

Cao, P., Shan, X., Zhao, D., Huang, M., and Zaiane, O. (2017). Sparse shared structure based multi-task learning for MRI based cognitive performance prediction of Alzheimer's disease. *Pattern Recognit.* 72, 219–235. doi: 10.1016/j.patcog.2017.07.018

Cheng, B., Liu, M., Zhang, D., Munsell, B. C., and Shen, D. (2015). Domain transfer learning for MCI conversion prediction. *IEEE Trans. Biomed. Eng.* 62, 1805–1817. doi: 10.1109/TBME.2015.2404809

Coupé, P., Eskildsen, S. F., Manjón, J. V., Fonov, V. S., Collins, D. L., and Alzheimer's Disease Neuroimaging Initiative (2012). Simultaneous segmentation and grading of anatomical structures for patient's classification: application to Alzheimer's disease. *Neuroimage* 59, 3736–3747. doi: 10.1016/j.neuroimage.2011.10.080

Coupe, P., Eskildsen, S. F., Manjon, J. V., Fonov, V. S., Pruessner, J. C., Allard, M., et al. (2012). Scoring by nonlocal image patch estimator for early detection of Alzheimer's disease. *Neuroimage* 1, 141–152. doi: 10.1016/j.nicl.2012.10.002

Cuingnet, R., Gerardin, E., Tessieras, J., Auzias, G., Lehéricy, S., Habert, M.-O., et al. (2011). Automatic classification of patients with Alzheimer's disease from structural MRI: a comparison of ten methods using the ADNI database. *Neuroimage* 56, 766–781. doi: 10.1016/j.neuroimage.2010.06.013

Desikan, R. S., Ségonne, F., Fischl, B., Quinn, B. T., Dickerson, B. C., Blacker, D., et al. (2006). An automated labeling system for subdividing the human cerebral cortex on MRI scans into gyral based regions of interest. *Neuroimage* 31, 968–980. doi: 10.1016/j.neuroimage.2006.01.021

Du, X., Qu, X., He, Y., and Guo, D. (2018). Single image super-resolution based on multi-scale competitive convolutional neural network. *Sensors* 18:789. doi: 10.3390/s18030789

Dukart, J., Schroeter, M. L., Mueller, K., and Alzheimer's Disease Neuroimaging. (2011). Age correction in dementia–matching to a healthy brain. *PLoS One* 6:e22193. doi: 10.1371/journal.pone.0022193

Efron, B., Hastie, T., Johnstone, I., and Tibshirani, R. (2004). Least angle regression. *Ann. Stat.* 32, 407–499. doi: 10.1214/009053604000000067

Eskildsen, S. F., Coupe, P., Fonov, V. S., Pruessner, J. C., Collins, D. L., and Alzheimer's Disease Neuroimaging (2015). Structural imaging biomarkers of Alzheimer's disease: predicting disease progression. *Neurobiol. Aging* 36(Suppl. 1), S23–S31. doi: 10.1016/j.neurobiolaging.2014.04.034

Fischl, B., and Dale, A. M. (2000). Measuring the thickness of the human cerebral cortex from magnetic resonance images. *Proc. Natl. Acad. Sci. U.S.A.* 97, 11050–11055. doi: 10.1073/pnas.200033797

Fischl, B., van der Kouwe, A., Destrieux, C., Halgren, E., Segonne, F., Salat, D. H., et al. (2004). Automatically parcellating the human cerebral cortex. *Cereb. Cortex* 14, 11–22. doi: 10.1093/cercor/bhg087

Giorgio, A., Santelli, L., Tomassini, V., Bosnell, R., Smith, S., De Stefano, N., et al. (2010). Age-related changes in grey and white matter structure throughout adulthood. *Neuroimage* 51, 943–951. doi: 10.1016/j.neuroimage.2010.03.004

Grundman, M., Petersen, R. C., Ferris, S. H., Thomas, R. G., Aisen, P. S., Bennett, D. A., et al. (2004). Mild cognitive impairment can be distinguished from Alzheimer disease and normal aging for clinical trials. *Arch. Neurol.* 61, 59–66. doi: 10.1001/archneur.61.1.59

Guerrero, R., Schmidt-Richberg, A., Ledig, C., Tong, T., Wolz, R., Rueckert, D., et al. (2016). Instantiated mixed effects modeling of Alzheimer's disease markers. *Neuroimage* 142, 113–125. doi: 10.1016/j.neuroimage.2016.06.049

Guerrero, R., Wolz, R., Rao, A., Rueckert, D., and Alzheimer's Disease Neuroimaging Initiative (2014). Manifold population modeling as a neuro-imaging biomarker: application to ADNI and ADNI-GO. *Neuroimage* 94, 275–286. doi: 10.1016/j.neuroimage.2014.03.036

Gulshan, V., Peng, L., Coram, M., Stumpe, M. C., Wu, D., Narayanaswamy, A., et al. (2016). Development and validation of a deep learning algorithm for detection of diabetic retinopathy in retinal fundus photographs. *JAMA* 316, 2402–2410. doi: 10.1001/jama.2016.17216

Han, X., Jovicich, J., Salat, D., van der Kouwe, A., Quinn, B., Czanner, S., et al. (2006). Reliability of MRI-derived measurements of human cerebral cortical thickness: the effects of field strength, scanner upgrade and manufacturer. *Neuroimage* 32, 180–194. doi: 10.1016/j.neuroimage.2006.02.051

Huang, G. B., Zhou, H., Ding, X., and Zhang, R. (2012). Extreme learning machine for regression and multiclass classification. *IEEE Trans. Syst. Man Cybern.* 42, 513–529. doi: 10.1109/TSMCB.2011.2168604

Karas, G. B., Scheltens, P., Rombouts, S. A., Visser, P. J., van Schijndel, R. A., Fox, N. C., et al. (2004). Global and local gray matter loss in mild cognitive impairment and Alzheimer's disease. *Neuroimage* 23, 708–716. doi: 10.1016/j.neuroimage.2004.07.006

Kukreja, S. L., Löfberg, J., and Brenner, M. J. (2006). A least absolute shrinkage and selection operator (LASSO) for nonlinear system identification. *IFAC Proc. Vol.* 39, 814–819. doi: 10.3182/20060329-3-AU-2901.00128

Ledig, C., Heckemann, R. A., Hammers, A., Lopez, J. C., Newcombe, V. F., Makropoulos, A., et al. (2015). Robust whole-brain segmentation: application to traumatic brain injury. *Med. Image Anal.* 21, 40–58. doi: 10.1016/j.media.2014.12.003

Leung, K. K., Barnes, J., Modat, M., Ridgway, G. R., Bartlett, J. W., Fox, N. C., et al. (2011). Brain MAPS: an automated, accurate and robust brain extraction technique using a template library. *Neuroimage* 55, 1091–1108. doi: 10.1016/j.neuroimage.2010.12.067

Li, F., Tran, L., Thung, K. H., Ji, S., Shen, D., and Li, J. (2015). A robust deep model for improved classification of AD/MCI patients. *IEEE J. Biomed. Health Inform.* 19, 1610–1616. doi: 10.1109/JBHI.2015.2429556

Liu, S., Liu, S., Cai, W., Che, H., Pujol, S., Kikinis, R., et al. (2015). Multimodal neuroimaging feature learning for multiclass diagnosis of Alzheimer's disease. *IEEE Trans. Biomed. Eng.* 62, 1132–1140. doi: 10.1109/TBME.2014.2372011

Lu, D., Popuri, K., Ding, G. W., Balachandar, R., and Beg, M. F. (2018a). Multimodal and multiscale deep neural networks for the early diagnosis of Alzheimer's disease using structural MR and FDG-PET images. *Sci. Rep.* 8:5697. doi: 10.1038/s41598-018-22871-z

Lu, D., Popuri, K., Ding, G. W., Balachandar, R., Beg, M. F., and Alzheimer's Disease Neuroimaging Initiative (2018b). Multiscale deep neural network based analysis of FDG-PET images for the early diagnosis of Alzheimer's disease. *Med. Image Anal.* 46, 26–34. doi: 10.1016/j.media.2018.02.002

Markesbery, W. R. (2010). Neuropathologic alterations in mild cognitive impairment: a review. *J. Alzheimers Dis.* 19, 221–228. doi: 10.3233/JAD-2010-1220

Moradi, E., Pepe, A., Gaser, C., Huttunen, H., Tohka, J., and Alzheimer's Disease Neuroimaging, I. (2015). Machine learning framework for early MRI-based Alzheimer's conversion prediction in MCI subjects. *Neuroimage* 104, 398–412. doi: 10.1016/j.neuroimage.2014.10.002

Nie, D., Wang, L., Gao, Y., and Shen, D. (2016). "Fully convolutional networks for multi-modality isointense infant brain image segmentation," in *Proceedings IEEE International Symposium Biomedical Imaging*, (Prague: IEEE), 1342–1345. doi: 10.1109/ISBI.2016.7493515

Nyul, L. G., and Udupa, J. K. (1999). On standardizing the MR image intensity scale. *Magn. Reson. Med.* 42, 1072–1081. doi: 10.1002/(SICI)1522-2594(199912)42:6<1072::AID-MRM11>3.0.CO;2-M

Ortiz, A., Munilla, J., Gorriz, J. M., and Ramirez, J. (2016). Ensembles of deep learning architectures for the early diagnosis of the Alzheimer's disease. *Int. J. Neural Syst.* 26:1650025. doi: 10.1142/S0129065716500258

Rajkomar, A., Lingam, S., Taylor, A. G., Blum, M., and Mongan, J. (2017). High-throughput classification of radiographs using deep convolutional neural networks. *J. Digit. Imaging* 30, 95–101. doi: 10.1007/s10278-016-9914-9

Rueckert, D., Sonoda, L. I., Hayes, C., Hill, D. L., Leach, M. O., and Hawkes, D. J. (1999). Nonrigid registration using free-form deformations: application to breast MR images. *IEEE Trans. Med. Imaging* 18, 712–721. doi: 10.1109/42.796284

Shi, J., Zheng, X., Li, Y., Zhang, Q., and Ying, S. (2018). Multimodal neuroimaging feature learning with multimodal stacked deep polynomial networks for diagnosis of Alzheimer's disease. *IEEE J. Biomed. Health Inform.* 22, 173–183. doi: 10.1109/JBHI.2017.2655720

Shin, H. C., Roth, H. R., Gao, M., Lu, L., Xu, Z., Nogues, I., et al. (2016). Deep convolutional neural networks for computer-aided detection: CNN architectures, dataset characteristics and transfer learning. *IEEE Trans. Med. Imaging* 35, 1285–1298. doi: 10.1109/TMI.2016.2528162

Singh, S., Srivastava, A., Mi, L., Caselli, R. J., Chen, K., Goradia, D., et al. (2017). "Deep-learning-based classification of FDG-PET data for Alzheimer's disease categories," in *Proceedings of the 13th International Conference on Medical Information Processing and Analysis*, (Bellingham, WA: International Society for Optics and Photonics). doi: 10.1117/12.2294537

Suk, H. I., Lee, S. W., Shen, D., and Alzheimer's Disease Neuroimaging (2014). Hierarchical feature representation and multimodal fusion with deep learning for AD/MCI diagnosis. *Neuroimage* 101, 569–582. doi: 10.1016/j.neuroimage.2014.06.077

Tong, T., Gao, Q., Guerrero, R., Ledig, C., Chen, L., Rueckert, D., et al. (2017). A novel grading biomarker for the prediction of conversion from mild cognitive impairment to Alzheimer's disease. *IEEE Trans. Biomed. Eng.* 64, 155–165. doi: 10.1109/TBME.2016.2549363

Tong, T., Wolz, R., Gao, Q., Hajnal, J. V., and Rueckert, D. (2013). Multiple instance learning for classification of dementia in brain MRI. *Med. Image Anal.* 16(Pt 2), 599–606. doi: 10.1007/978-3-642-40763-5_74

Usai, M. G., Goddard, M. E., and Hayes, B. J. (2009). LASSO with cross-validation for genomic selection. *Genet. Res.* 91, 427–436. doi: 10.1017/S0016672309990334

van de Pol, L. A., Hensel, A., van der Flier, W. M., Visser, P. J., Pijnenburg, Y. A., Barkhof, F., et al. (2006). Hippocampal atrophy on MRI in frontotemporal lobar degeneration and Alzheimer's disease. *J. Neurol. Neurosurg. Psychiatry* 77, 439–442. doi: 10.1136/jnnp.2005.075341

Wee, C. Y., Yap, P. T., and Shen, D. (2013). Prediction of Alzheimer's disease and mild cognitive impairment using cortical morphological patterns. *Hum. Brain Mapp.* 34, 3411–3425. doi: 10.1002/hbm.22156

Wu, P. H., Chen, C. C., Ding, J. J., Hsu, C. Y., and Huang, Y. W. (2013). Salient region detection improved by principle component analysis and boundary information. *IEEE Trans. Image Process.* 22, 3614–3624. doi: 10.1109/TIP.2013.2266099

Wyman, B. T., Harvey, D. J., Crawford, K., Bernstein, M. A., Carmichael, O., Cole, P. E., et al. (2013). Standardization of analysis sets for reporting results from ADNI MRI data. *Alzheimers Dement.* 9, 332–337. doi: 10.1016/j.jalz.2012.06.004

Xie, Q., Wang, S., Zhu, J., Zhang, X., and Alzheimer's Disease Neuroimaging Initiative (2016). Modeling and predicting AD progression by regression analysis of sequential clinical data. *Neurocomputing* 195, 50–55. doi: 10.1016/j.neucom.2015.07.145

Yamada, M., Jitkrittum, W., Sigal, L., Xing, E. P., and Sugiyama, M. (2014). High-dimensional feature selection by feature-wise kernelized Lasso. *Neural Comput.* 26, 185–207. doi: 10.1162/NECO_a_00537

Ye, J., Farnum, M., Yang, E., Verbeeck, R., Lobanov, V., Raghavan, N., et al. (2012). Sparse learning and stability selection for predicting MCI to AD conversion using baseline ADNI data. *BMC Neurol.* 12:46. doi: 10.1186/1471-2377-12-46

Young, J., Modat, M., Cardoso, M. J., Mendelson, A., Cash, D., Ourselin, S., et al. (2013). Accurate multimodal probabilistic prediction of conversion to Alzheimer's disease in patients with mild cognitive impairment. *Neuroimage* 2, 735–745. doi: 10.1016/j.nicl.2013.05.004

Zeng, N., Wang, Z., Zhang, H., Liu, W., and Alsaadi, F. E. (2016). Deep belief networks for quantitative analysis of a gold immunochromatographic strip. *Cogn. Comput.* 8, 684–692. doi: 10.1007/s12559-016-9404-x

Zeng, N., Zhang, H., Liu, W., Liang, J., and Alsaadi, F. E. (2017). A switching delayed PSO optimized extreme learning machine for short-term load forecasting. *Neurocomputing* 240, 175–182. doi: 10.1016/j.neucom.2017.01.090

Zeng, N., Zhang, H., Song, B., Liu, W., Li, Y., and Dobaie, A. M. (2018). Facial expression recognition via learning deep sparse autoencoders. *Neurocomputing* 273, 643–649. doi: 10.1016/j.neucom.2017.08.043

Zhang, D., Shen, D., and Alzheimer's Disease Neuroimaging Initiative (2012). Predicting future clinical changes of MCI patients using longitudinal and multimodal biomarkers. *PLoS One* 7:e33182. doi: 10.1371/journal.pone.0033182

Zhang, D., Wang, Y., Zhou, L., Yuan, H., Shen, D., and Alzheimer's Disease Neuroimaging (2011). Multimodal classification of Alzheimer's disease and mild cognitive impairment. *Neuroimage* 55, 856–867. doi: 10.1016/j.neuroimage.2011.01.008

17

Brain Differences Between Men and Women: Evidence From Deep Learning

Jiang Xin [1], *Yaoxue Zhang* [1], *Yan Tang* [1,2*] *and Yuan Yang* [3*]

[1] *School of Computer Science and Engineering, Central South University, Changsha, China,* [2] *Department of Neurology, Xiangya Hospital, Central South University, Changsha, China,* [3] *Department of Physical Therapy and Human Movement Sciences, Feinberg School of Medicine, Northwestern University, Chicago, IL, United States*

***Correspondence:**
Yan Tang
tangyan@csu.edu.cn
Yuan Yang
yuan.yang@northwestern.edu

Do men and women have different brains? Previous neuroimage studies sought to answer this question based on morphological difference between specific brain regions, reporting unfortunately conflicting results. In the present study, we aim to use a deep learning technique to address this challenge based on a large open-access, diffusion MRI database recorded from 1,065 young healthy subjects, including 490 men and 575 women healthy subjects. Different from commonly used 2D Convolutional Neural Network (CNN), we proposed a 3D CNN method with a newly designed structure including three hidden layers in cascade with a linear layer and a terminal Softmax layer. The proposed 3D CNN was applied to the maps of factional anisotropy (FA) in the whole-brain as well as specific brain regions. The entropy measure was applied to the lowest-level image features extracted from the first hidden layer to examine the difference of brain structure complexity between men and women. The obtained results compared with the results from using the Support Vector Machine (SVM) and Tract-Based Spatial Statistics (TBSS). The proposed 3D CNN yielded a better classification result (93.3%) than the SVM (78.2%) on the whole-brain FA images, indicating gender-related differences likely exist in the whole-brain range. Moreover, high classification accuracies are also shown in several specific brain regions including the left precuneus, the left postcentral gyrus, the left cingulate gyrus, the right orbital gyrus of frontal lobe, and the left occipital thalamus in the gray matter, and middle cerebellum peduncle, genu of corpus callosum, the right anterior corona radiata, the right superior corona radiata and the left anterior limb of internal capsule in the while matter. This study provides a new insight into the structure difference between men and women, which highlights the importance of considering sex as a biological variable in brain research.

Keywords: gender difference, deep learning, neural network, diffusion MRI, entropy

INTRODUCTION

Recent studies indicate that gender may have a substantial influence on human cognitive functions, including emotion, memory, perception, etc., (Cahill, 2006). Men and women appear to have different ways to encode memories, sense emotions, recognize faces, solve certain problems, and make decisions. Since the brain controls cognition and behaviors, these gender-related functional differences may be associated with the gender-specific structure of the brain (Cosgrove et al., 2007).

Diffusion tensor imaging (DTI) is an effective tool for characterizing nerve fibers architecture. By computing fractional anisotropy (FA) parameters in DTI, the anisotropy of nerve fibers can be quantitatively evaluated (Lasi et al., 2014). Differences in FA values are thought to associate with developmental processes of axon caliber, myelination, and/or fiber organization of nerve fibers pathways. By computing FA, researchers has revealed subtle changes related to normal brain development (Westlye et al., 2009), learning (Golestani et al., 2006), and healthy aging (Kochunov et al., 2007). Nevertheless, existing studies are yet to provide consistent results on exploring the difference of brain structure between men and women. Ingalhalikar et al. (2014) argued that the men have greater intra-hemispheric connection via the corpus callosum while women have greater interhemispheric connectivity. However, other studies reported no significant gender difference in brain structure (Raz et al., 2001; Salat et al., 2005). A recent critical opinion article suggested that more research is needed to investigate whether men and women really have different brain structures (Joel and Tarrasch, 2014).

Most existing DTI studies used the group-level statistical methods such as Tract-Based Spatial Statistics (TBSS) (Thatcher et al., 2010; Mueller et al., 2011; Shiino et al., 2017). However, recent studies indicated that machine learning techniques may provide us with a more powerful tool for analyzing brain images (Shen et al., 2010; Lu et al., 2017; Tang et al., 2018). Especially, deep learning can extract non-linear network structure, realize approximation of complex function, characterize distributed representation of input data, and demonstrate the powerful ability to learn the essential features of datasets based on a small size of samples (Zeng et al., 2016, 2018a; Tian et al., 2018; Wen et al., 2018). In particular, the deep convolutional neural network (CNN) uses the convolution kernels to extract the features of image and can find the characteristic spatial difference in brain images, which may promise a better result than using other conventional machine learning and statistical methods (Cole et al., 2017).

In this study, we performed CNN-based analyses on the FA images and extracts the features of the hidden layers to investigate the difference between man and woman brains. Different from commonly used 2D CNN model, we innovatively proposed a 3D CNN model with a new structure including 3 hidden layers, a linear layer and a softmax layer. Each hidden layer is comprised of a convolutional layer, a batch normalization layer, an activation layer and followed by a pooling layer. This novel CNN model allows using the whole 3D brain image (i.e., DTI) as the input to the model. The linear layer between the hidden layers and the softmax layer reduces the number of parameters and therefore avoids over-fitting problems.

MATERIALS AND METHODS

MRI Data Acquisition and Preprocessing

The database used in this work is from the Human Connectome Project (HCP) (Van Essen et al., 2013). This open-access database contains data from 1,065 subjects, including 490 men and 575 women. The ages range is from 22 to 36. This database represents a relatively large sample size compared to most neuroimaging studies. Using this open-access dataset allows replication and extension of this work by other researchers.

We performed DTI data preprocessing includes format conversion, b0 image extraction, brain extraction, eddy current correction, and tensor FA calculation. The first four steps were processed with the HCP diffusion pipeline, including diffusion weighting (bvals), direction (bvecs), time series, brain mask, a file (grad_dev.nii.gz) for gradient non-linearities during model fitting, and log files of EDDY processing. In the final step we use dtifit to calculate the tensors to get the FA, as well as mean diffusivity (MD), axial diffusivity (AD), and radial diffusivity (RD) values.

The original data were too large to train the model and it would cause RESOURCE EXAUSTED problem while training due to the insufficient of GPU memory. The GPU we used in the experiment is NVIDIAN TITAN_XP with 12G memory each. To solve the problem, we scaled the size of FA image to [58 × 70 × 58]. This procedure may lead to a better classification result, since a smaller size of the input image can provide a larger receptive field to the CNN model. In order to perform the image scaling, "dipy" (http://nipy.org/dipy/) was used to read the .nii data of FA. Then "ndimage" in the SciPy (http://www.scipy.org) was used to reduce the size of the data. Scaled data was written into the TFRecord files (http://www.tensorflow.org) with the corresponding labels. TFRecord file format is a simple record oriented binary format that is widely used in Tensorflow application for the training data to get a high performance of input efficiency. The labels were processed into the format of one-hot. We implemented a pipeline to read data asynchronously from TFRecord according to the interface specification provided by Tensorflow (Abadi et al., 2016). The pipeline included the reading of TFRecord files, data decoding, data type conversion, and reshape of data.

CNN Model

We did the experiments on a GPU work station, which has four NVIDIA TITAN Xp GPUs. The operation system of the GPU work station was Ubutnu16.04. We used FSL to preprocess the data. The CNN model was designed using the open source machine learning framework Tensorflow (Abadi et al., 2016).

Model Design

The commonly used CNN structures are based on 2D images. When using a 2D CNN to process 3D MRI images, it needs to map the original image from different directions to get 2D images, which will lose the spatial structure information of the image. In this study, we designed a 3D CNN with 3D convolutional kernels, which allowed us to extract 3D structural features from FA images. Besides, traditional CNN model usually uses several fully connected layers to connect the hidden layers and the output layer. The fully connected layer may be prone to the over-fitting problem in binary classification when the number of samples is limited (like our data). To address this problem, we used a linear layer to replace the fully connected layer. The linear layer integrates the outputs of hidden layers (i.e., a 3D matrix comprised of multiple featuremaps) into the inputs (i.e., a 1D vector) of the output layer which is a softmax classifier. Moreover, we performed a Batch Normalization (Ioffe and Szegedy, 2015) after each convolution operation. The Batch Normalization is used to avoid internal covariate shift problem in training the CNN model. Therefore, our designed model is a 3D "pure" CNN (3D PCNN). The architecture of the 3D PCNN model is shown in **Figure 1**. The 3D PCNN consists of three hidden layers, a linear layer and a softmax layer. Each of the hidden layer contains a convolutional layer, a Batch Normalization layer, an activation layer, a pooling layer with several feature maps as the outputs.

Convolutional layer

The process of convolutional layer is to convolve the input vector I with the convolution kernel K, represented by $I \otimes K$. The shape of the input vector in our 3D PCNN model was $[n, d, \ w, \ h, \ c]$, where d, w, h, c represent the depth, width, height and channel numbers (which is 1 for a grayscale image) of the input vector, respectively, and n is the batch size which is a hyperparameter that was set to 45 (an empirical value) in this paper. In the first layer, the input size was $58 \ \times 70 \times 58 \times 1$, which was the 3D size ($58 \times 70 \times 58$) of the input image plus a single channel (grayscale image). The shape of the convolution kernel was $[d_k, w_{k,} \ h_k, \ c_{in}, c_{out}]$, where $d_k, w_{k,} \ h_k$ represents the depth, width, and height of the convolution kernel, respectively. In all three hidden layers, the kernel size was set to3 $\times \ 3 \times \ 3$, which means that $d_k \ = \ w_k \ = \ \ h_k \ = \ 3$. The c_{in} is the number of input channels which is equal to the channel number of the input vector. The c_{out} is the number of output channels. As each kernel has an output channel, c_{out} is equal to the number of convolution kernels, and is also the same as the number of input channels for the next hidden layer. In all convolution layers, the moving stride of the kernel was set to 1 and padding mode was to "SAME."

Batch normalization layer

Batch normalization was performed after the convolutional layer. Batch normalization is a kind of training trick which normalizes the data of each mini-batch (with zero mean and variance of one) in the hidden layers of the network. To alleviate the gradient internal covariate shift phenomenon and speed up the CNN training, an Adam Gradient Decent method was used to train the model (Kingma and Ba, 2015).

Activation layer

After the batch normalization operation, an activation function was used to non-linearize the convolution result. The activation function we used in the model was the Rectified linear unit, ReLU (Nair and Hinton, 2010).

Pooling layer

Pooling layer was added after the activation layer. Pooling layers in the CNN summarize the outputs of neighboring groups of neurons in the same kernel map (Krizhevsky et al., 2012). Max-pooling method was used in this layer.

The outputs of each hidden layer were feature maps, which were the features extracted from the input images to the hidden layer. The outputs from the previous hidden layer were the inputs to the next layer. In our model, the first hidden layer generated 32 feature maps, the second hidden layer produced 64 feature maps, and the third hidden layer yielded 128 feature maps. Finally, we integrated the last 128 feature maps into the input of the softmax layer through a linear layer, and then got the final classification results from the softmax layer.

In our model, the input $X \ \in \ \{x^{(1)}, \ x^{(2)}, \ \ldots \ , \ x^{(n)}\}$, $x^{(i)}$ was the *ith* subject's FA value. $Y \ \in \ \{y^{(1)}, \ y^{(2)}, \ \ldots \ , \ y^{(n)}\}$, $y^{(i)}$ was the *ith* subject's label that were processed to one-hot vector where [1 0] represents man and [0 1] woman. We used $h(\theta, \ x)$ to represent the proposed 3D PCNN model. Then we had:

$$\hat{y} = h(\theta, x) \quad (1)$$

where $\hat{y}$ represents the predicted value obtained using the 3D PCNN on a sample x.

Parameters Optimization

The initial values of the weights of the convolution kernels were random values selected from a truncated normal distribution with standard deviation of 0.1. We defined a cost function to adjust these weights based on the softmax cross entropy (Dunne and Campbell, 1997):

$$J(\theta, x) = -\sum_{i=1}^{n} \hat{y}^{(i)} \log P\left(\hat{y}^{(i)} = y^{(i)} \,\middle|\, x = x^{(i)} \right) \quad (2)$$

As such, the task of adjusting the weight value became an optimization problem with $J(\theta, x)$ as the optimization goal, where a small penalty was given if the classification result was correct, and vice versa. We used the Adam Gradient Descent (Kingma and Ba, 2015) optimization algorithm to achieve this goal in the model training. All parameters in the Adam algorithm were set to the empirical values recommended by Kingma and Ba (2015), i.e., learning rate was $\alpha \ = \ 0.001$, exponential decay rates for the moment estimates were $\beta_1 \ = \ 0.9$, $\beta_1 \ = \ 0.999$, $\varepsilon \ = \ 10^{-8}$.

Cross-Validation

To ensure the independent training and testing in the cross-validation. The process of cross-validation is shown in **Figure 2**. We implemented a two-loop nested cross-validation scheme (Varoquaux et al., 2017). We divided the data set into three parts, i.e., 80% of the data as the training set for model training, 10% as the verification set for parameter selection, and 10% as the testing set for evaluating the generalization ability of the model. To eliminate the random error of model training, we run 10 fold cross validation and then took the average of classification accuracies as the final result.

Features in First Hidden Layer

CNN has an advantage that it can extract key features by itself (Zeng et al., 2018c). However, these features may be difficult to interpret since they are highly abstract features. Thus, in this

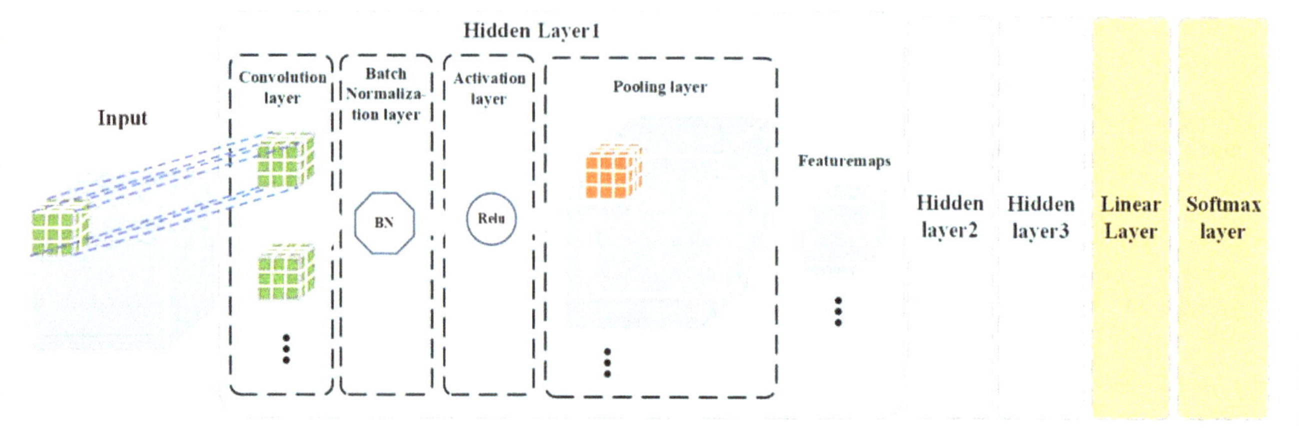

FIGURE 1 | 3D PCNN architecture.

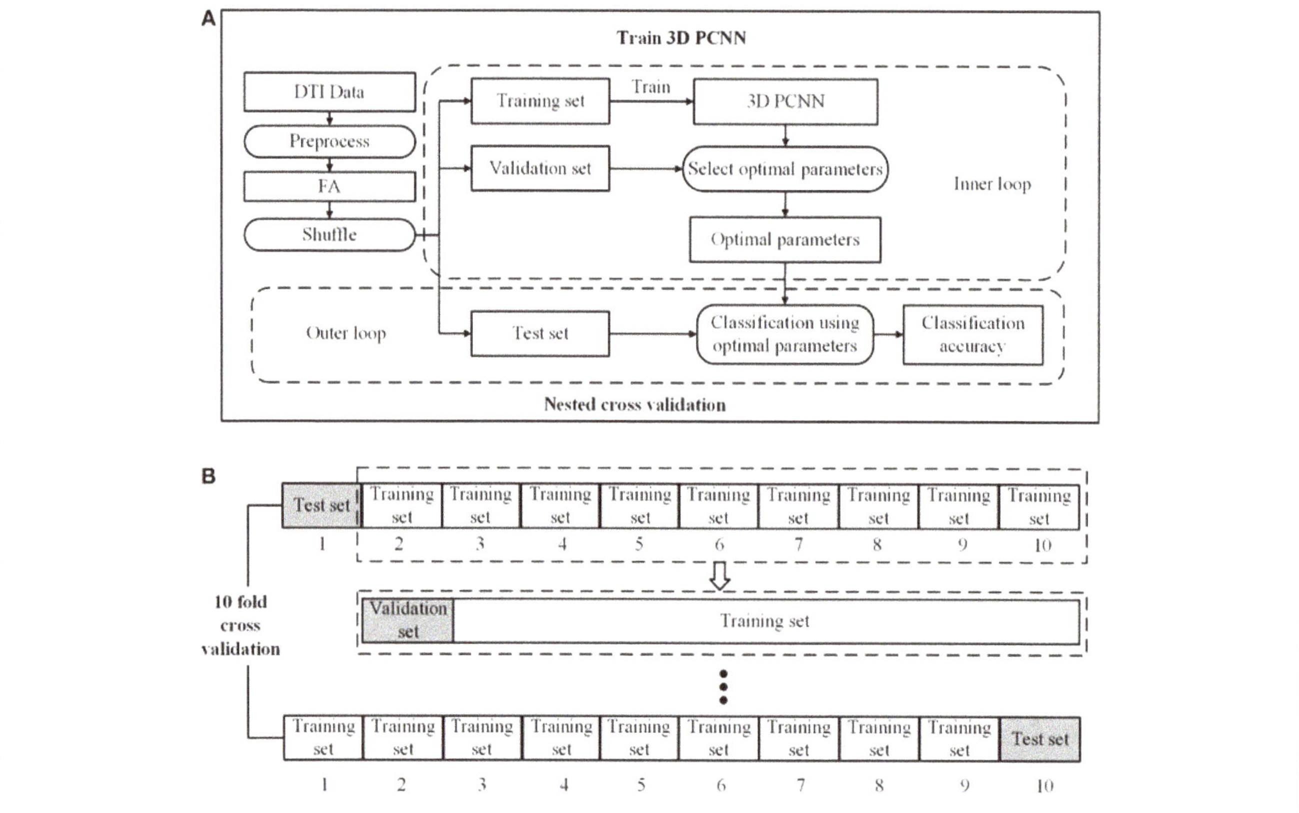

FIGURE 2 | Model training and nested cross validation. **(A)** General overview. **(B)** 10 fold cross validation.

study, we only analyzed the features obtained in the first hidden layer, since they are the direct outputs from the convolution on the grayscale FA images. In this case, the convolution operation of the first layer is equivalent to applying a convolution kernel based spatial filter on the FA images. The obtained features are less abstractive than those from the second and three hidden layers. There are totally 32 features in the first hidden layer. These features are the lowest-level features which may represent the structural features of FA images. We firstly computed the mean of voxel values across all subjects in each group (man vs. woman) for each feature and then evaluated their group-level difference using a two-sample t-test. Besides, we also computed the entropy on each feature for each individual:

$$H = -\sum_{i=0}^{255} p_i \log p_i \tag{3}$$

where p_i indicates the frequency of pixel with value i appears in the image. The entropy of each feature likely indicates the complexity of brain structural encoded in that feature.

We also performed a two-sample t-test on entropy results to explore the differences between men and women. A strict Bonferroni correction was applied for multiple comparisons with the threshold of $0.05/32 = 1.56 \times 10^{-3}$ to remove spurious significance.

Discriminative Power of Brain Regions

In order to determine which brain regions may play important role in gender-related brain structural differences, we repeated the same 3D PCNN-based classification on each specific brain region. We segmented each FA image into 246 gray matter regions of interests (ROIs) according to the Human Brainnetome Atlas (Fan et al., 2016) and 48 white matter ROIs according to the ICBM-DTI-81 White-Matter Labels Atlas (Mori et al., 2005). The classification accuracy was then obtained for each ROIs. A higher accuracy indicates a more important role of that ROI in gender-related difference. A map was then obtained based on the classification accuracies of different ROIs to show their distribution in the brain.

Comparisons With Tract Based Spatial Statistics and Support Vector Machine

To justify the effectiveness of our method, the Tract Based Spatial Statistics (TBSS) and Support Vector Machine (SVM) were applied to our dataset as comparisons, since these are two popular methods for data analysis in neuroimaging studies (Bach et al., 2014; Zeng et al., 2018b). We compared the results in following two conditions: (1) We used the SVM as the classifier while keeping the same preprocessing procedure in order to compare its results with our 3D PCNN method. We flatten each sample from the 3D FA matrix into a vector, and then fed the SVM with the vector. (2) We used the TBSS to identify the brain regions where are shown the statistically significant gender-related difference.

RESULTS

Classification Results on the Whole-Brain FA Images

Using our 3D PCNN methods on the whole-brain FA images, we can well-distinguish men and women with the classification accuracy of 93.3%. This result is much better than using the SVM, whose classification accuracy is only 78.2%.

As comparisons, we also used MD, AD, and RD to repeat the same analysis. The classification accuracy of MD is 65.8%, AD is 69.9%, and RD is 67.8%. All of them are lower than the classification accuracy obtained by using FA.

Feature Analysis in the First Hidden Layer of 3D PCNN

The result of two-sample t-test of 32 features of men and women shows that there are 25 features had significant gender differences including 13 features that women have larger values and 12 features that men have larger values (see **Figure 3**). Interestingly, men have significantly higher entropy than women for all features (see **Figure 4**).

Classification on Each Specific ROI

TBSS could not detect any statistically significant gender-related difference in this dataset. However, using 3D PCNN, we did find gender-related differences in all ROIs in the both gray and white matters, as the classification accuracies (>75%) are much higher than the chance level (50%) for all ROIs. The maps of classification accuracies for different ROIs are shown in **Figure 5**. The detail classification results are provided in the supplement (see **Table S1** for gray matter and **Table S2** for white matter). In the gray matter, the top 5 regions with highest classification accuracies are the left precuneus (Broadman area, BA 31, 87.2%), the left postcentral gyrus (BA 1/2/3 trunk region, 87.2%), the left cingulate gyrus (BA 32 subgenual area, 87.2%), the right orbital gyrus of frontal lobe (BA 13, 87.1%) and the left occipital thalamus (86.9%). In the white matter, the top 5 regions with highest classification accuracies are middle cerebellum peduncle (89.7%), genu of corpus callosum (88.4%), the right anterior corona radiata (88.3%), the right superior corona radiata (86%), and the left anterior limb of internal capsule (85.4%).

DISCUSSIONS

Classification on the Whole-Brain FA

The proposed 3D PCNN model achieved 93.3% classification accuracy in the whole-brain FA. The high classification accuracy rate indicates that the proposed model can accurately find the brain structure difference between men and women, which is the basis of subsequent feature analysis and subreginal analysis. Most existing classification, regression, and other machine learning methods are shallow learning algorithms, such as the SVM, Boosting, maximum entropy, and Logistic Regression. When complex functions need to be expressed, the models obtained by these algorithms will then have a limitation with small size of samples and limited computational resources. Thus, the generalization ability will be deteriorated as we demonstrated in the results from the SVM. The benefit of deep learning algorithms, using multiple layers in the artificial neural network, is that one can represent complex functions with few parameters. The CNN is one of the widely used deep learning algorithms. In compared to the method like SVM, which is just a classifier, 3D CNN is a method that can extract the 3D spatial structure features of the input image. Through constructing the 3D PCNN model, we extracted highly abstract features from FA images, which may, thusly, improve the classification accuracy. FA describes the partial anisotropy index, which indicates the difference between one direction and others (Feldman et al., 2010). It can reflect alterations in various tissue properties including axonal size, axonal packing density, and degree of myelination (Chung et al., 2016). In this study, we also run the same analysis using MD, AD, and RD images for comparisons. All their results are lower than that of FA, indicating that using FA is more effective to find the

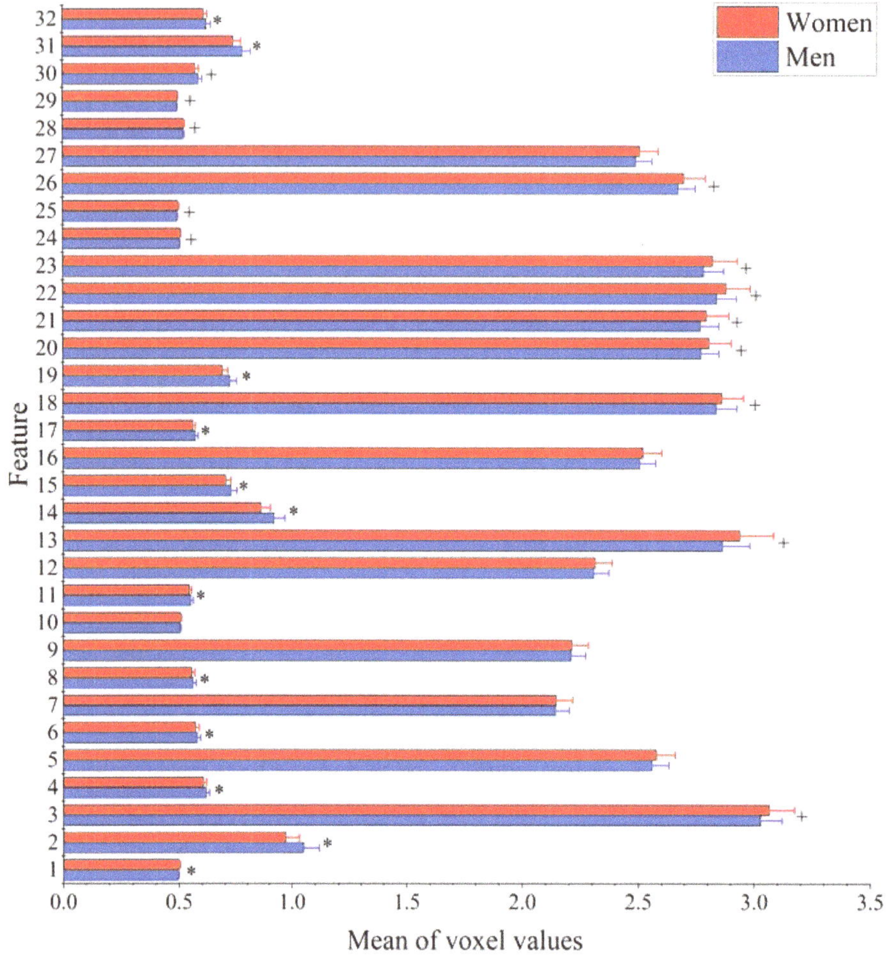

FIGURE 3 | Between-group differences of 32 features in voxel values. The mean (bar height) and standard deviation (error bars) of voxel values across all subjects in each group were evaluated for each feature. Their group-level difference was examined using a two-sample *t*-test. Bonferroni correction was applied for multiple comparisons with the threshold equal to $0.05/32 = 1.56 \times 10^{-3}$ to remove spurious significance. The features with significantly larger mean voxel values for men are marked out with*, while features with significantly larger mean voxel values for women are indicated by +.

structure difference between men and women's brain than using other images.

Feature Analysis in the First Hidden Layer of 3D PCNN

The degree of the macroscopic diffusion anisotropy is often quantified by the FA (Lasi et al., 2014). Previous studies found that wider skeleton of white matter in woman's brain but wider region of gray matter in man's brain (Witelson et al., 1995; Zaidi, 2010; Gong et al., 2011; Menzler et al., 2011). These mean that men appear to have more gray matter, made up of active neurons, while women may have more white matter for the neuronal communication between different areas of the brain. Furthermore, a recent study found that men had higher FA values than women in middle aged to elderly (between 44 and 77 years old) people by using a statistical analysis (Ritchie et al., 2018). This study focuses on the young healthy individuals with the age range between 22 and 36 years old. The structural features extracted from 3D PCNN reflect the brain structure difference between men and women. In the first hidden layer of 3D PCNN model, we found 25 features that have significant difference between men and women in voxels value. Moreover, using entropy measure, we found that men's brains likely have more complex features as reflected by significantly higher entropy. These results indicated that the gender-related differences likely exist in the whole-brain range including both white and gray matters.

Most Discriminative Brain Regions

Using FA images from each specific brain region as the input to the 3D PCNN, we found all tested brain regions may have gender-related difference, though the TBSS analysis cannot detect these differences. The brain regions with high classification accuracies include the left precuneus (Broadman area, BA 31, 87.2%), the left postcentral gyrus (BA 1/2/3 trunk region, 87.2%), the left cingulate gyrus (BA 32 subgenual area, 87.2%), the right orbital

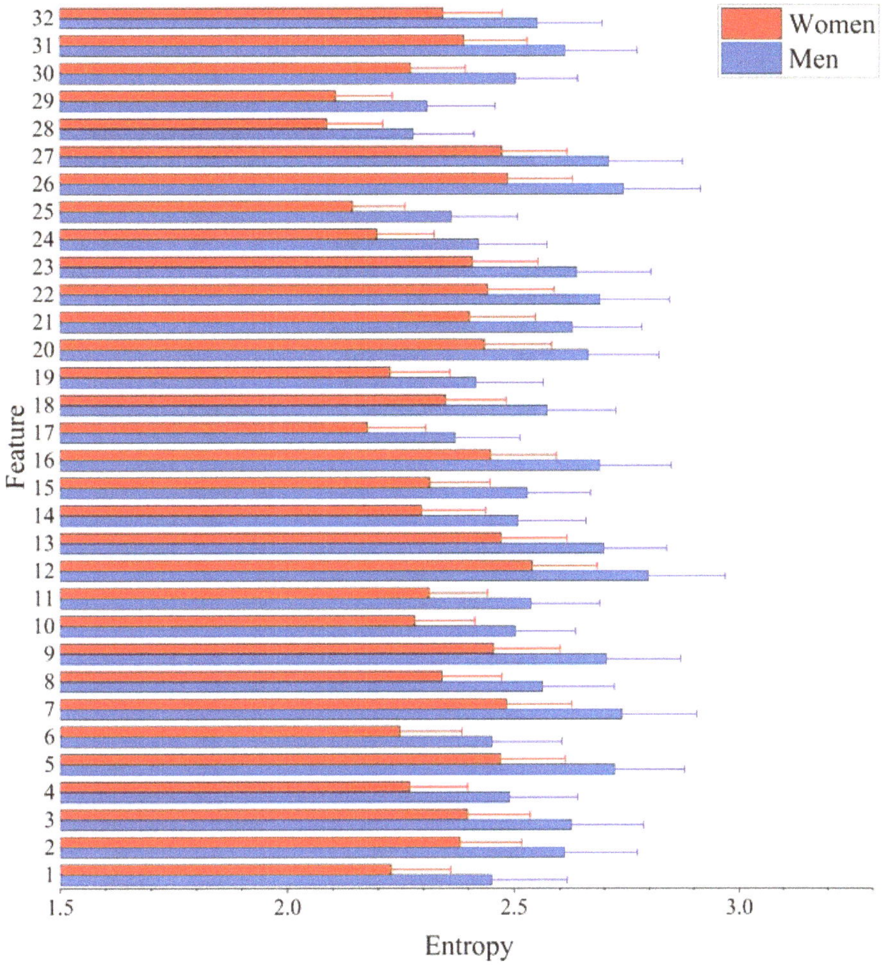

FIGURE 4 | Between-group differences of 32 features in entropy values. The mean (bar height) and standard deviation (error bars) of entropy value were computed across all subjects in each group for each feature. Their group-level difference was evaulated using a two-sample t-test. Bonferroni correction was applied for multiple comparisons with the threshold equal to $0.05/32 = 1.56 \times 10^{-3}$ to remove spurious significance. The entropy values are significantly larger in men than in women for features.

gyrus of frontal lobe (BA 13, 87.1%), and the left occipital thalamus (86.9%) in the gray matter, and middle cerebellum peduncle (89.7%), genu of corpus callosum (88.4%), the right anterior corona radiata (88.3%), the right superior corona radiata (86%), and the left anterior limb of internal capsule (85.4%).

The gender-related morphological difference at the corpus callosum has been previously reported, which may be associated with interhemispheric interaction (Sullivan et al., 2001; Luders et al., 2003; Prendergast et al., 2015). However, likely due to the limitation of applied methods, not all previous studies have reported this difference (Abe et al., 2002). Those likely results in the inconsistent findings were across different studies. Through 3D PCNN model, our results confirm that there is likely a morphological difference at the genu of corpus callosum between man and women.

The middle cerebellum peduncle is the brain area connected to the pons and receiving the inputs mainly from the pontine nuclei (Glickstein and Doron, 2008), which are the nuclei of the pons involved in motor activity (Wiesendanger et al., 1979). Raz et al. (2001) found larger volume in the cerebellum of men than women. The cerebellar cells release diffusible substances that promote the survival of thalamic neurons (Tracey et al., 1980; Hisanaga and Sharp, 1990). Previous studies have reported gender-difference differences in the basic glucose metabolism in the thalamus of young subjects between the ages of 20 and 40 (Fujimoto et al., 2008). Beside the thalamus and cerebellum, the postcentral gyrus was also found in our results as the brain region with high classification accuracy. Thus, there is very likely a gender-related difference in the cerebellar-thalamic-cortical circuitry. This difference may also be related to the reported gender differences in neurological degenerative diseases such as Parkinson's Disease (Lyons et al., 1998; Dluzen and Mcdermott, 2000; Miller and Cronin-Golomb, 2010), where the pathological changes are usually found in the cerebellar-thalamic-cortical circuitry.

The findings of the current study also indicated the gender-related difference in the limbic-thalamo-cortical circuitry. Anterior corona radiata is part of the limbic-thalamo-cortical

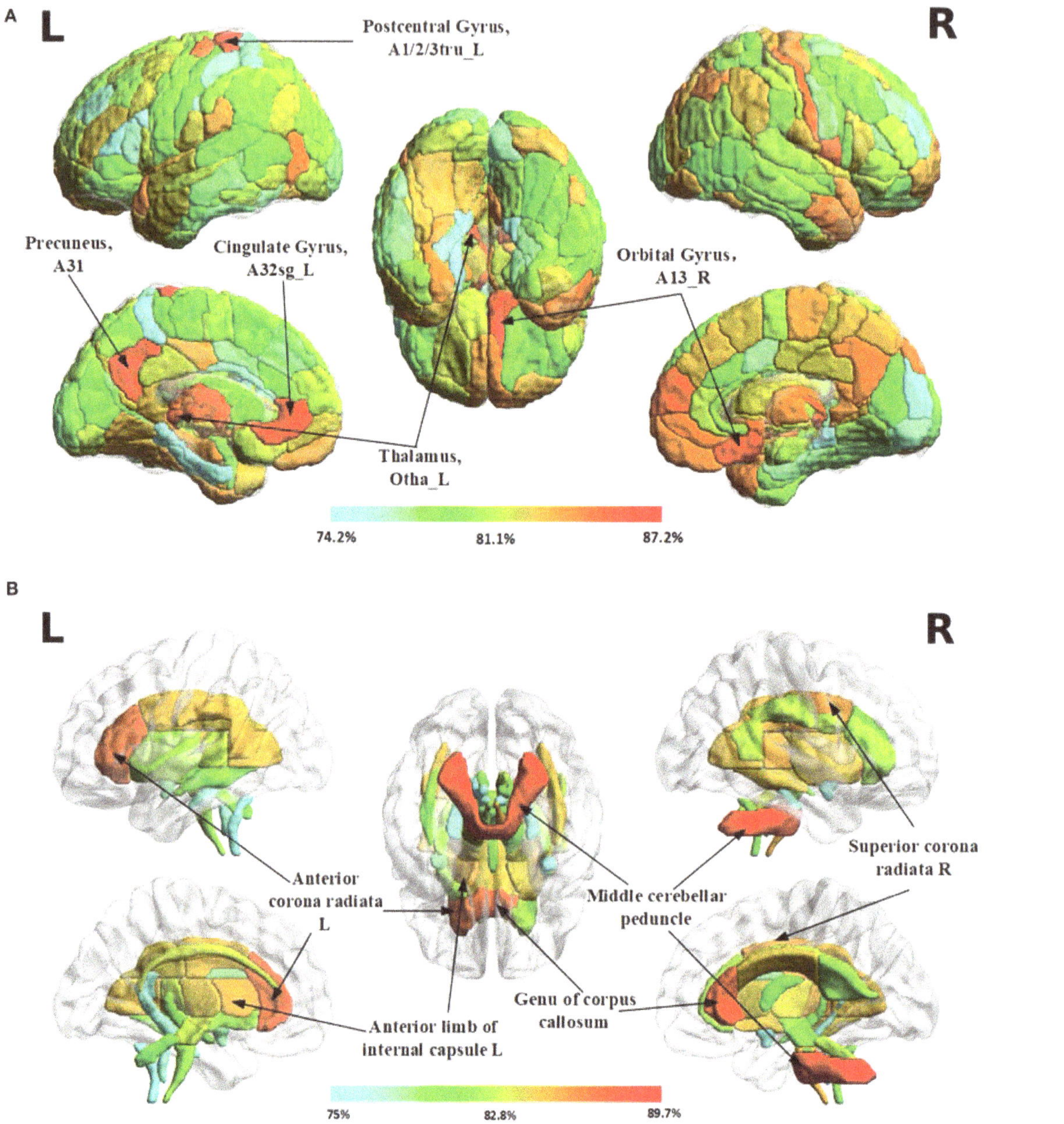

FIGURE 5 | Maps of classification accuracies for different ROIs in the gray and white matter of the brain. **(A)** Results in 246 gray matter regions of interests (ROIs) according to the Human Brainnetome Atlas **(B)** Results in 48 white matter ROIs according to the ICBM-DTI-81 White-Matter Labels Atlas.

circuitry and includes thalamic projections from the internal capsule to the prefrontal cortex. White matter changes in the anterior corona radiata could result in many of the cognitive and emotion regulation disturbances (Drevets, 2001). The orbital gyrus of frontal cortex gray matter areas and cingulate gyrus have also been reported to be associated with the emotion regulation system (Fan et al., 2005). Thus, the gender-related difference in the limbic-thalamo-cortical circuitry may explain the gender differences in thalamic activation during the processing of emotional stimuli or unpleasant linguistic information concerning interpersonal difficulties as demonstrated by previous fMRI (Lee and Kondziolka, 2005; Shirao et al., 2005).

In summary, by using the designed 3D PCNN algorithm, we confirmed that the gender-related differences exist in the whole-brain FA images as well as in each specific brain regions. These gender-related brain structural differences might be related to gender differences in cognition, emotional control as well as neurological disorders.

AUTHOR CONTRIBUTIONS

JX, YT, and YY contributed to the conception and design of the study. YT, JX, and YZ performed data analysis. YT and JX drafted manuscript. YT and YY participated in editing the manuscript.

FUNDING

JX and YZ are supported by 111 Project (No. B18059). YT is supported by grant 2016JJ4090 from the Natural Science Foundation of Hunan Province and grants 2017T100613 and 2016M592452 from the China Postdoctoral Science Foundation, China. YY is supported by the Dixon Translational Research Grants Initiative (PI: YY) from the Northwestern Memorial Foundation (NMF) and the Northwestern University Clinical and Translational Sciences (NUCATS) Institute.

REFERENCES

Abadi, M., Barham, P., Chen, J., Chen, Z., Davis, A., Dean, J., et al. (2016). "Tensorflow: a system for large-scale machine learning," in *12th USENIX Symposium on Operating Systems Design and Implementation (OSDI 16)*, (Savannah, GA), 265–283.

Abe, O., Aoki, S., Hayashi, N., Yamada, H., Kunimatsu, A., Mori, H., et al. (2002). Normal aging in the central nervous system: quantitative MR diffusion-tensor analysis. *Neurobiol. Aging* 23, 433–441. doi: 10.1016/S0197-4580(01)00318-9

Bach, M., Laun, F. B., Leemans, A., Tax, C. M., Biessels, G. J., Stieltjes, B., et al. (2014). Methodological considerations on tract-based spatial statistics (TBSS). *Neuroimage* 100, 358–369. doi: 10.1016/j.neuroimage.2014.06.021

Cahill, L. (2006). Why sex matters for neuroscience. *Nat. Rev. Neurosci.* 7, 477–484. doi: 10.1038/nrn1909

Chung, A. W., Seunarine, K. K., and Clark, C. A. (2016). NODDI reproducibility and variability with magnetic field strength: a comparison between 1.5 T and 3 T. *Human Brain Mapp.* 37, 4550–4565. doi: 10.1002/hbm.23328

Cole, J. H., Poudel R. P. K., Tsagkrasoulis, D., Mwa, C., Steves, C., Spector, T. D., et al. (2017). Predicting brain age with deep learning from raw imaging data results in a reliable and heritable biomarker. *Neuroimage* 163, 115–124. doi: 10.1016/j.neuroimage.2017.07.059

Cosgrove, K. P., Mazure, C. M., and Staley, J. K. (2007). Evolving knowledge of sex differences in brain structure, function, and chemistry. *Biol. Psychiatry* 62, 847–855. doi: 10.1016/j.biopsych.2007.03.001

Dluzen, D. E., and Mcdermott, J. L., (2000). Gender differences in neurotoxicity of the nigrostriatal dopaminergic system: implications for Parkinson's disease. *J. Gender Spec. Med.* 3, 36–42.

Drevets, W. C. (2001). Neuroimaging and neuropathological studies of depression: implications for the cognitive-emotional features of mood disorders. *Curr. Opin. Neurobiol.* 11, 240–249. doi: 10.1016/S0959-4388(00)00203-8

Dunne, R. A., and Campbell, N. A. (1997). "On the pairing of the softmax activation and cross-entropy penalty functions and the derivation of the softmax activation function," in *Proc. 8th Aust. Conf. on the Neural Networks*, (Melbourne, VIC: Citeseer), 185.

Fan, J., Mccandliss, B. D., Fossella, J., Flombaum, J. I., and Posner, M. I. (2005). The activation of attentional networks. *Neuroimage* 26, 471–479. doi: 10.1016/j.neuroimage.2005.02.004

Fan, L., Li H., Zhuo, J., Zhang, Y., Wang, J., Chen, L., et al. (2016). The human brainnetome atlas: a new brain atlas based on connectional architecture. *Cereb. Cortex* 26, 3508–3526. doi: 10.1093/cercor/bhw157

Feldman, H. M., Yeatman, J. D., Lee, E. S., Barde, L. H., and Gaman-Bean, S. (2010). Diffusion tensor imaging: a review for pediatric researchers and clinicians. *J. Dev. Behav. Pediatr.* 31, 346–356. doi: 10.1097/DBP.0b013e3181dcaa8b

Fujimoto, T., Matsumoto, T., Fujita, S., Takeuchi, K., Nakamura, K., Mitsuyama, Y., et al. (2008). Changes in glucose metabolism due to aging and gender-related differences in the healthy human brain. *Psychiatry Res.* 164, 58–72. doi: 10.1016/j.pscychresns.2006.12.014

Glickstein, M., and Doron, K. (2008). Cerebellum: connections and functions. *Cerebellum* 7, 589–594. doi: 10.1007/s12311-008-0074-4

Golestani, N., Molko, N., Dehaene, S., Lebihan, D., and Pallier, C. (2006). Brain structure predicts the learning of foreign speech sounds. *Cereb. Cortex* 17, 575–582. doi: 10.1093/cercor/bhk001

Gong, G., He, Y., and Evans, A. C. (2011). Brain connectivity: gender makes a difference. *Neuroscientist* 17, 575–591. doi: 10.1177/1073858410386492

Hisanaga, K., and Sharp, F. R. (1990). Diffusible neurotrophic factors for thalamic neurons are released from target neocortex and non-target cerebellum. *Progr. Brain Res.* 82, 67–71. doi: 10.1016/S0079-6123(08)62591-1

Ingalhalikar, M., Smith, A., Parker, D., Satterthwaite, T. D., Elliott, M. A., Ruparel, K., et al. (2014). Sex differences in the structural connectome of the human brain. *Proc. Natl. Acad. Sci. U.S.A.* 111, 823–828. doi: 10.1073/pnas.1316909110

Ioffe, S., and Szegedy, C. (2015). "Batch normalization: accelerating deep network training by reducing internal covariate shift," in *Proceedings of the 32nd International Conference on Machine Learning*, Vol. 37 (Lille), 448–456.

Joel, D., and Tarrasch, R. (2014). On the mis-presentation and misinterpretation of gender-related data: the case of Ingalhalikar's human connectome study. *Proc. Natl. Acad. Sci. U.S.A.* 111, E637–E637. doi: 10.1073%2Fpnas.1323319111

Kingma, D. P., and Ba, L. J. (2015). "Adam: A method for stochastic optimization," in *Proceedings of the 3rd International Conference on Learning Representations* (San Diego, CA).

Kochunov, P. M., Thompson, P., Lancaster, J. L., Bartzokis, G., Smith, S., Coyle, T., et al. (2007). Relationship between white matter fractional anisotropy and other indices of cerebral health in normal aging: tract-based spatial statistics study of aging. *Neuroimage* 35, 478–487. doi: 10.1016/j.neuroimage.2006.12.021

Krizhevsky, A., Sutskever, I., and Hinton, G. E. (2012). "Imagenet classification with deep convolutional neural networks," in *Advances in Neural Information Processing Systems 25 (NIPS 2012)* (Lake Tahoe, NV), 1097–1105.

Lasi, S., Szczepankiewicz, F., Eriksson, S., Nilsson, M., and Topgaard, D. (2014). Microanisotropy imaging: quantification of microscopic diffusion anisotropy and orientational order parameter by diffusion MRI with magic-angle spinning of the q-vector. *Front. Phys.* 2:11. doi: 10.3389/fphy.2014.00011

Lee, J. Y., and Kondziolka, D. (2005). Thalamic deep brain stimulation for management of essential tremor. *J. Neurosurgery* 103, 400–403. doi: 10.3171/jns.2005.103.3.0400

Lu, Y., Yi, S., Zeng, N., Liu, Y., and Zhang, Y. (2017). Identification of rice diseases using deep convolutional neural networks. *Neurocomputing* 267, 378–384. doi: 10.1016/j.neucom.2017.06.023

Luders, E., Rex, D. E., Narr, K. L., Woods, R. P., Jancke, L., Thompson, P. M., et al. (2003). Relationships between sulcal asymmetries and corpus callosum size: gender and handedness effects. *Cereb. Cortex* 13, 1084–1093. doi: 10.1093/cercor/13.10.1084

Lyons, K. E., Hubble, J. P., Troster, A. I., Pahwa, R., and Koller, W. C. (1998). Gender differences in Parkinson's disease. *Clin. Neuropharmacol.* 21, 118–121.

Menzler, K., Belke, M., Wehrmann, E., Krakow, K., Lengler, U., Jansen, A., et al. (2011). Men and women are different: diffusion tensor imaging reveals sexual dimorphism in the microstructure of the thalamus, corpus callosum and cingulum. *Neuroimage* 54, 2557–2562. doi: 10.1016/j.neuroimage.2010.11.029

Miller, I. N., and Cronin-Golomb, A. (2010). Gender differences in Parkinson's disease: clinical characteristics and cognition. *Movem. Disord.* 25, 2695–2703. doi: 10.1002/mds.23388

Mori, S., Al, S. M., Wakana, S., and Zijl, V. (2005). *MRI Atlas of Human White Matter.* London, UK: Elsevier/Academic Press.

Mueller K., Anwander A., Möller, H. E., Horstmann, A., Lepsien, J., Busse, F. et al. (2011). Sex-dependent influences of obesity on cerebral white matter investigated by diffusion-tensor imaging. *PloS ONE* 6:e18544. doi: 10.1371/journal.pone.0018544

Nair, V., and Hinton, G. E. (2010). "Rectified linear units improve restricted boltzmann machines," in *Proceedings of the 27th International Conference on Machine Learning (ICML-10)* (Haifa), 807–814.

Prendergast, D. M., Ardekani, B., Ikuta, T., John, M., Peters, B., Derosse, P., et al. (2015). Age and sex effects on corpus callosum morphology across the lifespan. *Human Brain Mapp.* 36, 2691–2702. doi: 10.1002/hbm.22800

Raz, N., Gunning-Dixon, F., Head, D., Williamson, A., and Acker, J. D. (2001). Age and sex differences in the cerebellum and the ventral pons: a prospective MR study of healthy adults. *Am. J. Neuroradiol.* 22, 1161–1167.

Ritchie, S. J., Cox, S. R., Shen, X., Lombardo, M. V., Reus, L. M., Alloza, C., et al. (2018). Sex differences in the adult human brain: evidence from 5216 UK Biobank participants. *Cereb. Cortex* 28, 2959–2975. doi: 10.1093/cercor/bhy109

Salat, D. H., Tuch, D. S., Greve, D. N., Van Der Kouwe, A. J., Hevelone, N. D., Zaleta, A. K., et al. (2005). Age-related alterations in white matter microstructure measured by diffusion tensor imaging. *Neurobiol. Aging* 26, 1215–1227. doi: 10.1016/j.neurobiolaging.2004.09.017

Shen, H., Wang, L., Liu, Y., and Hu, D. (2010). Discriminative analysis of resting-state functional connectivity patterns of schizophrenia using low dimensional embedding of fMRI. *Neuroimage* 49, 3110–3121. doi: 10.1016/j.neuroimage.2009.11.011

Shiino, A., Chen, Y. W., Tanigaki, K., Yamada, A., Vigers, P., Watanabe, T., et al. (2017). Sex-related difference in human white matter volumes studied: inspection of the corpus callosum and other white matter by VBM. *Sci. Rep.* 7:39818. doi: 10.1038/srep39818

Shirao, N., Okamoto, Y., Okada, G., Ueda, K., and Yamawaki, S. (2005). Gender differences in brain activity toward unpleasant linguistic stimuli concerning interpersonal relationships: an fMRI study. *Eur. Arch. Psychiatr. Clin.* 255, 327–333. doi: 10.1007/s00406-005-0566-x

Sullivan, E. V., Rosenbloom, M. J., Desmond, J. E., and Pfefferbaum, A. (2001). Sex differences in corpus callosum size: relationship to age and intracranial size. *Neurobiol. Aging* 22, 603–611. doi: 10.1016/S0197-4580(01)00232-9

Tang, Y., Liu, B., Yang, Y., Wang, C.-M., Meng, L., Tang, B.-S., et al. (2018). Identifying mild-moderate Parkinson's disease using whole-brain functional connectivity. *Clin. Nerophysiol.* 129, 2507–2516. doi: 10.1016/j.clinph.2018.09.006

Thatcher, D. L., Pajtek, S., Chung, T., Terwilliger, R. A., and Clark, D. B. (2010). Gender differences in the relationship between white matter organization and adolescent substance use disorders. *Drug Alcohol. Depend.* 110, 55–61. doi: 10.1016/j.drugalcdep.2010.02.004

Tian, R., Yang, Y., Van Der Helm, FCT and Dewald, JPA. (2018). A novel approach for modeling neural responses to joint perturbations using the NARMAX method and a hierarchical neural network. *Front. Comput. Neurosci.* 12:96. doi: 10.3389/fncom.2018.00096

Tracey, D., Asanuma, C. G., Jones, E., and Porter, R. (1980). Thalamic relay to motor cortex: Afferent pathways from brain stem, cerebellum, and spinal cord in monkeys. *J. Neurophysiol.* 44, 532–554. doi: 10.1152/jn.1980.44.3.532

Van Essen, D. C., Smith, S. M., Barch, D. M., Behrens, T. E., Yacoub, E., Ugurbil, K., et al. (2013). The WU-Minn human connectome project: an overview. *Neuroimage* 80, 62–79. doi: 10.1016/j.neuroimage.2013.05.041

Varoquaux, G., Raamana, P. R., Engemann, D. A., Hoyos-Idrobo, A., Schwartz, Y., and Thirion, B. (2017). Assessing and tuning brain decoders: cross-validation, caveats, and guidelines. *NeuroImage* 145, 166–179. doi: 10.1016/j.neuroimage.2016.10.038

Wen, D., Wei, Z., Zhou, Y., Li, G., Zhang, X., and Han, W. (2018). Deep learning methods to process fMRI data and their application in the diagnosis of cognitive impairment: a brief overview and our opinion. *Front. Neuroinform.* 12:23. doi: 10.3389/fninf.2018.00023

Westlye, L. T., Walhovd, K. B., Dale, A. M., Bjørnerud, A., Due-Tønnessen, P., Engvig, A., et al. (2009). Life-span changes of the human brain white matter: diffusion tensor imaging (DTI) and volumetry. *Cereb. Cortex* 20, 2055–2068. doi: 10.1093/cercor/bhp280

Wiesendanger, R., Wiesendanger, M., and Ru, D. (1979). An anatomical investigation of the corticopontine projection in the primate (*Macaca fascicularis* and *Saimiri sciureus*)—II. The projection from frontal and parietal association areas. *Neuroscience* 4, 747–765. doi: 10.1016/0306-4522(79)90004-6

Witelson, S. F., Glezer, I. I., and Kigar, D. L. (1995). Women have greater density of neurons in posterior temporal cortex. *J. Neurosci.* 15, 3418–3428. doi: 10.1523/JNEUROSCI.15-05-03418.1995

Zaidi, Z. F. (2010). Gender differences in human brain: a review. *Open Anat. J.* 2, 37–55. doi: 10.2174/1877609401002010037

Zeng, L. L., Wang, H., Hu, P., Yang, B., Pu, W., Shen, H., et al. (2018a). Multi-site diagnostic classification of schizophrenia using discriminant deep learning with functional connectivity MRI. *Ebiomedicine* 30, 74–85. doi: 10.1016/j.ebiom.2018.03.017

Zeng, N., Qiu, H., Wang, Z., Liu, W., Zhang, H., and Li, Y. (2018b). A new switching-delayed-PSO-based optimized SVM algorithm for diagnosis of Alzheimer's disease. *Neurocomputing* 320, 195–202. doi: 10.1016/j.neucom.2018.09.001

Zeng, N., Wang, Z., Zhang, H., Liu, W., and Alsaadi, F. E. (2016). Deep belief networks for quantitative analysis of a gold immunochromatographic strip. *Cogn. Comput.* 8, 684–692. doi: 10.1007/s12559-016-9404-x

Zeng, N., Zhang, H., Song, B., Liu, W., Li, Y., and Dobaie, A. M. (2018c). Facial expression recognition via learning deep sparse autoencoders. *Neurocomputing* 273, 643–649. doi: 10.1016/j.neucom.2017.08.043

18

Diagnosis of Alzheimer's Disease via Multi-Modality 3D Convolutional Neural Network

Yechong Huang[1], Jiahang Xu[1], Yuncheng Zhou[1], Tong Tong[2] and Xiahai Zhuang[1]*

[1] School of Data Science, Fudan University, Shanghai, China, [2] Fujian Provincial Key Laboratory of Medical Instrument and Pharmaceutical Technology, Fuzhou, China

***Correspondence:**
Xiahai Zhuang
zxh@fudan.edu.cn

† Data used in preparation of this article were obtained from the Alzheimer's Disease Neuroimaging Initiative (ADNI) database (adni.loni.usc.edu). As such, the investigators within the ADNI contributed to the design and implementation of ADNI and/or provided data but did not participate in analysis or writing of this report. A complete listing of ADNI investigators can be found at: http://adni.loni.usc.edu/wp-content/uploads/how_to_apply/ADNI_Acknowledgement_List.pdf

Alzheimer's disease (AD) is one of the most common neurodegenerative diseases. In the last decade, studies on AD diagnosis has attached great significance to artificial intelligence-based diagnostic algorithms. Among the diverse modalities of imaging data, T1-weighted MR and FDG-PET are widely used for this task. In this paper, we propose a convolutional neural network (CNN) to integrate all the multi-modality information included in both T1-MR and FDG-PET images of the hippocampal area, for the diagnosis of AD. Different from the traditional machine learning algorithms, this method does not require manually extracted features, instead, it utilizes 3D image-processing CNNs to learn features for the diagnosis or prognosis of AD. To test the performance of the proposed network, we trained the classifier with paired T1-MR and FDG-PET images in the ADNI datasets, including 731 cognitively unimpaired (labeled as CN) subjects, 647 subjects with AD, 441 subjects with stable mild cognitive impairment (sMCI) and 326 subjects with progressive mild cognitive impairment (pMCI). We obtained higher accuracies of 90.10% for CN vs. AD task, 87.46% for CN vs. pMCI task, and 76.90% for sMCI vs. pMCI task. The proposed framework yields a state-of-the-art performance. Finally, the results have demonstrated that (1) segmentation is not a prerequisite when using a CNN for the classification, (2) the combination of two modality imaging data generates better results.

Keywords: Alzheimer's disease, multi-modality, image classification, CNN, deep learning, hippocampal

INTRODUCTION

Aging of the global population results in an increasing number of people with dementia. Recent studies indicate that 50 million people are living with dementia (Patterson, 2018), of whom 60–70% have Alzheimer's Disease (AD) (World Health Organization, 2012). Known as one of the most common neurodegenerative diseases, AD can result in severe cognitive impairment and behavioral issues.

Mild cognitive impairment (MCI) is a neurological disorder, which may occur as a transitional stage between normal aging and the preclinical phase of dementia. MCI causes cognitive impairments with a minimal impact on instrumental activities of daily life (Petersen et al., 1999, 2018). MCI is a heterogeneous group and can be classified according to its various clinical outcomes (Huang et al., 2003). In this work, we partitioned MCI into progressive MCI (pMCI) and stable MCI (sMCI), which are retrospective diagnostic terms based on the clinical follow-up according to the DSM-5 criteria (American Psychiatric Association, 2013). The term pMCI, refers to MCI patients who develop dementia in a 36-month follow-up, while sMCI is assigned to MCI patients when they do not convert. Distinguishing between pMCI and sMCI plays an important role in the early diagnosis of dementia, which can assist clinicians in proposing effective therapeutic interventions for the disease process (Samper-González et al., 2018).

With the progression of MCI and AD, the structure and metabolic rate of the brain changes accordingly. The phenotypes include the shrinkage of cerebral cortices and hippocampi, the enlargement of ventricles, and the change of regional glucose uptake. These changes could be quantified with the help of medical imaging techniques such as magnetic resonance (MR) and positron-emission tomography (PET) (Correa et al., 2009). For instance, T1-weighted magnetic resonance image (T1-MRI) provides high-resolution information for the brain structure, making it possible to accurately measure structural metrics like thickness, volume and shape. Meanwhile, 18-Fluoro-DeoxyGlucose PET (^{18}F-FDG-PET or FDG-PET) indicates the regional cerebral metabolic rate of glucose, making it possible to evaluate the metabolic activity of the tissues. Other tracers, such as ^{11}C-PiB and ^{18}F-THK, are also widely used in AD diagnosis (Jack et al., 2008b; Harada et al., 2013), as they are sensitive to the pathology of AD as well. By analyzing these medical images, one can obtain important references to assist the diagnosis and prediction of AD (Desikan et al., 2009).

This work aims at distinguishing AD or potential AD patients from cognitively unimpaired (labeled as CN) subjects accurately and automatically using medical images of the hippocampal area and recent techniques in deep learning, as it facilitates a fast-preclinical diagnosis. The method is further extended for the classification between sMCI and pMCI so that an early diagnosis of dementia would be possible. Data of two modalities were used. i.e., the T1-MRI and ^{18}F-FDG-PET, as they provide complementary information.

Numerous studies have been published on diagnosing AD by utilizing these two methods. Using T1-MRI, Sorensen et al. segmented the brains and extracted features of thickness and volumetry in the selected regions of interest (ROIs) (Sorensen et al., 2017). A linear discriminant analysis (LDA) was used to classify AD, MCI, and CN. David et al. implemented the kernel metric learning method in the classification (Cárdenas-Peña et al., 2017). Another popular machine learning method is the random forest. Lebedeva et al. (2017) extracted the structural features of MRI and used mini-mental state examination (MMSE) as a cognitive measure. Ardekani et al. (2017) took the hippocampal volumetric integrity of MRI and neuropsychological scores as the selected features. Both studies used the random forest. As for ^{18}F-FDG-PET, Silveira and Marques (2010) proposed a boosting learning method that used a mixture of simple classifiers to perform voxel-wise feature selections. Cabral and Silveira (2013) used favorite class ensembles to form ensembled support vector machine (SVM) and random forest.

In addition to the single modality classifications, taking both T1-MRI and ^{18}F-FDG-PET into consideration is also a major concern for research on AD diagnosis. Gray et al. (2013) took regional MRI volumes, PET intensities, cerebrospinal fluid (CSF) biomarkers and genetic information as features and implemented random-forest based classification. Additionally, Zhang et al. (2011) conducted a classification based on MRI, PET, and CSF biomarkers . Moreover, other imaging modalities or PET tracers can be considered, as Rondina et al. (2018) used T1-MRI, ^{18}F-FDG-PET and rCBF-SPECT as the imaging modalities while Wang et al. (2016) used ^{18}F-FDG and ^{18}F-florbetapir as tracers of PET.

The studies mentioned above mostly follow three basic steps in the diagnosis algorithms, namely segmentation, feature extraction and classification. During segmentation, data are manually or automatically partitioned into multiple segments based on anatomy or physiology. In this way, the ROIs are well-defined, making it possible to extract features from them. Finally, these features will be fed to the classification step so that the classifiers are able to learn useful diagnostic information and propose predictions for given test subjects. Among them, segmentation plays an important role as it is used to measure the structural metrics in the feature extraction step. However, it is hard to obtain a segmentation automatically and accurately, which leads to a low efficiency. As a result, we proposed an end-to-end diagnosis without segmentation in the following work. What is more, though highly reliable and explainable, these steps could be integrated weakly, as different platforms are used in different steps of these algorithms. The above considerations lead to our attempt to use a neural network in AD diagnosis.

Benefited by the rapid development of computer science and the accumulation of clinical data, deep learning has become a popular and useful method in the field of medical imaging recently. The general applications of deep learning in medical imaging are mainly feature extraction, image classification, object detection, segmentation and registration (Litjens et al., 2017). Among the deep learning networks, convolutional neural networks (CNNs) are common choices. Hosseini-Asl et al. (2016) built a 3D-CNN based on a 3D convolutional auto-encoder, which takes functional MRI (fMRI) images as input and gives the prediction for the AD vs. MCI vs. CN task, while Sarraf and Tofighi (2016) used a CNN structured like LeNet-5 to classify AD from CN based on fMRI. Liu et al. (2018) conducted a T1-MRI and FDG-PET based cascaded CNN, which utilized a 3D CNN to extract features and adopted another 2D CNN to combine multi-modality features for task-specific classification. Previous studies showed a promising potential of AD diagnosis, and thus we propose to use a deep learning framework in our work to complete the feature extraction and classification steps simultaneously.

In this work, we propose a multi-modality AD classifier. It takes both MR and PET images of the hippocampal area as the inputs, and provides predictions in the CN vs. AD task, the CN vs. pMCI task and the sMCI vs. pMCI task. The main contributions of our work are listed below:

(1) We show that segmentation of the key substructures, such as hippocampi, is not a prerequisite in CNN-based classification.

(2) We show that the high-resolution information in the hippocampal area can make up the gap between ROIs of different sizes.
(3) We construct a 3D VGG-variant CNN to implement a single modality AD diagnosis.
(4) We introduce a new framework to combine complementary information from multiple modalities in our proposed network, for the classification tasks of CN vs. AD, CN vs. pMCI and sMCI vs. pMCI.

MATERIALS AND METHODS

Studies of biomarkers for AD diagnosis are of great interest in the research fields. Among these bio markers, the shrinkage of the hippocampi is the best-established MRI biomarker to stage the progression of AD (Jack et al., 2011a), and by now the only MRI biomarker qualified for the enrichment of clinical trials (Hill et al., 2014). Therefore, the hippocampi are the most studied organs for MRI based AD diagnosis, and the hippocampal area is chosen to be the ROI of MRI in this work. As for PET images, published studies indicated that AD may cause the decline of $^{[18]}$F-FDG uptake in both hippocampi and cortices (Mosconi et al., 2006; Mosconi et al., 2008; Jack et al., 2011b). Hence, when dealing with PET images, we tried different ROIs, i.e., containing only hippocampi, and containing both hippocampi and cortices.

Image Acquisition

Data used in the preparation of this article were obtained from the Alzheimer's Disease Neuroimaging Initiative (ADNI) database[1]. The ADNI was launched in 2003 as a public-private partnership, led by Principal Investigator Michael W. Weiner, MD. The primary goal of ADNI has been to test whether serial magnetic resonance imaging (MRI), positron emission tomography (PET), other biological markers, and clinical and neuropsychological assessment can be combined to measure the progression of mild cognitive impairment (MCI) and early Alzheimer's disease (AD). In this work, we used the T1-MRI and the FDG-PET from the baseline and follow-up visit in ADNI, as these two modalities have the greatest number of images. The details about the data acquisition are interpreted on the ADNI website (Jack et al., 2008a). We generated two datasets in this work. The Segmented dataset, containing MR images and corresponding segmentation results, was chosen to verify the effect of the segmentation, and the Paired dataset, containing MR and PET images, to verify the effect of multi-modality images.

In the Segmented dataset, we picked 2861 T1-MR images, including AD and cognitively unimpaired subjects. Basic information of the Segmented dataset is summarized in **Table 1**. All images in the Segmented dataset were segmented using multi-atlas label propagation with the expectation-maximization (MALP-EM) framework[2] (Ledig et al., 2015). MALP-EM is a framework for the fully automatic segmentation of MR brain images. The approach is based on multi-atlas label fusion and intensity-based label refinement, using an expectation-maximization (EM) algorithm. Through the MALP-EM framework, we obtained 138 anatomical regions with fixed boundaries, including the hippocampi of interest.

TABLE 1 | Summary of the studied subjects from Segmented dataset.

Diagnosis	Number	Age	Gender(M/F)	MMSE
AD	1355	76.13 ± 7.50	772/583	21.89 ± 4.33
CN	1506	76.04 ± 5.81	776/730	29.04 ± 1.20

TABLE 2 | Summary of the studied subjects from the Paired dataset.

Diagnosis	Number	Age	Gender(M/F)	MMSE
AD	647	76.36 ± 7.21	361/287	24.84 ± 2.65
pMCI	326	75.00 ± 7.06	212/114	27.22 ± 1.74
sMCI	441	74.37 ± 7.40	297/144	28.15 ± 1.55
CN	731	76.16 ± 6.02	421/310	28.99 ± 1.20

As for the Paired dataset, we used the following steps to generate it. For the same subject, we paired the MRI with the PET with (a) closest acquisition dates, (b) within 1 year since the MRI scan, and (c) at the time of the scan with the same diagnosis as the MRI. Among the acquired data, the MCI subjects were classified into pMCI and sMCI according to the DSM-5 criteria, that is, MCI should be defined as pMCI if it develops into AD within 3 years, or be defined as sMCI if it does not. Subjects without follow-up data for more than 3 years were ignored. Finally, we acquired 647 AD, 767 MCI (326 pMCI and 441 sMCI) and 731 cognitively unimpaired subjects over 1211 ADNI participants. All the information for these subjects is summarized in **Table 2**.

Data Processing

The pre-processing of images was implemented by *zxhtools*[3] (Zhuang et al., 2011). In this work, MR images were re-oriented and resampled to a resolution of 221 × 257 × 221 and with a 1 mm isotropic spacing using *zxhreg* and *zxhtransform* from *zxhtools*. Furthermore, in the Paired dataset, each PET image was rigid-registered to a respective MR image for the proceeding process.

The hippocampal area was selected to be the region of interest (ROI) because of its great significance in AD diagnosis. In addition, due to limited computation ability, we cropped the ROI centered in the hippocampi. For the Segmented dataset, which includes the segmentation results, we directly calculated the center of the hippocampi as it has been shown in the segmentation results. For the Paired dataset, we acquired the central points of the MR images as follows. First, we randomly chose one MR image from the Paired dataset as a template. Then we registered the images from the Segmented dataset to the template image by affine-registration, thus calculating the average indices of the center in the template image. After that, we registered the template image to other MR images in the Paired dataset using affine-transformation and used the corresponding affine matrix to determine the center for each MR image. Finally, each PET image was rigid-registered to a respective MR image for the identification of the hippocampi's

[1] http://adni.loni.usc.edu

[2] https://biomedia.doc.ic.ac.uk/software/malp-em/

[3] http://www.sdspeople.fudan.edu.cn/zhuangxiahai/0/zxhproj/

center. After the registration, PET images were transformed into a uniform isotropic spacing of 1 mm.

After the centers of the ROIs were located, we dilated and cropped the ROIs to a region of size 96 × 96 × 48 in voxels from the center of hippocampi for MR images (see the red rectangles in **Figures 1A–C**). In the experiment on the Segmented dataset, we processed the cropped ROI and corresponding labels in three different ways. Three slightly different groups were obtained: ImageOnly, MaskedImage and Mask. The ImageOnly group contains MR raw images and maintains all the imaging information of the hippocampi and surrounding areas. The MaskedImage group is made up of MR images masked by binary labels, it considers both the original images and the segmentation results for the hippocampi as the inputs. The Mask group is made up of binary hippocampi segmentation labels, only indicating information about the shape and volume of the hippocampi. By comparing the classification performance using these three datasets, it can be judged whether the segmentation results have an important effect on AD diagnosis. The information for the three groups from the Segmented dataset is shown in **Figures 1D–F**. When it comes to the Paired dataset, we used two different methods to generate the patches of PET images. The group generated using the first method is called the Small Reception Field (SmallRF) group, which has the same reception field as the ROI of MR images with 1 mm isotropic spacing. The group generated using the second method is called the Big Reception Field (BigRF) group, which has the same orientation and ROI center but has a 2 mm isotropic spacing for each dimension, thus having a larger reception field but a lower spatial resolution. The information for the two groups from the Paired dataset is shown in **Figures 1H,I** as a sample of the original PET image is shown in **Figure 1G**.

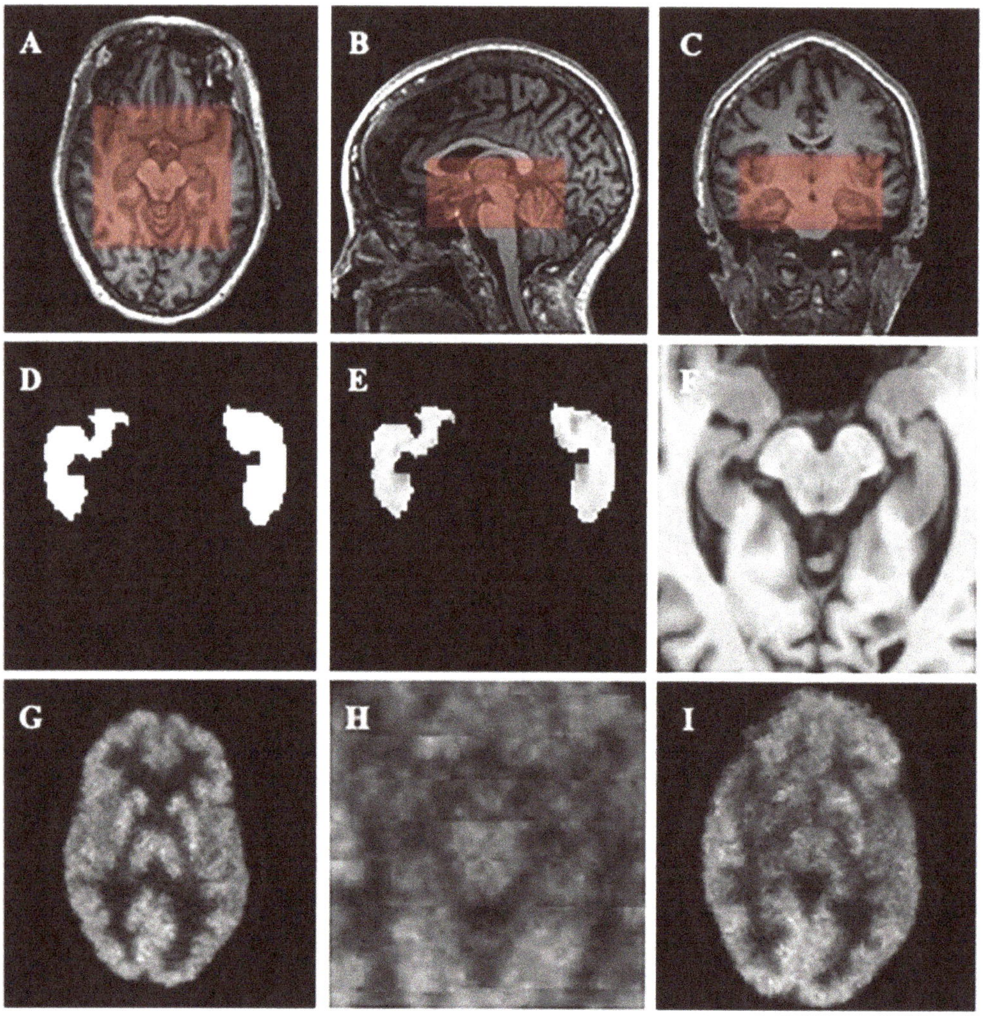

FIGURE 1 | Demonstrations of the datasets and ROIs. **(A–C)** demonstrate the selected ROI of MR images. **(A)** is an axial slice, **(B)** is a sagittal slice, and **(C)** is a coronal slice. **(D–F)** are generated from the same MR image to demonstrate the Mask **(D)**, MaskedImage **(E)**, and ImageOnly **(F)** groups. **(D)** is a mask image of the segmentation of hippocampi. **(E)** is a image masked by hippocampal segmentation. **(F)** is a cropped image. **(G–I)** are generated from the same PET image to demonstrate the images in the SmallRF **(H)** and BigRF **(I)** groups, while **(G)** is the corresponding PET image. Among them, **(H)** is cropped from **(G)**, and **(I)** is downsampled from **(G)**.

After the data processing, the datasets were randomly split into training sets, validation sets, and testing sets according to the patient IDs to ensure that all subjects of the same patient only appear in one set. Finally, 70% of a dataset was used as the training set, 10% as the validation set, and 20% as the testing set by random sampling. Details of these subsets were shown in **Supplementary Tables S1** and **S2**.

Methodology

Convolutional neural network (LeCun et al., 1995) is a deep feedforward neural network composed of multi-layer artificial neurons, with excellent performance in large-scale image processing. Unlike traditional methods which use manually extracted features of radiological images, CNNs are used to learn general features automatically. CNNs are trained with a back propagation algorithm while it usually consists of multiple convolutional layers, pooling layers and fully connected layers and connects to the output units through fully connected layers or other kinds of layers. Compared to other deep feedforward networks, CNNs have fewer connections and a smaller number of parameters, due to the sharing of the convolution kernel among pixels and are therefore easier to train and more popular.

With CNNs prospering in the field of computer vision, a number of attempts have been made to improve the original network structure to achieve better accuracy. VGG (Simonyan and Zisserman, 2014) is a neural network based on AlexNet (Krizhevsky et al., 2012) and it achieved a 7.3% error rate in the 2014 ILSVRC competition (Russakovsky et al., 2015) as one of the Top-5 winners. VGGs further deepen the network based on AlexNet by adding more convolutional layers and pooling layers. Different from traditional CNNs, VGGs evaluate very deep convolutional networks for large-scale image classification, which come up with significantly more accurate CNN architectures and can achieve excellent performance even when used as a part of relatively simple pipelines. In this work, we built our network with reference to the structure of VGG.

EXPERIMENTS

In the Section "Data Type Analysis", we determined the proper types of data and ROIs through two experiments. In the Section "Multi-Modality AD Classifier", we constructed a set of VGG-like multi-modality AD classifiers, which considers both T1-MRI and FDG-PET data as inputs and provides predictions. In the Section "Classification of sMCI vs. pMCI and CN vs. pMCI Tasks", we trained and tested our networks with the pMCI and sMCI data. Finally, in the Section "Comparison With Other Methods" we compared our proposed method with state-of-the-art methods.

Implementation Details

All the networks mentioned above were programmed based on TensorFlow (Abadi et al., 2016). Training procedures of the networks were conducted on a personal computer with a Nvidia GTX1080Ti GPU. During the training, batch normalization (Ioffe and Szegedy, 2015) was deployed in the convolutional layers and dropout (Hinton et al., 2015) was deployed in fully connected layers to avoid overfitting. To accelerate the training process and to avoid local minima, we used an ADAM optimizer (Kingma and Ba, 2014) to train. The batch size was set to 16 when we trained single modality networks and to eight when we trained multi-modality networks. The number of epochs was set to 150, though the loss would generally converge after 30 epochs. Each training epoch took several minutes. During training, the parameters of the networks were saved every 10 epochs. The resulting models were tested using the validation data set. The accuracies and receiver operating characteristic (ROC) curves of the classification on the validation data were then calculated, and the model with the best accuracy was chosen to be the final classifier.

Data Type Analysis

In order to determine the proper data type for network training, we designed two experiments and evaluated the classification performances of models when they were fed with different data types.

(1) Testing whether segmentation is needed in the MR images. We used three different groups from the Segmented Dataset, with or without segmentation, to show that segmentation is not necessary for a CNN.
(2) Finding a proper PET ROI. Different spacings for PET images, i.e., the SmallRF and the BigRF groups from the Paired Dataset, were tested and we found that the classification model with the SmallRF group is similar to the model with the BigRF group in performance.

All the models mentioned above were trained in the same network, as shown in **Figure 2**. The input resolution is $96 \times 96 \times 48$ in voxels, and the network contains eight convolutional layers, five max-pooling layers, and three fully connected layers. The output was given through a softmax layer.

The Influence of Segmentation

As mentioned above, segmentation plays an important role in traditional classification methods. However, segmentation is also known to be time-consuming. Additionally, CNN can extract useful features directly from raw images, as CNNs show a strong ability to locate key points in object detection tasks for natural images (Ren et al., 2015; He et al., 2017).

To verify the effect of segmentation, we segmented the AD and cognitively unimpaired subjects of T1-MR images with the MALP-EM algorithm (Ledig et al., 2015) and obtained the Segmented datasets, including 2861 subjects and containing both MR images and the corresponding segmentation. In our assumption, segmentation can indicate the shapes, volumes, textures and relative locations of hippocampal areas. Therefore, the data obtained from the subjects formed three different groups, as shown in **Figures 1D–F**. The ImageOnly group contains raw MR images only; the Mask group is made up of binary hippocampal segmentation labels and the MaskedImage group is made up of MR images masked by the binary labels.

For each model trained from these groups, accuracy and AUC were evaluated, as listed in **Table 3**. Among all the three models, the model trained by the Mask group provided a favorable prediction, though inferior to those trained by the ImageOnly and the MaskedImage group. The results indicate

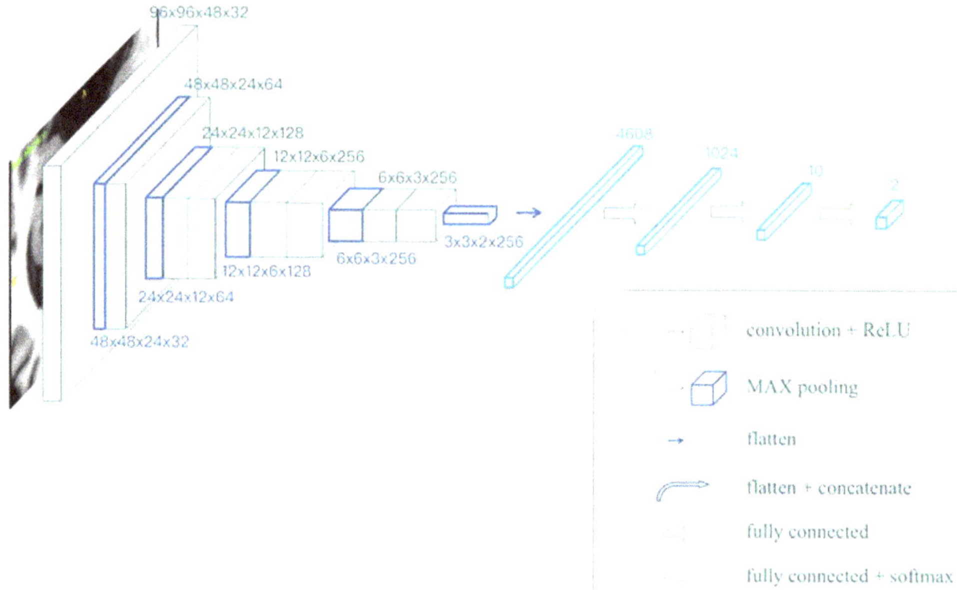

FIGURE 2 | The architecture of the single modality classifier.

TABLE 3 | Summary of the models trained from the Mask, MaskedImage, and ImageOnly groups for CN vs. AD task.

MRI ROI	ACC[1]	SEN	SPE	AUC
Mask	76.57%	83.87%	71.51%	84.24%
MaskedImage	79.21%	76.61%	81.01%	84.63%
ImageOnly	84.82%	87.90%	82.68%	87.47%

The Segmented dataset was used. [1]ACC, SEN, SPE, AUC denotes accuracy, sensitivity, specificity and area under curve, respectively. When testing, the numbers of true positive (TP), true negative (TN), false negative (FP), and false negative (FN) subjects were counted, as ACC = (TP+TN)/(TP+TN+FP+FN), SEN = TP/(TP+FN), SPE = TN/(TN+FP). AUC is obtained through calculating the area under the receiver operating characteristic (ROC) curve. For all four metrics, the values are between 0 and 100%, the higher, the better.

that segmentation results do contain information needed for the classification, however, it is not necessary for the classification task since CNN is able to learn useful features without labeling the voxels. In addition, features from the region out of the hippocampi also provide further information to separate AD patients from normal ones.

ROI Determination for PET Images

Due to the limitation of GPU RAM and its computational ability, it was difficult to consider the entire image as the network input, as our proposed network only considered a region of 96 × 96 × 48 in voxels, which was still 2.91 times the input size of the original VGG (224 × 224 pixels × 3 channels). Hence, the selection of the ROI was of great importance, as only the features in the ROI were considered. As for the MR images, the selection of the ROI was of little doubt, because the hippocampal area was long enough to be the main concern of AD research (Jack et al., 2011b; Hill et al., 2014). However, the ROIs of PET images varied, as studies also attached great significance to metabolic changes in cortices, e.g., temporal lobes (Mosconi et al., 2006, 2008).

To verify the effects of cortices on the classification, we generated two groups from all PET images from the Paired dataset, the SmallRF and the BigRF groups, as shown in **Figures 1H,I**. The SmallRF group uses exactly the same reception field with the MRI ROI; the images in the BigRF group are eight times the volume of the images in the SmallRF group but have a lower spatial resolution.

Two models were trained using these two groups, and their performance was evaluated by some metrics, as listed in **Table 4**. The result showed that the two models behaved similarly. This is because although the SmallRF group has a higher spatial resolution, the BigRF group contains more features. Furthermore, in terms of multi-modality classification tasks, the SmallRF group might be better, because PET images in the SmallRF group were voxel-wisely aligned with paired MR images, which could help better locate the spatial features. Therefore, we chose the same ROI for both MR and PET images in the following experiments (see the red rectangles in **Figures 1A–C**).

Multi-Modality AD Classifier

The information a classifier can obtain, by using a single modality, is limited, as one medical imaging method can only profile one or several aspects of AD pathological changes, which is far from being complete. For example, T1-MR images provide a high-resolution brain structure but give little information about the functional information of the brain. Meanwhile, FDG-PET images are fuzzy but are better in revealing the metabolic activity of glucose in the brain. In order to take as much information of the brain as possible, we introduced a classification framework to integrate multi-modality information.

TABLE 4 | Summary of the models trained from the SmallRF and the BigRF groups for CN vs. AD task.

PET ROI	ACC	SEN	SPE	AUC
SmallRF PET	89.11%	90.24%	87.77%	92.69%
BigRF PET	89.44%	87.20%	92.09%	90.35%

The Paired dataset was used.

To prepare the dataset, we first matched MR with PET images and transformed them into same world coordinates. After that, paired images of MR and PET were aligned by rigid registration to ensure that the voxels of the same indices in the paired images represent the same part of the brain. After the paired images were cropped with reference to the center point of MR images, the Paired dataset was obtained.

To implement the multi-modality classifier, we proposed two different network architectures, as shown in **Figure 3**. In **Figure 3A**, MR and PET images were used as two parallel channels, in which paired images were stacked into 4D images. In these 4D images, the first three dimensions represent the three spatial dimensions, and the fourth one represents the channels. In **Figure 3B**, MR and PET images have separate entrances, as they are convolved, respectively, in two separate VGG-11s, and the extracted features are concatenated. This network was trained in two strategies, denoted by B1 and B2. B1 was to train the model with weights shared for the convolutional layers. Meanwhile, B2 usedwas to update the weights of two VGG-11s separately.

We trained five models based on the Paired dataset, that is, two single modality models (for MRI and PET respectively), and three multi-modality models (A, B1, and B2). The results are shown in **Table 5** and **Figure 4A**. As shown in **Table 5**, multi-modality classifiers had better performance than single modality classifiers. Additionally, among the three multi-modality models, the model trained with strategy B1 had the highest accuracy and sensitivity, while the model trained with strategy B2 had the highest specificity and AUC.

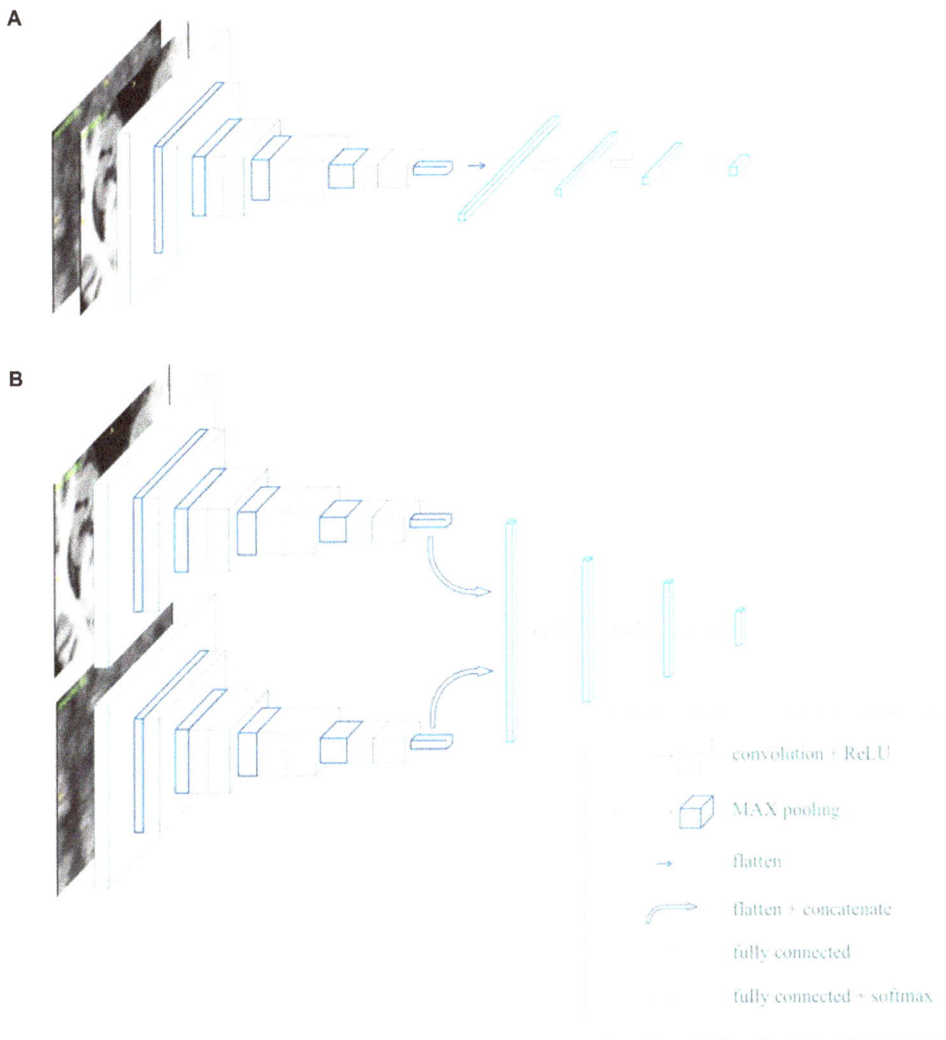

FIGURE 3 | The architecture of the multi-modality network **(A,B)**.

TABLE 5 | Summary of the models trained from single modality protocols and three multi-modality protocols for CN vs. AD task.

Method	ACC	SEN	SPE	AUC
MRI	81.19%	79.27%	83.45%	83.67%
PET	89.11%	90.24%	87.77%	**92.69%**
A	87.79%	85.98%	**89.93%**	89.42%
B1	**90.10%**	**90.85%**	89.21%	90.84%
B2	89.44%	89.02%	**89.93%**	92.01%

The Paired dataset was used. The best results were indicated in bold.

Classification of sMCI vs. pMCI and CN vs. pMCI Tasks

Simply classifying AD patients from normal controls is relatively easy but of little significance, as the development of AD can be observed easily by the behaviors of the patients. In addition, there are a lot of alternative indicators in clinical diagnosis. Therefore, the prediction of AD seems to be more meaningful, as one of the main concerns is telling pMCI from sMCI and normal individuals. As pMCI would progress to AD while the other two would not, identifying pMCI could give a prediction of the development of MCI, and thus have high reference value and clinical meaning.

According to Lin et al. (2018), the models that were trained by the CN vs. AD training set performed better than the models trained by the sMCI vs. pMCI training set in the sMCI vs. pMCI task. Therefore, we trained models with the CN vs. AD training set and tested the models with the CN vs. pMCI testing set and the sMCI vs. pMCI testing set, with the results shown in **Table 6** and **Figures 4B,C**. Though B1 performed slightly better in CN vs. AD task, B2 was superior in CN vs. pMCI and sMCI vs. pMCI tasks. These results indicate that features of MRI and PET tend to be more consistent when dementia is highly developed, since convolutional kernels of model B1 shared the weight, while those of B2 did not.

Comparison With Other Methods

In this part, we compared our method with those that were used in previous literature. We first compared our method with state-of-the-art research using 3D CNN-based multi-modality models as well (Lin et al., 2018). Liu et al. (2015) proposed a multi-modality cascaded CNN. They used the patch-based information of a whole brain to train or test their models and they integrated the information from the two modalities by concatenating the feature maps(Liu et al., 2015). **Table 7** shows the results of the method in comparison to our work. Note that our models used the data from multiple facilities and that our models only used the hippocampal area as the input. These would influence the behavior of our method.

Moreover, Lin et al. (2018), chose to reduce the amount of input by slicing the data (in different directions) instead of

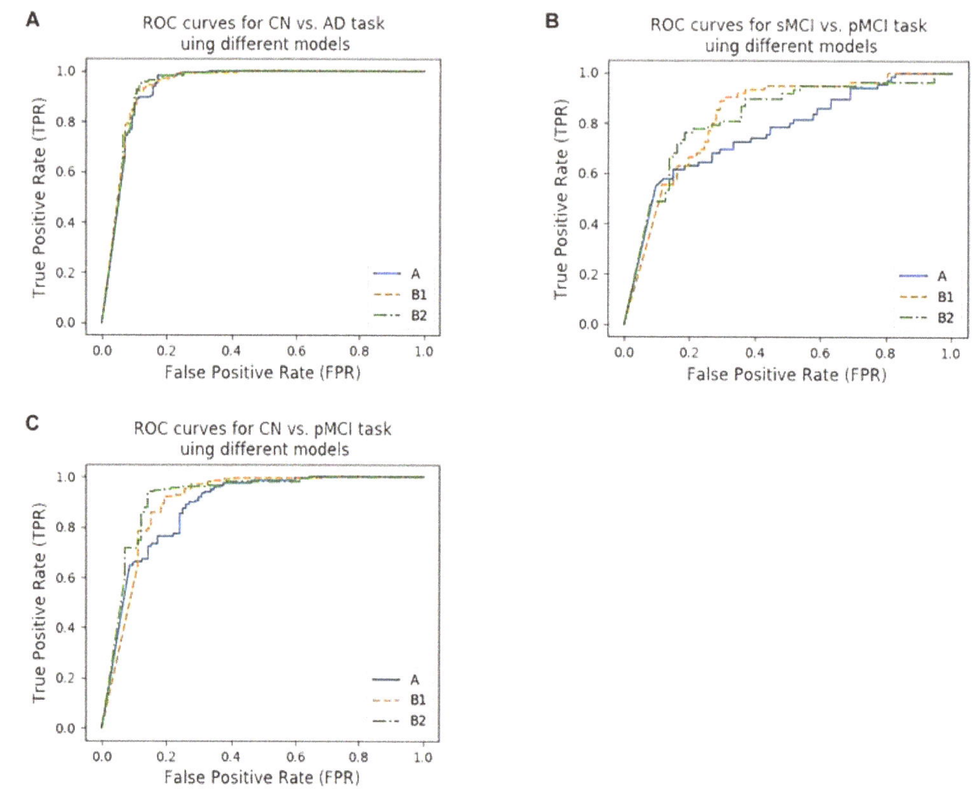

FIGURE 4 | ROC curves of different models. **(A–C)** show the ROC curves for three tasks using different models. **(A)** shows the ROC curves for CN vs. AD task using model trained from protocol A, B1, and B2, while **(B)** shows the ROC curves for CN vs. pMCI task, **(C)** shows the ROC curves for sMCI vs. pMCI task, respectively.

TABLE 6 | Summary of the models trained from three multi-modality protocols for CN vs. AD.

Method	A				B1				B2			
	ACC	SEN	SPE	AUC	ACC	SEN	SPE	AUC	ACC	SEN	SPE	AUC
CN/AD	87.79%	85.98%	**89.93%**	89.42%	**90.10%**	**90.85%**	89.21%	90.84%	89.44%	89.02%	**89.93%**	**92.01%**
CN/pMCI	70.49%	73.17%	65.00%	71.63%	79.10%	**87.80%**	61.25%	76.84%	**82.38%**	87.20%	**72.50%**	**81.64%**
sMCI/pMCI	65.28%	65.63%	65.00%	65.81%	65.28%	54.69%	**73.75%**	66.82%	**72.22%**	**73.44%**	71.25%	**77.49%**

The best results were indicated in bold.

TABLE 7 | Comparison of our proposed method and Liu's multi-modality method.

Method	Subjects	Modality	CN vs. AD				CN vs. pMCI			
			ACC	SEN	SPE	AUC	ACC	SEN	SPE	AUC
Liu et al., 2018	93 AD + 204 MCI + 100 CN	MRI	84.97%	82.65%	87.37%	90.63%	77.84%	76.81%	78.59%	82.72%
		PET	88.08%	90.70%	85.98%	94.51%	78.41%	77.94%	78.70%	85.96%
		Both	**93.26%**	**92.55%**	**93.94%**	**95.68%**	82.95%	81.08%	**84.31%**	**88.43%**
Proposed method	465 AD + 567 MCI + 480 CN	MRI	81.19%	79.27%	83.45%	83.67%	–	–	–	–
		PET	89.11%	90.24%	87.77%	92.69%	–	–	–	–
		Both	90.10%[1]	90.85%	89.21%	90.84%	82.38%[2]	87.20%	72.50%	81.64%
		Both	–	–	–	–	**87.46%**[3]	**90.73%**	80.61%	87.61%

[1]*Using B1 protocol, the CN vs. AD training set and the CN vs. AD testing set.* [2]*Using B2 protocol, the CN vs. pMCI training set and the CN vs. pMCI testing set.* [3]*Using B1 protocol, the CN vs. AD training but the CN vs. pMCI testing set. See* ***Table 9*** *for reference. The best results were indicated in bold.*

TABLE 8 | Comparison of our proposed method and published AD diagnosis methods.

Method	Subjects	CN vs. AD				sMCI vs. pMCI			
		ACC	SEN	SPE	AUC	ACC	SEN	SPE	AUC
Lin et al., 2018	93 AD + 204 MCI + 100 CN	88.79%	–	–	–	73.04%	–	–	–
Tong et al., 2017	37 AD + 75 MCI + 35 CN	88.6%	–	–	94.8%	–	–	–	–
Zu et al., 2016	51 AD + 99MCI + 52 CN	**95.95%**	–	–	–	69.78%	–	–	–
Liu et al., 2015	85 AD + 168 MCI + 77 CN	91.40%	92.32%	90.42%	–	–	–	–	–
Jie et al., 2015	51 AD + 99 MCI + 52 CN	95.03%	–	–	–	68.94%	–	–	–
Li et al., 2014	93 AD + 204 MCI + 101 CN	92.87%	–	–	89.82%	72.44%	–	–	70.14%
Proposed method	465 AD + 567 MCI + 480 CN	90.10%[1]	90.85%	89.21%	90.84%	72.22%[2]	**73.44%**	71.25%	77.49%
		–	–	–	–	**76.90%**[3]	68.15%	**83.93%**	**79.61%**

[1]*Using B1 protocol, the CN vs. AD training set and the CN vs. AD testing set.* [2]*Using B2 protocol, the CN vs. sMCI training set and the CN vs. sMCI testing set.* [3]*Using B2 protocol, the CN vs. AD training but the CN vs. sMCI testing set. See* ***Table 9*** *for reference. The best results were indicated in bold.*

TABLE 9 | Comparison of the performance of models trained from the CN vs. AD training set and the tasks' own training set.

Task	Training Set	Testing Set	B1				B2			
			ACC	SEN	SPE	AUC	ACC	SEN	SPE	AUC
CN/pMCI	CN/AD	CN/pMCI	87.46%	90.73%	80.61%	87.61%	87.13%	87.80%	85.71%	90.31%
CN/pMCI	CN/pMCI	CN/pMCI	79.10%	87.80%	61.25%	76.84%	82.38%	87.20%	72.50%	81.64%
sMCI/pMCI	CN/AD	sMCI/pMCI	73.60%	66.67%	79.17%	75.59%	76.90%	68.15%	83.93%	79.61%
sMCI/pMCI	sMCI/pMCI	sMCI/pMCI	65.28%	54.69%	73.75%	66.82%	72.22%	73.44%	71.25%	77.49%

The Paired dataset was used.

cropping the hippocampi out as we did. Tong et al. (2017) used non-linear graph fusion to join the features of different modalities. In Zu et al.'s (2016) study, the feature selection from multiple modalities were treated as different learning tasks. Liu et al. (2015) used stacked autoencoders (SAE) with a masking training strategy. Jie et al. (2015) used a manifold regularized multitask feature learning method to preserve both the relations among modalities of data and the distribution in each modality.

Li et al. (2014) used a deep learning framework to predict the missing data. **Table 8** compares the previous multi-modality models with our proposed models. Among all the results listed below, our results are favorable in the CN vs. AD task and are the best in the sMCI vs. pMCI task.

DISCUSSION

In this work, we proposed a VGG-like framework, with several instances, to implement a T1-MRI and FDG-PET based multi-modality AD diagnosing system. The ROI of MRI was selected to be the hippocampal area, as it is the most frequently studied and is thought to be of the highest clinical value. Through the experiments, we proved that segmentation is not necessary for a CNN-based diagnosing system, which is different from the traditional machine learning based methods. However, registration is still needed, as the images we used were taken from different facilities and had different spacings and orientations. Although models obtained from the SmallRF and BigRF groups had similar performances, the ROI of PET was chosen to be the same as the MRI's, because the ROI of SmallRF was voxel-wisely aligned with the ROI of the paired MRI. In short, only hippocampal areas were used as ROIs in our proposed methods, which is the main difference between our study and previous studies. Thus, we constructed a deeper neural network and fed it with medical images of higher resolution, as we supposed that the hippocampal area itself can serve as a favorable reference in AD diagnosis.

"Since the ROI was selected, we introduced a multi-modality method to the classifier. Two networks and three types of models were proposed as listed in **Table 6**. Among these three types of models, the model trained using strategy B1, which means that the MR and PET images were separately input for the convolutional layers, but with their convolutional kernels shared, performed the best in the CN vs. AD task. One possible explanation is that MR and PET images have some common features, and sharing weight helped the model to extract these features during the training process. Furthermore, we used proposed networks to train CN vs. pMCI and sMCI vs. pMCI classifiers, both of them indicated the potential of preclinical diagnosis using our proposed methods.

We also followed Lin et al.'s (2018) lead and used the model trained by CN vs. AD subjects to distinguish sMCI and pMCI. The results were better than that of the model trained by sMCI and pMCI themselves, as shown in **Table 9**. This is reasonable because the features of sMCI and pMCI are close to each other in the feature space and are difficult to differentiate, while those of CN and AD are widely spread making the classification a lot easier. The same conclusion can be obtained by testing the CN vs. AD model on the CN vs. pMCI dataset. Specifically, when the CN vs. AD model was used, the accuracy reached 76.90% for sMCI vs. pMCI and 87.46% for CN vs. pMCI, which was about 5% higher than the accuracy obtained using their own models. These results are also better than those of Lin et al.'s (2018).

As for the future work, we only used two modalities (T1-MRI and FDG-PET) as inputs for this work. However, new modalities can easily be implemented based on the proposed networks. The interested new imaging modalities include T2-MRI (Rombouts et al., 2005), ^{11}C-PIB-PET (Zhang et al., 2014), and other PET agents such as amyloid protein imaging (Glenner and Wong, 1984). Also, the features extracted by CNN are hard for human beings to comprehend, while some methods like attention mechanisms (Jetley et al., 2018) are able to visualize and analyze the activation maps of the model, in which future work could be done to improve the classification performance and to discover new medical imaging biomarkers.

CONCLUSION

To conclude, we have proposed a multi-modality CNN-based classifier for AD diagnosis and prognosis. VGG backbone, which is deeper than most similar studies, has been used and explored. The accuracy of models reached 90.10% for the CN vs. AD task, 87.46% for the CN vs. pMCI task and 76.90% for the sMCI vs. pMCI task. Our work also indicates that the hippocampal area with no segmentation can be chosen as the input.

ETHICS STATEMENT

Data used in the preparation of this article were obtained from the Alzheimer's Disease Neuroimaging Initiative (ADNI) database (adni.loni.usc.edu). The ADNI was launched in 2003 as a public-private partnership, led by Principal Investigator Michael W. Weiner, MD. The primary goal of ADNI has been to test whether serial magnetic resonance imaging (MRI), positron emission tomography (PET), other biological markers, and clinical and neuropsychological assessment can be combined to measure the progression of mild cognitive impairment (MCI) and early Alzheimer's disease (AD). Since its launch more than a decade ago, the landmark public-private partnership has made major contributions to AD research, enabling the sharing of data between researchers around the world. For up-to-date information, see www.adni-info.org.

AUTHOR CONTRIBUTIONS

XZ is the corresponding author. XZ proposed the idea, supervised and managed the research, and revised the manuscript. YH lead the implementations, experiments, and wrote the manuscript. JX co-lead the work and wrote the manuscript. YZ provided the support to the work of coding, experiments, and wrote the manuscript. TT co-investigated the work and revised the manuscript.

FUNDING

This work was supported by the Science and Technology Commission of Shanghai Municipality (17JC1401600) and the Key Projects of Technological Department in Fujian Province (321192016Y0069201615).

ACKNOWLEDGMENTS

Data collection and sharing for this project was funded by the Alzheimer's Disease Neuroimaging Initiative (ADNI) (National Institutes of Health Grant U01 AG024904) and DOD ADNI (Department of Defense award number W81XWH-12-2-0012). ADNI is funded by the National Institute on Aging, the National Institute of Biomedical Imaging and Bioengineering, and through generous contributions from the following: AbbVie, Alzheimer's Association; Alzheimer's Drug Discovery Foundation; Araclon Biotech; BioClinica, Inc.; Biogen; Bristol-Myers Squibb Company; CereSpir, Inc.; Cogstate; Eisai Inc.; Elan Pharmaceuticals, Inc.; Eli Lilly and Company; EuroImmun; F. Hoffmann-La Roche Ltd. and its affiliated company Genentech, Inc.; Fujirebio; GE Healthcare; IXICO Ltd.; Janssen Alzheimer Immunotherapy Research & Development, LLC.; Johnson & Johnson Pharmaceutical Research & Development LLC.; Lumosity; Lundbeck; Merck & Co., Inc.; Meso Scale Diagnostics, LLC.; NeuroRx Research; Neurotrack Technologies; Novartis Pharmaceuticals Corporation; Pfizer Inc.; Piramal Imaging; Servier; Takeda Pharmaceutical Company; and Transition Therapeutics. The Canadian Institutes of Health Research is providing funds to support ADNI clinical sites in Canada. Private sector contributions are facilitated by the Foundation for the National Institutes of Health (www.fnih.org). The grantee organization is the Northern California Institute for Research and Education, and the study is coordinated by the Alzheimer's Therapeutic Research Institute at the University of Southern California. ADNI data are disseminated by the Laboratory for Neuro Imaging at the University of Southern California.

REFERENCES

Abadi, M., Barham, P., Chen, J., Chen, Z., Davis, A., Dean, J., et al. (2016). "Tensorflow: a system for large-scale machine learning," in *Proceedings of the 12th USENIX Conference on Operating Systems Design and Implementation OSDI'16*, Savannah, GA, 265–283.

American Psychiatric Association (2013). *Diagnostic and Statistical Manual of Mental Disorders (DSM-5)*. Philadelphia: American Psychiatric Pub.

Ardekani, B. A., Bermudez, E., Mubeen, A. M., Bachman, A. H., and Alzheimer's Disease Neuroimaging Initiative. (2017). Prediction of incipient Alzheimer's disease dementia in patients with mild cognitive impairment. *J. Alzheimer's Dis.* 55, 269–281.

Cabral, C., and Silveira, M. (2013). "Classification of Alzheimer's disease from FDG-PET images using favourite class ensembles," in *Proceedings of the 35th Annual International Conference of the IEEE Engineering in Medicine and Biology Society (EMBC)*, (Osaka: IEEE), 2477–2480.

Cárdenas-Peña, D., Collazos-Huertas, D., and Castellanos-Dominguez, G. (2017). Enhanced data representation by kernel metric learning for dementia diagnosis. *Front. Neurosci.* 11:413. doi: 10.3389/fnins.2017.00413

Correa, N. M., Li, Y. O., Adali, T., and Calhoun, V. D. (2009). "Fusion of fMRI, sMRI, and EEG data using canonical correlation analysis," in *Proceedings of the 2009 IEEE International Conference on Acoustics, Speech and Signal Processing*, (Taipei: IEEE), 385–388.

Desikan, R. S., Cabral, H. J., Hess, C. P., Dillon, W. P., Glastonbury, C. M., Weiner, M. W., et al. (2009). Automated MRI measures identify individuals with mild cognitive impairment and Alzheimer's disease. *Brain* 132, 2048–2057. doi: 10.1093/brain/awp123

Glenner, G., and Wong, C. W. (1984). Alzheimer's disease: initial report of the purification and characterization of a novel cerebrovascular amyloid protein. *Biochem. Biophys. Res. Commun.* 120, 885–890. doi: 10.1016/s0006-291x(84)80190-4

Gray, K. R., Aljabar, P., Heckemann, R. A., Hammers, A., and Rueckert, D. (2013). Random forest-based similarity measures for multi-modal classification of Alzheimer's disease. *NeuroImage* 65, 167–175. doi: 10.1016/j.neuroimage.2012.09.065

Harada, R., Okamura, N., Furumoto, S., Tago, T., Maruyama, M., Higuchi, M., et al. (2013). Comparison of the binding characteristics of [18 F] THK-523 and other amyloid imaging tracers to Alzheimer's disease pathology. *Eur. J. Nucl. Med. Mol. Imaging* 40, 125–132. doi: 10.1007/s00259-012-2261-2

He, K., Gkioxari, G., Dollár, P., and Girshick, R. (2017). Mask r-cnn. *arXiv*

Hill, D. L. G., Schwarz, A. J., Isaac, M., Pani, L., Vamvakas, S., Hemmings, R., et al. (2014). Coalition against major diseases/european medicines agency biomarker qualification of hippocampal volume for enrichment of clinical trials in predementia stages of Alzheimer's disease. *Alzheimer's Dement.* 10, 421–429. doi: 10.1016/j.jalz.2013.07.003

Hinton, G. E., Srivastava, N., Krizhevsky, A., Sutskever, I., and Salakhutdinov, R. R. (2015). Improving neural networks by preventing co-adaptation of feature detectors. *arXiv*

Hosseini-Asl, E., Gimel'farb, G., and El-Baz, A. (2016). Alzheimer's disease diagnostics by a deeply supervised adaptable 3d convolutional network. *arXiv*

Huang, C., Wahlund, L. O., Almkvist, O., Elehu, D., Svensson, L., Jonsson, T., et al. (2003). Voxel-and VOI-based analysis of SPECT CBF in relation to clinical and psychological heterogeneity of mild cognitive impairment. *Neuroimage* 19, 1137–1144. doi: 10.1016/s1053-8119(03)00168-x

Ioffe, S., and Szegedy, C. (2015). Batch normalization: accelerating deep network training by reducing internal covariate shift. *arXiv*

Jack, C. R. Jr., Albert, M. S., Knopman, D. S., McKhann, G. M., Sperling, R. A., Carrillo, M. C., et al. (2011a). Introduction to the recommendations from the national institute on aging-alzheimer's association workgroups on diagnostic guidelines for alzheimer's disease. *Alzheimer's Dement.* 7, 257–262. doi: 10.1016/j.jalz.2011.03.004

Jack, C. R. Jr., Barkhof, F., Bernstein, M. A., Cantillon, M., Cole, P. E., DeCarli, C., et al. (2011b). Steps to standardization and validation of hippocampal volumetry as a biomarker in clinical trials and diagnostic criterion for Alzheimer's disease. *Alzheimer's Dement.* 7, 474–485.

Jack, C. R. Jr., Bernstein, M. A., Fox, N. C., Thompson, P., Alexander, G., Harvey, D., et al. (2008a). The Alzheimer's disease neuroimaging initiative (ADNI): MRI methods. *J. Mag. Reson. Imag.* 27, 685–691.

Jack, C. R. Jr., Lowe, V. J., Senjem, M. L., Weigand, S. D., Kemp, B. J., Shiung, M. M., et al. (2008b). 11C PiB and structural MRI provide complementary information in imaging of Alzheimer's disease and amnestic mild cognitive impairment. *Brain* 131, 665–680. doi: 10.1093/brain/awm336

Jetley, S., Lord, N. A., Lee, N., and Torr, P. H. S. (2018). Learn to pay attention. *arXiv*

Jie, B., Zhang, D., Cheng, B., and Shen, D. (2015). Manifold regularized multitask feature learning for multimodality disease classification. *Hum. Brain Mapp.* 36, 489–507. doi: 10.1002/hbm.22642

Kingma, D. P., and Ba, J. (2014). Adam: a method for stochastic optimization. *arXiv* doi: 10.1002/mp.13112

Krizhevsky, A., Sutskever, I., and Hinton, G. E. (2012). Imagenet classification with deep convolutional neural networks. *Adv. Neural Inform. Process. Syst.* 25, 1097–1105.

Lebedeva, A. K., Westman, E., Borza, T., Beyer, M. K., Engedal, K., Aarsland, D., et al. (2017). MRI-based classification models in prediction of mild cognitive impairment and dementia in late-life depression. *Front. Aging Neurosci.* 9:13. doi: 10.3389/fnagi.2017.00013

LeCun, Y., Jackel, L. D., Bottou, L., Cortes, C., Denker, J. S., Drucker, H., et al. (1995). "Learning algorithms for classification: A comparison on handwritten digit recognition," in *Neural Networks: The Statistical Mechanics Perspective* eds J. H. Oh, C. Kwon, and S. Cho (Singapore: World Scientific), 261–276.

Ledig, C., Heckemann, R. A., Hammers, A., Lopez, J. C., Newcombe, V. F. J., Makropoulos, A., et al. (2015). Robust whole-brain segmentation: application to traumatic brain injury. *Med. Image Anal.* 21, 40–58. doi: 10.1016/j.media.2014.12.003

Li, R., Zhang, W., Suk, H. I., Wang, L., Li, J., Shen, D., et al. (2014). "Deep learning based imaging data completion for improved brain disease diagnosis," in *Proceedings of the International Conference on Medical Image Computing and Computer-Assisted Intervention*, (Cham: Springer), 305–312. doi: 10.1007/978-3-319-10443-0_39

Lin, W., Tong, T., Gao, Q., Guo, D., Du, X., Yang, Y., et al. (2018). Convolutional neural networks-based MRI image analysis for the alzheimer's disease prediction from mild cognitive impairment. *Front. Neurosci.* 12:777. doi: 10.3389/fnins.2018.00777

Litjens, G., Kooi, T., Bejnordi, B. E., Adiyoso Setio, A. A., Ciompi, F., Ghafoorian, M., et al. (2017). A survey on deep learning in medical image analysis. *Med. Image Anal.* 42, 60–88. doi: 10.1016/j.media.2017.07.005

Liu, M., Cheng, D., Wang, K., and Wang, Y. (2018). Multi-modality cascaded convolutional neural networks for alzheimer's disease diagnosis. *Neuroinformatics* 16, 295–308. doi: 10.1007/s12021-018-9370-4

Liu, S., Liu, S., Cai, W., Che, H., Pujol, S., Kikinis, R., et al. (2015). Multimodal neuroimaging feature learning for multiclass diagnosis of Alzheimer's disease. *IEEE Trans. Biomed. Eng.* 62, 1132–1140. doi: 10.1109/tbme.2014.2372011

Mosconi, L., De Santi, S., Li, Y., Zhan, J., Tsui, W. H., Boppana, M., et al. (2006). Visual rating of medial temporal lobe metabolism in mild cognitive impairment and Alzheimer's disease using FDG-PET. *Eur. J. Nucl. Med. Mol. Imaging* 33, 210–221. doi: 10.1007/s00259-005-1956-z

Mosconi, L., Tsui, W. H., Herholz, K., Pupi, A., Drzezga, A., Lucignani, G., et al. (2008). Multicenter standardized 18F-FDG PET diagnosis of mild cognitive impairment, Alzheimer's disease, and other dementias. *J. Nuclear Med.* 49:390. doi: 10.2967/jnumed.107.045385

Patterson, C. (2018). *World Alzheimer Report 2018, The State of the Art of Dementia Research: New frontiers*. London: Alzheimer's Disease International (ADI).

Petersen, R. C., Lopez, O., Armstrong, M. J., Getchius, T. S. D., Ganguli, M., Gloss, D., et al. (2018). Practice guideline update summary: mild cognitive impairment: report of the guideline development, dissemination, and implementation subcommittee of the American academy of neurology. *Neurology* 90, 126–135. doi: 10.1212/wnl.0000000000004826

Petersen, R. C., Smith, G. E., and Waring, S. C. (1999). Mild cognitive impairment: clinical characterization and outcome. *Arch. Neurol.* 56, 303–308.

Ren, S., He, K., Girshick, R., and Sun, J. (2015). "Faster r-cnn: Towards real-time object detection with region proposal networks," in *Proceedings of the IEEE Transactions on Pattern Analysis and Machine Intelligence*, (Piscataway: IEEE).

Rombouts, S. A. R. B., Barkhof, F., Goekoop, R., Stam, C. J., and Scheltens, P. (2005). Altered resting state networks in mild cognitive impairment and mild Alzheimer's disease: an fMRI study. *Hum. Brain Mapp.* 26, 231–239. doi: 10.1002/hbm.20160

Rondina, J. M., Ferreira, L. K., de Souza Duran, F. L., Kubo, R., Ono, C. R., Leite, C. C., et al. (2018). Selecting the most relevant brain regions to discriminate Alzheimer's disease patients from healthy controls using multiple kernel learning: a comparison across functional and structural imaging modalities and atlases. *NeuroImage Clin.* 17, 628–641. doi: 10.1016/j.nicl.2017.10.026

Russakovsky, O., Deng, J., Su, H., Krause, J., Satheesh, S., Ma, S., et al. (2015). Imagenet large scale visual recognition challenge. *Int. J. Comp. Vis.* 115, 211–252. doi: 10.1007/s11263-015-0816-y

Samper-González, J., Burgos, N., Bottani, S., Fontanella, S., Lu, P., Marcoux, A., et al. (2018). Reproducible evaluation of classification methods in Alzheimer's disease: framework and application to MRI and PET data. *bioRxiv*

Sarraf, S., and Tofighi, G. (2016). Classification of alzheimer's disease using fmri data and deep learning convolutional neural networks. *arXiv*

Silveira, M., and Marques, J. (2010). "Boosting Alzheimer disease diagnosis using PET images," in *Proceedings of the 2010 20th International Conference on Pattern Recognition*, (Istanbul: IEEE), 2556–2559.

Simonyan, K., and Zisserman, A. (2014). Very deep convolutional networks for large-scale image recognition. *arXiv*

Sorensen, L., Igel, C., Pai, A., Balas, I., Anker, C., Lillholm, M., et al. (2017). Differential diagnosis of mild cognitive impairment and Alzheimer's disease using structural MRI cortical thickness, hippocampal shape, hippocampal texture, and volumetry. *NeuroImage Clin.* 13, 470–482. doi: 10.1016/j.nicl.2016.11.025

Tong, T., Gray, K., Gao, Q., Chen, L., and Rueckert, D. (2017). Multi-modal classification of Alzheimer's disease using nonlinear graph fusion. *Patt. Recogn.* 63, 171–181. doi: 10.1016/j.patcog.2016.10.009

Wang, P., Chen, K., Yao, L., Hu, B., Wu, X., Zhang, J., et al. (2016). Multimodal classification of mild cognitive impairment based on partial least squares. *J. Alzheimer's Dis.* 54, 359–371. doi: 10.3233/jad-160102

World Health Organization (2012). *Dementia: a Public Health Priority*. Geneva: World Health Organization.

Zhang, D., Wang, Y., Zhou, L., Yuan, H., and Shen, D. (2011). Multimodal classification of Alzheimer's disease and mild cognitive impairment. *Neuroimage* 55, 856–867. doi: 10.1016/j.neuroimage.2011.01.008

Zhang, S., Smailagic, N., Hyde, C., Noel-Storr, A. H., Takwoingi, Y., McShane, R., et al. (2014). 11 C-PIB-PET for the early diagnosis of Alzheimer's disease dementia and other dementias in people with mild cognitive impairment (MCI). *Coch. Database Syst. Rev.* 2014:CD010386.

Zhuang, X., Arridge, S., Hawkes, D. J., and Ourselin, S. (2011). A nonrigid registration framework using spatially encoded mutual information and free-form deformations. *IEEE Trans. Med. Imaging* 30, 1819–1828. doi: 10.1109/TMI.2011.2150240

Zu, C., Jie, B., Liu, M., Chen, S., Shen, D., and Zhang, D. (2016). Label-aligned multi-task feature learning for multimodal classification of Alzheimer's disease and mild cognitive impairment. *Brain Imaging Behav.* 10, 1148–1159. doi: 10.1007/s11682-015-9480-7

19

A New Pulse Coupled Neural Network (PCNN) for Brain Medical Image Fusion Empowered by Shuffled Frog Leaping Algorithm

Chenxi Huang[1]*, Ganxun Tian*[1]*, Yisha Lan*[1]*, Yonghong Peng*[2]*, E. Y. K. Ng*[3]*, Yongtao Hao*[1]**,*
Yongqiang Cheng[4]* *and Wenliang Che*[5]*

[1] Department of Computer Science and Technology, Tongji University, Shanghai, China, [2] Faculty of Computer Science, University of Sunderland, Sunderland, United Kingdom, [3] School of Mechanical and Aerospace Engineering, Nanyang Technological University, Singapore, Singapore, [4] School of Engineering and Computer Science, University of Hull, Kingston upon Hull, United Kingdom, [5] Department of Cardiology, Shanghai Tenth People's Hospital, Tongji University School of Medicine, Shanghai, China

***Correspondence:**
Yongtao Hao
hao0yt@163.com
Yongqiang Cheng
Y.Cheng@hull.ac.uk
Wenliang Che
chewenliang@tongji.edu.cn

Recent research has reported the application of image fusion technologies in medical images in a wide range of aspects, such as in the diagnosis of brain diseases, the detection of glioma and the diagnosis of Alzheimer's disease. In our study, a new fusion method based on the combination of the shuffled frog leaping algorithm (SFLA) and the pulse coupled neural network (PCNN) is proposed for the fusion of SPECT and CT images to improve the quality of fused brain images. First, the intensity-hue-saturation (IHS) of a SPECT and CT image are decomposed using a non-subsampled contourlet transform (NSCT) independently, where both low-frequency and high-frequency images, using NSCT, are obtained. We then used the combined SFLA and PCNN to fuse the high-frequency sub-band images and low-frequency images. The SFLA is considered to optimize the PCNN network parameters. Finally, the fused image was produced from the reversed NSCT and reversed IHS transforms. We evaluated our algorithms against standard deviation (SD), mean gradient ($\bar{G}$), spatial frequency (SF) and information entropy (E) using three different sets of brain images. The experimental results demonstrated the superior performance of the proposed fusion method to enhance both precision and spatial resolution significantly.

Keywords: single-photon emission computed tomography image, computed tomography image, image fusion, pulse coupled neural network, shuffled frog leaping

INTRODUCTION

In 1895 Rontgen obtained the first human medical image by X-ray, after which research of medical images gained momentum, laying the foundation for medical image fusion. With the development of both medical imaging technology and hardware facilities, a series of medical images with different characteristics and information were obtained, contributing to a key source of information for disease diagnosis. At present, clinical medical images mainly include Computed Tomography (CT) images, Magnetic Resonance Imaging (MRI) images, Single-Photon Emission Computed

Tomography (SPECT) images, Dynamic Single-Photon Emission Computed Tomography (DSPECT) and ultrasonic images, etc. (Jodoin et al., 2015; Hansen et al., 2017; Zhang J. et al., 2017). It is necessary to fuse different modes of medical images into more informative images based on fusion algorithms, in order to provide doctors with more reliable information during clinical diagnosis (Kavitha and Chellamuthu, 2014; Zeng et al., 2014). At present, medical image fusion has been considered in many aspects, such as the localization of brain diseases, the detection of glioma, the diagnosis of AD (Alzheimer's disease), etc. (Huang, 1996; Singh et al., 2015; Zeng et al., 2018).

Image fusion is the synthesis of images into a new image using a specific algorithm. The space-time relativity and complementarity of information in fused images can be fully used in the process of image fusion, contributing to a more comprehensive expression of the scene (Wu et al., 2005; Choi, 2006). Conventional methods of SPECT and CT fusion images mainly include component substitution and multi-resolution analysis (Amolins et al., 2007; Huang and Du, 2008; Huang and Jiang, 2012). Component substitution mainly refers to intensity-hue-saturation (IHS) transform, with the advantage of improving the spatial resolution of SPECT images (Huang, 1999; Rahmani et al., 2010). The limitation of transform invariance leads to difficulty in extracting both image contour and edge details. In order to solve this problem, contourlet transform was proposed by Da et al. (2006), Zhao et al. (2012), Xin and Deng (2013). Moreover, non-subsampled contourlet transform (NSCT) was also proposed to fully extract the directional information of SPECT images and CT images to be fused, providing better performance in image decomposition (Da et al., 2006; Wang and Zhou, 2010; Yang et al., 2016).

The Pulse Coupled Neural Network (PCNN) was discovered by Eckhorn et al. (1989) in the 1990s while studying the imaging mechanisms of the visual cortex of small mammals. No training process is required in the PCNN and useful information can be obtained from a complex background through the PCNN. Nevertheless, the PCNN has its shortcomings, such as the numerous parameters and the complicated process of setting parameters. Thus, novel algorithms to optimize the PCNN parameters has been introduced to improve the calculation speed of PCNN (Huang, 2004; Huang et al., 2004; Jiang et al., 2014; Xiang et al., 2015). SFLA is a new heuristic algorithm first presented by Eusuff and Lansey, which combines the advantages of the memetic algorithm and particle swarm optimization. The algorithm can search and analyze the optimal value in a complex space with fewer parameters and has a higher performance and robustness (Samuel and Asir Rajan, 2015; Sapkheyli et al., 2015; Kaur and Mehta, 2017).

In our study, a new fusion approach based on the SFLA and PCNN is proposed to address the limitations discussed above. Our proposed method not only innovatively uses SFLA optimization to effectively learn the PCNN parameters, but also produces high quality fused images. A series of contrasting experiments are discussed in view of image quality and objective evaluations.

The remaining part of the paper is organized as follows. Related work is introduced in Section "Related Works." The fusion method is proposed in Section "Materials and Methods." The experimental results are presented in Sections "Result" and "Conclusion" concludes the paper with an outlook on future work.

RELATED WORKS

Image fusion involves a wide range of disciplines and can be classified under the category of information fusion, where a series of methods have been presented. A novel fusion method, for multi-scale images has been presented by Zhang X. et al. (2017) using Empirical Wavelet Transform (EWT). In the proposed method, simultaneous empirical wavelet transforms (SEWT) were used for one-dimensional and two-dimensional signals, to ensure the optimal wavelets for processed signals. A satisfying visual perception was achieved through a series of experiments and in terms of objective evaluations, it was demonstrated that the method was superior to other traditional algorithms. However, time consumption of the proposed method is high, mainly during the process of image decomposition, causing application difficulties in a real time system. Noised images should also be considered in future work where the process of generating optimal wavelets may be affected (Zeng et al., 2016b; Zhang X. et al., 2017).

Aishwarya and Thangammal (2017) also proposed a fusion method based on a supervised dictionary learning approach. During the dictionary training, in order to reduce the number of input patches, gradient information was first obtained for every patch in the training set. Second, both the information content and edge strength was measured for each gradient patch. Finally, the patches with better focus features were selected by a selection rule, to train the over complete dictionary. Additionally, in the process of fusion, the globally learned dictionary was used to achieve better visual quality. Nevertheless, high computational costs also exist in this proposed approach during the process of sparse coding and final fusion performance, which may be affected by high frequency noise (Zeng et al., 2016a; Aishwarya and Thangammal, 2017).

Moreover, an algorithm for the fusion of thermal and visual images was introduced by M Kanmani et al. in order to obtain a single comprehensive fused image. A novel method called self tuning particle swarm optimization (STPSO) was presented to calculate the optimal weights. A weighted averaging fusion rule was also used to fuse the low frequency- and high frequency coefficients, obtained through Dual Tree Discrete Wavelet Transform (DT-DWT) (Kanmani and Narasimhan, 2017; Zeng et al., 2017a). Xinxia Ji et al. proposed a new fusion algorithm based on an adaptive weighted method in combination with the idea of fuzzy theory. In the algorithm, a membership function with fuzzy logic variables were designed to achieve the transformation of different leveled coefficients by different weights. Experimental results indicated that the proposed algorithm outperformed existing algorithms in aspects of visual quality and objective measures (Ji and Zhang, 2017; Zeng et al., 2017b).

MATERIALS AND METHODS

The Image Fusion Method Based on PCNN and SFLA

The algorithm 3.1 represents an image fusion algorithm based on the PCNN and SFLA, where SPECT and CT images are fused. In our proposed algorithm, a SPECT image is first decomposed on three components using IHS transform, which include saturation S, hue H and intensity I. Component I is then decomposed to a low-frequency and high-frequency image through NSCT decomposition. Additionally, a CT image is decomposed into a low-frequency and high-frequency image through NSCT decomposition. Moreover, the two low-frequency images obtained above are fused in a new low-frequency image through the SFLA and PCNN combination fusion rules, while the two high-frequency images obtained above are fused into a new high-frequency image through the SFLA and PCNN combination fusion rules. Next, the new low-frequency and new high-frequency images are fused to generate a new image with intensity I' using reversed NSCT. Finally, the target image is achieved by using reversed IHS transform to integrate the three components S, H and I'.

Algorithm 1: An image fusion algorithm based on PCNN and SFLA

Input: A SPECT image A and a CT image B

Output: A fused image F

Step 1: Obtain three components of image A using IHS transform; saturation S, hue H and intensity I.

Step 2: Image decomposition

(1) Decompose the component I of image A to a low-frequency image AL and high-frequency image AH through NSCT decomposition.

(2) Decompose image B to a low-frequency image BL and high-frequency image BH through NSCT decomposition.

Step 3: Image fusion

(1) Fuse the low-frequency images AL and BL to a new low-frequency image CL through the SFLA and PCNN combination fusion rules.

(2) Fuse the high-frequency images AH and BH to form a new high-frequency image CH through the SFLA and PCNN combination fusion rules.

Step 4: Inverse transform

Fuse the low-frequency image CL and high-frequency image CH to a new image with intensity I' using reversed NSCT.

Step 5: Reversed IHS transform

Through the reversed IHS transform, integrate the three components S, H and I', then obtain the target image F.

The overall method of the proposed algorithm for the fusion of a SPECT and CT image is outlined in **Figure 1**.

Decomposition Rule

In our proposed method, the SPECT image and CT image are decomposed into a low-frequency and high-frequency image using NSCT.

Non-subsampled contourlet transform (Huang, 1999; Rahmani et al., 2010) is composed of a non-subsampled pyramid filter bank (NSPFB) and a non-subsampled directional filter bank (NSDFB). The source image is decomposed into a high-frequency sub-band and a low-frequency sub-band by NSPFB. The high-frequency sub-band is then decomposed into a sub-band of each direction by NSDFB. The structure diagram of the two-level decomposition of NSCT is shown in **Figure 2**.

An analysis filter $\{H_1(z), H_2(z)\}$ and a synthesis filter $\{G_1(z), G_2(z)\}$ are used when using NSCT to decompose images and the two filters satisfy $H_1(z)G_1(z) + H_2(z)G_2(z) = 1$. The source image can generate low-frequency and high-frequency sub-band images when it is decomposed by NSP. The next level of NSP decomposition is performed on low-frequency components obtained by the upper-level decomposition. An analysis filter $\{U_1(z), U_2(z)\}$ and synthesis filters $\{V_1(z), V_2(z)\}$ are contained in the design structure of NSDFB with the requirement of $U_1(z)V_1(z) + U_2(z)V_2(z) = 1$. The high-pass sub-band image decomposed by J-level NSP is decomposed by L-level NSDFB, and the high-frequency sub-band coefficients can be obtained at the number of 2^n, where n is an integer higher than 0. A fused image with clearer contours and translation invariants can be obtained through the fusion method based on NSCT (Xin and Deng, 2013).

Fusion Rule

Fusion rules affect image performance, so the selection of fusion rules largely determines the quality of the final fused image. In this section, the PCNN fusion algorithm based on SFLA is introduced for low-frequency and high-frequency sub-band images decomposed by NSCT.

Pulse Coupled Neural Network

The PCNN is a neural network model of single-cortex feedback, to simulate the processing mechanism of visual signals in the cerebral cortex of cats. It consists of several neurons connected to each other, where each neuron is composed of three parts: the receiving domain, the coupled linking modulation domain and the pulse generator. In image fusion using the PCNN, the M * N neurons of a two-dimensional PCNN network correspond to the M * N pixels of the two-dimensional input image, and the gray value of the pixel is taken as the external stimulus of the network neuron. Initially, the internal activation of neurons is equal to the external stimulation. When the external stimulus is greater than the threshold value, a natural ignition will occur. When a neuron ignites, its threshold will increase sharply and then decay exponentially with time. When the threshold attenuates to less than the corresponding internal activation, the neuron will ignite again, and the neuron will generate a pulse sequence signal. The ignited neurons stimulate the ignition of adjacent neurons by interacting with adjacent neurons, thereby generating an automatic wave in the activation region to propagate outward (Ge et al., 2009).

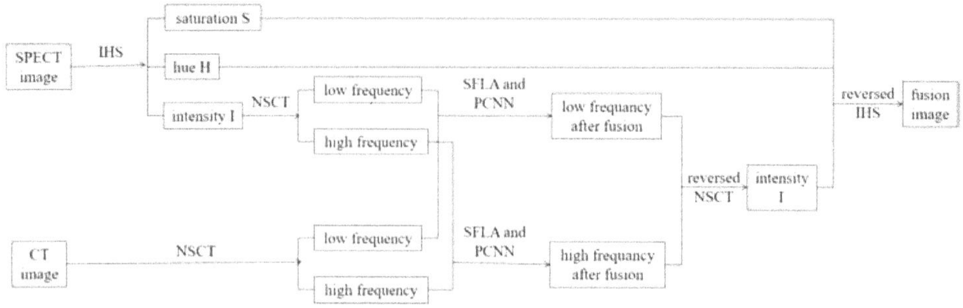

FIGURE 1 | The proposed method for the process of fusion.

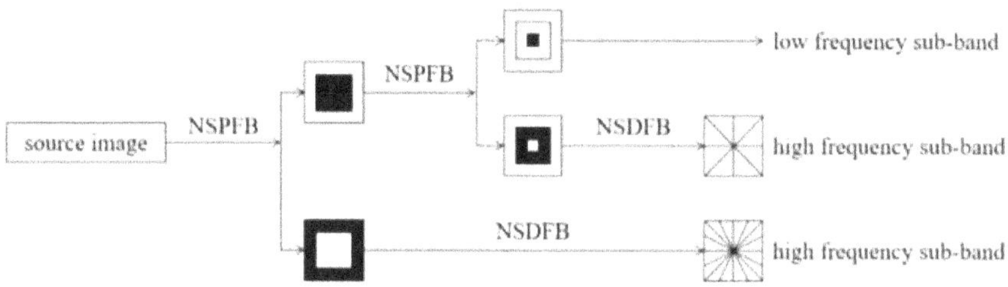

FIGURE 2 | The structure diagram of the two-level decomposition of NSCT.

The parameters of the PCNN affect the quality of image fusion, and most current research uses the method of regressively exploring the values of parameters, which is subjective to a certain degree. Therefore, how to reasonably set the parameters of the PCNN is the key to improving its performance. In our paper, SFLA is used to optimize the PCNN network parameters.

Shuffled Frog Leaping Algorithm

Shuffled frog leaping algorithm is a particle swarm search method based on groups to obtain optimal results. The flowchart of SFLA is shown in **Figure 3**. First, the population size F, the number of sub populations m, the maximum iterations of local search for each sub population N and the number of frogs in each sub population n were defined. Second, a population was initialed, and the fitness value of each frog was calculated and sorted in a descending order. A memetic algorithm is used in the process of the search, and the search is carried out in groups. All groups are then fused, and the frogs are sorted according to an established rule. Moreover, the frog population is divided based on the established rules, and the overall information exchange is achieved using this method until the number of iterations are equal to the maximum iterations N (Li et al., 2018).

F(x) is defined as a fitness function and Ω is a feasible domain. In each iteration, P_g is the best frog for a frog population, P_b represents the best frog for each group and P_w is the worst frog for each group. The algorithm adopts the following update strategy to carry out a local search in each group:

$$\begin{cases} S_j = rand() \cdot (P_b - P_w), \quad -S_{max} \leq S_j \leq S_{max} \\ P_{w,new} = P_w + S_j \end{cases} \tag{1}$$

where S_j represents the updated value of frog leaping, rand () is defined as the random number between 0 and 1, S_{max} is described as the maximum leaping value, and $P_{w,new}$ is the worst frog of updated group. If $P_{w,new} \in \Omega$ and $F(P_{w,new}) > F(P_w)$, P_w can be replaced by $P_{w,new}$, otherwise, P_b will be replaced by P_g. At the same time, if $P'_{w,new} \in \Omega$ and $F(P'_{w,new}) > F(P_w)$, P_w can be replaced by $P'_{w,new}$, otherwise P_w can be replaced by a new frog and then the process of iteration will continue until the maximum iterations is reached.

PCNN Fusion Algorithm Based on SFLA

Three parameters α_θ, β and V_θ in PCNN are essential for the results of image fusion. Therefore, as it is shown in **Figure 4**, in our study, the SFLA is used to optimize the PCNN in order to achieve the optimal solution of the PCNN parameters. Each frog is defined as a spatial solution $X(\alpha_\theta, \beta, V_\theta)$ and the optimal configuration scheme of the PCNN parameters can finally be obtained by searching for the best frog $X_b(\alpha_\theta, \beta, V_\theta)$.

In our proposed method, possible configuration schemes of parameters are defined, which constitute a solution space for the parameter optimization. After generating an initial frog solution space, F frogs in the population are divided into m groups, and each group is dependent on one another. Starting from the initial solution, the frogs in each group first carry out an intraclass optimization by a local search, thereby continuously updating their own fitness values. In N iterations of local optimization, the quality of the whole frog population is optimized with the improvement of the quality of frogs in all groups. The frogs of the population are then fused and regrouped according to the established rule, and local optimization within the group is

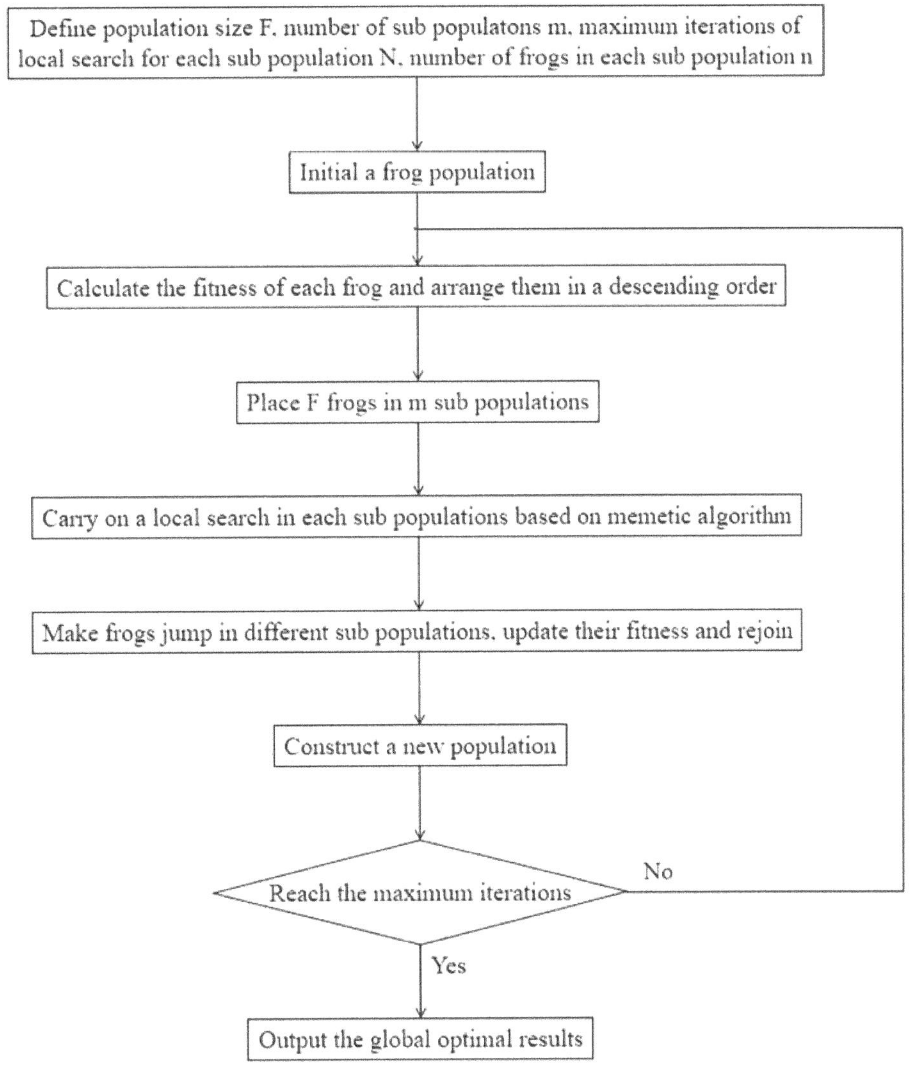

FIGURE 3 | The flowchart of the shuffled frog leaping algorithm.

carried out until reaching the final iteration conditions. Finally, the global optimal solution of the frog population is defined as the optimal PCNN parameter configuration. The final fusion image is thus obtained using the optimal parameter configuration above.

RESULTS

In order to verify the accuracy and preservation of the edge details in our proposed method, three sets of CT and SPECT images were fused based on our method. The results of each set were compared with four fusion methods; IHS, NSCT+FL, DWT, NSCT+PCNN. In the method of NSCT+FL, images are first decomposed by NSCT to obtain high-frequency and low-frequency coefficients, and then fusion images are obtained by taking large value high-frequency coefficients and taking average value low-frequency coefficients. In NSCT+PCNN, images are decomposed by NSCT and fused by the PCNN.

Subjective Evaluations of Experimental Results

Experiments were implemented on the image database from the Whole Brain Web Site of Harvard Medical School (Johnson and Becker, 2001) which contains two groups of images including CT and SPECT images. Each group has three examples including normal brain images, glioma brain images and brain images of patients diagnosed with Alzheimer's disease. The testing images have been used in many related papers (Du et al., 2016a,b,c) and the platform is MATLAB R2018a.

A series of fusion results of SPECT and CT images, based on different methods including IHS, NSCT+FL, DWT, NSCT+PCNN, and our proposed method is shown in **Figures 5–7**. The fusion results of a set of normal brain images are shown in **Figure 5**, the fusion results of a set of glioma brain images are presented in **Figure 6**, while a set of brain images of patients diagnosed with Alzheimer's disease are shown

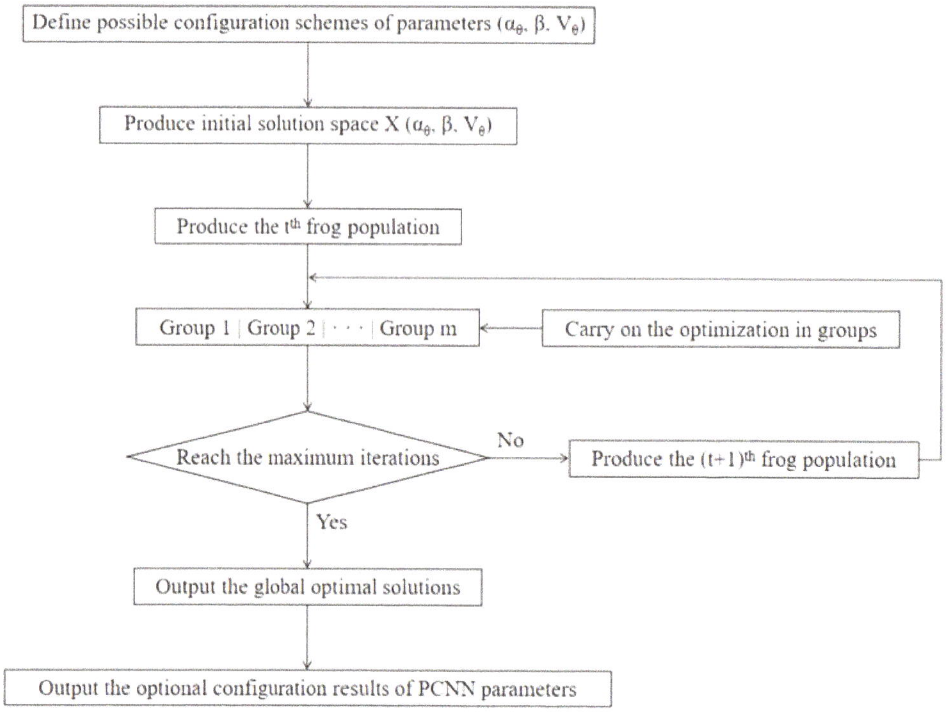

FIGURE 4 | The process of PCNN parameter optimization based on SFLA.

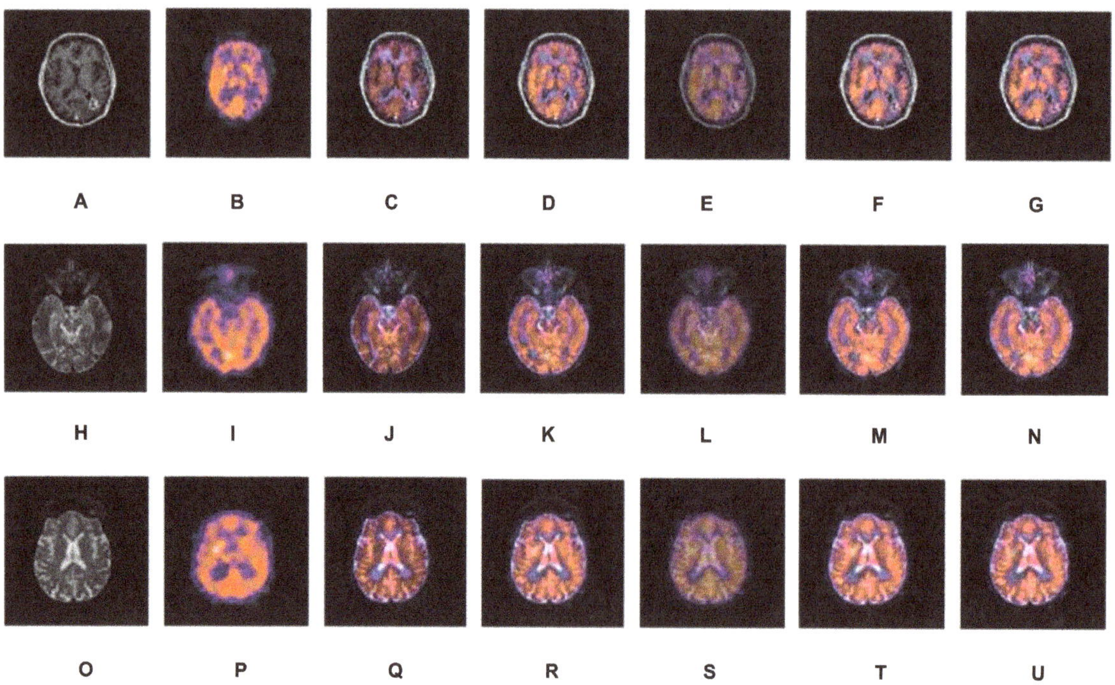

FIGURE 5 | A series of contrasting experiments for normal brain images on fusion images based on different fusion methods (set 1). **(A,H,O)** are source CT images; **(B,I,P)** are source SPECT images; **(C,J,Q)** are fused images based on IHS; **(D,K,R)** are fused images based on NSCT+FL; **(E,L,S)** are fused images based on DWT; **(F,M,T)** are fused images based on the combination of NSCT+PCNN; **(G,N,U)** are fused images based on the proposed method.

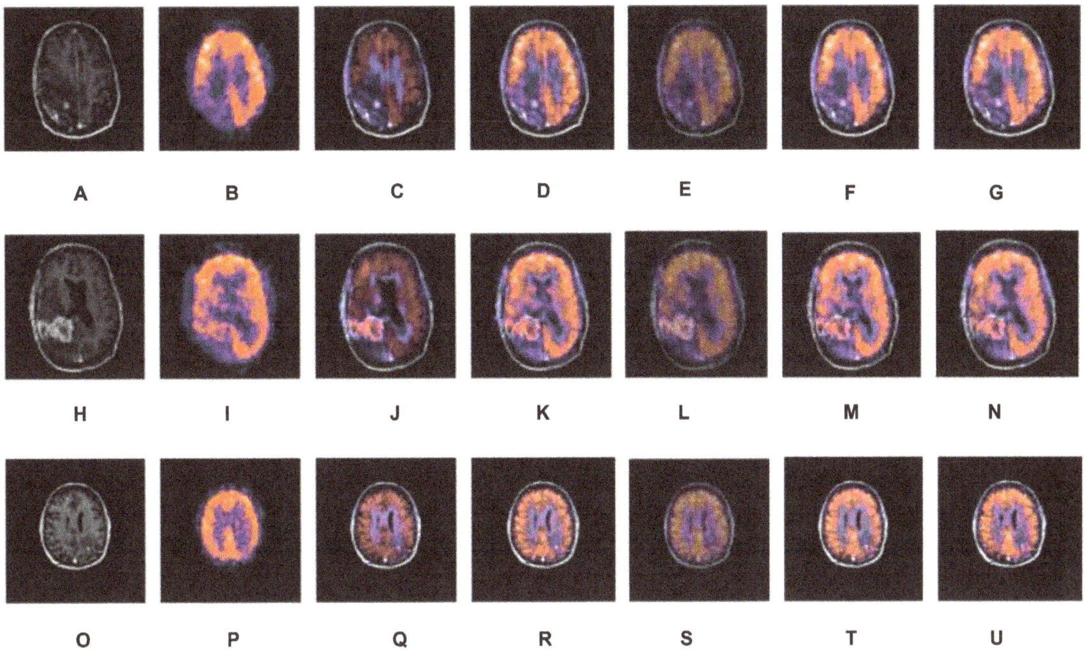

FIGURE 6 | A series of contrasting experiments for glioma brain images on fusion images based on different fusion methods (set 2). **(A,H,O)** are source CT images; **(B,I,P)** are source SPECT images; **(C,J,Q)** are fused images based on IHS; **(D,K,R)** are fused images based on NSCT+FL; **(E,L,S)** are fused images based on DWT; **(F,M,T)** are fused images based on the combination of NSCT+PCNN; **(G,N,U)** are fused images based on the proposed method.

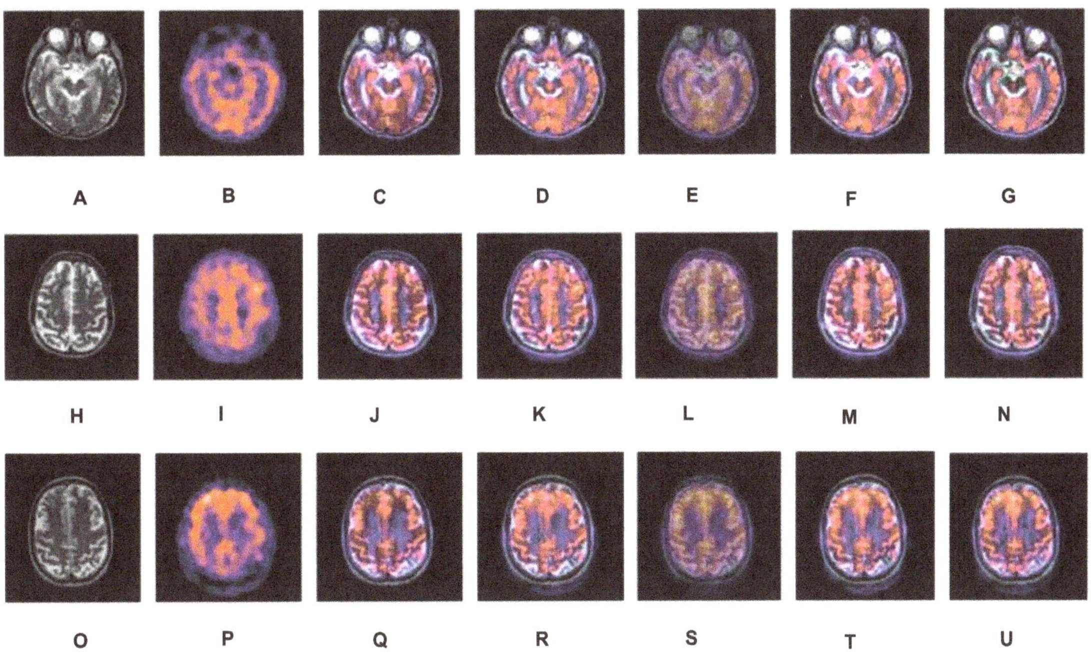

FIGURE 7 | A series of contrasting experiments for brain images of patients diagnosed with Alzheimer's disease on fusion images based on different fusion methods (set 3). **(A,H,O)** are source CT images; **(B,I,P)** are source SPECT images; **(C,J,Q)** are fused images based on IHS; **(D,K,R)** are fused images based on NSCT+FL; **(E,L,S)** are fused images based on DWT; **(F,M,T)** are fused images based on the combination of NSCT+PCNN; **(G,N,U)** are fused images based on the proposed method.

in **Figure 7**. In **Figures 5–7**, (a), (h) and (o) are source CT images; (b), (i), (p) are source SPECT images; (c), (j) and (q) are fused images based on IHS; (d), (k) and (r) are fused images based on NSCT+FL; (e), (l) and (s) are fused images based on DWT; (f), (m) and (t) are fused images based on the combination of NSCT+PCNN; (g), (n) and (u) are fused images based on the proposed method. It can be seen that the fusion results based on our proposed method are more accurate and clearer than those based on various other methods. Our proposed method contributes to a higher brightness of fusion images and more information on the edge details.

Objective Evaluations of Experimental Results

A set of metrics is used to compare the performance of the fusion methods including IHS, DWT, NSCT, PCNN, a combination of NSCT and the PCNN, and our proposed method. The evaluation metrics including standard deviation (SD), mean gradient ($\bar{G}$), spatial frequency (SF) and information entropy (E) are entailed as follows (Huang et al., 2018):

(1) Standard deviation

Standard deviation is used to evaluate the contrast of the fused image, which is defined as

$$\sigma = \sqrt{\sum_{i=1}^{M}\sum_{j=1}^{N}(Z(i,j)-\bar{Z})^2/(M\times N)} \quad (2)$$

where $Z(i,j)$ represents the pixel value of the fused image and $\bar{Z}$ is the mean value of the pixel values of the image. The SD reflects the discrete image gray scale relative to the mean value of gray scale. And a higher value of SD demonstrates the performance of a fused image.

(2) Mean gradient ($\bar{G}$)

$\bar{G}$ corresponds to the ability of a fused image to represent the contrast of tiny details sensitively. It can be mathematically described as

$$\bar{G} = \frac{1}{(M-1)(N-1)}\sum_{i=1}^{M-1}\sum_{j=1}^{N-1} \times\sqrt{((\frac{\partial Z(x_i,y_j)}{\partial x_i})^2+(\frac{\partial Z(x_i,y_j)}{\partial y_i})^2)/2} \quad (3)$$

The fused image is clearer when the value of mean gradient is higher.

(3) Spatial frequency (SF)

Spatial frequency is the measure of the overall activity in a fused image. For an image with a gray value $Z(x_i, y_j)$ at position (x_i, y_j), the spatial frequency is defined as

$$SF = \sqrt{RF^2 + CF^2} \quad (4)$$

Where row frequency

$$RF = \sqrt{\frac{1}{M\times N}\sum_{i=1}^{M}\sum_{j=2}^{N}[Z(x_i,y_j)-Z(x_i,y_{j-1})]^2} \quad (5)$$

Column frequency

$$CF = \sqrt{\frac{1}{M\times N}\sum_{i=2}^{M}\sum_{j=1}^{N}[Z(x_i,y_j)-Z(x_{i-1},y_j)]^2} \quad (6)$$

The higher the value of frequency, the better the fused image quality.

(4) Information entropy (E)

Information entropy is provided by the below equation

$$E = -\sum_{i=0}^{L-1} p_i \log_2 p_i \quad (7)$$

TABLE 1 | Performance evaluations on normal brain fused images based on different methods.

	Metric	IHS	NSCT+FL	DWT	NSCT+PCNN	Proposed
Set 1	Standard deviation	51.6141	55.2178	42.5312	57.1188	57.2258
	Mean gradient	8.8561	8.714	6.2027	8.8568	8.8071
	Spatial frequency	33.5851	33.2324	22.0093	33.7566	33.6546
	Information entropy	2.6859	2.7565	3.0483	2.7729	3.0621
Set 2	Standard deviation	43.278	49.5989	43.0915	52.9246	53.1691
	Mean gradient	6.686	6.6633	4.5622	6.5672	6.7489
	Spatial frequency	20.3855	19.9558	12.7416	19.8214	20.0956
	Information entropy	3.6325	3.9243	4.2501	3.8386	3.9424
Set 3	Standard deviation	50.0926	55.7124	47.4476	57.1246	57.1268
	Mean gradient	6.2153	6.1775	4.1822	6.086	6.1796
	Spatial frequency	19.244	18.9682	12.0096	18.7269	18.7335
	Information entropy	3.6226	3.7122	4.0074	3.7139	3.7399

TABLE 2 | Performance evaluations on glioma brain fused images based on different methods.

	Metric	IHS	NSCT+FL	DWT	NSCT+PCNN	Proposed
Set 1	Standard deviation	41.7514	55.2055	39.8132	58.0374	58.3122
	Mean gradient	5.2953	5.5442	3.8166	5.459	5.5678
	Spatial frequency	16.2064	16.5277	10.1649	16.466	16.4776
	Information entropy	3.9255	4.1433	4.6303	4.08	4.1788
Set 2	Standard deviation	44.154	55.5879	42.436	57.7284	57.775
	Mean gradient	6.2881	6.6316	4.595	6.535	6.7276
	Spatial frequency	17.6675	17.9369	11.359	17.9359	17.9095
	Information entropy	4.3966	4.7513	5.1901	4.6312	4.837
Set 3	Standard deviation	48.6572	54.0708	41.78	56.2065	56.3546
	Mean gradient	6.8855	6.8515	4.8166	6.774	6.7977
	Spatial frequency	27.8964	27.8583	17.8725	27.7365	27.7654
	Information entropy	2.4852	2.5749	2.8442	2.5239	2.658

TABLE 3 | Performance evaluations on fused brain images of patients diagnosed with Alzheimer's disease, based on different methods.

	Metric	IHS	NSCT+FL	DWT	NSCT+PCNN	Proposed
Set 1	Standard deviation	66.1357	65.3766	51.0336	69.5392	66.5782
	Mean gradient	9.9938	10.0303	6.509	10.0089	10.2068
	Spatial frequency	26.7087	26.7329	16.1614	26.6568	27.1771
	Information entropy	4.7735	4.834	5.4105	4.8036	4.8966
Set 2	Standard deviation	59.1931	59.2093	52.0837	61.4981	60.6457
	Mean gradient	6.7482	7.0266	4.5756	7	7.0461
	Spatial frequency	19.0263	19.3264	11.8249	19.3257	19.512
	Information entropy	3.9901	4.1834	4.5922	4.0985	4.2156
Set 3	Standard deviation	56.0974	58.787	47.6032	56.0943	57.7578
	Mean gradient	7.9023	8.111	5.4579	7.9592	7.966
	Spatial frequency	22.2846	22.4084	13.907	21.9421	22.0022
	Information entropy	3.895	4.1058	5.1943	4.2228	4.2897

where L is image gray scale and Pi is the proportion of the pixel of the gray value i in whole pixels. A higher value of entropy indicates more information contained in the fused image.

Experiment results on fused images of SPECT images and CT images are shown in **Tables 1–3**. The fusion results of a set of normal brain images are shown in **Table 1**, the fusion results of a set of glioma brain images are presented in **Table 2**, while a set of brain images of patients diagnosed with Alzheimer's disease are shown **Table 3**. It can be seen that compared to other fusion methods, our proposed method generally has higher values in SD, $\bar{G}$, SF and E. The experimental results demonstrate that information of fusion images obtained by our proposed method is more abundant, the inheritance of detail information performs better, while the resolution is significantly improved.

CONCLUSION

In this paper, a new fusion method for SPECT brain and CT brain images was put forward. First, NSCT was used to decompose the IHS transform of a SPECT and CT image. The fusion rules, based on the regional average energy, was then used for low-frequency coefficients and the combination of SFLA and the PCNN was used for high-frequency sub-bands. Finally, the fused image was produced by reversed NSCT and reversed IHS transform. Both subjective evaluations and objective evaluations were used to analyze the quality of the fused images. The results demonstrated that the method we put forward can retain the information of source images better and reveal more details in integration. It can be seen that the proposed method is valid and effective in achieving satisfactory fusion results, leading to a wide range of applications in practice.

The paper focuses on multi-mode medical image fusion. However, there is a negative correlation between the real-time processing speed and the effectiveness of medical image fusion. Under the premise of ensuring the quality of fusion results, how to improve the efficiency of the method should be considered in the future.

AUTHOR CONTRIBUTIONS

CH conceived the study. GT and CH designed the model. YC and YP analyzed the data. YL and WC wrote the draft. EN and YH interpreted the results. All authors gave critical revision and consent for this submission.

FUNDING

This work was supported in part by the Tongji University Short-term Study Abroad Program under Grant 2018020017, National Science and Technology Support Program under Grant 2015BAF10B01, and National Natural Science Foundation of China under Grants 81670403, 81500381, and 81201069. CH acknowledges support from Tongji University for the exchange with Nanyang Technological University.

REFERENCES

Aishwarya, N., and Thangammal, C. B. (2017). An image fusion framework using novel dictionary based sparse representation. *Multimed. Tools Appl.* 76, 21869–21888. doi: 10.1007/s11042-016-4030-x

Amolins, K., Zhang, Y., and Dare, P. (2007). Wavelet based image fusion techniques- an introduction, review and comparison. *ISPRS J. Photogramm. Remote Sens.* 62, 249–263. doi: 10.1016/j.isprsjprs.2007.05.009

Choi, M. (2006). A new intensity-hue-saturation fusion approach to image fusion with a tradeoff parameter. *IEEE Trans. Geosci. Remote Sens.* 44, 1672–1682. doi: 10.1109/TGRS.2006.869923

Da, C., Zhou, J., and Do, M. (2006). "The non-subsampled contourlet transform: theory, design, and applications," in *Proceedings of the IEEE Transaction on Image Processing*, Vol. 15 (Piscataway, NJ: IEEE), 3089–3101. doi: 10.1109/TIP.2006.877507

Du, J., Li, W., Xiao, B., and Nawaz, Q. (2016a). An overview of multi-modal medical image fusion. *Knowl. Based Syst.* 215, 3–20.

Du, J., Li, W., Xiao, B., and Nawaz, Q. (2016b). Medical image fusion by combining parallel features on multi-scale local extrema scheme. *Knowl. Based Syst.* 113, 4–12. doi: 10.1016/j.knosys.2016.09.008

Du, J., Li, W., Xiao, B., and Nawaz, Q. (2016c). Union Laplacian pyramid with multiple features for medical image fusion. *Neurocomputing* 194, 326–339. doi: 10.1016/j.neucom.2016.02.047

Eckhorn, R., Reitboeck, H. J., Arndt, M., and Dicke, P. (1989). "A neural network for feature linking via synchronous activity: results from cat visual cortex and from simulations," in *Models of Brain Function*, ed. R. M. J. Cotterill (Cambridge: Cambridge University Press), 255–272. doi: 10.1139/w00-039

Ge, J., Wang, Y., Zhang, H., and Zhou, B. (2009). Study of intelligent inspection machine based on modified pulse coupled neural network. *Chin. J. Sci. Instrum.* 30, 1866–1873.

Hansen, N. L., Koo, B. C., Gallagher, F. A., Warren, A. Y., Doble, A., Gnanapragasam, V., et al. (2017). Comparison of initial and tertiary centre second opinion reads of multiparametric magnetic resonance imaging of the prostate prior to repeat biopsy. *Eur. Radiol.* 27, 2259–2266. doi: 10.1007/s00330-016-4635-5

Huang, C., Xie, Y., Lan, Y., Hao, Y., Chen, F., Cheng, Y., et al. (2018). A new framework for the integrative analytics of intravascular ultrasound and optical coherence tomography images. *IEEE Access* 6, 36408–36419. doi: 10.1109/ACCESS.2018.2839694

Huang, D. (1999). Radial basis probabilistic neural networks: model and application. *Int. J. Pattern Recogn.* 13, 1083–1101. doi: 10.1109/LGRS.2010.2046715

Huang, D. (2004). A constructive approach for finding arbitrary roots of polynomials by neural networks. *IEEE Trans. Neural Netw.* 15, 477–491. doi: 10.1109/TNN.2004.824424

Huang, D., and Du, J. (2008). A constructive hybrid structure optimization methodology for radial basis probabilistic neural networks. *IEEE Trans. Neural Netw.* 19, 2099–2115. doi: 10.1109/TNN.2008.2004370

Huang, D., Horace, H., and Chi, Z. (2004). A neural root finder of polynomials based on root moments. *Neural Comput.* 16, 1721–1762. doi: 10.1162/089976604774201668

Huang, D., and Jiang, W. (2012). A general CPL-AdS methodology for fixing dynamic parameters in dual environments. *IEEE Trans. Syst. Man Cybern. B Cybern.* 42, 1489–1500. doi: 10.1109/TSMCB.2012.2192475

Huang, S. (1996). *Systematic Theory of Neural Networks for Pattern Recognition (in Chinese).* Beijing: Publishing House of Electronic Industry of China.

Ji, X., and Zhang, G. (2017). Image fusion method of SAR and infrared image based on Curvelet transform with adaptive weighting. *Multimed. Tools Appl.* 76, 17633–17649. doi: 10.1007/s11042-016-4030-x

Jiang, P., Zhang, Q., Li, J., and Zhang, J. (2014). Fusion algorithm for infrared and visible image based on NSST and adaptive PCNN. *Laser Infrared* 44, 108–113.

Jodoin, P. M., Pinheiro, F., Oudot, A., and Lalande, A. (2015). Left-ventricle segmentation of SPECT images of rats. *IEEE Trans. Biomed. Eng.* 5, 2260–2268. doi: 10.1109/TBME.2015.2422263

Johnson, K. A., and Becker, J. A. (2001). *The Whole Brain Altas.* Available at: http://www.med.harvard.edu/aanlib/

Kanmani, M., and Narasimhan, V. (2017). An optimal weighted averaging fusion strategy for thermal and visible images using dual tree discrete wavelet transform and self tunning particle swarm optimization. *Multimed. Tools Appl.* 76, 20989–21010. doi: 10.1007/s11042-016-4030-x

Kaur, P., and Mehta, S. (2017). Resource provisioning and work flow scheduling in clouds using augmented shuffled frog leaping algorithm. *J. Parallel Distrib. Comput.* 101, 41–50. doi: 10.1016/j.jpdc.2016.11.003

Kavitha, C. T., and Chellamuthu, C. (2014). Fusion of SPECT and MRI images using integer wavelet transform in combination with curvelet transform. *Imaging Sci. J.* 63, 17–24. doi: 10.1179/1743131X14Y.0000000092

Li, R., Ji, C., Sun, P., Liu, D., Zhang, P., and Li, J. (2018). Optimizing operation of cascade reservoirs based on improved shuffled frog leaping algorithm. *J. Yangtze River Sci. Res. Inst.* 35, 30–35.

Rahmani, S., Strait, M., Merkurjev, D., Moeller, M., and Wittman, T. (2010). An adaptive IHS pan-sharpening method. *IEEE Geosci. Remote Sens. Lett.* 7, 746–750. doi: 10.1109/LGRS.2010.2046715

Samuel, G. C., and Asir Rajan, C. C. (2015). Hybrid: particle swarm optimization-genetic algorithm and particle swarm optimization-shuffled frog leaping algorithm for long-term generator maintenance scheduling. *Int. J. Elec. Power* 65, 432–442. doi: 10.1016/j.ijepes.2014.10.042

Sapkheyli, A., Zain, A. M., and Sharif, S. (2015). The role of basic, modified and hybrid shuffled frog leaping algorithm on optimization problems: a review. *Soft Comput.* 19, 2011–2038. doi: 10.1007/s00500-014-1388-4

Singh, S., Gupta, D., Anand, R. S., and Kumar, V. (2015). Nonsubsampled shearlet based CT and MRI medical image fusion using biologically inspired spiking neural network. *Biomed. Signal Process. Control* 18, 91–101. doi: 10.1016/j.bspc.2014.11.009

Wang, D., and Zhou, J. (2010). Image fusion algorithm based on the nonsubsampled contourlet transform. *Comput. Syst. Appl.* 19, 220–224. doi: 10.1109/ICFCC.2010.5497801

Wu, J., Huang, H., Qiu, Y., Wu, H., Tian, J., and Liu, J. (2005). "Remote sensing image fusion based on average gradient of wavelet transform," in *Proccedings of the 2005 IEEE International Conference on Mechatronics and Automation*, Vol. 4 (Niagara Falls, ON: IEEE), 1817–1821. doi: 10.1109/ICMA.2005.1626836

Xiang, T., Yan, L., and Gao, R. (2015). A fusion algorithm for infrared and visible images based on adaptive dual-channel unit-linking PCNN in NSCT domain. *Infrared Phys. Technol.* 69, 53–61. doi: 10.1016/j.infrared.2015.01.002

Xin, Y., and Deng, L. (2013). An improved remote sensing image fusion method based on wavelet transform. *Laser Optoelectron. Prog.* 15, 133–138.

Yang, J., Wu, Y., Wang, Y., and Xiong, Y. (2016). "A novel fusion technique for CT and MRI medical image based on NSST," in *Proccedings of the Chinese Control and Decision Conference* (Yinchuan: IEEE), 4367–4372. doi: 10.1109/CCDC.2016.7531752

Zeng, N., Qiu, H., Wang, Z., Liu, W., Zhang, H., and Li, Y. (2018). A new switching-delayed-PSO-based optimized SVM algorithm for diagnosis of Alzheimer's disease. *Neurocomputing* 320, 195–202. doi: 10.1016/j.neucom.2018.09.001

Zeng, N., Wang, H., Liu, W., Liang, J., and Alsaadi, F. E. (2017a). A switching delayed PSO optimized extreme learning machine for short-term load forecasting. *Neurocomputing* 240, 175–182. doi: 10.1016/j.neucom.2017.01.090

Zeng, N., Zhang, H., Li, Y., Liang, J., and Dobaie, A. M. (2017b). Denoising and deblurring gold immunochromatographic strip images via gradient projection algorithms. *Neurocomputing* 247, 165–172. doi: 10.1016/j.neucom.2017.03.056

Zeng, N., Wang, Z., and Zhang, H. (2016a). Inferring nonlinear lateral flow immunoassay state-space models via an unscented Kalman filter. *Sci. China Inform. Sci.* 59:112204. doi: 10.1007/s11432-016-0280-9

Zeng, N., Wang, Z., Zhang, H., and Alsaadi, F. E. (2016b). A novel switching delayed PSO algorithm for estimating unknown parameters of lateral flow immunoassay. *Cogn. Comput.* 8, 143–152. doi: 10.1007/s12559-016-9396-6

Zeng, N., Wang, Z., Zineddin, B., Li, Y., Du, M., Xiao, L., et al. (2014). Image-based quantitative analysis of gold immunochromato graphic strip via cellular neural network approach. *IEEE Trans. Med. Imaging* 33, 1129–1136. doi: 10.1109/TMI.2014.2305394

Zhang, J., Sun, Y., Zhang, Y., and Teng, J. (2017). Double regularization medical CT image blind restoration reconstruction based on proximal alternating direction method of multipliers. *EURASIP J. Image Video Process.* 2017:70. doi: 10.1186/s13640-017-0218-x

Zhang, X., Li, X., and Feng, Y. (2017). Image fusion based on simultaneous empirical wavelet transform. *Multimed. Tools Appl.* 76, 8175–8193. doi: 10.1007/s11042-016-4030-x

Zhao, Q., He, L., and Wen, P. (2012). Image fusion method based on average grads and wavelet contrast. *Comput. Eng. Appl.* 48, 165–168. doi: 10.3778/j.issn.1002-8331.2012.24.037

Permissions

All chapters in this book were first published by Frontiers; hereby published with permission under the Creative Commons Attribution License or equivalent. Every chapter published in this book has been scrutinized by our experts. Their significance has been extensively debated. The topics covered herein carry significant findings which will fuel the growth of the discipline. They may even be implemented as practical applications or may be referred to as a beginning point for another development.

The contributors of this book come from diverse backgrounds, making this book a truly international effort. This book will bring forth new frontiers with its revolutionizing research information and detailed analysis of the nascent developments around the world.

We would like to thank all the contributing authors for lending their expertise to make the book truly unique. They have played a crucial role in the development of this book. Without their invaluable contributions this book wouldn't have been possible. They have made vital efforts to compile up to date information on the varied aspects of this subject to make this book a valuable addition to the collection of many professionals and students.

This book was conceptualized with the vision of imparting up-to-date information and advanced data in this field. To ensure the same, a matchless editorial board was set up. Every individual on the board went through rigorous rounds of assessment to prove their worth. After which they invested a large part of their time researching and compiling the most relevant data for our readers.

The editorial board has been involved in producing this book since its inception. They have spent rigorous hours researching and exploring the diverse topics which have resulted in the successful publishing of this book. They have passed on their knowledge of decades through this book. To expedite this challenging task, the publisher supported the team at every step. A small team of assistant editors was also appointed to further simplify the editing procedure and attain best results for the readers.

Apart from the editorial board, the designing team has also invested a significant amount of their time in understanding the subject and creating the most relevant covers. They scrutinized every image to scout for the most suitable representation of the subject and create an appropriate cover for the book.

The publishing team has been an ardent support to the editorial, designing and production team. Their endless efforts to recruit the best for this project, has resulted in the accomplishment of this book. They are a veteran in the field of academics and their pool of knowledge is as vast as their experience in printing. Their expertise and guidance has proved useful at every step. Their uncompromising quality standards have made this book an exceptional effort. Their encouragement from time to time has been an inspiration for everyone.

The publisher and the editorial board hope that this book will prove to be a valuable piece of knowledge for researchers, students, practitioners and scholars across the globe.

List of Contributors

Shui-Hua Wang
School of Computer Science and Technology, Henan Polytechnic University, Jiaozuo, China
School of Architecture Building and Civil Engineering, Loughborough University, Loughborough, United Kingdom
Department of Informatics, University of Leicester, Leicester, United Kingdom

Chaosheng Tang and Junding Sun
School of Computer Science and Technology, Henan Polytechnic University, Jiaozuo, China

Jingyuan Yang
The Faculty of Computer Science and Engineering, Xi'an University of Technology, Xi'an, China

Chenxi Huang
Department of Computer Science and Technology, Tongji University, Shanghai, China

Preetha Phillips
West Virginia School of Osteopathic Medicine, Lewisburg, WV, United States

Yu-Dong Zhang
School of Computer Science and Technology, Henan Polytechnic University, Jiaozuo, China
Department of Informatics, University of Leicester, Leicester, United Kingdom

Junting Zhao and Ran Su
School of Computer Software, College of Intelligence and Computing, Tianjin University, Tianjin, China

Leyi Wei
School of Computer Science and Technology, College of Intelligence and Computing, Tianjin University, Tianjin, China

David S. Guttery
Department of Informatics, University of Leicester, Leicester, United Kingdom

Changming Sun
CSIRO Data61, Sydney, NSW, Australia

Quan Zou
Institute of Fundamental and Frontier Sciences, University of Electronic Science and Technology of China, Chengdu, China

Michelle Livne, Tabea Kossen and Vince I. Madai
Predictive Modelling in Medicine Research Group, Department of Neurosurgery, Charité - Universitätsmedizin Berlin, Berlin, Germany
Centre for Stroke Research Berlin, Charité - Universitätsmedizin Berlin, Berlin, Germany

Jana Rieger, Orhun Utku Aydin, Ela Marie Akay and Dietmar Frey
Predictive Modelling in Medicine Research Group, Department of Neurosurgery, Charité - Universitätsmedizin Berlin, Berlin, Germany

Abdel Aziz Taha
Research Studios Data Science, Research Studios Austria, Salzburg, Austria

Jan Sobesky
Centre for Stroke Research Berlin, Charité - Universitätsmedizin Berlin, Berlin, Germany
Department of Neurology, Johanna-Etienne Hospital Neuss, Neuss, Germany

John D. Kelleher
Information, Communication and Entertainment Institute (ICE), Dublin Institute of Technology, Dublin, Ireland

Yubraj Gupta, Ramesh Kumar Lama and Goo-Rak Kwon
Department of Information and Communication Engineering, Chosun University, Gwangju, South Korea

Zhaopeng Meng
School of Computer Software, College of Intelligence and Computing, Tianjin University, Tianjin, China
Tianjin University of Traditional Chinese Medicine, Tianjin, China

Fangyang Jiao
Department of Nuclear Medicine, Daping Hospital, Army Medical University, Chongqing, China

Kristian Hildebrand
Department VI Computer Science and Media, Beuth University of Applied Sciences, Berlin, Germany

Shipeng Xie
College of Telecommunications and Information Engineering, Nanjing University of Posts and Telecommunications, Nanjing, China,

Xianqing Chen
Department of Electrical Engineering, College of Engineering, Zhejiang Normal University, Jinhua, China

Chaosheng Tang and Junding Sun
School of Computer Science and Technology, Henan Polytechnic University, Jiaozuo, China

Yu-Dong Zhang
School of Computer Science and Technology, Henan Polytechnic University, Jiaozuo, China
Department of Informatics, University of Leicester, Leicester, United Kingdom
Guangxi Key Laboratory of Manufacturing System and Advanced Manufacturing Technology, Guilin, China

Claes Nøhr Ladefoged, Lisbeth Marner, Amalie Hindsholm, Ian Law, Liselotte Højgaard and Flemming Littrup Andersen
Department of Clinical Physiology, Nuclear Medicine and PET, Rigshospitalet, Copenhagen, Denmark

Zehua Zhang and Fei Guo
School of Computer Science and Technology, College of Intelligence and Computing, Tianjin University, Tianjin, China

Junhai Xu
School of Artificial Intelligence, College of Intelligence and Computing, Tianjin University, Tianjin, China

Jijun Tang
School of Computer Science and Technology, College of Intelligence and Computing, Tianjin University, Tianjin, China
Department of Computer Science and Engineering, University of South Carolina, Columbia, SC, United States

Quan Zou
Institute of Fundamental and Frontier Sciences, University of Electronic Science and Technology of China, Chengdu, China

Chih-Ying Gwo
Department of Information Management, Chien Hsin University of Science and Technology, Zhongli District, Taiwan

Weifeng Ding
The Chinese People's Liberation Army 118 Hospital, WenZhou, China

Jiahang Xu and Xiahai Zhuang
School of Data Science, Fudan University, Shanghai, China
Fudan-Xinzailing Joint Research Center for Big Data, Fudan University, Shanghai, China

Yechong Huang and Xinzhe Luo
School of Data Science, Fudan University, Shanghai, China

Qian Xu
Department of Nuclear Medicine, North Huashan Hospital, Fudan University, Shanghai, China

Ling Li, Chuantao Zuo and Ping Wu
PET Center, Huashan Hospital, Fudan University, Shanghai, China

Xueling Liu
Department of Radiology, Huashan Hospital, Fudan University, Shanghai, China

Xia-an Bi, Qian Xu, Qi Sun and Zhigang Wang
College of Information Science and Engineering, Hunan Normal University, Changsha, China

Xianhao Luo
College of Mathematics and Statistics, Hunan Normal University, Changsha, China

Chuanlu Lin, Yi Wang, Tianfu Wang and Dong Ni
National-Regional Key Technology Engineering Laboratory for Medical Ultrasound, Guangdong Provincial Key Laboratory of Biomedical Measurements and Ultrasound Imaging, Health Science Center, School of Biomedical Engineering, Shenzhen University, Shenzhen, China

David C. Zhu
Department of Radiology and Psychology, and Cognitive Imaging Research Center, Michigan State University, East Lansing, MI, United States

Rong Zhang
Department of Neurology and Neurotherapeutics, Department of Internal Medicine, University of Texas Southwestern Medical Center and Institute for Exercise and Environmental Medicine, Texas Health Presbyterian Hospital Dallas, Dallas, TX, United States

Tong Tong
Fujian Key Lab of Medical Instrumentation & Pharmaceutical Technology, Fuzhou, China
Imperial Vision Technology, Fuzhou, China

Amirali Kazeminejad
Hotchkiss Brain Institute, University of Calgary, Calgary, AB, Canada
Biomedical Engineering Graduate Program, University of Calgary, Calgary, AB, Canada

Roberto C. Sotero
Hotchkiss Brain Institute, University of Calgary, Calgary, AB, Canada
Biomedical Engineering Graduate Program, University of Calgary, Calgary, AB, Canada
Department of Radiology, University of Calgary, Calgary, AB, Canada

Yang Zhang
School of Information and Engineering, The First Affiliated Hospital of WenZhou Medical University, WenZhou Medical University, WenZhou, China

Zhifang Pan
School of Information and Engineering and Information Technology Centre, WenZhou Medical University, WenZhou, China

Jing Qin
School of Nursing, Hong Kong Polytechnic University, Kowloon, Hong Kong

Liansheng Wang and Yiping Chen
Fujian Key Laboratory of Sensing and Computing for Smart City, School of Information Science and Engineering, Xiamen University, Xiamen, China
Department of Computer Science, School of Information Science and Engineering, Xiamen University, Xiamen, China

Shuxin Wang, Rongzhen Chen and Shaohui Huang
Department of Computer Science, School of Information Science and Engineering, Xiamen University, Xiamen, China

Xiaobo Qu
Department of Electronic Science, Fujian Provincial Key Laboratory of Plasma and Magnetic Resonance, School of Electronic Science and Engineering (National Model Microelectronics College), Xiamen University, Xiamen, China

Changhua Liu
Department of Medical Imaging, Chenggong Hospital Affiliated to Xiamen University, Xiamen, China

Weiming Lin
College of Physics and Information Engineering, Fuzhou University, Fuzhou, China
School of Opto-Electronic and Communication Engineering, Xiamen University of Technology, Xiamen, China
Fujian Key Lab of Medical Instrumentation & Pharmaceutical Technology, Fuzhou, China

Qinquan Gao
College of Physics and Information Engineering, Fuzhou University, Fuzhou, China
Fujian Key Lab of Medical Instrumentation & Pharmaceutical Technology, Fuzhou, China
Imperial Vision Technology, Fuzhou, China

Di Guo and Xiaofeng Du
Schoolof Computer & Information Engineering, Xiamen University of Technology, Xiamen, China

Yonggui Yang and Gang Guo
Department of Radiology, Xiamen 2nd Hospital, Xiamen, China

Min Xiao
School of Opto-Electronic and Communication Engineering, Xiamen University of Technology, Xiamen, China

Min Du
College of Physics and Information Engineering, Fuzhou University, Fuzhou, China
Fujian Provincial Key Laboratory of Eco-Industrial Green Technology, Nanping, China

Xiaobo Qu
Department of Electronic Science, Xiamen University, Xiamen, China

Jiang Xin and Yaoxue Zhang
School of Computer Science and Engineering, Central South University, Changsha, China

Yan Tang
School of Computer Science and Engineering, Central South University, Changsha, China
Department of Neurology, Xiangya Hospital, Central South University, Changsha, China

Yuan Yang
Department of Physical Therapy and Human Movement Sciences, Feinberg School of Medicine, Northwestern University, Chicago, IL, United States

Yechong Huang, Jiahang Xu, Yuncheng Zhou and Xiahai Zhuang
School of Data Science, Fudan University, Shanghai, China

Tong Tong
Fujian Provincial Key Laboratory of Medical Instrument and Pharmaceutical Technology, Fuzhou, China

Chenxi Huang, Ganxun Tian, Yisha Lan and Yongtao Hao
Department of Computer Science and Technology, Tongji University, Shanghai, China

Yonghong Peng
Faculty of Computer Science, University of Sunderland, Sunderland, United Kingdom

E. Y. K. Ng
School of Mechanical and Aerospace Engineering, Nanyang Technological University, Singapore, Singapore

Yongqiang Cheng
School of Engineering and Computer Science, University of Hull, Kingston upon Hull, United Kingdom

Wenliang Che
Department of Cardiology, Shanghai Tenth People's Hospital, Tongji University School of Medicine, Shanghai, China

Index

www.ingramcontent.com/pod-product-compliance
Lightning Source LLC
LaVergne TN
LVHW082223200926
848484LV00008B/2296